Guide to Medical Billing

An Honors Certification™ Book

ICDC Publishing, Inc.

Los Angeles

Publisher: ICDC Publishing, Inc.
Editor-in-Chief: Sharon E. Brown
Editor: Caitlind L. Alexander
Copyeditor: Teresa Aguilar
Layout & Design: Anita Garcia
Technical Consultant: CarolAnn Jeffries, PA-C, MHS

Sixth Edition

Printed in the United States of America

ICDC Publishing, Inc.
4123 Lankershim Blvd.
North Hollywood, CA 91602
Phone: (818) 487-1199
Fax: (818) 487-1186
www.ICDCPublishing.com

International Standard Book Number 0-13-171849-5

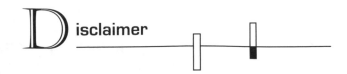

Disclaimer

This text is a guide for learning the medical billing field. Decisions should not be based solely on information within this guide. Decisions impacting the practice of medical billing must be based on individual circumstances including legal/ethical considerations, local conditions and payor policies.

The information contained in this text is based on experience and research. However, in the complex, rapidly changing medical environment, this information may not always prove correct. Data used are widely variable and can change at any time. Readers should follow current coding regulations outlined by official coding organizations.

Any five-digit numeric Physicians' *Current Procedural Terminology*, fourth edition (CPT®) codes, services, and descriptions, instructions and/or guidelines are copyright 2004 (or such other date of publication of CPT® as defined in the federal copyright laws) American Medical Association. All Rights Reserved.

CPT® is a listing of descriptive terms and five-digit numeric identifying codes and modifiers for reporting medical services performed by physicians. This presentation includes only CPT® descriptive terms, numeric identifying codes, and modifiers for reporting medical services and procedures that were selected by ICDC Publishing, Inc. (ICDC) for inclusion in this publication. The most current CPT® is available from the American Medical Association. No fee schedules, basic unit values, relative value goods conversion factors or scales or components thereof are included in CPT®.

ICDC has selected certain CPT® codes and service/procedure descriptions and assigned them to various specialty groups. The listing of a CPT® service or procedure description and its code number in this publication does not restrict its use to a particular specialty group. Any procedure or service in this publication may be used to designate the services rendered by any qualified physician.

The American Medical Association assumes no responsibility for the consequences attributable or related to any use or interpretation of any information or views contained in or not contained in this publication.

The publisher and author do not accept responsibility for any adverse outcome from undetected errors, opinion and analysis contained in this text that may prove inaccurate or incorrect, or the reader's misunderstanding of an extremely complex topic. All names used in this book are completely fictitious. Any resemblance to persons or to companies, current or no longer existing, is purely coincidental.

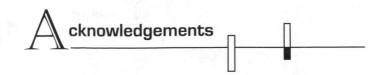Acknowledgements

Many people have contributed to the development and success of *Guide to Medical Billing*. We extend our thanks and deep appreciation to the many students and classroom instructors who have provided us with helpful suggestions for this edition of the text.

We would like to express our thanks to the following individuals:

Linda Jepson
Janet Grossfeld, Adelante Career Institute, Van Nuys, CA
Hollis Anglin and Michael Coffin, Dawn Training Institute, New Castle, DE
Michael Williams, 4-D Success Academy, Colton, CA
Anna McCracken, **Lynn Russell**, American Career College, Los Angeles, CA
Lowell P. Theard, PH.D, MD, Culver Healthcare Associates, Culver City, CA
Tabari Jeffries

Thanks to the CPA firm of Miller, Kaplan, Arase and Company, LLP:

Mannon Kaplan, C.P.A.
George Nadel Rivin, C.P.A.
Joseph C. Cahn, C.P.A.
Edwin Kanemaru, C.P.A.
Kenneth R. Holmer, C.P.A.
Douglas S. Waite, C.P.A.
Charles Schnaid, C.P.A.
Donald G. Garrett, C.P.A.
Catherine C. Gardner, C.P.A.
Jeffrey L. Goss, C.P.A.

And finally to:

Sean Adams
Sydney Adams
Floree Brown
Nathaniel Brown Sr.

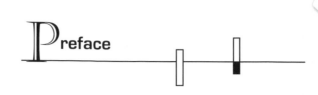Preface

Medical billing is one of the fastest-growing employment opportunities in the United States today. Insurance companies, medical offices, hospitals, and other health care providers are in great need of trained personnel to create medical claims.

With the aid of this textbook, you can learn the skills necessary to become a successful medical claims biller. The material has been designed to be comprehensive, yet user-friendly. The text follows a logical learning format by beginning with a broad base of information and then, step by step, following the course for creation of a medical claim.

This text may be used with ICDC Publishing, Inc.'s Medical Biller Curriculum Program, which is divided into five modules consisting of 90 hours each.

Special Features
Some special features of the text enhance understanding and retention of the material covered:

Each chapter begins with **learning objectives** to focus the student on the most pertinent topics covered in that chapter. The straightforward, **easy-to-understand writing style** presents information clearly and concisely. **Questions for Review** at the end of the chapter reinforce key concepts. Answering questions without looking back into the chapter will help students determine if they have grasped the principles within the chapter or if there is a need for further study. They also serve to prepare students for exams. Answers are contained in the instructor materials for this course. **Exercises** provided with most chapters give students the opportunity to put their knowledge into practice. These hands-on, real-life exercises will ensure competence in medical billing.

The most important ingredient to success in this course is the desire to learn, without which the learning process is ineffective. The desire to learn can lead you to a rewarding career in the medical billing field.

Table of Contents

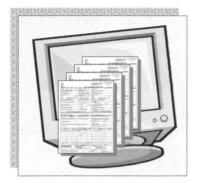

1

Introduction

After completion of this chapter you will be able to:

- List the job responsibilities of a medical biller.
- Describe the duties of each member of the medical team.
- Discuss how technology has affected the medical biller's job.
- State the attitudes that make a successful medical biller.
- Describe professional behaviors in an office setting.
- List the interpersonal skills that will help establish relationships in an office setting.
- State the symptoms of stress.
- List things that can help a person deal with stress.

Key words and concepts you will learn in this chapter:

Detail Orientation – The ability to spot very small differences in items and understand their significance.

Health Maintenance Organizations (HMOs) – Groups that provide services in exchange for premiums.

Innovation – The act of introducing something new.

Job Stress – The harmful physical and emotional responses that occur when the requirements of the job do not match the capabilities, resources or needs of the worker.

Left-brained People – Often those who tend to focus on the smaller details.

Office Politics – Negative interaction among people in an office setting.

Professionalism – A set of values and approaches to learning and doing business characterized by respect for others, commitment to quality, active learning, and personal integrity.

Provider – The person or entity that provides health care services. This can be a doctor, chiropractor, hospital, emergency facility, x-ray technician, or any certified professional who is licensed to provide health care services.

Right-brained People – People who tend to focus on the big picture and overall relationships between items.

The medical biller is an important part of the medical environment. As a medical biller, it is your responsibility to properly bill for services received by patients. Since most of the revenues generated by a medical office involve patient care, billing and collecting the revenue generated from patient care is one of the vital functions of the medical biller.

As such, the medical biller is an integral part of the medical team. Their contribution is essential to running the medical office.

Medical billers may also handle such thing as filling out claim forms, corresponding with patients, managing office supplies, and handling minor accounting for the office. The scope of a medical biller's duties will often depend on the size of the office. Larger offices may have multiple personnel responsible for running the office, setting appointments and handling the clients. Smaller offices may assign more of these duties to a medical biller/ receptionist.

For purposes of this course, we will cover all duties that a medical biller may perform in a smaller practice setting.

The Historical Perspective

In the past, people only sought medical treatment when seriously ill. As medical technology has advanced no longer is it routine to call a doctor only for serious illnesses. Preventative care has become a priority in the well being of society. People also realize that seeing a doctor early in their illness could mean a better and faster chance of recovery.

As more and more people began seeking medical care, doctors recognized the need for assistants to help with their patients and to handle some of the office duties. These duties often included billing patients and their insurance companies for the procedures performed.

With the advent of the personal computer and access to the Internet, the front office position, and the health care field in general changed dramatically. Making changes to documents became much quicker and easier, and transmission of information became more efficient. Eventually, government and world health officials would begin using computers to help track worldwide health statistics using standardized health codes. These codes would eventually be adopted for billing purposes by health providers.

Although computer technology has brought many conveniences, it has also increased the work load. Depending on the number of patients a provider had, it could often take more than one person to manage an office.

The specialized and autonomous profession of medical biller arose to satisfy many of those needs. Today, in addition to one or more medical assistants, many offices also employ a medical biller to handle patient accounts.

Job Roles and Duties

Medical billers play a diversified role in the medical office. The most common duties associated with medical billing include:
- Billing insurance carriers for services performed,
- Billing patients for any amounts not covered by the insurance carrier,
- Performing basic accounting,
- Handling collections on overdue accounts,
- Scheduling appointments for patients,
- Greeting patients,
- Maintaining and updating patient files; filing and retrieving files when needed,
- Answering the office phones,
- Ordering general office supplies, and
- Keeping abreast of, and utilizing appropriate computer programs for billing, correspondence, and accounting.

Job Titles
While the main purpose of this course it to teach medical billing and coding, students who successfully pass this course often qualify for other jobs as well. The most common job titles include:
- Medical Coder,
- Medical Coding Specialist,
- Hospital Biller, and
- Patient Account Manager.

The Medical Team

With any medical office there are a number of people who work together to provide complete health care to the patient. While the doctor may be the main provider, without the ancillary people it would be difficult for the office to function. Each member of the team is vital to providing overall patient care.

In a medical office setting there are often several team members. These include:
- The Provider,
- The Office Manager,
- The Medical Assistants,
- The Medical Biller, and
- Receptionist.

Medical assistants assist the provider with the care of the patient and may also handle some minor procedures. They are often responsible for sterilization of equipment, room preparation, setting up the patient, and administering injections.

The medical biller and/or receptionist also have their important duties. These can include ensuring that the provider has patients scheduled in an appropriate manner and billing and collecting revenues.

The office manager supervises the staff and handles the day to day organization of the medical office. The office manager may also be responsible for scheduling staff, payroll, and management of office expenses.

In a hospital setting the same levels of patient care exist with some minor differences. The doctors usually provide the direction of care by giving verbal or written orders to the nursing staff. The nurses and other medical personnel provide most of the direct patient care. The billing department is often separate from the other departments and simply handles the billing of patients and the collecting of revenues. However, in a hospital setting there are additional administrative, reception and other departments.

Regardless of the number of departments a medical provider has, each department is a necessary part of the whole operation. Without any one department, the facility could easily cease to exist.

Types of Healthcare Settings

There are several places a medical biller can work, depending on their experience and their preferences. The most common places include those listed below:

Provider's Office
There are many areas in a provider's office a medical biller may work. In addition to handling the billing, a medical biller may perform other front office duties such as greeting clients and handling patient intake. They will often be responsible for scheduling patient appointments and maintaining patient files.

Billing Company
Some medical billers work for independent billing companies. These companies usually perform the billing for a number of doctors. Doctors who only have a small practice may not need a full-time medical biller. If the provider only sees ten or 15

patients a day, performing the billing for those ten to 15 patients may only take an hour. Having a full-time medical biller would probably not be cost effective. In smaller medical offices the medical assistant may handle the tasks of greeting patients, and making appointments. However, the billing information regarding the patients seen and the procedures performed may be sent to a medical billing company for handling.

The medical billing company will create the claims and will often handle patient accounting. They will input any information regarding payments received onto the account, and then bill the patient for any balance remaining. Some billing companies have the capacity to transmit information directly into the provider's computer. Thus, the provider's office has information that is fairly current regarding each patient and their account.

Hospital
Hospitals need billers who can make sure that every item the patient uses is accounted for and billed. In a hospital setting, billers will have little contact with the patients. The only exception is when a patient or the parent of a patient comes to the billing office to make a payment on their account. Most often this happens when a portion of the fee is payable before the services are rendered.

Health Maintenance Organization
Health Maintenance Organizations (HMOs) are groups that provide services in exchange for premiums. Unlike traditional insurance, many HMOs act as both the insurance carrier and the provider of services. However, there are always times when an HMO facility sees a patient that is not one of their members. This most often occurs during a medical emergency when the patient is transferred to the nearest facility. If a patient is treated at an HMO facility, but they are not a member of that HMO, the HMO facility will bill the patient and/or their insurance carrier for the services provided.

An HMO facility may have to bill another insurance carrier when a patient with a work-related injury sees their regular HMO provider for treatment. Since most workers are covered by Workers' Compensation insurance, the HMO will bill the Worker's Compensation carrier for the services.

Pharmacy

More and more insurance plans are covering prescription drugs. While a few pharmacies will rely on the patient to file their own claim, most pharmacies have direct access to insurance carriers. This is especially true since Medicare now provides drug coverage benefits.

Medical Equipment Provider

Companies which supply medical equipment for patient use outside the hospital (i.e. a wheelchair), will sometimes have billers on staff. However, some companies may rely on the patient to file their own insurance claim. However, equipment providers are realizing that it can be a wonderful marketing tool to file insurance claims for patients.

Other Care Facilities

Numerous other types of facilities need medical billers on staff. These can include nursing homes, convalescent homes, hospices, rehabilitation centers, or any place that provides medical services.

Within each of the above settings there are numerous specialties. For example, an individual provider may specialize in general practice, cardiology, pediatric medicine, or any number of other specialties. Medical billers, however, are needed and may find employment at all of the above listed facilities.

Technology and the Medical Biller

While technology may continue to entrench itself further and further within the medical world, it can never completely replace the human element.

In the same way that machines can never fully replace medical assistants, computers can never fully replace medical billers. Computers, rather than replacing, have enhanced and facilitated many of the jobs associated with medical billing. Now that data can be stored it is not necessary to type in a patient's name, address and other information every time you generate a bill. Instead you can just access the previously entered information from a database and enter any newly acquired information such as the corresponding diagnosis and treatment provided.

However, since governments decided that the computer would be a wonderful way to collect all kinds of statistical data, some aspects of the job have become more difficult. It is no longer enough to type in the name of the procedure the doctor performed. Instead, every procedure has been assigned a code. Medical billers must locate the correct procedure code from a listing of over 30,000 codes. As a result, the medical billing profession has become more specialized.

Providers will continue to look for personnel who have the skills to bill patients and bring in the revenues for the services they provide. Good medical billers are always in demand to perform this specialized function.

Attitudes that Make a Successful Medical Biller

As in all professions, a good attitude is one key factor to a successful career. A good attitude makes a better employee, and it also benefits the company as a whole by improving the productivity of the work environment. By contributing to a more efficient workplace, an employee makes himself more valuable to the company, and in doing so, improves their chances of success in the field.

Thus, learning and applying the right attitudes in the workplace can help improve the workplace for you and your co-workers, and increases your chances for advancement.

Promotable Attitudes

Many people seem to think that you should get promoted just because you have stayed with a company for years and years. Advancement is often seen as a right, not as a reward.

This simply is not true. Research has shown that people who get promoted often share certain characteristics and do certain things that ensure their advancement in a company. Those that simply perform their job, no matter how well they perform it, may be promoted in the initial stages, but may be passed over when it comes to being promoted above a certain level.

Listed below are the attitudes that have been found to aid in making a successful medical biller.

Be willing to try new things. The medical billing job market is constantly changing. No matter how much you learn in school or on the job, you may be asked to do something for which you have not been formally trained Those people who are willing to try new things and accept new challenges will be the most successful. Because of this you should never utter words such as, "That is not in my job description."

Be creative. Innovation is the act of introducing something new. Try to find different ways of doing things, and then have the confidence to place your creations or ideas in front of your supervisors to seek their input. Supervisors are nearly always supportive of people who find easier, faster and less expensive ways of performing tasks. Learn to embrace innovation.

Be willing to upgrade your skills. Since the medical biller's role changes with new software and services that come on the market, you need to be willing to take the time and effort to keep your skills upgraded. This may mean learning things on your own time and at your own expense. However, if you do not learn new skills, you may soon find yourself outdated, and your skills will be in far less demand than those of others who have continued to develop their skills.

Think back to what worked. When things are not going well, think back to what worked before the current technology being used existed. You will often run into little glitches in the workplace. Just when you need it, the Internet will not connect, or the printer will not work, or the software program will crash. Before software programs were designed to cut and paste, people did it manually. Before faxes, people mailed items. These methods still work today. If you run into a roadblock when doing things the new way, revert back to the old way in which they were done until you can solve the problem.

Learn how to handle more than one task at a time. A medical biller is rarely ever doing just one thing. You may be working primarily on one project, but at the same time you may be constantly interrupted by the telephone, by people, and by new demands that come along.

Be willing to middle-manage. More and more medical billers are called on to assume the middle-management role scheduling co-workers, and organizing office functions, etc. Take the initiative. The more responsibility you are willing to assume, and the better your managerial skills, the further you will progress in this career.

Be flexible and know your limitations. Although it is important to make yourself as useful as possible, it is also necessary to learn how to manage your responsibilities, and to learn to recognize when you have reached your limit.

When working on a project, other projects may constantly come along with a higher priority than the one you are working on. You may often need to stop what you are doing, complete the urgent project, and then return to your previous assignment. Learn to be flexible enough to handle this type of situation without getting frustrated.

But more important than learning to manage multiple tasks, you need to learn to recognize your limitations. If you are handed ten urgent projects it may be impossible to do all of them immediately unless you have help. Be willing to admit when you need assistance, and when you can handle things on your own. If you take on too many projects, you will invariably end up not doing a good job on some of them.

Try to do as much as you can, but do not go beyond your abilities. Medical billers are not trained in patient care and should never attempt to treat a patient or even assist in patient treatment.

Be responsible. Knowing they can count on you to do what you say you will do, and perform it well, is very important to your supervisor. This includes both your actions and your attendance. You made a promise to be available for your employer when they hired you for the position. It is a promise you need to keep. Most employers consider being absent more than once a month to be too frequent.

Remember that it is your responsibility to do your absolute best at each task. If you can be counted on to turn in quality work, your supervisors are more likely to trust you with important work. If you turn in work that is sloppy or filled with errors, you will be given only unimportant assignments. Let your work speak for itself.

In addition to fulfilling your duties to the best of your ability, being responsible also means accepting your mistakes. If you make a mistake, accept it, apologize and move on. Denying a mistake or blaming it on someone else can damage your credibility.

Be a team player. When things need to get done, do them. Do not use excuses such as it's not in my job description, I am not in the mood, or any other number of excuses. Consider everything your job. People who are unwilling to work as part of the team, hinders both the productivity of the office and their opportunity for advancement.

Be productive. Although doing your best work is important, you must remember not to spend too much time trying to make things absolutely perfect. Projects need to get done.

Sometimes people can get bogged down in making minute changes that no one else may notice. Belaboring a project may give you the appearance of being a slow worker. This is a fast paced world; therefore, your productivity level needs to match the rhythm of the workplace.

Be logical, not emotional. Everyone has problems and things that go wrong in their lives. Constantly complaining about life is not only non-productive, it is a good way to get people to avoid you. After all, people prefer to be around those who make them happy, rather than those who make them depressed.

The business world runs on logic, not emotion. If you resort to emotional tactics to feel important, you may limit your ability for advancement. Constantly talking about yourself, your feelings and your needs, or manipulating others with your emotions may provide a momentary bit of esteem but using these tactics may also get you labeled as someone the company cannot count.

Meeting your emotional needs should be something you do on your own time, not company time. Remember, your boss is paying you to meet his needs, not for others to meet yours.

Strive for knowledge recognition rather than social recognition. Are you the kind of person who gains a feeling of self-worth by your social interactions with others or by the skills and knowledge you possess? People who depend on social interaction for their status will often bow to peer pressure or will pass up opportunities for advancement to stay with friends in comparable jobs. This does not mean they will overtly pass up a promotion. However, they will often make choices which will lead to this outcome.

While friendships are important, make sure they do not prevent you from doing those things that will give you the best chance for advancement.

Keep socializing to a minimum. While it is important to be friendly with others in the office and to let them know you care about them, it is also important to remember that you are on company time. The company has paid for your time and your mind during working hours. It is unfair to expect to be able to socialize and chat with friends (either inside or outside the company) excessively during this time.

Be self-motivated. Medical billers will often need to work alone, or may be given a task, then left to complete it. Being able to motivate yourself to begin the task and follow it through to completion is important.

The role of the medical biller is rapidly changing. If you are willing to accept the challenges and opportunities this job offers with a positive attitude, then an exciting career is waiting for you.

Workplace Professionalism

Professionalism is a set of values and approaches to learning and doing business. It is characterized by respect for others, commitment to quality, active learning, and personal integrity.

There are a number of components that define professionalism at work. These can include behavior and appearance.

It is important to note that professionalism is not only determined by your attire, but also by your attitude.

In fact, your attitudes and actions will often be judged as much as your appearance when someone is deciding whether or not to employ or promote you.

Office Politics and Diplomacy

Office politics is simply negative interaction among people in an office setting. This negative interaction can be in the form of gossiping about co-workers, playing games, manipulating people or not being completely honest.

Regardless of your reasons for doing so, it is important to remember that negative interaction does not work in your favor. Any time you treat a co-worker as less than a friend, you damage your relationship with that person as well as your professional image.

Some companies are caught up with a number of people who play the "office politics" game. For example, one person may start negative gossip about another co-worker. This may remind another person of some previous negative gossip about that co-worker tempting them to possibly add their negative piece to the conversation.

While chiming in is tempting, remember to ask yourself:

1. How would you feel if that co-worker overheard what you were saying?
2. How would you feel if you were that co-worker and heard those things said about you?

If you can answer positively to the above questions, you are spreading goodwill among employees. If you cannot, you are engaging in office politics.

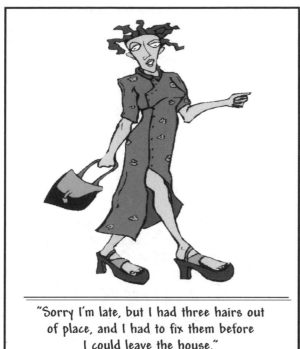

"Sorry I'm late, but I had three hairs out of place, and I had to fix them before I could leave the house."

Tips For on the Job Behavior

Employers are expecting you to conform to their workplace. The general guidelines for professional behavior are typically as follows:

- Be on time or call if you will be late or absent,
- Call in promptly if you are ill, and be sure to inform anyone with whom you have scheduled meetings,
- Do not leave early without your supervisor's approval,
- Do not perform personal business on company time,
- Do not use your employer's equipment (including computers, fax machines and telephones) or supplies (including mail, paper, etc.) for personal use, and
- Do not let your personal life intrude into the workplace.

Interpersonal Skills

The following interpersonal skills will help you to get along harmoniously with others in the workplace.

Place the company ahead of yourself. Give your absolute best at work. Establish a reputation that shows people they can rely on you to do good work on time.

Be willing to admit when you are wrong. Rather than losing face, people will appreciate your honesty.

Speak well of others whenever possible. Remember to praise people for a job well done, both to them and to their superiors.

Show an interest in what others say. Take the time to listen to others. If you cannot spare the time, politely find a way to postpone the conversation. For example, "Unfortunately I am under a deadline. How about if we discuss this further over lunch?"

Give credit where credit is due. If someone else helps you with a project, even in a small way, do not take the credit for their work. Be sure that the superiors know who actually did the work. If you try to take credit for work that someone else has done, you will eventually be exposed and people will be less willing to help or trust you in the future.

Compromise. Sometimes you may disagree with a co-worker. In such cases a compromise can work wonders toward keeping the relationship intact and resolving the conflict. Try to find a solution where each of you gain something. Allow them to win one point, while you win another.

Make others look good, especially your supervisor. If you are asked to help with a project, do your best work. Go the extra mile in finding solutions for a problem, and then allow the responsible person to turn in the project and take credit for their share. If they take credit for your work, do not refute it. You do not know if something was said at a different time. If you start jumping in and insisting that you helped, you appear to lack confidence in others and yourself.

Introduce yourself to new people. The office environment will often change quickly. Taking the time to learn the names of those you work with lets them know that they are important to you. Take the time to make small talk and find out something about them.

Build networks. Be willing to refer work to others who can do a better job than you can. Also, take work from others that they want you to try.

Talk to people about non-work related matters during lunch hours or break times. Get to know them a little better, and let them get to know you.

Smile and be positive. Positive people are more pleasant to be around. No one wants to spend time with someone that brings out the worst in everyone. Maintain a positive attitude. If you're positive, it makes other people positive as well.

Try to keep your personal problems to yourself. Constantly discussing personal problems at work can make others feel uncomfortable and will often strain your relationship since they may be reluctant to engage in conversation with you.

Keep your mouth shut. If someone passes information on to you, do not share it with others unless you are specifically asked to do so.

Confirm rumors before acting on them. Often things get twisted around in the office grapevine and bear no resemblance to the truth after it has gone through the twentieth telling.

Actions to Avoid
There are several actions which should be avoided on the job. These include:
- Having loud phone conversations,
- Not cleaning up after yourself in common areas such as the kitchen or lounge,
- Looking over a co-workers shoulder,
- Going through a co-worker's desk,
- Neglecting to say please and thank you,
- Wearing too much perfume or cologne,
- Not being clean, especially in your work area. The appearance of your work area reveals a lot about a person,
- Smoking,
- Talking behind someone's back,
- Asking someone else to tell a lie or to be dishonest,
- Blaming someone else when you are at fault,
- Asking someone, especially a subordinate to do an errand that is not work related,
- Telling offensive jokes or making sexist or politically incorrect comments,
- Complaining about another person, and
- Being condescending toward others.

Professional Appearance

Although your attitude is very important, attire also counts. Many companies have a formal dress code that employees must adhere to.

During your interview, it is important to look your best. You should take the time to notice the attire of the employees at the company, especially those in the same position or department as you. This can give you a general idea of the dress code. However, during the first few weeks on the job it is important to dress up a bit more. It is always easier to relax your style after having made a good impression than to try to upgrade your style after making a poor impression.

Above all else, always make sure that your clothes are clean, pressed, and well-maintained. Taking pride in your appearance lets your employer know that you take pride in yourself and in the work that you do.

Business Casual
Many companies have instituted a business casual dress code. Unfortunately, there is no single description of what comprises business casual. For some companies business casual may mean wearing a tie but no jacket. Other companies may define business casual as a nice shirt (not necessarily a button-down shirt) and slacks.

If a company has a business casual dress code, find out what they mean by this phrase before deciding on your wardrobe. For most medical billers, business casual usually means nice slacks, nice blouses and low-heeled shoes for ladies, and nice shirts, nice slacks and soft-soled shoes for men.

Inappropriate Clothing
Regardless of the type of company, there are some forms of attire that are generally considered inappropriate. These usually include:
- Jeans,
- Baggy styled clothing,
- Sweatshirts or other exercise attire,
- Shirts which expose the midriff,
- Clothing which is sheer enough to reveal underclothing,
- Clothing which prevents you from doing the job effectively and safely, and
- Clothing which is too tight, too revealing, or is otherwise considered sexual in nature.

Dress Code Regulations
Dress codes are legal as long as they do not discriminate based on age, gender, race or even position within the company. Gender discrimination can sometimes be difficult to define. It is legal for a company to require that

female employees wear different clothing than male employees if male employees are also required to meet the same level of attire. Thus, if female employees must wear a dress, male employees must be required to wear a suit and tie.

Dressing for Success

If you want to advance within a company, take notice of what those in higher management are wearing. If it does not conflict with your job duties, try to match this style. If most of the supervisors are wearing ties, but most of the employees are not, wear a tie. It will signal your willingness to move up to the supervisory level.

Sometimes the attire of supervisors in your company will conflict with your job requirements. For example, if you work in a medical practice, the provider may wear a lab coat but prefer that you dress in regular clothing.

Even if dressing like those above you does conflict with your job, you can still make yourself stand out. Try to dress a little more professionally than those in the same position as you. This may mean wearing a dress shirt instead of a tee shirt, or wearing a better quality of clothing.

Stress

Job stress is defined as the harmful physical and emotional responses that occur when the requirements of the job do not match the capabilities, resources or needs of the worker.

Often people will say, "A little bit of stress is good for you." However, this often depends on your definition of stress, and how much is a "little bit." What people often mean is that a challenge can be good for you.

Challenges energize us psychologically and physically and help motivate us to learn new skills. When a challenge is met, we feel relaxed and satisfied. Thus, challenges can be an important ingredient for healthy and productive work.

While challenges can be good for you, stress is not. Stress causes negative physiological reactions such as an increase in adrenaline and heart rate, without the physical ability to expend and use the adrenaline.

Symptoms of Stress

Stress can cause a variety of symptoms that can inhibit your ability to function properly, both at work and in your daily life. The most common symptoms of stress include:

- Headaches,
- Anxiety,
- High blood pressure,
- Trouble falling asleep or other sleep disturbances,
- Difficulty concentrating,
- Short temper,
- Upset stomach,
- Job dissatisfaction,
- Low morale,
- Hyperventilation, and
- Clenching or grinding of the teeth.

Pent-up stress can also cause emotional outbursts, ranging from intense anger to tears and self-pity. Chronic stress can cause problems in relationships, heart problems, and immune system deficiencies.

Handling Stress

While stress is a part of everyday life, it is important to deal with stress appropriately so that it does not accumulate and overwhelm you. Handling stress is an important part of being able to function in the working world.

Quick stress relievers can include:

- Exercising vigorously,
- A massage,
- Deep, slow breathing,
- Getting more sleep,
- Skipping extra caffeine in items such as coffee, cola and chocolate, and
- Eating properly and regularly.

Other means of handling stress may take a bit longer, but can be more effective. These include:

Finding the humor in life. Learn to laugh at the mistakes you make and things that go wrong. Laughter is a great stress reliever.

Creating a new attitude. Try to see each problem as a challenge. Think of it as a chance for you to go up against an imaginary adversary and come out victorious by conquering the problem. By changing your attitude toward problems you can create an aura of excitement, thus giving yourself the energy to tackle and handle them.

Giving yourself opportunities to relax. You should spend at least half an hour every day doing something that helps to relax your body and mind. This can be reading a book, exercising, socializing with friends, or whatever helps you work off stress and relax. Remember, these should be activities that give you pleasure, not those that give you stress of a different nature.

Creating a stress barrier. Do not bring your family or life problems to work, and do not take your work problems home with you. Establishing a routine that provides a break between the two environments can help. Some people create this barrier by having a long commute home, others will take a few minutes upon arriving home to relax before tackling home activities, and others will stop off on the way home to do something else.

Such habits can help you keep the troubles of work and home from interfering with each other.

Making a "To Do" list. We often get overwhelmed thinking of all the things we need to accomplish, and sometimes everything we think of leads to something else. Like trying to remember the names of the seven dwarves, we suddenly start renaming them until we have ten dwarfs instead of seven. Even then we keep thinking in the back of our minds that we have forgotten something.

Tasks are like dwarfs. You can end up naming and renaming lots of things you have to do, and still feel like you have not remembered everything. However, if you take the time to write down the tasks you are facing, suddenly many of them seem more manageable. Now you have a goal in mind and a clear direction of what needs to be accomplished. You will feel good knowing what you have to do, and you will feel even better when you start to accomplish some of them and scratch them off the list.

Also remember to do one thing at a time. Multi-tasking doesn't mean doing everything at once. Performing the items on your list one at a time allows you to concentrate on each item and be more productive, giving you the opportunity to complete them more efficiently.

Ask others not to disturb you. If you have a time-sensitive project or a fast approaching deadline, ask not to be disturbed. Hang a sign on your desk with the words "Please Do Not Disturb, Important Deadline Looming." In some companies notifying others that you do not want to be disturbed can be easily accomplished by closing your door.

Ask the receptionist to hold your calls, or if you have voice mail, switch to a greeting that informs people that you are working on a very important project. Include in your message when you will be available and ask them to leave a message or call you back at a later time.

Other people are busy too and they understand the need to buckle down and focus on a project. Most people are more than willing to respect your request.

Pre-Vacation Work Planning

Taking a vacation can be great for you, but stressful for your co-workers. Taking a vacation means the rest are left with one less person to carry on the work.

While many people think only of themselves when planning a vacation, good medical billers also think of their company. Following are some guidelines to use when planning a vacation.

Take your vacation during the company's slow period. Nearly all companies have one or two seasons that are busier than others. Schedule your vacation around these times so that you are there when you are most needed. Co-workers and especially your bosses will appreciate your thoughtfulness.

Some people may think that scheduling a vacation during the busy time will reveal how valuable they are. Unfortunately, the negative impression that they are thinking only of themselves and not of the company will outweigh any thoughts of how important their skills are.

Before leaving, be sure that your desk is in order. All paperwork and folders should be filed appropriately. This allows anyone who needs something to find it while you are away. All work with a due date prior to your vacation should be completed and turned in. Sometimes, this means working through lunch or working harder to make sure things are accomplished. Others can get a negative impression of you if you leave without completing assignments or without properly filing things away.

Let others know two weeks in advance that you are leaving. This gives your supervisors and others enough advance notice for any projects that need your input for completion.

Leave a number with a trusted co-worker for emergencies. Providing a number where you can be reached in case of emergency shows those in your office that you care. A brief word such as "So-and-so knows how to reach me if it is an emergency," should be enough to let people know of your whereabouts.

Enjoy your vacation. Ignore what is happening at work. Give your mind and body a break. This will allow you to come back and face work with a fresh outlook because you will be more rested, refreshed, and ready to take on new challenges.

Detail Orientation

It is imperative that a medical biller pay particular attention to detail. **Detail orientation** is the ability to spot very small differences in items and understand their significance. In a business setting, the little details can make a big difference.

For example, if a check arrives and you are not paying attention to detail, you could end up applying the check to the wrong invoice. This small error will have an effect on many other items in the accounting system

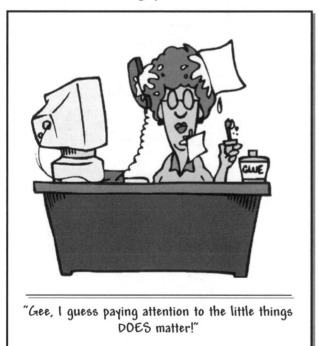

"Gee, I guess paying attention to the little things DOES matter!"

Many people tend to be either right-brained or left-brained. As a general rule, **right-brained** people focus on the big picture and overall relationships between items. **Left-brained** people tend to focus on the smaller details. Both viewpoints are important in your work. It is possible to cultivate the ability to work with both parts of your brain simultaneously; however, it often takes practice.

If you need more practice in being detail oriented be aware of when opportunities are presented to work on this skill. This can include things such as working on word puzzles, jigsaw puzzles, comparison puzzles (find six differences between these pictures), etc. Even though these are games that might not necessarily relate directly to your job, the skill of being able to spot details will carry over.

Following are additional items that will help you to focus on details:

- Concentrate on the specifics of a subject when taking notes.
- Number or bullet details to call attention to them.
- When setting up a schedule or project, list all main ideas or items to be accomplished on one side of a paper, and all the details to accomplish that item on the opposite side of the paper. This will help to ensure that you are looking at the details for each item, not just at subsections of the overall project.
- Force yourself to write down ten details about completing each assignment that you work on. For example, rather than say you will proofread a document, make up a style sheet listing all the items to look for (i.e., are all main headers centered in bold caps; all secondary headers non-caps, bolded, on the left; all figures consecutively numbered, etc.). Then force yourself to go through the project looking only for one item on the list before moving on to the next item.
- Make an outline of a project with a numbered heading for each of the main items, and at least three detail items indented under each numbered heading. By listing each item to be accomplished, you learn to focus on the little things that help you do the job well.

For an example of the importance of paying attention to small details, consider the following: You are given two invoices one has a shipper tracking number on it and the other does not. What does this one little detail tell you about this invoice? It should tell you that one of the orders has been shipped out already, and the other has not. By tracing the tracking number you can find out if and when the order was delivered and who signed for it.

At first it may be difficult to focus on details, however, with practice it will become easier. The information that can be obtained by looking at the details of a document can ensure that the item is handled properly.

Certification Programs for Medical Billers

Currently there is no state or federal certification or licensing requirement for medical billers. However, more and more employers are requesting or requiring certification of their medical billing and coding applicants.

Certification offers increased job security, income, prestige, advancement and recognition as well as professional affiliation.

There are several different certification programs as of this writing. They are:

- Certified Procedural Coder (CPC) – awarded by the American Academy of Professional Coders (AAPC).
- Certified Coding Associate (CCA) and Certified Coding Specialist (CCS) both awarded by American Health Information Management Association (AHIMA).

For further information on coding certification, contact these organizations.

Summary

Medical billers handle everything from billing patients to scheduling appointments and handling charts. Technology has made the lives of medical billers a lot easier. However, the medical biller must stay abreast of the latest technology to stay competitive.

A positive attitude goes a long way. Possessing the right attitude not only helps you work better, it also helps you get ahead. Being professional in the work place is an additional attribute that will aid in the advancement of your career. Understanding and implementing these simple principles can assist you in being successful at the job of medical billing.

While stress is a part of everyday life, it is important to deal with stress appropriately so that it does not accumulate and overwhelm you. Handling stress is an important part of being able to function in the working world.

It is not always easy to know how to act in the workplace. Only time and experience will help you to develop into a professional.

Assignments

Complete the Questions for Review.
Complete Exercises 1 – 1 through 1 – 3.

Questions for Review

Directions: Answer the following questions without looking back into the material just covered. Write your answers in the space provided.

1. List three job responsibilities of the medical biller.

    1. _____

    2. _____

    3. _____

2. What are eight promotable attitudes that will make a successful medical biller?

    1. _____

    2. _____

    3. _____

    4. _____

    5. _____

    6. _____

    7. _____

    8. _____

3. (True or False?) A professional appearance is only determined by your attire. _____

4. What is job stress? _____

    _____

    _____

5. List five stress relievers.

    1. _____

    2. _____

    3. _____

    4. _____

    5. _____

If you were unable to answer any of the questions, refer back to that section, and then fill in the answers.

Exercise 1 – 1

Directions: Rate yourself on the following attitudes. 1 = Never, 2 = Occasionally, 3= Sometimes, 4 = Almost Always, 5 = Always.

Are you or do you:

1.	Willing to try new things	1	2	3	4	5
2.	Willing to upgrade your skills	1	2	3	4	5
3.	Willing to accept a challenge	1	2	3	4	5
4.	Creative	1	2	3	4	5
5.	Willing to use prior technology	1	2	3	4	5
6.	Handle more than one task at a time	1	2	3	4	5
7.	Flexible	1	2	3	4	5
8.	Productive	1	2	3	4	5
9.	Willing to middle manage	1	2	3	4	5
10.	Self-motivated	1	2	3	4	5
11.	A non-complainer	1	2	3	4	5
12.	Not use excuses	1	2	3	4	5
13.	Responsible	1	2	3	4	5
14.	Accepting of your mistakes	1	2	3	4	5
15.	Understanding of your limitations	1	2	3	4	5
16.	Limit your socializing	1	2	3	4	5

Look back over the above items. Which ones are you good at? _____

_____

_____

Which ones do you need more work on? _____

_____

_____

What do you think you can do to improve those areas you need more work on? _____

_____

_____

_____

_____

Exercise 1 – 2

Directions: Make a sign with the following (or similar) phrase, "Please Do Not Disturb, Important Deadline Looming!" Be creative and make it attractive, but do not take so long that it becomes a major project. Consider making it a tri-fold sign, which will stand on your desk or one you can easily hang from the side of your desk. Use this sign when necessary.

Exercise 1 – 3

Directions: Rate yourself on each of the qualities listed below, and then answer the following questions. 1 = Never, 2 = Almost Never,   3 = Sometimes,   4 = Almost Always,   5 = Always.

Do you:

Embrace innovation?	1 2 3 4 5
Take the initiative?	1 2 3 4 5
Consider everything within your job title?	1 2 3 4 5
Strive for knowledge recognition rather than social recognition?	1 2 3 4 5
Let your work speak for itself or take pride in the quality of your work?	1 2 3 4 5
Like to learn new skills?	1 2 3 4 5
Ally yourself with powerful people?	1 2 3 4 5
Have high morale?	1 2 3 4 5

Are you:

Willing to learn and do someone else's job?	1 2 3 4 5
Logical, not emotional?	1 2 3 4 5
Self-confident?	1 2 3 4 5
Willing to take on more than your responsibilities?	1 2 3 4 5

1. For what assets did you circle a 5? _____

_____

2. For what assets did you circle a 4? _____

_____

3. For what assets did you circle a 1, 2 or 3? _____

_____

4. What can you do to improve each of those assets that you ranked yourself 1, 2 or 3? _____

_____

_____

_____

_____

_____

Honors Certification™

The work for your honors certificate begins immediately. Read through the following items to determine what the requirements are for the subjects covered in this chapter. The requirements for each honors certification challenge will be included at the end of each chapter. You must complete all honors certification challenges to successfully achieve your honors certificate.

This will be among the hardest certificate challenges in the book. For many people it will require breaking habits they have lived with their entire lives. However, learning the correct behaviors to exhibit on the job will help you throughout your working life to get and keep the best jobs, and to make those jobs a satisfying place to work.

To achieve your certificate, from this point forward you will need to do the following:

Attitude

Begin exhibiting those attitudes which make a successful medical biller. Make a conscious effort to improve those areas which you may be deficient in, and begin treating your class experience as if it were a work experience. Your attitude in class each day should reflect the proper attitude you would have on the job.

Beginning immediately, any time you exhibit an attitude which is contrary to those listed in this chapter you will receive a violation. You are allowed only five attitude violations before you are in danger of not qualifying for your certificate. If you commit a sixth violation, you must perform a make up exercise given by the instructor. You are allowed only one makeup exercise for an attitude violation. If you commit a seventh violation you no longer qualify for certification.

Attitudes which will earn you a violation include:
- Not being willing to try new things.
- Not being willing to learn and upgrade your skills.
- Not accepting a challenge.
- Not being creative.
- Only handling one task at a time, being unable to multi-task.
- Not being flexible.
- Not being productive.
- Not being willing to middle manage.
- Not being self-motivated.
- Complaining.
- Giving excuses.
- Not being responsible.
- Not accepting responsibility for your mistakes.
- Not understanding your limitations.
- Not limiting your socializing.
- Refusing to do something.

Additionally, your instructor may designate other attitudes which will earn you a violation. This is similar to the working world where your supervisor will request that you act a certain way, and will expect you to do so.

Your attitude is perhaps the most important factor in getting and keeping a job. More people are fired for attitude problems than for most other problems on the job.

No more than five instances of improper attitude will be allowed.

Properly Completing Assignments

When each class assignment is given, you will be told when it is due. All class assignments must be turned in when due. If an assignment is due at the beginning of the class, and you complete it during the class, you have not completed the assignment on time.

All assignments should be completed in a professional manner. This includes:
- Assignments should be neat in appearance (not sloppy).
- Assignments should be fully completed, rather than partially completed.
- Proper punctuation, spelling and grammar should be used.

You are allowed up to three improperly completed assignment violations.

You will be allowed one late assignment which is not counted against your record if you speak with the instructor prior to the deadline and ask for an extension of that deadline. If the instructor grants the extension, the new deadline will be considered the due date you must meet.

Dress

Dress appropriately. Your instructor will dictate appropriate dress; however, casual business dress or higher is expected. If you do not have appropriate clothing in your wardrobe, speak with your instructor. The instructor may, at their discretion, give you up to two weeks to acquire appropriate dress. If you show up in inappropriate dress more than three times you will not gain your certificate.

Inappropriate attire includes:

- Inappropriate hats or caps.
- Clothing that is dirty, wrinkled or not properly maintained.
- Clothing with tears, rips or holes.
- Clothing that is excessively revealing or sexual in nature.
- Clothing that is too tight.
- Any clothing not suitable for business.

No more than three instances of showing up in inappropriate attire will be allowed in a semester.

Acting Professionally

You are expected to act in a professional manner at all times. You are allowed up to five total violations (not five violations per item). If you receive more than five violations you will not be eligible to receive certification.

Violations will be given for:

- Not doing your best work.
- Not being willing to admit when you are wrong.
- Not speaking well of others.
- Not showing an interest in what others say.
- Not giving credit where credit is due.
- Taking credit for someone else's work.
- Not compromising.
- Not making others look good, especially your instructor.
- Not building networks.
- Not learning a fellow student's name.
- Not putting the company/school ahead of yourself.
- Not smiling and keeping a positive attitude.
- Not introducing yourself to new people.
- Not keeping your mouth shut, when appropriate.
- Passing on rumors, gossip or other information.
- Acting on rumors before confirming them.
- Entering into secret deals.
- Not keeping your personal problems to yourself.
- Not being dependable or doing what you say you will.
- Disrespecting the instructor.
- Disrespecting a fellow student.
- Having loud conversations.
- Not cleaning up after yourself in common areas such as the kitchen or lounge.
- Looking over a co-worker's (other student's) shoulder.
- Going through a co-worker's (other student's) desk or bag.
- Neglecting to say please and thank you.
- Wearing too much perfume or cologne.
- Not being clean.

- Smoking (smoking may be permitted outside at your instructor's discretion).
- Talking behind someone's back.
- Asking someone else to tell a lie or to be dishonest.
- Blaming someone else when you are at fault.
- Telling offensive jokes or making sexist, racist or politically incorrect comments.
- Complaining about another person.
- Being condescending toward others.
- Showing up without required materials.
- Showing signs of stress.
- Not embracing innovation.
- Not being willing to learn new jobs.
- Striving for social recognition rather than knowledge recognition.
- Not taking the initiative.
- Not being willing to pitch in and consider everything your job/responsibility.
- Not letting your work speak for itself (i.e., bragging).
- Not learning new skills.
- Being emotional rather than logical.
- Not being self-confident.
- Not being willing to accept projects that have high visibility.
- Not having high morale.
- Not being patient.

If students are caught completing the assignment for a fellow student, both students will receive a violation.

Tardiness and Absences

Show up to class on time. This means in your seat, ready to begin work when the class begins. It does not mean walking in the door when class time starts. It also means that if there is a break period in the class, you return to your desk and are ready to work when the break period ends. Each time you are late it will count as 1/2 of an unexcused absence. Thus, two incidences of being tardy, regardless of the amount of time you are late, equals one unexcused absence. Even being one minute late counts as a tardy.

If you are going to be absent, you must call in to the office before the class begins or within 15 minutes of the start of your class. If you call in and have a reasonable excuse for not coming in (i.e., illness), it will count as an excused absence. If you do not call in, regardless of the reason for your absence, it will be counted as an unexcused absence.

If you leave class early without the instructor's permission, it will count as an unexcused absence.

You are allowed only two unexcused absences and three excused absences. Any absences or tardies beyond this amount will cause you to be ineligible for a certificate.

If you are aware that you are going to be tardy before class starts, you can lessen the effect by calling in and letting the school know that you will be late. The school will then note the time of your call on a tardy slip. This slip should be picked up at the office before entering class, and handed to the instructor.

By calling in prior to the start time of your class, the tardy will count as only 1/3 of an unexcused absence. Thus, it will take three times of being late but having called in to equal one unexcused absence.

Excused absences

Regardless of the reason, employers will not be happy with an employee who fails to show for work.

Valid reasons for not showing up to class include:
- Illness or severe injury (for yourself or an immediate family member), and
- National disaster which impacts the local area.

No more than three excused absences are allowed per semester.

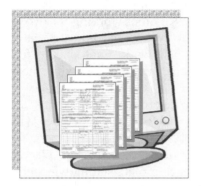

2

Time Management and Prioritizing

After completion of this chapter you will be able to:

- Properly prioritize a given set of projects.
- Describe how to prioritize projects.
- List ways that will help you handle pressure projects.
- List appropriate time management skills.
- Discuss ways of handling overlapping projects.

Key words and concepts you will learn in this chapter:

Overlapping Projects – Projects that are being performed by more than one person simultaneously but could actually be performed by one person, thus, eliminating the duplicate effort.

Prioritize – To arrange items in the order of importance.

Time Costs – The monetary calculation for the actual time needed to complete a project.

The ability to prioritize projects can be one of the most important assets a medical biller can develop. When expectations are high, deadlines are short, and resources are limited, you want to make sure that the most important projects get completed on time. To do so requires prioritizing.

Prioritize is to arrange items in order of importance. In most working environments you will be given a number of projects to complete. Prioritizing these projects can help to ensure that the most important ones get completed first, and that you keep the office running smoothly and efficiently.

When setting priorities, you need to balance the business benefit each item provides against its time cost and other costs. **Time costs** are the monetary calculation for the actual time needed to complete a project.

After analyzing the cost factors and the time needed to complete the project, you may find that the project is not worth the amount of time and effort that is involved. Perhaps, because of the time and effort involved it becomes a low priority project, or one to be worked on when there is nothing else to do.

Prioritization

Prioritizing means putting one item before another in time or importance. There are several ways to prioritize the projects you are given. One way is to simply determine the date the item must be completed and putting those projects that must be completed earliest first. While this is a form of prioritizing, it does not take into account those items that might be more important than others, or those items that, while they may not be important in and of themselves, may need to be done prior to another project. For example, if the boss wants you to make address labels for a mailing, you must first enter the addresses into the computer before you can print them on labels.

A second method of prioritizing projects is by assessing their importance. The reality of business life is that some projects are more important than others. Prioritizing in this manner ensures that those items which are the most important will get done first. However, this method may not take into account specific deadlines for items. For example, an item that is vital to the company may not need to be done for another 30 days while a lower priority item may need to be completed within a day or two.

Thus, the best method of prioritizing items is to use a combination of the two methods. Items are first grouped according to the date they must be accomplished. Then, a second look is taken to ensure that items of great importance have not been pushed so far down on the list that you are unable to complete them by their deadline. If they have been moved too far down on the list, they should be moved up so that sufficient time is allowed to complete them.

This may mean delaying or completely eliminating those items that are of a lesser priority; however, this is a business decision that often needs to be made.

Another common approach to prioritizing projects is to group items into three priority categories: high, medium and low. **High priority** items are critical and need to be completed as soon as possible. **Medium priority** items are important. Although they do not have to be completed immediately, they should not be put off for too long. **Low priority** items are enhancements or items that would be nice to have but are not essential, or items whose deadline is so far in advance that they are not important at the moment.

Once you have assigned each project a high, medium or low priority rating, simply take the high priority items and decide which is the most important item. This item should be worked on first. The next important item should be worked on next, and so on until all high priority items are completed. Then you move on to the medium priority items and do the same.

Of course, if you are working for more than one person you must make sure that each person is treated fairly. Double check your list to make sure

that one person is not getting all of her projects dropped into the low priority column while another person has all the high priority spots. One of your jobs as a medical biller working for two or more supervisors is to make each boss feel as if you are there to do their work. Each should feel like they are of equal importance with those around them.

So how do you determine which items are critical and which are not? Often this comes with experience on the job; however, you can ask for help from your supervisors. Ask them to place a note on the front of each project stating whether it is high, medium or low priority, and the date that it must be completed by. This will help you to prioritize effectively.

Of course, there will always be those times when everything lands in the high priority file, or people insist their projects always demand first priority. People naturally have their own interests at heart and are not always willing to compromise their needs or desires for someone else's benefit. When each boss thinks every item on his agenda is of the highest priority, you will have to make the final decision of which item you work on first.

Start by assessing how long each project will take, then do or ask yourself the following:
1. Can either of the projects be finished within about five minutes? If so, set aside the other project and quickly finish the five-minute project.
2. If one or both projects can be finished in less than 1/2 hour, determine the impact of that delay on the other project. For example, if the project for Mr. B will take 15 minutes, can Ms. A's project be held off for 15 minutes without causing a major problem? If the answer is yes, do Mr. B's project, and then return to Ms. A's project.
3. If neither project can be finished quickly or without impact to the other project, go back to the priority scale previously listed and decide which project is the most important. Complete that project first.

The best prioritization method takes into account all of the following items:
- Length of time needed to complete the project,
- High, medium, or low importance level,

- Visibility of the project. If it is highly visible and a poor or late job would reflect badly to a number of important people, the project's importance should be increased, and
- Length of time for approvals. If you will need to add in extra time for others to approve or change the work you have done, be sure to calculate and include this time when deciding when to schedule a project.

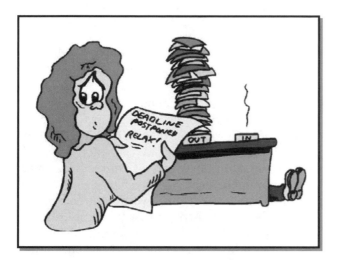

Discussing Your Work with Your Bosses
If you are in the middle of an urgent project for Mr. B and Ms. A approaches you and insists that you work on her project, let her know that you are already in the middle of an extremely urgent project for Mr. B and ask if it can wait. If she insists that it must be done immediately, perform the steps above.

As you can see, mentioning a current project you are working on is not a big issue. However, you want to be careful about telling a boss about projects you are currently working on for others. For example, if you were to go to Mr. B and say, "Your project will be delayed because Ms. A insists that I work on her project first," may be interpreted as you're inability to keep up with the assignments you are given and that you need others to prioritize them for you. Additionally, such a statement can cause resentment in the office since some people may be upset that their projects are not perceived as being as important as other people's projects.

While such situations can be difficult, it is important to remember that handling these types of problems is part of your job. Simply take care of the situation as best you can and move on.

Pressure Projects

At times you may be called upon to drop everything and deal with a project that needs to be completed immediately. If there is not enough time to complete a pressure project, it can cause stress. Here are some tips for handling rush projects.

Make sure you understand the assignment. When you and the person you are taking instructions from are stressed, there is a greater likelihood that important instructions will be miscommunicated or left out entirely. Be sure that you do not waste time going in the wrong direction.

Take a deep breath. When you feel yourself getting stressed, stop and take a deep breath, or even a quick stroll around the building. The more stressed you are the greater the likelihood you will make mistakes. By taking a moment to relax you can face the problem more efficiently.

Organize. Now is the time for creating "To Do" lists and charting the steps that need to be taken to get everything done. It is easy to forget one little detail when you have a huge project on your mind.

Do not be afraid to ask for help. This is especially true if you are not the first person to have tackled this project. If someone has done this type of project before, take a few minutes to ask for tips. Also be sure to ask for any examples, forms, lists or other items that might prove helpful.

If all you need is manpower, let your boss know as soon as possible. If you speak up soon enough it may only take one other person to help you complete the task. If you wait until the last minute you might require everyone in the office to drop what they are doing and come to your aid, potentially creating other emergency situations within the office.

Get the resources you need. Find out if you can use the conference room or some other work area if you need peace and quiet or a larger working area. Ask for any office supplies you need so that they are available when you need them.

Once you have completed each step, double check your work. Or better yet, have someone else check it. It is easy to make mistakes when you are rushing. Take the time to make sure you have done the work properly, and you will not risk having to redo everything that comes after a major mistake.

Time Management

A good medical biller must become an expert in the efficient management of time. If you do not keep up with the pace of office life you may quickly be replaced by someone who can. Therefore, it is of the utmost importance to manage your time effectively.

Without time management, tasks cannot be completed and things back up, which causes stress in our lives.

Following are ten time management guidelines:

1. **Make a daily list of "Things to Do."** List daily goals and set priorities to make sure those unimportant trivial tasks are not being attempted when there are items that are near their deadline.

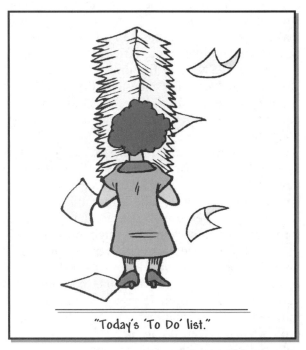

"Today's 'To Do' list."

2. **Determine what the best use of your time is right now.** Are you currently working on something that is best done by someone else? If so and if you can, delegate the task to that person. Focus your energies on the task at hand. Decide what you want from your time, determine how you will use it, and use it wisely.

3. **Use your calendar as a follow-up system.** Make notations on calendar days to indicate when follow-up calls are to be made, when follow-up letters are to be sent, and when deadlines are approaching.

4. **Begin and end each day.** Begin each day with the above "Things to Do" list, prioritizing the most important items at the top of the list and eliminating or putting trivial tasks at the bottom of the list. End your day by going over your list to determine which tasks were not accomplished. Those tasks should be put at the top of the list for the next day, unless they are trivial. Make a rule to move forward trivial items only a maximum of three days. On the third day it must be completed. By doing this, you avoid turning trivial matters into urgent tasks.

5. **Organize calls.** Determine which calls should be made first, and at what time they should be made. Take into consideration the area of the country you are calling. If you are calling from the West Coast to the East Coast, since there is a three hours time difference, making a call after 2 p.m. is probably a waste of time since most businesses close around 5 p.m.

6. **Organize your work area.** Place frequently used items within arms' reach to prevent wasting time looking for them.

7. **Handle it now.** Spend 20 seconds filing that important paper now rather than spending 30 minutes later searching for it. Take a moment to jot down that phone number on your permanent list instead of spending ten minutes tracking it down later.

8. **Be realistic.** One way to set yourself up for a panic situation is to plan an unrealistic amount of work for one day/week/etc. Use common sense to recognize when you have over-scheduled yourself. Enthusiasm is wonderful, but it does not add more hours to the day.

9. **Schedule time for yourself.** If someone wants to see you during the time you have scheduled for yourself, just say, "I am sorry, I have an appointment then." Whether you use this time for personal reflection or as a few quiet minutes to catch your breath or simply to think, it is a legitimate use of time. You will still get as much, if not more, done.

10. **Consider when your energy level peaks.** Do you hit your highest energy level at 10 a.m. or mid-afternoon? Schedule your most important project during your peak energy periods.

Use of the previous guidelines will help you to effectively and efficiently manage your time, and to reach your goals and maintain all standards set before you as a medical biller.

Counting Time Backwards

Sometimes time management involves counting time backwards. Actually this happens in business more often than you may think.

Counting time backwards involves three steps as follows:

- Setting a goal date for the finishing of the project,
- Determining what steps you will need to take before you reach the goal date, and
- Determining the dates that these steps must be accomplished.

For example, if a company wants to put out a catalog of their books in time for the summer, they might set a date of May 5th to mail out the catalogs.

Once you have the date of May 5th, you can start counting backwards. How long will it take the printer to print the catalogs? If the answer is one week, then you know that you have to get the catalog to the printer by April 28th. Before you can get the catalog to the printer you have to allow time for the layout, which includes time to figure out the fonts, the styles and everything else that goes into laying out a catalog. If this takes a week, you need to have all the copy (words and pictures) for layout by April 21st.

It will take about a week to shoot pictures of the books, or to scan in pictures of the books, so the covers on the books will need to be completed by April 14th. It will take about two weeks to design the covers, so this will need to begin on April 1st. The copy for the catalog can be written at the same time the covers are being created and the pictures scanned in, so writing the copy also needs to be scheduled to start on April 1st.

Being able to count time backwards is an important skill for a medical biller. If projects are not started on time they will not be finished on time, and this can cause numerous problems.

When counting time backwards you also need to take into account any holidays, non-working days or other things such as meetings that may cut

into the project time. It is also wise to schedule in a bit of time for unexpected problems. It always seems as though the tighter a schedule is, the more mistakes happen. This is partly due to the stress of focusing on the deadline rather than the project at hand, but it can also be caused from making simple mistakes. By scheduling a few extra days into the project you can give yourself and others the chance to relax and focus.

Overlapping Projects

Overlapping projects are those projects that are being performed by more than one person simultaneously but could actually be performed by one person, thus, eliminating the duplicate effort. Take a moment to look at your project list. Are there any items that can be overlapped? Are there things that can be done at the same time by two different people? Are there two things that can be done at the same time by the same person? For example, if someone is scanning in photos of the speakers for a convention, you may ask them to scan in other pictures for the convention. Scanning in one or two extra items when you already have the program up and running is a lot more time efficient than doing it at two separate times.

One of the best ways to handle this type of situation is to have "ready folders" near some of your projects. For example, if you need some photos scanned in, but it is not important at the moment, just place them in a folder right next to the scanner (or even on the scanner screen). Then, the next time you need to scan in documents you will have available all of the other items that you also need scanned.

The same situation applies to just about any machine, but especially those that take a bit of time to get warmed up. For example, if the fax machine is on a different floor, put a ready folder near the door. Then, the next time you find that you need to go to the floor where the fax is located, you can simply check the ready folder, and fax the document while you are on that floor.

One company had the same system set up for the entire company. They put a couple of hanging file folders beside the elevator. If you had a document that needed to be delivered to someone on a different floor, you put the person's name on the item and dropped it in the hanging folder for that floor. Whenever anyone went to a different floor they would check the folder while waiting for the elevator. If they were passing by anyone who had an item in the folder, they would simply pick up the item and deliver it on their way. At least once a day the person handling the mail would take everything out of these folders and deliver it with the mail. The combined effort of having numerous people make endless trips up and down the stairs just to deliver a piece of paper or two was eliminated, saving the company thousands of dollars a year.

You can set up the same type of system for your desk. Have a folder or specified area for items that need to go to a different floor. Place items in it that need to be delivered to a different work area. Then handle everything on a given floor at a single time.

behind. It is also important to learn to schedule projects in such a way that allow an adequate amount of time to perform them properly. This often requires determining your goal date and working backwards from there to determine the starting date for each portion of the project.

There will always be those projects that are high priority and those that are not. Your job is to make sure that the most important projects are completed in a timely manner. Completing projects in order of priority is the best way to accomplish this.

When you are faced with a pressure situation make sure you understand the assignment, take a deep breath, organize yourself, do not be afraid to ask for help, get the resources you need, and double check your work. Following these steps can help prevent many problems before they start.

Summary

In order to be a good medical biller, you need to manage your time efficiently. If you do not, you will find yourself getting further and further

Assignments

Complete the Questions for Review.
Complete Exercises 2 – 1 through 2 – 2.

Questions for Review

Directions: Answer the following questions without looking back into the material just covered. Write your answer in the space provided.

1. Define prioritize. _____

_____

_____

2. Explain the best method of prioritizing projects._____

_____

_____

_____

3. Before attacking a pressure project what must you make sure you understand? _____

_____

_____

4. When setting priorities, you need to balance the _____ each item provides

   against the _____ and any _____.

5. (True or False?) When you are in a pressure situation do not waste time relaxing to relieve stress. ____

6. What three steps do counting time backwards involve?

   1. _____

   2. _____

   3. _____

7. What are the ten time management guidelines?

   1. _____

   2. _____

   3. _____

   4. _____

   5. _____

   6. _____

   7. _____

   8. _____

   9. _____

   10. _____

8. What are overlapping projects? _____

   _____

   _____

9. What types of machines should be especially used for overlapping projects? _____

   _____

10. What must you do in order to be a good medical biller? _____

   _____

   _____

If you were unable to answer any of the questions, refer back to that section, and then fill in the answers.

Exercise 2 – 1

Directions: Prioritize the following projects by writing the order in the space provided.

	Description	Due Date	Priority Level	Time Needed
_____	Create Lender's Letter	ASAP	High	30 minutes
_____	Gather Information on Statistics	ASAP	Medium	3 hours
_____	Order Word Processing Software	6 weeks	Low	15 minutes
_____	Update Office Policy Memo	2 weeks	Medium	45 minutes
_____	Check and Catalog Diskettes	4 weeks	Low	60 minutes
_____	Register Domain Name	ASAP	High	20 minutes
_____	Enter Invoices	2 months	High	5 hours
_____	Complete Website	3 months	Medium	1 week
_____	Send Mailing	2 months	Medium	2 days
_____	Order Office Supplies	4 weeks	High	1 hour
_____	Call Vendor for New Account #	ASAP	High	5 minutes
_____	File Completed Files	1 week	Medium	4 hours
_____	Update Client List	3 weeks	Low	2 hours
_____	Type Monthly Checks	2 weeks	High	90 minutes
_____	Schedule Staff Meeting	1 week	High	1 hour

Exercise 2 – 2

Directions: Put the following items in the proper order and then show the dates they need to be started and finished.

1. The company is planning a weekend conference for all its employees on June 25th and 26th. It is being planned as a retreat at a nice hotel/resort in Los Angeles. For three hours each morning there will be meetings. One keynote speaker will speak in the morning during breakfast and then there will be four one-hour classes, of which the participants will choose two, to attend. The afternoons will be spent visiting local attractions.

    The following items need to be completed:

    Get speakers (2 weeks to contact, confirm, sign contracts).

    Locate resort (10 days to check out facilities, sign contracts).

    Catering (3 days to plan menus, sign contracts).

    Determine the best events to see (1 week to gather information and make plans and schedule).

    Produce information on the conference for the employees (3 weeks for layout, pictures, biographies, etc.).

    Print the information packets (1 week).

    Create labels of employees name and address and send invitations out (5 days).

2. Craig and Carla Conyers are planning a wedding for July 4th. They want to get married at the Elvis Chapel and honeymoon at the Blue Suede Shoe Hotel in Las Vegas, NV. They plan to invite 50 guests and would like to hire an Elvis impersonator to sing "You Ain't Nothing but a Hound Dog," as well as conduct the ceremony.

    The following items need to be completed:

Reserve blue limousine (3 weeks before wedding date).
Order food for the reception (2 months before wedding date).
Fitting for bridal gown and tuxedo (each 1 week before wedding date).
Find and book Elvis impersonator (4 months before wedding date).
Order invitations for the wedding (12 weeks before wedding date).
Wedding rehearsal at the Chapel (schedule 2 weeks in advance, but rehearsal must be within 5 days of wedding).
Send wedding invitations to guests (must be sent 8 weeks prior to wedding).
Order wedding cake with "Love Me Tender, Love Me Sweet" on it (2 weeks before wedding date).
Deposit for Elvis Chapel (Due 2 months before wedding date).
Find bridal gown (6 weeks before wedding date).
Reserve the Elvis Chapel (6 months before wedding date).
Find tuxedo "Elvis Style" (4 weeks before wedding date).
Make reservations for 7 days at the Blue Suede Shoe Hotel (7 weeks before wedding date).

3. Create your own scenario and list the steps needed to complete it, along with start and finish times for each task. Scenarios must have at least five steps to complete. The scenario should have a completion date of January 5th.

Honors Certification™

Prioritizing
The honors certification for this section is a written test. You will be given a list of items and asked to prioritize them. Each incorrect prioritization will result in a deduction of up to 5% from your grade. You must achieve a score of 85% or higher to pass this test. If you fail the test on your first attempt you may retake the test one additional time. The items included in the second test may be different from those in the first test.

Counting Time Backwards
The honors certification for this section is a written test. You will be given a list of activities similar to those found in Exercise 2 – 2, along with a calendar, and asked to list the date that you should begin working on each of the items. Each incorrect answer will result in a deduction of up to 5% from your grade. You must achieve a score of 85% or higher to pass this test. If you fail the test on your first attempt you may retake the test one additional time. The items included in the second test may be different from those in the first test.

Overall Chapter Test
You will also be given a written test of the information contained in this chapter. Each incorrect answer will result in a deduction of up to 5% from your grade. You must achieve a score of 85% or higher to pass this test. If you fail the test on your first attempt you may retake the test one additional time. The items included in the second test may be different from those in the first test.

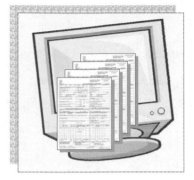

3

Legal Issues

After completion of this chapter you will be able to:

- List the general guidelines to be followed to maintain patient privacy.
- Describe how to maintain patient privacy when faxing information.
- List exceptions to the privacy guidelines.
- List some of the most common instances of fraud in the medical environment.
- Describe HIPAA and its relationship to fraud and abuse.
- Define embezzlement and give several examples.
- Explain what disclaimers are and how to use them appropriately.
- Define and explain the two types of damages that can be awarded in a bad faith action.
- Define malice, fraud and oppression.
- State the ethics guidelines medical billers should adhere to.
- List the appropriate procedures to be followed when handed a records subpoena.
- List and describe instances in which the patient should be notified and the patient chart notated.

Key words and concepts you will learn in this chapter:

Disclaimers – Statements such as "It appears that," or "This may be...." These words allow a general answer to the question without making any type of promise.

Embezzlement – The act of an employee illegally taking funds from a company they work for.

Fraud – Intentional misrepresentation of a fact with the intent to deprive a person of property or legal rights.

Legal Damages – Monetary awards that a plan member may attempt to recover, which are above and beyond the benefits provided by the group plan.

Malice – Intentional conduct to cause injury or conduct that is carried on with the conscious disregard of the rights of others.

Oppression – Putting a person through cruel and unjust hardships with conscious disregard of rights.

There are several legal issues that affect the medical biller on a daily basis. These include privacy regulations, rules and regulations regarding allowable collections procedures, and fraud.

Privacy Guidelines

The very nature of health care requires a great deal of personal information to be gathered and maintained about many individuals. Therefore, the needs of the company must be carefully weighed against the person's right to privacy so as to avoid unwarranted invasions of that right.

In particular, medical information is considered to be privileged and confidential in the context of the physician/patient relationship. Unauthorized disclosure of information may represent a violation of that confidentiality.

The confidentiality of medical records has assumed a new importance for several reasons:

1. People are becoming more litigation-minded.
2. Health plans are reimbursing for more sensitive services that were excluded in the past, for example, alcohol detoxification, mental health treatment, and AIDS-related illnesses.
3. More employers are self-administering or self-funding their health plans, which means that highly personal medical information is, in some instances, routinely handled by fellow employees.
4. New HIPAA regulations require that all personnel involved in the health care process respect the patient's right to privacy and confidentiality.

HIPAA

In 1996, President William Clinton signed into law the **Health Insurance Portability and Accountability Act (HIPAA)**.The portability issues refer to persons being covered by insurance when they transfer from one job to another. These issues are most important to the health claims examiner. However, the privacy issues and the health insurance fraud and abuse issues are vitally important for the medical biller to understand.

HIPAA encompasses two main issues:

1. Portability, or the ability to transfer insurance companies and still be covered for pre-existing conditions, and
2. Accountability, generally dealing with the patient's right to privacy from the medical provider, health insurer, and any other parties required in the health care process (i.e., billers, clearinghouses, etc.), and the lack of fraud and abuse when dealing with health care.

Regarding the Privacy section of HIPAA, the Department of Health and Human Services states:

"The privacy requirements limit the release of patient Protected Health Information (PHI) without the patient's knowledge and consent beyond that required for patient care. Patient's personal information must be more securely guarded and more carefully handled when conducting the business of health care."

All health care entities were required to meet the standards set in the privacy issues section of HIPAA on April 14, 2003.

General Rules

Following are the general rules for ensuring that privacy guidelines are met:

1. Always obtain an authorization to release information before releasing any information. Most releases routinely signed in the medical practice only authorize the physician to release information necessary to process a patient's claim. Additional authorization should be obtained to release any information to other parties. These releases should state exactly what information is to be released, the dates of any services provided which fall within the release, the person to whom the information may be released, the signature of the patient, the date of the signature, and the date the release expires.
2. Gather only the information that is necessary and relevant to the billing or processing of the claim.
3. Use only legal and ethical means to collect the information required. Whenever permission is necessary, obtain written authorization from the insured or patient (guardian or parent if the patient is a minor).
4. When requested, and subject to any applicable legal or ethical prohibition or privilege, the insured or patient concerned should be advised of the nature and general uses to be made of the information.
5. Make every reasonable effort to ensure that the information upon which an action is based is accurate, relevant, timely, and complete.
7. Upon request, the patient or insured should be given the opportunity to correct or clarify the information given by or about he or she, and the file should be amended to the extent that it is fair to both the provider and the patient or insured. Requests for review or clarification of medical information will be accepted only from the person from whom the information was obtained.

8. In general, disclosures of information to a third party (other than those described to the insured or patient) should be made only with the written authorization of the patient or insured. This includes disclosure to employers, family members or former spouses.

9. All practical precautions should be taken to ensure that medical files are physically secure and that access to the use of such files is limited to authorized personnel. This includes not leaving files out, locking all files, and even turning your computer screen away from where it might be seen by other persons. Security passwords and other security measures may also be required, depending on your office situation.

10. All personnel involved in the keeping of medical records should be advised of the need to protect the Right of Privacy in obtaining required information and the need to treat all individually identifiable information as confidential. Willful abuse of the privacy of any insured or patient by the employee may be cause for dismissal.

11. The disclosure of a diagnosis should never be made to an insured or his or her family. If the insured requests this information, refer the insured to the physician. There may be a reason the patient does not know his or her diagnosis.

12. Never release any information to an ex-spouse. This includes the patient's address, phone number, when services were rendered, to whom, and other information. The ex-spouse should be instructed to contact the patient directly.

13. Do not leave files, patients' records or appointment books open on your desk or in an area where they may be seen by others. This includes patient's files or information that may be displayed on a computer screen. The best way to handle this is to be sure that all files are closed or are turned over on your desk. Computer screens must be placed in such a way that they cannot be seen by anyone passing by. If necessary, use a screen saver or other unrestricted document that can be clicked on to replace the one you are working on instantaneously.

14. If a minor patient has the legal right to authorize treatment for services, disclosure to the parents, legal guardians of the minor, or to other persons may be a violation of HIPAA and/or the confidentiality of Medical Information Privacy and Security Act (MIPSA).

15. Be cautious about releasing information to a patient's employer, even if an authorization to release information has been obtained.

If in doubt as to whether specific information should be released, check with your supervisor before, not after, releasing it.

These guidelines cover some of the basic aspects of HIPAA privacy regulations. For detailed information regarding HIPAA guidelines, complete rules and regulations regarding HIPAA are printed in the Federal Register.

Faxing

When faxing items, be aware of sensitive information on a fax. All faxes should contain a cover sheet which announces who the fax is to, who it is from, and a notation that the enclosed information is personal and confidential. Information regarding diagnosis, treatments, sexually transmitted diseases, HIV, drug or alcohol abuse or financial information should never be faxed. Following is sample wording for the fax confidentiality statement:

The enclosed information is intended exclusively for the individual or entity to which it is addressed and contains information which is privileged, confidential or exempt from disclosure under federal or state laws. If the reader of this message is not the recipient or the agent or employee responsible for delivering this facsimile transmission to the intended recipient you are hereby notified that any dissemination, distribution or copying of the information contained in this facsimile is strictly prohibited. If you have received this facsimile in error, please notify our office immediately by telephone and return the original facsimile to us at the above address.

When faxing other information, consider asking the receiving party for a code number (i.e., the patient's ID number or birthdate), then black out all pertinent information on the patient and replace it with the code number.

Items should only be faxed in an emergency. Otherwise, regular or certified mail should be used.

The guidelines listed are just that. The final decisions are up to you. Use common sense and put yourself in the place of the patient or insured.

Exceptions

There are a few exceptions to the privacy laws. In the following instances the privacy guidelines may be considered less stringent, or the patient may be deemed to have waived their rights to confidentiality:

1. Less stringent guidelines apply for physicians who are employed by insurance companies. Disclosure to their employers of patient records and information is more routine.
2. Cases of gunshot wounds, stabbings resulting from criminal actions, and suspected child abuse which must be reported to the local police department or child care agency. Some states also require that incidents of spousal abuse be reported.
3. Reports of communicable diseases and some diseases and illnesses of infants and newborns. These are most often used for compiling statistics and attempting to stop the spread of communicable diseases.
4. Information obtained by the Medicare insurance carrier which pertains to a patient may be reported directly to that patient's beneficiary or his representative. The Medicare insurance specialist cannot accept or withhold information they receive regarding a patient, even if the information is marked "confidential."
5. If a patient is seen at the request of a third party who is covering the bill (i.e., workers compensation cases), limited confidentiality is waived and the information may be provided to the person or company ordering the procedures.
6. If records are subpoenaed or a search warrant is issued, records may be turned over to the court or their representatives.

Fraud

Fraud is defined as intentional misrepresentation of a fact with the intent to deprive a person of property or legal rights. The most common instance of fraud that occurs in the health claims industry is doctors or other providers of service billing for goods or services that were not actually provided.

Because of the high incidence of abuse, all billed services must be documented in the medical record to prove that they were actually provided. The "law of documentation" states that "if it wasn't documented, it didn't happen." Billing for services not provided is a serious offense and constitutes fraud. If a person is convicted the penalties are extremely stiff. In addition, both the physician and the medical biller can be held liable for the filing of fraudulent claims.

The most common cases of fraud include:

1. Overbilling or billing for services not rendered.
2. Altering records or claims to upgrade the service presented (i.e., billing for a high complexity office visit when the services provided were for a low complexity visit).
3. Changing dates on services or splitting procedures (i.e., placing different dates on services that were actually performed on the same date, changing the date to make it appear as if treatment were rendered after the surgery follow-up days, rather than during the follow-up days).
4. Unbundling of charges (i.e., listing lab charges as though a number of separate tests were done when several tests were done simultaneously from the same sample).
5. Allowing a patient to use the medical coverage card for another patient, or billing services under an incorrect patient name (i.e., Sally Smith, 23 and not covered under her parents insurance is billed as Sandy Smith, her 16 year old sister who is covered).
6. Allowing, offering, soliciting or accepting a kickback or return of monies for a referral or for use of a specific product.
7. Altering the diagnosis to substantiate procedures performed.
8. Billing twice for the same services.
9. Billing group services as if they were individual services (i.e., a psychiatrist visits several patients in a group session, but billing as if each patient was seen individually).
10. Ordering or billing for services that were performed, but were not medically necessary.

11. Accepting payment in full from insurance carriers. Such practice is considered fraudulent (especially with Medicare) because the insurance is actually paying 100% of the services, not the 80% (or other coinsurance percent) which they contracted with the patient to pay. Such a practice often leads physicians to increase their bills to make up the difference, and can lead patients to over utilizing services since there is no financial incentive to limit visits.

    If occasional cases are written off due to hardship, this should be documented in the records, along with an explanation of the hardship circumstances and the reasoning for the dismissal of the debt.

12. Billing different patients at different rates (i.e., one charge for Medicare patients and a different charge for uninsured patients for the same services).

13. Requiring patients to pay balances in excess of Medicare, Medicaid or HMO limits.

14. Requiring Medicare patients to pay for services which should be covered by Medicare, thus not being limited by the Medicare approved amount.

15. Failing to refund copayments and deductible charges for Medicare patients whose charges have been deemed by Medicare to be not medically necessary.

16. Submitting claims to two or more insurers without disclosing that more than one insurance may cover the charges.

17. Billing Medicare or other insurance carriers when bills should be submitted to a third party (i.e., workers compensation coverage, a third party that may be liable in the case of an accident).

If the physician is engaging in such practices and it can be shown that the biller participated, or even if they merely knew about the fraudulent acts and did nothing, the medical biller can be charged as an accomplice, even if they received no money themselves. As a precautionary measure, having billers initial the claims they create and/or submit for payment can help to track down the guilty party.

Since a physician is considered ultimately responsible for everything that goes on in his or her practice, the physician may be considered guilty of fraud even if they had no knowledge of the crime. The physician may be criminally sentenced, or may merely have to reimburse the insurance carrier for all fraudulently submitted claims.

If a person, either a physician or a biller, is found guilty of Medicare or Medicaid fraud, they are excluded from ever participating in the program again.

HIPAA and Fraud and Abuse

The new HIPAA fraud statutes have greatly broadened the scope of the federal government for prosecuting fraud and abuse in the health care industry. HIPAA defines four new criminal health care fraud offenses: Health Care Fraud, Theft or Embezzlement in Connection with Health Care, False Statements Relating to Health Care Matters, and Obstruction of Criminal Investigations of Health Care Offenses.

HIPAA now defines a health care benefit program as "any public or private plan or contract, affecting commerce, under which any medical benefit, item, or service is provided to any individual, and includes any individual or entity who is providing a medical benefit, item, or service for which payment may be made under the plan or contract." By including private health benefit plans and any individual or entity, they have effectively given themselves the right to prosecute anyone involved in the health care industry for fraud or abuse.

The following four sections further define the HIPAA statutes:

Health Care Fraud (18 USC 1347): Whoever knowingly and willfully executes, or attempts to execute, a scheme or artifice to defraud any health care benefit program; or to obtain, by means of false or fraudulent pretenses, representations, or promises, any of the money or property owned by, or under the custody or control of, any health care benefit program, in connection with the delivery of or payment for health care benefits, items, or services, shall be fined under this title [up to $250,000 per offense] or imprisoned not more than 10 years, or both.

The medical biller needs to keep in mind that if he creates or submits a health claim which he knows to be fraudulent he may be held liable under this portion of the statute.

<u>Theft or Embezzlement in Connection with Health Care (18 USC 669)</u>: Whoever knowingly and willfully embezzles, steals, or otherwise without authority converts to the use of any person other than the rightful owner, or intentionally misapplies any of the moneys, funds, securities, premiums, credits, property, or other assets of a health care benefit program, shall be fined under this title or imprisoned not more than 10 years, or both; but if the value of such property does not exceed the sum of $100 the defendant shall be fined under this title or imprisoned not more than one year, or both.

Any medical biller that does any of the following: accepts payment on claims which they know to be fraudulent; misapplies medical payments to the wrong account; takes home office supplies, equipment or other items with the intent to keep; and drafts unauthorized checks to himself or others, may be held liable under this portion of the statute.

<u>False Statements Relating to Health Care Matters (18 USC 1035)</u>: Whoever, in any matter involving a health care benefit program, knowingly and willfully falsifies, conceals, or covers up by any trick, scheme, or device a material fact; or makes any materially false, fictitious, or fraudulent statements or representations, or makes or uses any materially false writing or document knowing the same to contain any materially false, fictitious, or fraudulent statement or entry, in connection with the delivery of or payment for health care benefits, items, or services, shall be fined under this title or imprisoned not more than 5 years, or both.

A medical biller that creates false claims and/or claim documents, alters and/or falsifies claim information, lies about claims situations, and does not come forward to disclose fraudulent situations that they are aware of, may be held liable under this portion of the statute.

<u>Obstruction of Criminal Investigations of Health Care Offenses (18 USC 1518)</u>: (a) Whoever willfully prevents, obstructs, misleads, delays or attempts to prevent, obstruct, mislead or delay the communication of information or records relating to a violation of a Federal health care offense to a criminal investigator shall be fined under this title or imprisoned not more than 5 years, or both. (b) As used in this section the term criminal investigator means any individual duly authorized by a department, agency, or armed force of the United States to conduct or engage in investigations for prosecutions for violations of health care offenses.

Destroying records, not turning over files or documents when asked, lying to investigators and generally being uncooperative during an investigation may cause a medical biller to be liable under this portion of the statute.

It is important for the medical biller to be aware of these issues. If you discover a possibly fraudulent claim, it is important to bring it to your supervisor's attention as soon as possible. Additionally, if an investigation is initiated you should cooperate fully with the investigators. Not doing so could be construed as hindering their investigation, making you liable for fines and imprisonment up to five years. It is important to note that the statutes are written in such a way that you can be found guilty of hindering an investigation, even if that investigation later fails to turn up fraud.

Additionally, medical billers need to be cautious about the statements or comments they make regarding a claim, especially written comments which are placed in a file. If those comments turn out to be fraudulent, the medical biller may be held liable.

Embezzlement

Embezzlement is the act of an employee illegally taking funds from a company they work for. Embezzlement can be committed by anyone in a firm, including the receptionist, the biller, or the physician.

To protect against embezzlement:
1. Accurate records must be kept of all transactions. Be sure to issue a receipt for all amounts received and to accurately record these amounts against the patient's account.
2. Any amounts removed should be notated and a receipt given for them. This is not only true for amounts that may have been taken from the cash drawer to pay for office supplies, but for amounts a physician may remove. Even if the physician is the sole owner of the practice, he or she should never be allowed to take money from the cash drawer without issuing a receipt. Such

a practice helps keep accurate records for financial accounting purposes, and protects the keeper of the cash drawer from being charged with removing the money.

3. All checks should be immediately stamped FOR DEPOSIT ONLY with the account number. The bank should be given instructtions that they are never to cash a check made payable to the practice and cash back should never be given from a deposit.

4. All monthly bank statements should be matched with the daily and monthly journals for the office. Total deposits should tally with the total of all daily journals. Any discrepancies should be reported immediately to a supervisor.

5. If embezzlement is suspected, the proper person should be notified. In the case of a co-worker, this is usually their supervisor. If a worker knows of embezzlement by a co-worker and say nothing, they are guilty of being an accomplice to the crime.

6. A bond (insurance against embezzlement) should be obtained for each member of the practice who deals directly with the practice's receipts. These bonds can be issued on individual persons, on a job position, or for the entire office staff.

7. If you notice poor bookkeeping or inaccurate records which were kept by a previous employee or a current co-worker, this should be brought to the attention of your supervisor or employer. You should then document the problems in writing and ask the supervisor or employer to initial a copy for you to keep. This may provide minimal protection in case the problems with the records were found to conceal embezzlement or mismanagement of funds.

As with fraud, a physician is considered ultimately responsible for everything that goes on in his or her practice. If embezzlement is found, the physician may be considered guilty and may be responsible for monies embezzled by their employees.

Disclaimers

One of the best ways to protect yourself from possible legal action is to use disclaimers. **Disclaimers** are statements such as "It appears that," or "This may be...." These words allow a

general answer to the question without making any type of promise. If the biller or examiner makes a statement that is later found to be in error, it can cause numerous problems, both in customer satisfaction and in possible legal issues.

All medical billers and claims examiners should practice using disclaimers in their conversations.

When confirming a subscriber's eligibility and benefits, disclaimers should always be included. The following are disclaimers that could possibly be used in your verbal and written responses:

Eligibility. "We show that _____ is currently effective on group_____. However, in order to receive benefits, he/she must be eligible at the time services are rendered."

Benefit. "These are the benefits now in effect for this contract. In order to receive benefits, your membership must be in good standing on the dates services are rendered."

Legal Damages

Legal damages are monetary awards that a plan member may attempt to recover, which are above and beyond the benefits provided by the group plan.

In the legal climate today, it is not uncommon for plan members to seek legal channels to obtain benefits or to obtain greater benefits than provided by a plan of benefits. Usually, such cases are based on what is known as "bad faith."

An insurance policy or a health and welfare plan is considered a legal contract. Under contract law, the patient can only recover benefits up to the policy or plan limits.

However, with the development of consumerism the courts have become more liberal. In some states there has developed a body of law that says that there is an implied obligation of good faith and fair dealings in every contract. If this obligation is breached, it is termed as "bad faith." Generally, the law of bad faith allows an insured to attempt to recover various types of damages above and beyond the benefits provided by the plan. The courts will look at two concepts to determine whether a plan has met the obligation of good faith and fair dealing:

1. Did the plan give the patient's interest equal consideration with that given the company's interest?

2. Was the claim handled or denied in accordance with the plan provisions and in a timely manner?

The following are examples of how courts often view policy interpretations:

- The meaning of a plan of benefits is determined by the member's reasonable expectations of coverage.
- Uncertain wording that could be subject to more than one interpretation will usually be resolved against the plan and in favor of the insured.
- When two equally believable interpretations may be made, the one that gives the greatest amount of protection to the insured will prevail.

There are two types of damages that a court may award: compensatory damages and punitive damages.

Compensatory damages are designed to compensate an insured for all of the actual losses or damages to make that person whole again. For example, if a person has not been able to pay his or her home mortgage or car payment because they did not receive a monthly disability check and, therefore, the person's home and car are repossessed, he or she may be able to recover equity in the home and car as well as attorney fees and also possible damages for emotional stress.

Punitive damages are often the larger of the two awards and are intended primarily to punish a wrongdoing defendant and set them up as an example to help deter such actions in the future. Unlike compensatory damages, punitive damages are not automatically recoverable if bad faith is found. In addition to bad faith, a plan member in California, for example, must prove the plan to be guilty of oppression, fraud, or malice.

Bad Faith Awards

The dollar amount of a bad faith award is based on two concepts: (1) the degree of wrongfulness and (2) the wealth of the defendant.

All lawsuits are expensive not only in the dollar cost of the damages, but in other costs as well. These costs remain even if the case is settled out of court. If the case is settled out of court, the plaintiff's attorney's costs, miscellaneous costs, the attorney costs for the plan, and the benefit not originally paid must be paid and, finally, substantial "pain and suffering" costs may be included. The value of the claim usually has no correlation to the amount of restitution (award) sought.

Part of the reason for the continuing escalation of premium costs is the necessity to be prepared for lawsuits, because whether the case is settled in court or out of court, the monetary damage to the plan is usually significant and often preventable.

In light of the foregoing information, it is important that every claim be handled quickly, correctly, and fairly. This responsibility falls on each and every medical biller and claims examiner. To fulfill this responsibility, the following four guidelines should be incorporated into the routine handling and processing of claims:

1. Every customer and patient is entitled to courteous, fair and just treatment. An acknowledgment of all communications with respect to a claim or bill should be received with reasonable promptness.
2. Customers and patients should be treated equally and without outside considerations other than those dictated by the office policy or plan provisions.
3. Every claim is entitled to a prompt investigation of all pertinent facts and objective evaluation in the fair and equitable settlement of the claim.
4. Recognize the obligation to pay all just claims promptly.

Medical Ethics

Ethics is defined as the rules or standards governing the conduct of members of a profession. In general, medical ethics defines a right and proper way of treating patients.

The American Medical Association has created a set of standards that all physicians are expected to uphold. These standards include the following:

- Providing competent service with compassion and respect for the patients,
- Dealing honestly with people,
- Being a law-abiding citizen, but also working to change those laws that may not be in the best interests of the patient,
- Respecting the rights of others,
- Continuing to study and upgrade skills with the latest in medical advancement,
- Providing emergency medical treatment to anyone who is in need, and
- Working to improve the community.

Although the medical biller has not sworn an oath to uphold these principles he or she should realize that the physician he or she works with upholds this oath. As an adjunct to the physician, the medical biller should do the best to also uphold these standards and to assist the physician in doing so.

Among other things, ethics guidelines include:

1. Not making critical remarks about your physician, another physician, or any treatment given or not given.

2. If you discover that a patient is being treated by more than one physician for the same ailment, notify your physician immediately. It is not only unethical for two physicians to treat a patient for the same condition, but it can be potentially dangerous. Prescription overdose or complications between treatment plans could result if one physician is unaware of treatment given by another physician.

3. Respecting the dignity of others. This includes calling patients and co-workers by their appropriate title and last name (i.e., Dr. Smith, Mrs. Hall), not using slang terms in reference to someone, (i.e., honey, dear, sweetie), making no references to race, religion, creed, color, sex, or ethnic origin unless it is medically necessary for the treatment of the patient, refraining from touching a patient or co-worker unless it is medically necessary.

4. Refusing to participate in illegal or unethical acts or to conceal the illegal or unethical acts of others.

Subpoenas

Occasionally, the medical records of a patient may be needed in a court action. In such a case a subpoena is issued requesting the records. A **subpoena** is a demand for a witness to appear. Sometimes a witness will need to turn the records over to the court personally, at other times they may be mailed.

One person in the office should be designated in charge of medical records. This person should be the only person to accept a subpoena of medical records. If you are designated that person, the subpoena must be served in person. It cannot be laid on a desk or sent through the mail. No one else should accept the subpoena in your absence.

A witness fee or mileage amount may be given to a witness. You should request any payable fees at the time the subpoena is served.

If the subpoena is only for the records, not for the records and for the record keeper as a witness, you should call the attorney who sent the subpoena and ask if the records can be sent. If so, send the records by certified mail, return receipt requested.

Usually, you are given a specified amount of time to produce the records. Occasionally the records will need to be turned over at the time of the subpoena. In all cases, consult with the physician before turning over the records. If the physician is unavailable, let the server know that you are unable to turn over the records without proper authorization and let them know when they can come back and serve the subpoena directly on the physician. This will give you time to be sure that the records are complete, accurate and in good order. Also be sure all signatures are identifiable and make copies.

In most cases the original record must be sent. Always keep a copy of all records sent. This allows you to check for changes in the records and protects against loss on information if the records are lost. Number the pages before copying so you can determine if any pages are missing.

If there is more than one physician in your office be sure the subpoena is served on the record keeper for that physician or to that physician directly.

If you are unable to accept the subpoena and no one is present who is authorized to accept it, explain the situation to the person serving the subpoena. Suggest a time when they can come back or ask them to contact the doctor's attorney. Then inform the doctor and/or their attorney of the situation.

Once a subpoena has been served, ask the doctor to check over the medical records to be sure they are accurate and complete, then number the pages and make a complete copy. The original file should then be sent out immediately (if delivery by certified mail is allowed) or placed under lock and key to avoid tampering. Find out the day of the trial and comply with all orders given by the court. Be sure not to allow anyone to see the records or tamper with them. The records should be turned over only to the judge and should only be left in the care of the judge or jury, never in the care of an attorney. Be sure to obtain a receipt for the records if leaving them.

Subpoena Notification

If a subpoena is served to request medical records, many offices will notify the patient in writing that the records have been requested. This allows the patient's attorney to file papers with the court to block the subpoena.

If there is very little time between the date the subpoena was served and the date the records have been requested, the letter may be faxed or the patient may be contacted by telephone. In either case, be sure to let the patient know that they do not have the authority to stop you from releasing the records. They must have their attorney file a petition with the court in order to have the subpoena rescinded. A sample of a subpoena notification follows:

PATIENT NOTIFICATION OF SUBPOENA

Date: _____
To: _____
Address: _____

Dear Patient and your Attorney of Record:

Please note that a subpoena for records pertaining to you are being sought by/from_____ as shown in the subpoena attached to this Notice.

If you object to us furnishing any part of the records described in this action, you must file papers with the court prior to our release of these records. This subpoena requires that we furnish the records on or by _____ (date).

You or your attorney of record may contact the attorney for the party seeking to examine such records and determine whether they are willing to agree to cancel or limit this subpoena. If no such agreement is reached and you are not already represented by an attorney in this action, **you should consult an attorney to advise you of your rights in this matter.**

If we do not have notification in writing regarding the cancellation or limitation of this subpoena at least 24 hours prior to the above date, we will assume you have no objection to us releasing this information.

Signed: _____ Date: _____

Instances in Which the Patient Should be Notified and the File Notated

The following sections include situations which may warrant the sending of a letter to the patient. In each case the letters are samples and should be modified to fit the circumstances of the individual situation.

A copy of the letter should always be placed in the patient's file. The physician may choose to have the patient sign this letter and return it, acknowledging receipt of the letter and the information it contains. This is a further step protecting the physician against a lawsuit.

If a signature is requested, two copies of the letter should be sent to the patient and a third copy placed in the file. The patient should keep one of the copies they receive, sign the other one and return it. If a letter is not returned with a signature within two weeks of having been mailed, call the patient and discuss the situation with them, then document the phone conversation in the patient's medical file.

Patient Who Fails to Keep an Appointment

If a patient fails to keep an appointment when their condition is serious and/or needs constant monitoring, a letter should be sent advising the patient of the need for treatment or monitoring. The patient may not realize the seriousness of their condition, and may hold the doctor liable for this lack of knowledge if consequences arise from not being treated.

ON LETTERHEAD

Date:
Dear _____:

An appointment was scheduled for you on (date)_____ at _____ a.m./p.m. which you failed to keep. Please be advised that I consider your condition to be serious and in need of further medical treatment and/or monitoring.

Please contact my office for another appointment as soon as possible. If you choose to be treated by another physician, I urge you to seek an appointment with him or her without delay. With your authorization, I would be happy to share any test results or medical records with such a physician.

Two copies of this letter are enclosed. One is for your files. Please sign the second copy and return it to our office in the enclosed envelope.

Please understand my purpose in writing this letter is concern for your overall medical health.

Sincerely,

Doctor, M.D.

Patient Signature: _____Date: _____

Patient Left Facility Against Medical Advice

Occasionally, a patient will leave the hospital against medical advice, or will refuse to follow the advice given by the doctor. In such cases, the medical practice needs to be protected against lawsuits stemming from the lack of proper treatment.

In the case of a patient that leaves a treatment facility against the advice of their doctor, the facility will often ask the patient to sign a form stating that they are leaving even though they understand the doctor advises against it. A patient cannot be restrained from leaving or forced to sign the waiver. If the patient refuses to sign the waiver a notation should be made on the form of the refusal to sign and the form should then be signed and dated by two witnesses.

Most facilities have a standard form to use for this purpose. A copy of a form follows.

STATEMENT OF PATIENT LEAVING XXX TREATMENT CENTER AGAINST MEDICAL ADVICE

Date: _____

This letter is to certify that I, (patient name) am leaving the above-named facility at my own insistence and against the advice of my attending physician and other treatment facility authorities. I understand the dangers of my leaving at this time. This letter hereby releases the facility, its employees and officers and any attending physicians from any and all liability which may be caused as a result of my departure.

This letter may also be construed as an agreement to hold harmless the above facility, its employees and officers and any attending physicians from any and all liability which may be caused as a result of my departure.

Patient Signature: _____ Date: _____

Parent/Guardian Signature: _____ Date: _____

Witness: _____ Date: _____

___ If the patient refuses to sign this form, place an X in the space at left, fill out the form, and have it signed by two treatment center personnel. The words SIGNATURE REFUSED should be placed on the line reserved for the patient signature.

Refusal to Follow Treatment

At times there are patients who refuse to follow the advice of their physician. This can be anything from a decision not to give up smoking for improving overall health, to a patient refusing to take the prescribed medication which could save their life.

In all cases, the practice should be protected as much as possible by having the patient sign a letter. The letter should state the condition of the patient, the medical advice, and the possible consequences of not following the advice. Having a signed copy of this letter in the patient's file helps to protect against a lawsuit in which the patient states they were not informed of the consequences of not following the medical advice. A letter similar to the following could be written:

ON LETTERHEAD

Date:

Dear _____:

Two weeks ago you were diagnosed with hypertension (high blood pressure). At that time I prescribed a dosage of 500 mg of Diuril (Chlorothiazide) to be taken twice daily. It has come to our attention that you are not taking your medication as prescribed. I strongly urge you to take your medication as prescribed and return to my office for another checkup in two weeks to monitor your condition. If you choose to seek care from another physician, we will be happy to provide him or her with any test results or records.

Please understand that not taking your medication can result in severe damage to your kidneys, heart, circulatory system and other organs. Not getting your hypertension under control can lead to a heart attack, stroke or even death.

Please sign the bottom of this letter and return it in the enclosed envelope to attest that you have read it and are aware of the consequences that may result from not following the medical advice given to you.

Sincerely,

Doctor, M.D.

Patient Signature: _____ Date: _____

Termination of Treatment

It sometimes becomes necessary for a patient to terminate their care with a physician. This most often happens at the request of the patient and is often due to circumstances beyond their control (i.e., relocation out of the area).

To protect the practice, it is best to ask the patient to complete a letter of termination of care. If a patient is not currently under treatment for a condition, the following letter will usually suffice:

ON LETTERHEAD

Letter Confirming Termination of Treatment

Date: _____

Dear: _____

This letter is to confirm our understanding that as of _____ (date) you wish to discharge Donald Doctor, M.D. as your physician. We will be sorry to see you go.

Please know that we have enjoyed the opportunity to serve you and will be happy to provide your medical records, with your authorization, to any new physician you choose.

Please sign the bottom of this letter to confirm termination of treatment and return it to our office in the enclosed envelope.

Thank you very much.

Sincerely,

Doctor, M.D.

I hereby acknowledge receipt of this letter and agree to termination of treatment on the above date.

Patient Signature: _____ Date: _____

When a Physician Terminates Care

Occasionally, a physician will feel the need to terminate the care of a patient when the patient continually refuses to follow medical advice. Termination of treatment should occur only after the patient has been fully advised of the consequences of not following the prescribed medical advice.

ON LETTERHEAD

Date:

Dear Mr. _____:

I find it necessary to terminate any further care of your case due to your repeated refusal to follow medical advice. It is my opinion that your condition requires further treatment or serious consequences may develop. I strongly urge you to seek the care of another physician immediately.

I would be happy to provide, upon your authorization, any test results or medical records needed by the new physician.

If you desire, I shall continue to provide your medical care for the next _____ days, until _____. This should give you ample time to secure the services of a new physician.

Please sign one copy of this letter and return it to our office to acknowledge that you have read and understand this information. The second copy is for your records.

Sincerely,

Doctor, M.D.

Patient Signature: _____ Date: _____

Summary

The medical biller needs to be aware of numerous legal and ethical issues. These include being aware of what it means to file a fraudulent claim, knowing possible damages that could be assessed, understanding the Right to Privacy Act, and agreeing to abide by the basic principles of medical ethics.

Additionally, there are numerous instances or situations in which the patient should be notified and the patient's chart notated. There are a number of forms and letters to cover many of these situations. The medical biller should be aware of these situations and the proper information to be included in these forms and letters.

Assignments

Complete the Questions for Review.

Questions for Review

Directions: Answer the following questions without looking back into the material just covered. Write your answers in the space provided.

1. What are the two concepts that a court will usually look at to determine whether a health insurance plan has met the obligation of good faith and fair dealing?

    1. _____

    2. _____

2. When two equally believable interpretations may be made, the one which gives _____
   _____ will prevail.

3. Name and explain the two types of damages that may be awarded in bad faith actions.

    1. _____

    2. _____

4. _____ is intentional misrepresentation of a fact with the intent to deprive a person of legal rights.

5. _____ is intentional conduct to cause injury, or conduct that is carried on with the conscious disregard of the rights of others.

6. _____ is to put a person through cruel and unjust hardships with conscious disregard of rights.

7. The dollar amount of a bad faith award is based on two concepts:

    1. _____and

    2. _____.

8. (True or False?)The diagnosis or disclosure of an illness should never be made to the patient even if he or she asks for this information._____

9. Name three instances in which the patient should be notified and a notation made in the patient's chart.

    1. _____

    2. _____

    3. _____

10. What are disclaimers and when should you use them? _____
    _____
    _____

If you were unable to answer any of the questions, refer back to that section, and then fill in the answers.

Honors Certification™

The certification challenge for this chapter will be a written test of the information contained in this chapter. Each incorrect answer will result in a deduction of up to 5% from your grade. You must achieve a score of 85% or higher to pass this test.   If you fail the test on your first attempt you may retake the test one additional time. The items included in the second test may be different from those in the first test.

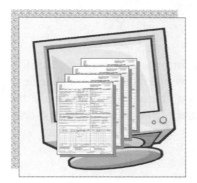

4

Clinical Records Management

After completion of this chapter you will be able to:

- Describe how a medical chart is put together.
- Describe how charts for pediatric and emergency patients are different from other medical charts.
- Show how to file x-rays in a chart.
- Properly file a patient chart.
- List the rules for proper medical charting.
- Properly complete a signature card.
- Describe the use of a signature card.
- Explain why and for how long records should be retained.
- Describe the process for storing medical records.
- Describe features available with electronic medical charting.
- Discuss the pros and cons of computerized medical charting.
- Properly complete a records transfer request.

Key words and concepts you will learn in this chapter:

Alphabetical Filing – Filing medical charts alphabetically by the first letter of the patient's last name.

Altering – Changing or amending the information contained in a record or chart.

Children's Chart – A medical file specifically for children.

Correction Fluid – A liquid that covers over the writing on paper.

Electronic Prescriptions – Prescriptions that are entered into the provider's computer, then electronically sent to the computer at the patient's pharmacy.

Maintaining Records – Keeping the information in a record updated and filing the chart or record in a manner that makes it easy to locate if you should need it at a later date.

Non-compliance – Not following the instructions given by the provider.

Pediatric Chart – A patient file for a child.

Keeping accurate patient charts is essential to the running of a good medical practice. Without accurate patient charts the provider may find it difficult to properly treat the patient's condition. Additionally, it can be difficult to bill insurance companies and/or the patient for treatment that was performed.

Medical charts contain a number of forms. Some of these forms are needed at each visit. Other forms, such as those authorizing treatment, are completed once and merely stored in the patient's file.

Maintaining records means keeping the information in a record updated and filing the chart or record in a manner that makes it easy to locate if you should need it at a later date. In this chapter we will cover the general practices in maintaining patient charts. The actual forms within a chart will be covered in other chapters in this text.

Medical Charts

In most medical offices, a separate chart is kept on each and every patient. While this can often necessitate the repetition of some information, it is necessary to insure compliance with HIPAA guidelines and to keep the information separate for each patient.

Medical billers are often responsible for creating new patient charts. This means completing or having the patient complete the initial forms and putting them in the charts in the proper order. If the patient has an insurance card or other proof of coverage, a photocopy of this information is included with the above forms.

Often the medical biller or receptionist is the first person who sees a new patient. At that time they often ask the patient (or their parent or guardian in the case of a minor) to complete a number of forms. It helps to have the required forms already placed together on a clipboard so the patient can complete them easily. These forms then need to be placed in the patient's chart in the proper order. If forms are not in the proper order a lot of time may be spent searching for the right information.

There are many different types of forms used in the medical office, and the style of the forms varies from provider to provider. There are also a number of companies that create and produce medical forms. The actual creation of the chart will therefore be different from provider to provider.

Additionally, some providers will use a single fold manila folder for charts, while others will use a multi-page chart.

The easiest way to determine the order the medical office puts patient charts into is to look at an existing chart. Below is an example of the types of forms and the order that a medical office might use with a multi-page chart.

Page 1 of the Patient Chart:
- Acknowledgement of Receipt of Privacy Practices Notice
- Registration
- Medical History/Physicals

Page 2 of the Patient Chart:
- Examination/Treatment Forms
- Pathology/Laboratory/X-ray Reports
- Operative Reports
- Discharge Summaries

Page 3 of the Patient Chart:
- Billing Forms for Previous Visits

Page 4 of the Patient Chart:
- Consent Form
- Signature on File
- Financial Arrangements
- Correspondence Log
- Letters To/From Provider

Some charts contain a fifth page or a back pocket for other information.

During the course of treatment the physician may add additional forms to the patient chart, such as a History and Physical Form, Progress Notes, or a Medication Flow Sheet for tracking prescribed medicine. If the patient is a child, a pediatric chart should be assembled.

After the patient has become established and has had several visits, lab and x-ray results and consultation reports may be submitted from other providers. These results should be reviewed by the physician or, in some offices, by a nurse. If reviewed by a nurse, abnormal lab, x-ray or urgent results or requests will be forwarded directly to the physician for an immediate response. After review, these results should be stamped with the date and signed by the physician prior to being filed in the patient chart.

Items should be grouped together (i.e., all pathology reports together, followed by all laboratory reports, etc.). They should then be in order by date, with the most recent one on top. Having a specific order allows the doctor to find the data he needs quickly and easily.

Items should be placed in the patient's file as soon as they are received from the doctor. If a report comes in from an outside entity (i.e., results of lab tests from an outside lab), the report should immediately be given to the doctor with the patient's file. The doctor should initial the report to indicate that he has looked at it prior to the report being placed in the file. Reports should not be placed in a medical record without first being initialed by the provider.

To facilitate finding the forms within the charts quickly and easily, many companies create forms of different lengths. Additionally, the name of the form is printed on the bottom. This allows you to see the bottom of each form, and the name of the form, when the forms are properly stacked in the medical chart.

Some of the charts may also be duplicated on each side. This allows the provider to use the same form for multiple visits without creating excess paper in the chart. Once one side of the form has been completed, the form can be turned over and additional information placed on the reverse side.

If you are preparing a chart for a patient's visit, be sure that the provider has space on the necessary forms for recording their examination, treatment plans and progress notes. If necessary, add additional forms to the chart. Most medical offices add additional forms on top of the existing forms, rather than underneath them. This places the most current information on the top where it is easily found.

Under no circumstances should you remove the old information from a chart, no matter how full the chart has become. Medical treatment plans can extend over a length of time. At any point in the treatment plan the provider may need to refer back to the initial examination or treatment plan to fully understand the patient's situation.

Pediatric Charts

Some medical offices use a different type of chart for children. These are called children's charts or **pediatric charts**. Pediatric charts may have additional or different forms. For example, a Children's Medical History form would eliminate information that is not appropriate for children, such as pregnancy history.

Pediatric charts also require additional forms such as an Immunization Record to track immunizations and forms for hearing and vision exams. These records are often needed by a parent before they are allowed to enter their child into a public school.

Some medical offices may also use restraints on young children to prevent them from moving and causing themselves injury during medical treatment. The use of these restraints must be authorized by a parent or guardian.

Emergency Patients

Medical offices may see patients on a one-time, emergency basis. These may be people from out of town who have a medical emergency or simply patients who need a procedure done and are unable or unwilling to see their normal provider for treatment. Or they may be a patient who is seeking a second opinion on the treatment plan suggested by their normal provider.

Many medical offices have a separate chart for these patients. Because these patients will not be receiving extended treatment, many of the documents in a normal chart such as call-back and telephone records will not be needed. However, even these patients need to give the provider information regarding their medical history.

The forms that are normally included in an emergency patient record include:

- Registration,
- Medical History,
- Doctor's Notes (or Treatment Plan), and
- Release and Consent Forms.

Because there are far fewer forms for emergency or one-time patients, many medical offices will use a simple manila folder for these patients, rather than a multi-page chart.

Radiology

Many offices also take radiological films (x-rays) of patients. Because x-rays are often the same size as the body part being x-rayed, they can be rather large. Because of this, x-rays are often stored separately from the patient files.

X-rays are often placed in a large envelope and labeled with the name of the patient, the date the x-ray was taken, and the specific body part shown on the x-ray (i.e., right wrist). Many offices also label the x-ray itself with this information. Additionally, many medical offices include a birth date, account number, or other identifying number to insure that the x-rays for two people with similar names are not mixed up.

If you are writing on the envelope, write on it before placing the x-ray inside. This will prevent damage to the x-ray from pressing too hard on it.

Over time labels placed on x-ray or charts may lose their adhesion. This may cause labels to come lose from the x-ray or chart. If you notice any labels beginning to peel away from an x-ray or chart, it should be reaffixed as soon as possible, or a new label applied.

To make labeling easier, some medical offices use x-ray film that has a white covering in one corner for labeling the x-ray. This is put on by the manufacturer and usually solves the problem of missing labels.

Once the x-ray has been properly labeled, be sure to add the information to the patient chart. By documenting in the patient chart all the x-rays that have been taken, a provider can easily see if there was a prior x-ray on a body part he is treating. This can help show changes in the patient or their condition or disease.

X-rays are often kept in a back office, and are filed alphabetically by the last name of the patient.

It is important to remember not to place other items in the same pocket with the medical x-rays as these items may scratch the x-ray.

Some providers also take pictures of a patient to document conditions or situations. These pictures may be needed to verify the need for treatment to an insurance carrier, or for explanations provided to the patient. These pictures should be labeled and treated in the same manner as the x-rays. However, some medical offices will file pictures directly in the patient chart, since they are often small enough to fit.

Filing the Chart

Once the chart has been completed, it will need to be filed in such a way that it can easily be located. Medical offices are run in many different ways, and because of this there are several different filing methods. It will take time to determine which filing system is right for the work situation you find yourself in.

Due to the new HIPAA regulations, the name of the patient should not appear on the outside of the chart. This is especially true if the charts are kept in a place that is visible to other patients or to anyone entering the office. If at all possible, all patient charts should be placed in a locked room that is inaccessible to anyone who is not authorized to enter. If this is not possible, charts should only contain information on the outside which is considered to be non-personal information. Thus, charts should be identified with a number, rather than with the patient's name. Some medical offices will use an account number that is alphanumeric (a combination of numbers and letters). In such cases care should be taken to

preserve the patient's identity. The letters used should not be those which could indicate the patient's name.

Having a numerical or alphanumeric filing system will often necessitate having a master list with the patients' names in alphabetical order. This will allow you to quickly and easily find the correct patient chart.

When creating a new chart for a patient, be sure to label the chart as soon as it is put together. If the practice is using a numeric or alphanumeric filing system, the chart information should be added to the master list immediately.

Many times a master list is computerized. Even when the list is on the computer, a printed list should always be kept available. This will allow you to access patient charts when the computer is down, or is in use by another person.

Adding a file to a computerized master list can be quick and easy. If the master list is not computerized, or if you are unable to add the information to the master list immediately, you can write the information on the printed master list.

Alphabetical Filing

If a practice keeps its charts in an area that is not accessible or viewable by unauthorized personnel, then an alphabetical filing system may be used. **Alphabetical filing** simply means filing the charts alphabetically by the first letter of the patient's last name.

Many medical offices use color coded tabs for alphabetical filing. Depending on the number of patients and/or files, the color coding may be broken down into the first letter of the last name, or the first two letters of the last name.

Many medical supply companies sell labels with letters in a multitude of colors. It is not uncommon to have nine or ten colors used. For example; A is red, B is orange, C is yellow, D is green, etc.

By placing the proper label or labels on the outside of the chart, you can easily see any charts that are out of order. Additionally, it is much easier to find a chart since you have only a few to look through, rather than a large number of them.

Each practice will have a specific area for the letter to be placed on the outside of the chart. Keeping the letters in the proper area will also help you spot charts that may be out of order.

Medical Documentation Rules

Regardless of the type of medical practitioner you work for, there are some important factors to include when documenting in a medical chart.

Often a patient's chart will include notations from three or more different people within the medical office:

- Medical biller/receptionist,
- Medical assistant (or nurse in a hospital), and
- Medical Provider (physician, surgeon, anesthesiologist, etc.).

There is much more litigation in the world today. Because of that, everyone who touches a medical chart needs to think about what they are writing in the chart before a lawsuit is filed.

The following rules are important to remember when performing medical charting:

Document only in your area of responsibility. You are not the provider or medical assistant. Therefore, your notations on the chart should be limited to those areas which are your responsibility for the patient. This can include appointment setting, follow-up phone calls, and encounters in the reception area. Under no circumstances should you make any notations regarding the patient's treatment, even when asked by the provider.

Never use correction fluid on a chart or obscure any writing. Correction fluid, "white-out" or any liquid which covers over the writing on paper should never be used. If you make a mistake, draw a single line through the error in such a way that the original entry can still be read. Then write the correction directly next to the crossed out entry and initial it. If a malpractice lawsuit is ever filed, correction fluid always makes people wonder what was removed. By drawing a single line through the entry there is no question about what was there previously. This enables the viewing of the initial documentation.

Use standard abbreviations and terms. Each office should have a set of standard abbreviations and terms to be used in medical documentation. Using different abbreviations and terms can cause confusion in the records. These confusions can be detrimental to the treatment of a patient, or can lead to confusion during a law suit, which may mean a higher damage award. A chart of standard abbreviations and terms should be available to all office staff...

Do not write in the margins. If most material written in the chart falls within the margins, but one sentence is outside the margins, it can appear as though that sentence was added at a later time and inserted into the available space. If you run out of room, write on the next line. If there is no next line, use an additional form and continue writing on it. Paying for an additional form is much less costly than having a lawyer argue that the material was on the chart from the beginning.

Never alter the information on a chart. To **alter** means to change or amend (add to) the information contained in a record or chart. If there is information in a chart that has changed or needs to be corrected, the information should be documented on the next available line, with the date of documentation.

Never write information in a patient chart that you do not want them to see. Patient charts legally belong to both the patient and the provider. However, the provider is considered to be the legal custodian of the records. Thus, a patient is allowed to see their records any time they. However, they may not remove the records from the provider's office.

Document anything the patient says with quotation marks. Juries automatically believe that anything that is put in quotation marks was a direct quote. This can work to the provider's advantage if the patient had originally said something good, then later sues. This is especially true when you are listing the details of a follow-up phone call. Since there is no face to face contact in which observations can be made, words can carry a greater impact.

Take the time to document non-compliance. Non-compliance means not following the instructions given by the provider. If the provider has suggested that the patient perform a certain action (i.e., physical therapy exercises twice a day, etc.), ask if the patient is performing such actions during a follow-up call. If the patient indicates that they are not doing so, make sure that it is recorded in the chart. This will protect the provider in case the patient sues. Juries will wonder if the patient's outcome would have been different if the patient had followed the provider's advice.

Be specific when documenting. The more specific you can be in a reasonable period of time, the better. For example, instead of saying "Patient was referred to a specialist," include the name, title, and address of the specialist and what the patient was referred for. This person may be able to testify for the provider if the patient never followed up on the referral.

If you see something in the chart that could be a potential problem, bring it to the attention of the provider. The provider is ultimately responsible for the information contained in a patient chart. While the provider should not alter the record, they can add additional information which can help counter something that should not have been said.

Document in ink. Many states require that information contained in the patient chart be documented in ink. Pencil is not acceptable. If you have difficulty expressing yourself without reworking the wording, write the information on a piece of scratch paper first, then write it into the patient's chart.

Be sure that any change to a patient's appointment is documented. If the patient calls and says that they will be late, be sure it is noted on the patient's chart. If the patient calls to cancel or reschedule the appointment, be sure it is notated. If the patient later sues the provider, you can show documentation that the patient repeatedly changed or cancelled appointments. The argument can then be made that the patient's condition could have been better taken care of if they had sought treatment for the problem earlier. Document changes in an appointment can also fend off accusations of sloppy documentation if the patient chart no longer matches the appointment book. For example, if the patient postponed an appointment for a week, the chart may have one date, and the appointment book a different date.

When documenting an appointment, include the reason for the appointment. If the patient indicates that they are having a problem, this should be notated on both the appointment calendar and the patient's chart. This not only helps the provider know what to look for, but also helps protect the provider if the patient then cancels an appointment. The provider will have a better understanding of how urgently the patient may need care.

Make detailed notes of follow-up calls. If the proper follow-up call is not performed, the provider may be considered guilty of "patient

abandonment." This can carry a high price tag in the event of a law suit. Many providers have the medical biller or receptionist make follow-up calls. This is completely legal. However, if the procedure was extraordinarily difficult or the results were not those anticipated, it might be better if the provider herself made the follow-up call. This will often show more concern for the patient.

Update the patient's medical history at each visit. This is not as complicated as it might sound. Simply asking the patient if there have been any changes to their medical history or to their drug/medication use is sufficient. If the patient indicates that there has been no change, simply note on the chart the date and "No Change in Medical History" (sometimes abbreviated as NCMH).

Signature Cards

It is important that all pertinent data regarding a patient's condition and treatment be added to the medical record. This record not only helps the doctor to track the patient's progress and determine what treatment is best, but also helps to verify the services which were done and the need for those services.

Because of the importance of maintaining proper records, only certain authorized persons should ever be allowed to make notations or changes to a patient's medical records. Each change or notation should be initialed or signed and dated. If reports or other data are received from outside entities (i.e., a lab report from an outside lab), the report should be presented to the doctor along with the patient's chart. The doctor should then initial the report indicating that he has seen it, before it is placed in the patient's medical record.

The appropriate people will be different for each office, and for the jobs within an office. For example, a biller may be allowed to make changes to a patient's insurance information or account, but not to any of their medical data. The best way to track those authorized to make notations or changes is by use of signature cards.

A **signature card** shows the person authorized to make changes, the dates they are authorized, and the scope of the changes they are allowed to make (see Figure 4 – 1). These cards should be kept in the billing office.

```
┌─────────────────────────────────────────────────┐
│ SIGNATURE CARD        Date Created _____  │
│                                                   │
│ A copy of this card shall be maintained on file at all times and updated as │
│ needed. The following person is authorized to make notations and/or │
│ changes to the patient medical records as indicated. │
│                                                   │
│ Name _____  Title _____   │
│                                                   │
│ Authorized From _____ to _____         │
│                                                   │
│ Signature: _____ Initials: Printed ____ Signed ____ │
│                                                   │
│ Scope of authorization (i.e. all records and files, insurance data only, etc.) │
│ _____   │
│ _____   │
│ _____   │
└─────────────────────────────────────────────────┘
```

Figure 4 – 1: Signature Card

If a change is to be made to a person's authority or scope of the records they may change, an ending date should be placed in the "Authorized date: ... to:" space. A new signature card should be completed with the new data. The old signature card should be kept on file. Then, if an auditor or other person is looking through older medical records and needs to know whose signature was signed on a certain date with the authority, the old signature card can be pulled.

Some medical offices choose to have a signature log on file. A signature log contains the information from several signature cards on a single sheet of paper. The disadvantage of signature logs is that some data on a signature log can be outdated while other data is still current. Since several people are listed on a single paper, if one person leaves the practice, then their name is no longer valid but the other signatures still are. Such a system makes it much more difficult to track authority. You may need to go through any number of signature logs to find the signature you are looking for.

Signature cards have the advantage of allowing each authorized person to be listed on a separate card. This can be neater in an office which has a high turnover rate or for whom the job status and authority for notations often changes. The current cards are kept in a card file in front of a divider in alphabetical order by last name. The outdated cards are kept behind the divider in alphabetical order.

If an authorized person's initials are different than their full name (i.e., full name Charles Smith-Lyton, M.D., but they go by Charles Lyton and sign

their initials CL, MD) then a notation should be placed under the letter "S", and the card placed under "L". This allows you to find the card quickly and easily.

Retention of Records

Storing medical charts can become a huge undertaking for a medical practice, especially if it is large and has been in operation for a number of years. However, it is important to maintain patients' medical charts for an extended period of time.

All records should be kept as long as they are needed. However, since many conditions are linked to previous episodes of care, records may be needed on patients long after they have been treated for a condition. For example:

1. Pediatric records may be needed for a 30 year old pregnant woman to determine if she had measles as a child.
2. Scarlet fever in a young child can cause damage to the heart that may not show up until the patient is 50 or 60 years old.
3. Hereditary links are being found in numerous conditions, providing a need for the doctors of children and even grandchildren to see the medical records of a patient.

For these reasons, many medical offices are putting their medical records on microfiche, microfilm or computer files and keeping them indefinitely.

The laws vary from state to state; however, many states require medical offices to keep records for several years after the patient has died. This can essentially mean keeping medical records forever, especially if the practice treats a number of young patients.

One of the main reasons for keeping records so long is the way the laws are written. Many states allow patients to sue a provider five or even ten years after the patient discovers a problem. If they do not discover a problem until 30 years after treatment has ended, they still have the right to sue for five more years. In effect, you cannot be certain that a patient will not sue, and that the records will not be needed, until five to ten years after the patient is dead.

This means that there is a tremendous amount of paperwork that a medical office must maintain. To make it easier, records of patients who are no longer seen by the medical office will often be placed in storage.

Additionally, federal regulations mandate that records on Medicare and Medicaid patients be retained for at least seven years after treatment. At any time during this seven year period, the medical practice can be audited and must provide substantiation for their charges and receipts.

For tax purposes, records should be kept for at least four years after the tax return is filed. However, documents regarding the purchase of a building or equipment should be kept for at least four years after the selling or disposal of the building or equipment.

Storing Medical Records

When storing medical records, it is important to keep them in a manageable order in order to locate the records if you should need them at a later date. This often means creating lists of the items that are included in the storage boxes, and properly labeling these boxes.

Many companies use numerical or alphabetical labels on their boxes. For example, the labeling on a box might be shown as "Medical Charts, 2000, A – K." This could mean that charts for all patients who terminated care in the year 2000 whose last names began with A – K would be found in this box. However, a master list would still be needed to easily find a chart since it may be difficult to determine which year a patient terminated treatment.

Labeling boxes with a clear label can allow them to be stored in a logical sequence. This makes them much easier to locate when a file is needed.

When medical providers store their records they often use a storage service. The files will be placed in specified storage boxes and placed in a specific location. The storage company will then pick up the boxes and take them to their facility for storage.

If a file needs to be retrieved from storage, the storage company is contacted and is told to retrieve the needed box and return it to the medical office. The practice then pulls the file from the box.

Since the storage company will often charge for each box brought back or forth, it is important to have a master list that tells you exactly which box a file is located in. You do not want to spend several days shipping the wrong box back and forth.

Since many patients may have the same or similar names, it is important to create a master list that will give you the detail you need to locate the correct medical chart. This is often done by listing the name of the box at the top of the master list page **(see Figure 4 – 2)**. The medical charts included in that box are then listed in alphabetical order by the patient's last name. Another piece of identifying information is also included, such as the patient's birth date.

Box: Medical Charts 1999, A – L

Adams, Sean	10/01/68
Adams, Sydney	12/14/70
Adams, Thomas	06/05/56
Alexander, Betty	08/21/35
Alexander, Karen	11/03/60

Figure 4 – 2: Sample Master List for Box Contents

If the medical office has been around a while, they may have a large number of boxes in storage **(see Figure 4 – 3)**. In this case, listing the contents in each box may not be practical. These medical offices will often create a single list of all charts that are in storage. This list includes the name of the patient on the chart, the identifying information (i.e., birthday or account number), and the name of the box the chart is in.

Patient Name	Birth date	Box
Adams, Amy	03/15/48	Med Charts 2000 L-S
Adams, Sean	10/01/68	Med Charts 1999 A-L
Adams, Sydney	12/14/70	Med Charts 1999 A-L
Adams, Thomas	06/05/56	Med Charts 1999 A-L
Adamson, Kirk	05/10/63	Med Charts 2001 S-Z
Alexander, Betty	08/21/35	Med Charts 1999 A-L
Alexander, Karen	11/03/60	Med Charts 1999 A-L

Figure 4 – 3: Sample Master Storage List for Practice

Electronic Medical Charting

More and more computer programs are including electronic medical charting. Previous computer programs used by the medical office were often limited to billing software. Those that were considered "high tech" may have included the opportunity to submit the claims electronically, rather than just print them on paper and mail them to the insurance carrier.

However, new software programs include a much wider variety of features. Following are some of the most common features, and how these features could impact the job of the medical biller:

Patient Identification: In addition to the standard patient information included in software programs (i.e., name, address, employer, and insurance information, etc.), many new programs include the addition of a patient photograph. This photo allows the medical staff to insure they are working on the proper patient before services are rendered. It has the added benefits of decreasing fraud caused by one person seeking treatment under a different person's Medicaid or insurance coverage. Additionally, it can increase customer satisfaction since medical staff will be able to recognize more patients.

If this type of software is used in the medical office, it will often fall to the medical biller or receptionist to take a quick snapshot of the patient and download it into the computer program. Additionally, the patient's information will need to be added into the program.

Prescription Control: Some software programs allow the creation of electronic prescriptions. **Electronic prescriptions** are prescriptions that are entered into the provider's computer, and then electronically sent to the computer at the patient's pharmacy.

There are many advantages of electronic prescriptions over paper prescriptions. These include:

- Prescriptions can be sent immediately, without the patient having to carry a paper prescription to the pharmacist.
- There is no danger of the patient loosing the prescription like there is with a paper prescription.
- The prescription is typed rather than hand written, preventing errors from misinterpreting a provider's handwriting.
- There are fewer errors resulting from pharmacists entering the prescriptions into their computer.

- Provider computers can be tied to the patient's chart, thus alerting the provider if there is a possible complication with a patient's medical condition or other medications.

While electronic charting programs can provide enhancement to the medical practice, they do not take the place of the paper chart. It is still important to insure that the patient's chart is completely updated at all times. If the chart is subpoenaed by the courts, printing out and sending a computerized chart not only takes more time, but may be unacceptable as a court document. This is especially true since it is difficult to tell if any items on the chart have been altered, and if so, when.

Computerized Files

More and more medical offices are utilizing computerized files. In fact, there are now computer programs that allow a medical office to keep all their patient records, including x-rays, in a computerized file.

The provider is also able to display a patient's record from anywhere in the office. This can allow them to have the patient's records right next to them as they are treating the patient. They, or the medical assistant, can make notations on the medical record as the treatment is being done. This can prevent problems due to providers having to remember what treatment was provided. Sometimes providers will be working on several patients at the same time. It is easy to become confused regarding which patient had which treatment.

However, even when sophisticated computer records exist, it is important that the practice still maintains a full set of paper files. This is due to the complexity of medical records and for legal considerations.

The legality of electronically stored records has yet to be established in the courts. In a written record it is easier to determine when changes have been made to a document. The handwriting or ink color may be different. With computerized files there is no way to effectively determine when a specific notation was made into a patient's chart.

Additionally, most states require that any documentation in a medical record includes the signature or initials of the person making the notation, and the date. Many states also carry the provision that medical records must be written on paper or printed. Some states go so far as to say that medical records must be "written in ink" or that a "signature is required on each page". For example, Florida law says that the "caregiver's signature (not stamp or facsimile)," must be included on each page. In such cases, the entire record would need to be printed out and signed each time a change was made to the record.

Even if a state allows electronic record keeping, it is easy for a good attorney to claim that the records were altered after treatment to make them look more favorable to the provider. With electronic records, there is currently no way to prove this is not the case.

An additional problem with computer files is the issue of vulnerability. Computers, and the records on them, can be hacked into by outsiders. Allowing this information to be shared with anyone without the patient's approval is a violation of the HIPAA laws.

Additionally, computers get viruses and hard drives can become inoperable. Having all files stored on the computer allows the medical office to be vulnerable to such situations. If a computer crashes in the middle of treating a patient, written records will still leave the provider with a clear picture of the work that needs to be done.

Since much of the patient information is stored in electronic files it is important to insure the privacy of these files. This includes making sure that all files require a log-in and password to access them. Security levels also need to be in place to insure that people do not have access to records they do not need to do their job.

Everyone in the office must be made aware of the need to maintain the secrecy of their log-in name and password. To share this information with anyone, even inadvertently, could be considered a violation of HIPAA regulations.

Record Transfers

At times it may be necessary for a doctor to transfer records or medical information to another doctor. This is often the case when a patient transfers their care to a specialist, moves to another area, or begins treatment with another physician. In order to avoid legal complications, written permission should be obtained from the patient regarding the right to transfer information, specifically what information should be transferred, and when the transfer is to take place. Often a letter such as the following is used:

ON LETTERHEAD

I, ___(Patient's Name)___ request and authorize Donald Doolitle, M.D. to release the following medical information from the medical records of _____
___ (myself or patient name) to the physician or facility listed below.

Information to be released _____
_____
_____
_____

Dates of treatment: From: _____ To: _____
Information should be sent to:
Person: _____
Facility: _____
Address: _____
Street, City, Zip: _____
Phone: _____
Date information is to be sent: _____

I release you from all legal responsibility or liability that may arise from this authorization.

Signed _____ Date_____

When transferring records or data, do not send the original record or file. Instead, make a copy of all the data to be transferred. The envelope containing the records should be marked "**Personal and Confidential**." To ensure security, most medical offices will send the information via courier, or via registered mail, return receipt requested. The receipt can specify, if necessary, that the information be delivered only to the person to whom it is addressed (i.e., the doctor). This insures that it is not opened by others in the office and handled carelessly. A cover page should be included with the information which states that the information contained should be considered confidential and is for the express use of and dissemination to only the person to whom it is addressed.

Be sure that you transfer only that data which the patient has authorized. If data which has not been authorized is on the same page (i.e., information regarding two separate diagnoses), cover the non-pertinent information and make a copy. If it is not possible to cover the data, make a copy of the record, black out the non-pertinent information, and then copy the page again. This prevents the information from being revealed by holding the page up to the light or by other means.

Under no circumstances should a patient be allowed to take their records or any data from their records, to the doctor themselves. Doing so can allow the patient to alter the records, falsify the information, or remove data from the records. Such actions could put both the patient and the provider at risk. For example, a patient may remove the evidence that a certain drug was prescribed in order to get an additional supply of the drug. However, the new provider may prescribe a drug which is counteractive or could produce an adverse reaction when mixed with the first drug.

Summary

Maintaining patient files in a proper manner is one of a medical biller's most important jobs. Without properly maintained files, patient treatment can suffer. Additionally, should a provider be sued, improper maintenance of patient charts can add thousands of dollars in penalties to a judgment.

Three main people in a medical practice are usually responsible for the maintenance of patient charts. These people include the medical biller/receptionist, medical assistant, and the physician or other provider. It is important that everyone who makes notations 1n a patient chart follows the rules of proper medical charting.

Additionally, the medical biller should be aware of how to properly store charts, and to retrieve stored charts.

Assignments

Complete the Questions for Review.
Complete Exercise 4 – 1.

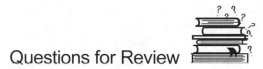

Questions for Review

Directions: Answer the following questions without looking back into the material just covered. Write your answers in the space provided.

1. What are ten of the 15 medical charting rules?

 1. _____

 2. _____

 3. _____

 4. _____

 5. _____

 6. _____

 7. _____

 8. _____

 9. _____

10. _____

11. _____

12. _____

13. _____

14. _____

15. _____

2. What information do you need on a master list when storing patient records? _____
_____
_____

3. Who is the legal owner of a patient's medical chart? _____
_____

4. How long should you keep medical records, and why? _____
_____
_____

5. What three people will often be involved in documenting a patient chart?

    1. _____

    2. _____

    3. _____

If you were unable to answer any of the questions, refer back to that section, and then fill in the answers.

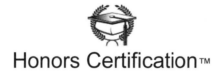

Honors Certification™

You will be given a written test of the information contained in this chapter. Each incorrect answer will result in a deduction of up to 5% from your grade. You must achieve a score of 85% or higher to pass this test. If you fail the test on your first attempt you may retake the test one additional time. The items included in the second test may be different from those in the first test.

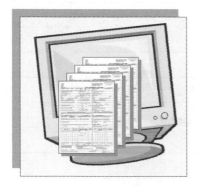

5

Medical Documentation Forms

Key words and concepts you will learn in this chapter:

Carrier – Insurance company.
Claim – A bill for services rendered by a provider.
Coverage – The act of being covered by an insurance plan; having an insurance policy.
Payor – Any entity that pays on a claim. This is usually used an insurance company.
Policy – A contractual agreement between an insurance carrier and a person or company. The agreement states items that the insurance carrier will cover or pay for, and the price they charge for covering those services.

Policyholder – The person or company who purchases an insurance policy.
Provider – The person or entity that provides health care services. This can be a doctor, chiropractor, hospital, emergency facility, x-ray technician, or any certified professional who is licensed to provide health care services.
Subscriber – An insured person.
Third Party Payor – Someone other than the insured or carrier who may be responsible for paying for services rendered. This may be a worker's compensation carrier if the patient was injured at work, someone else's auto insurance if they caused an auto accident the patient was injured in, etc.

Eventually almost everyone will visit a doctor's office or clinic or use the services of a hospital. This means that the services received will generate a claim or bill for processing or payment. Whether the patient has insurance coverage or will be responsible for payment of the services themselves, a claim or bill for the services will be prepared.

In this chapter we will walk you through the basic forms needed in a medical chart in order to properly bill the patient.

When a patient walks into a provider's office for the first time, a patient file must be established and several forms must be filled out. These forms provide all the information needed to treat and bill the patient. The most commonly used forms include the following:

- The Patient Information Sheet,
- The Release of Information Form,
- The Assignment of Benefits Form, and
- The Patient History Form.

Each form has a distinct purpose and, in one style or another, will be present in nearly every provider's office. However, sometimes two or more items are combined on a single form. This is most often true of the Release of Information Form, the Assignment of Benefits Form, and the Patient Information Sheet.

Filling out these forms is relatively simple since the information called for is self-explanatory.

Let's look at each of the forms in greater detail.

Patient Information Sheet

The Patient Information Sheet is used to collect general information regarding the patient (see Figure 5 – 1). The medical biller should always ensure that the information obtained on the Patient Information Sheet is complete and accurate, since this information will be used for billing and collection and for notifying family members in case of emergency. The Patient Information Sheet should be updated periodically to ensure its accuracy.

There are various versions of this form, but they all usually request the following basic information:

- Name: first, middle, and last,
- Address and telephone number,
- Business address, telephone number, and occupation,
- Date of birth,
- Social Security number,
- Person responsible, or insured's name,
- Spouse's name and occupation,
- Information about patient referral,
- Driver's license number,
- Close relative or friend to contact in case of emergency, and
- Insurance billing information.

Obtain the names, addresses, and policy and group numbers of all carriers insuring the patient. This is important because of coordination of benefits clauses included in most health insurance policies. If the patient has an insurance card, make a copy of the card to keep in the patient's file. Insurance coverage should be verified prior to rendering services. The insurance information should be rechecked every six months, since this information may change.

Release of Information Form

The Release of Information Form is used to allow the provider to request additional information from other providers of service or to share information with an insurance carrier (see Figure 5 – 2). If the doctor is submitting an insurance claim for the patient, the patient must sign a Release of Information Form before information may be given to an insurance company, attorney, or other third party. According to the Privacy Act, it is illegal to release any information regarding a patient without the patient's knowledge and written consent. Without this signature the provider's office is not allowed to submit a claim to the insurance carrier since disclosing the patient's diagnosis and other medical information to the insurance carrier would be a breach of the privacy laws.

The patient's signature is usually good for one year from the date the release is signed. If the patient is a child, the parent or guardian must sign the release. Often a release of information statement is included on the actual claim form describing treatment. This brief statement does not take the place of having a completed and signed release of information statement in the patient's file.

Assignment of Benefits Form

The Assignment of Benefits Form is a request for all insurance payments to be directed to the provider holding the assignment (see Figure 5 – 3). Most providers consider this a necessity for those patients who have insurance, because the assignment ensures that monies paid for services provided are issued directly to the provider and not to the patient or subscriber. Assignment of benefits indicates that the payor is authorized to send payment directly to the provider of services. The Assignment of Benefits Form should be signed, dated (preferably date stamped), and attached to the insurance verification form.

PATIENT INFORMATION SHEET

INSURED'S INFORMATION

Patient ID: _____ Assigned Provider: _____ Birth date: _____

Name: (Last, First, Middle) _____ Sex: _____

Address: (Inc City, State, Zip) _____

Home Phone: _____ Marital Status:_____ Social Security #: _____

Employer Name: _____ Work Phone: _____

Employer Address: _____

Employment Status: _____ Referred by: _____

Allergies/Medical conditions: _____

Primary Ins Name: _____ Address: _____

ID #: _____ Plan #/Name: _____ Policy Holder Name: _____

Secondary Ins Name: _____ Address: _____

ID #: _____ Plan #/Name: _____ Policy Holder Name: _____

SPOUSE'S INFORMATION

Patient ID: _____ Assigned Provider: _____ Birth date: _____

Name: (Last, First, Middle) _____ Sex: _____

Social Security #: _____ Employment Status:_____

Employer Name: _____ Work Phone: _____

Employer Address: _____

Allergies/Medical conditions: _____

Primary Ins Name: _____ Address: _____

ID #: _____ Plan #/Name: _____ Policy Holder Name: _____

Secondary Ins Name: _____ Address: _____

ID #: _____ Plan #/Name: _____ Policy Holder Name: _____

CHILD #1

Patient ID: _____ Assigned Provider: _____ Birth date: _____

Name of Minor Child: _____ Social Security #: _____

Sex: _____ Marital Status: _____ Relationship to Insured: _____

Allergies/Medical conditions: _____

Primary Ins Name: _____ Primary Insured: _____

Secondary Ins Name: _____ Secondary Insured: _____

CHILD #2

Patient ID: _____ Assigned Provider: _____ Birth date: _____

Name of Minor Child: _____ Social Security #: _____

Sex: _____ Marital Status: _____ Relationship to Insured: _____

Allergies/Medical conditions: _____

Primary Ins Name: _____ Primary Insured: _____

Secondary Ins Name: _____ Secondary Insured: _____

CHILD #3

Patient ID: _____ Assigned Provider: _____ Birth date: _____

Name of Minor Child: _____ Social Security #: _____

Sex: _____ Marital Status: _____ Relationship to Insured: _____

Allergies/Medical conditions: _____

Primary Ins Name: _____Primary Insured:_____

Secondary Ins Name: _____ Secondary Insured: _____

CHILD #4

Patient ID: _____ Assigned Provider: _____ Birth date: _____

Name of Minor Child: _____ Social Security #: _____

Sex: _____ Marital Status: _____ Relationship to Insured: _____

Allergies/Medical conditions: _____

Primary Ins Name: _____ Primary Insured: _____

Secondary Ins Name: _____ Secondary Insured: _____

EMERGENCY CONTACT

Name: _____ Home Phone: _____ Other Phone: _____

Address: (Inc City, State, Zip) _____

ACKNOWLEDGMENT AND AUTHORITY FOR TREATMENT AND PAYMENT

Initial

_____ I consent to treatment as necessary or desirable to the care of the patient named above, including but not restricted to whatever drugs, medicine, performance of operations and conduct of laboratory, x-ray, or other studies that may be used by the attending doctor, his/her nurse or qualified designate:

_____ I also acknowledge full responsibility for the payment of such services and agree to pay for them upon demand, in full, AT THE TIME OF SERVICE. If the physician must use a collection agency/attorney or court to collect its charges, then I will pay reasonable attorney fees and costs incurred in collecting same, regardless of insurance coverage.

_____ I hereby authorize payment directly to Consolidated Health Services of the medical expense benefits otherwise payable to me but not to exceed my indebtedness to said physician on account of the enclosed charge.

_____ I hereby authorize any medical practitioner, medical or medically related facility, insurance or reinsuring company, consumer reporting agency, or employer having information with respect to any physical or mental condition and/or treatment of me or my minor children and any other non-medical information of me and my minor children to give to the group policy holder, my employer, or its legal representative, any and all such information.

_____ I understand the information obtained by the use of the Authorization will be used to determine eligibility for insurance, and eligibility for benefits under any existing policy. Any information obtained will not be released by/to any organization EXCEPT to the group policyholder, my employer, reinsuring companies, the Medical Information Bureau, Inc., or other persons or organizations performing business or legal services in connection with my application, claim, or as may be otherwise lawfully required or as I may further authorize.

_____ I further agree that a photographic copy of this Authorization shall be valid as the original. This Authorization shall be valid for one year from the date shown below.

Signature of Insured: _____ Date: _____

Signature of Spouse: _____ Date: _____

Figure 5 – 1: Patient Information Sheet

Any Doctor's Office
1234 Drive Way ● Any City, Any State 56789 ● (555) 555-0000

AUTHORIZATION TO OBTAIN INFORMATION

I AUTHORIZE any physician, medical practitioner, hospital, clinic, or other medical or medically related facility, insurance or reinsurance company, the Medical Information Bureau, Inc., consumer reporting agency, or employer having information available as to diagnosis, treatment and prognosis with respect to any physical or mental condition and/or treatment of me or my minor children and any other non-medical information of me and my minor children to give to the group policy holder, my employer, or its legal representative, any and all such information.

I UNDERSTAND the information obtained by the use of this Authorization will be used to determine eligibility for insurance, and eligibility for benefits under any existing policy. Any information obtained will not be released by/to any person or organization EXCEPT to the group policyholder, my employer, reinsuring companies, or other persons or organizations performing business or legal services in connection with my application, claim, or as may be otherwise lawfully required or as I may further authorize.

I KNOW that I may request to receive a copy of this Authorization.

I AGREE that a photographic copy of this Authorization shall be as valid as the original.

I AGREE this Authorization shall be valid for one year from the date shown below.

Signature of Insured and/or Spouse _____ Date _____

Name(s) of minor child (ren) _____

Figure 5 – 2: Release of Information Form

Any Doctor's Office
1234 Drive Way ● Any City, Any State 56789 ● (555) 555-0000

ASSIGNMENT OF BENEFITS

I authorize payment directly to the above named provider of medical expense benefits otherwise payable to me but not to exceed my indebtedness to said provider for any services furnished to me by that provider.

The signature on this form or a photocopy is valid for one year from the date indicated.

Signature _____ Date _____

Figure 5 – 3: Assignment of Benefits Form

Patient History

Date _____

Patient Name _____ Age _____

Any allergies to food or medicine?   No Yes
If yes: Allergic to: _____

Have you ever been hospitalized?   No Yes
If yes: Indicate date and reason: _____

Have you ever been diagnosed or experienced:

Bladder Infections	_____	Underweight	_____	Anemia	_____
Ear Infections	_____	Epilepsy	_____	Overweight	_____
Sinus Infections	_____	Seizures	_____	Hay Fever	_____
Vision Problems	_____	Mumps	_____	Chickenpox	_____
Frequent Headaches	_____	Sickle Cell Anemia	_____	Heart Murmur	_____

Other _____

Are you currently taking any medication(s)?
If yes: Name of medication(s): _____

Date of last Tuberculosis and/or Tetanus shot: _____

Check any of the following that any blood relative has or has had:

Anemia	_____	Heart Disease	_____	Thyroid Problems	_____
Sickle Cell Anemia	_____	Heart Attack	_____	Diabetes	_____
Stroke	_____	Birth Defects	_____	Asthma	_____
Cancer	_____	Mental Retardation	_____	Kidney Disease	_____
Tuberculosis	_____	Alcoholism	_____	High Blood Pressure	_____

Patient Signature: _____Date: _____

Figure 5 – 4: Patient History Form

Patient History Form

The Patient History Form is important to the physician **(see Figure 5 – 4)**. It helps in identifying previous incidents of illness that may be important in treating the patient's present condition. This is usually a detailed form with basic health questions requiring only yes or no answers. The provider will give the patient a complete history and physical in the exam room. The provider will then complete a physical exam and include his findings. Some physicians may dictate a medical history report (see the Medical Reports chapter).

The Patient Information Sheet, Release of Information Form, Assignment of Benefits Form, and Patient History Form should all be completed by the patient at the time of the first visit. However, it is the job of the person receiving the forms from the patient to insure that they are complete. Each item should be completed. If the answer to a question is "no", the patient should write the word "no" in the field. If the information is not applicable, the patient should write "N/A" in the field. This insures that the patient has looked at each of the fields and responded to them. This can prevent problems when a patient mistakenly skips over a question when the answer could be important for their proper care.

Insurance Verification

Many practices will verify insurance coverage and collect the patient portion of the charges at the time service is rendered. Each office has a standard form for this verification of coverage. **Figure 5 – 5** shows a sample Insurance Coverage Form.

This form covers much of the pertinent information needed to determine the patient's portion of the claim, and to assist in gaining the maximum reimbursement for the patient. Maximum reimbursement may be obtained by following any requirements set forth in the contract, such as obtaining pre-authorization for certain services or taking advantage of benefits which might be paid at a higher percent (i.e., pre-admit testing, outpatient instead of inpatient surgeries, etc.).

Some forms will have room for information on other family members so that family deductible and coinsurance maximum amounts can be tracked.

You will need to contact the insurance carrier to accurately complete this form. Provide the insurance carrier with the name of the patient, the name of the insured, and the policy name/number. The carrier can then provide you with the information needed to complete each field.

Some carriers may prefer to have you fax the Insurance Coverage Sheet to them, rather than spend time with you on the phone. If this is the case, also fax the Release of Information Form with the patient's signature on it.

Additionally, some carriers may send you a copy of the contract. This will provide you with the information needed to properly complete the Insurance Coverage Sheet.

Additional Suggestions

There are a number of things to keep in mind when dealing with customers. Of course, customer service should always be your first and foremost concern, but at the same time you need to have regard for the medical office. It is important to obtain all necessary information from the patient. Remember that one of the primary objectives of the medical biller is to minimize the amount of time between the physician's service and the complete payment of the bill. The information that can facilitate this process may include the following:

1. Ask the patient to fill out all necessary forms for setting up the patient file. Give the patient sufficient time to fill out the forms and check that they are complete before accepting them. Many offices mail the forms to the patient prior to their first visit to ensure their completeness.
2. Be sure you understand the policies of the office you work for regarding the completion of forms and payment for bills. This way you can explain it accurately to the patient at the time of their first visit.
3. Use the office forms consistently and accurately so that the tracking of information runs smoothly, regardless of who enters the information.
4. Secure all the details of the insurance information. If the patient or insured has a card, make a copy of it for your files. Make sure the information contains the subscriber's name, the policy number, the effective date, the company that holds the policy or the name of the policy, and the insurance carrier's address.

Insurance Coverage Sheet

INSURED: _____ BIRTHDATE: _____

SSN: _____ EFFECTIVE DATE: _____

DEDUCTIBE AMOUNT: _____ 3 MO CARRYOVER: _____ COINSURANCE%: _____

FAMILY DEDUCTIBLE: _____ AGGREGATE/NON-AGGREGATE

DEPENDENT AGE LIMIT: _____

BENEFITS PAID AT OTHER THAN THE STANDARD COINSURANCE % [Including benefit, coinsurance amount and special circumstances, (i.e., SSO allowed at 100%, required for hysterectomy, coronary bypass, etc.)]:

_____

_____

_____

_____

PRE-AUTHORIZATION REQUIRED FOR: _____

_____

_____

ACCIDENT BENEFIT AMOUNT: _____ TREATMENT TO BE RECEIVED WITHIN _____ DAYS

OTHER NOTES/COMMENTS: _____

_____

_____

_____

_____

Total Payments (20XX)

Indicate below the names of the insured and their dependents. When any of the following information is received, write it in pencil followed by the date. This will help you to realize when a patient's deductible has been met and if they are nearing any maximum benefit.

	INSURED	DEPENDENT	DEPENDENT	DEPENDENT	DEPENDENT
NAME:	_____	_____	_____	_____	_____
DEDUCTIBE:	_____	_____	_____	_____	_____
COINS PD:	_____	_____	_____	_____	_____
LIFETIME:	_____	_____	_____	_____	_____

Figure 5 – 5: Insurance Coverage Sheet

5. Make sure the patient understands the provider's policy regarding any amounts that the insurance carrier does not pay or does not cover.

Summary

There are several forms which need to be included in all medical charts. These forms include the Patient Information Sheet, the Assignment of Benefits form, the Authorization to Release Information form, and the patient history. Many of these forms will need to be completed by the patient at the time of their first visit.

At this same time the patient's insurance information will need to be verified. Many practices use a specific form for this purpose so that all pertinent insurance information can be included in the patient's chart.

Assignments

Complete the Questions for Review.
Complete Exercise 5 – 1.

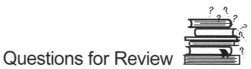

Questions for Review

Directions: Answer the following questions without looking back into the material just covered. Write your answers in the space provided.

1. List five of the items which should be included on the Patient Information Sheet.

    1. _____

    2. _____

    3. _____

    4. _____

    5. _____

2. What is the purpose of the Patient Information Sheet? _____

    _____

    _____

3. Name two instances in which financial responsibility for a bill does not lie with the patient.

    1. _____

    2. _____

4. What is the purpose of the Insurance Coverage Sheet? _____

    _____

    _____

5. What is an Assignment of Benefits Form? _____

    _____

    _____

If you were unable to answer any of the questions, refer back to that section, and then fill in the answers.

Exercise 5 – 1

Directions: Complete a Patient Information Sheet and set up charts for the following five patients. Individual folders may be used to keep information for each patient.

Patient #1 - Name: Abby Addison
5678 Any Avenue
Alverville, AK 99087
Home: (765) 555-4321 Work: (765) 555-4567
DOB: 12/12/68
Martial Status: Single
Social Security Number: 001-00-0001
Policy #: A001A
Referred by: Friend
Responsible Party: Self
Person to Contact in Emergency: Alice Avery (Friend) (765) 555-7689
Employer: Red Enterprises. 7677 Royal Road, Colter, CO 81369
Insurance Carrier: Rover Insurers, Inc. 5931 Rolling Road, Ronson, CO, 81369

Patient #2 - Name: Bobby Bumble
93485 Bumpkiss Court
Barkingville, DC 23456
(210) 555-4756
DOB: 1/1/44
Martial Status: Married
Social Security Number: 002-02-0020
Policy #: B10935B
Referred by: Spouse
Responsible Party: Self
Person to Contact in Emergency: Barbara Bumble (Spouse)
Employer: Blue Corporation, 9817 Bobcat Blvd., Bastion, CO 81319
Insurance Carrier: Ball Ins. Carriers, 3895 Bubble Blvd. Ste. 283, Boxwood, CO 85931

Patient #3 - Name: Cathy Crenshaw
9876 Cranbury Lane
Crabapple, CT 06192
(086) 555-3579
DOB: 2/4/43
Marital Status: Single
Social Security Number: 003-03-0030
Referred by: Friend
Responsible Party: Self
Person to Contact in Emergency: Carmen Castro (Sister)
Employer: (Part-time) Creative Creations Corp., 1234 Creature Lane, Crevise, CT 06192
Insurance Carrier: No insurance (Cash patient)

Patient #4 - Name: Daisy Doolittle
                      1234 Daffy Lane
                      Danbury, DE 19876
                      (098) 555-4311
                      DOB: 8/1/59
                      Marital Status: Married
                      Social Security Number: 004-04-0040
                      Policy #: DD0895627
                      Referred by: Dr. Daniel Dobby
                      Responsible Party: Self
                      Person to Contact in Emergency: Danny Doolittle (Spouse)
                      Employer: None
                      Insurance Carrier: Medicaid, P.O. Box 0098, Danbury, DE 19876

Patient #5 - Name: Edward Edmunds
                      8888 Every Lane
                      Evansville, CA 90012
                      (123) 555-7890
                      DOB: 1/10/27
                      Marital Status: Widow
                      Social Security Number: 508-12-3456
                      Medicare #: A508123456
                      Referred by: Edith Evan, M.D.
                      Responsible Party: Self
                      Person to Contact in Emergency: Edgar Edmunds (Brother)
                      Employer: Retired
                      Insurance Carrier: (Medicare) Blues of America, P.O. Box 1234, Evansville, CA 90012

Honors Certification™

The certification challenge for this chapter will be a written test of the information contained in this chapter. Each incorrect answer will result in a deduction of up to 5% from your grade. You must achieve a score of 85% or higher to pass this test. If you fail the test on your first attempt you may retake the test one additional time. The items included in the second test may be different from those in the first test.

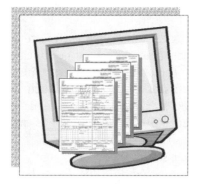

6 Contract Interpretation

After completion of this chapter you will be able to:

- Describe how Blue Cross/Blue Shield and other indemnity plans share expenses.
- Define the basic terms used in an insurance contract.
- Explain how the various elements of a contract can affect billing.
- Properly complete a Treatment Authorization Request form.
- Describe the common basic benefits that are included in a contract.
- Accurately calculate deductible amounts given a contract and scenario.
- Describe how major medical limits (i.e., coinsurance limits, lifetime maximums, etc.) can affect the insurance carrier's payment on a claim.
- Explain what COBRA is and how it affects coverage for pre-existing conditions.
- Explain how exclusions and allowed amounts can affect payment on a claim.
- Describe the pre-certification process.
- Describe what utilization review is and how it can affect benefit payments.
- List situations in which a surgery may be considered unnecessary.
- State the purposes of Second Surgical Opinions and how they can affect claim payments.
- Describe the two types of second surgical opinion programs.

Key words and concepts you will learn in this chapter:

Accident – An unintentional injury which has a specific time, date and place.

Allowed Amount – Is what the insurance company considers to be a reasonable charge for the procedure performed, and is often less than the amount which the doctor bills.

Basic Benefits – Benefits that are usually paid at 100% and are paid before major medical benefits are paid.

Coinsurance – The portion of covered expenses the member pays, and the portion the plan pays after any deductible amounts are met.

Deductible – The amount which the patient must pay prior to the insurance paying their benefits.

Eligibility – The qualifications which makes a person eligible for coverage.

Exclusions – These are items which the insurance carrier does not cover.

Indemnity Plans – The term often used to refer to health care plans that share the cost of health care between the insurance carrier and the patient.

Mental and Nervous Expenses – Claims submitted for psychiatric services, marriage and family counseling, and drug and alcohol treatment.

Pre-authorization – Is to gain approval of the services which are to be performed, and often to obtain an understanding of whether or not the insurance carrier will provide coverage for those services.

Pre-admission Testing – Testing done before the patient enters the hospital for surgery.

Pre-certify – To get pre-approval for admission on elective, non-emergency hospitalization.

Pre-existing Conditions – Conditions which existed prior to a patient being covered under a contract.

Unnecessary Surgery – Surgery that is recommended as an elective procedure when an alternative method of treatment may be preferable.

Interpreting and understanding contracts is one of the most important aspects of being a medical biller. The health care contract is the one document which is used to determine the benefits which the insurance carrier will pay for services rendered.

The wording and terminology of health insurance contracts can often be confusing to someone who is not well versed in the insurance field. For this reason, medical billers will often be called upon to interpret the provisions of a contract for billing purposes or to explain benefits to a patient.

Also, many medical practices prefer to collect the patient's portion of the bill (that portion not covered by insurance) at the time services are rendered. In order to properly calculate the amount due from the patient, it is important that medical billers be able to interpret the benefits covered in the contract.

Additionally, an astute medical biller can often suggest options to a patient or provider that will provide greater coverage under the terms of the contract. For example, a contract may provide 100% coverage for certain services which are performed on an outpatient basis. If a patient has in-patient surgery scheduled for a listed procedure, it can be beneficial for the medical biller to inform the provider of the increased payment for outpatient surgery. It is then up to the provider and the patient to determine if the increased coverage is beneficial to the patient in their particular circumstance or situation.

Blue Cross/ Blue Shield

There are many insurance carriers doing business within the United States. One of the largest of these is the Blue Cross/Blue Shield group. While many people consider Blue Cross/Blue Shield to be separate or different from many other companies, in truth their contracts cover many of the same procedures and have many of the same benefits as other indemnity plans.

Indemnity plans is the term often used to refer to health care plans that share the cost of health care between the insurance carrier and the patient. These plans often pay benefits at a set amount, such as 80% of the covered services. The patient is responsible for the remaining 20%, as well as any amounts not covered by the insurance carrier.

The concepts discussed in this chapter apply to all types of contracts, including Blue Cross/Blue Shield, managed care providers (discussed more fully in Chapter 10), and numerous other carriers.

Contract Provisions

If a biller is familiar with the provisions of a specific contract they may be able to provide added benefits due to the scheduling of a patient, or the manner in which a claim is filed.

We have provided you with three contracts at the end of this chapter: Ball Insurance Carrier (Blue Corporation), Rover Insurers, Inc. (Red Enterprises), and Winter Insurance Company (White Corporation). Each contract is different. Throughout this chapter we will refer to these contracts to help familiarize you with the provisions in each contract.

Eligibility

The first item which is considered on the contract is **eligibility**, or the qualifications which make the person eligible for coverage. Usually this includes items such as working full-time for a company, and the description of what is considered full time. For example, in the Winter Insurance Company contract, an employee must work a minimum of 30 hours per week to be covered by this contract. The contract also covers who is considered a dependent of the employee.

Of course, if a person has purchased individual coverage and is not covered by their place of work, there would be no minimum work requirements. However, there would still be qualifications to have coverage as a dependent under this plan.

Dependent eligibility is usually defined by the relationship to the employee and the age of the dependent. For example, in the Winter contract a child is covered until age 19, or to age 23 if they are a full-time student. If an eligible dependent becomes disabled before age 19, or if a student and the eligible dependent becomes disabled before age 23, dependent coverage would continue until age 23. Children include unmarried natural children, legally adopted children, foster children and those for whom the employee is considered the legal guardian.

Some contracts have provisions which state that if a husband and wife (or parent and child) work for the same employer and are covered under the same contract, the spouse or child cannot be covered as a dependent on the employee's policy. Also, some contracts state that if both spouses are working at the same company and are covered under the same contract, the children may be covered by one parent or the other, but not both. This prevents the insurance carrier from having to pay twice for the same patient and services rendered.

Effective Date

The next item to be considered is whether or not the contract was in force at the time the services were rendered. This is often defined as a minimum length of time an employee has worked for a company.

There is also an "actively-at-work" stipulation that is included in many contracts. This clause states that a person must be at work (or actively engaged in their normal activities, if a dependent) on the date coverage becomes effective. If he or she is not at work or actively engaged in their normal activities, the contract does not become effective until the employee or dependent returns to work.

As a medical biller, it is important that you ensure that a patient is eligible and is covered under an insurance policy in order to receive benefits. Many providers contact the insurance company prior to performing a procedure to be sure that the patient is covered. This is especially important when a patient is covered under an individual policy and pays a monthly premium for coverage.

Termination of Coverage

This section of a contract provides information regarding when coverage will terminate for both the employee and their dependents. It is important to note when coverage ceases as the insurance carrier will not pay benefits after this date. You should be

TREATMENT AUTHORIZATION REQUEST

Name of Patient: _____
Address: _____
City, State, Zip: _____
Sex: _____ Marital Status: _____ Date of Birth: _____
Insurance Policy Name/Group Number: _____
Name of Insured: _____
Diagnosis Description: _____
ICD-9 Code(s): _____
Reason for Services: _____

Specific Services you are requesting authorization for:
CPT Code: _____ Units: _____ Charges: _____

I hereby certify that the above information is true and correct to the best of my knowledge.

Signature: _____ Date: _____

Figure 6 – 1: Pre-authorization Request

aware that coverage will often continue until the end of the month in which an employee terminates. Knowing this, it is important to schedule any follow-up visits prior to the end of the month if you know that a patient's insurance is being terminated.

Pre-authorization

A number of insurance carriers will require that certain benefits be pre-authorized before the services are received. **Pre-authorization** means to gain approval of the services which are to be performed, and often to obtain an understanding of whether or not the insurance carrier will provide coverage for those services.

Many insurance carriers have a standard pre-authorization form **(see Figure 6 – 1)**. This form requests information regarding the patient, the diagnosis, and the procedures to be performed.

Following is a description of how to complete a Treatment Authorization Request:

Name of Patient: Enter the name of the patient that will receive the services.
Address: Enter the patient's address.
City, State, Zip: Enter the city, state and zip code of the patient.
Sex: Enter M for Male or F for female.
Marital Status: Enter the patient's marital status. This is especially important when the patient is a dependent of the insured.
Date of Birth: Enter the patient's date of birth.
Insurance Policy Name/Group Number: Enter the insurance policy name and/or number that the patient is insured under.
Name of Insured: Enter the name of the insured. This may be a spouse or parent of the patient. In rare instances it may be a different relation to the insured (i.e., the patient is a grandchild of the insured and the insured has custody).
Relationship to Insured: Check the appropriate relationship box.
Diagnosis Description: Enter the English-Language description of the patient's illness, injury or condition.
ICD-9 Code: Enter the ICD-9 code(s) associated with the patient's condition. These codes indicate the patient's diagnosis.
Reason for Services: Describe the reason or the medical justification for the services which will be rendered. If necessary, include any laboratory reports, x-rays, pictures, or other documentation to justify the need for services.

Specific Services: Enter the specific services that the provider is seeking authorization for. These should be identified by specific CPT® or HCPCS procedure codes (CPT® and HCPCS codes identify a procedure or service). Each service or item should be listed on a separate line.
Units: Enter the number of units or the number of times the provider feels this service should be performed (i.e., 10 for requesting 10 psychiatric visits).
Charges: Enter the charges for each service or item. This should be the charge for a single unit of service, not the total amount for all the units you are requesting.
Signature: The provider must sign the Treatment Authorization Request.

Contract Benefits

The next section of the contract usually details the benefits that the contract covers. These can include basic benefits and major medical benefits. Premiums are based upon the number and amount of benefits that a contract covers. The greater the coverage, the higher the cost of the premiums. For example, a contract which covers charges at 90% of the allowed amount (allowed amounts will be discussed later) and has a $100 deductible will usually cost more than a comparative contract which covers charges at 70% of the allowed amount and has a $250 deductible.

Basic Benefits

Basic benefits are those benefits usually paid at 100% and are paid before major medical benefits are paid. Therefore, it is possible for the insurance plan to pay basic benefits even when the patient has not yet met their deductible. Not all contracts will have basic benefits. Most basic benefit plans have been replaced with managed care plans.

Some contracts have a basic benefit which is based upon the unit value (a number based upon the difficulty of a procedure and the overhead needed, see Allowed Amount) being multiplied by a basic conversion factor (see Ball Insurance Carrier contract). This allows a small portion of most services to be paid at 100% with the remaining portion paid at the normal coinsurance percentage. These types of basic benefits do not cover all procedures.

Accident Benefits

One of the most common basic benefits is an accident benefit. An **accident** is defined as an unintentional injury which has a specific time, date and place. Under the Winter Insurance Company contract, the first $300 of services that are due to an accident occurrence are paid at 100%. After that, the remaining charges are paid at 90%. This benefit is for the first $300 of charges that are incurred within 120 days of the date of the accident, so follow-up care should be scheduled within that 120 day period in order to get the higher rate. Also, be aware that if other providers charge for the same accident, it is the first $300 of <u>all</u> charges that receives the 100% benefit. Therefore, if Tommy Tucker gets hit by a car, remember that there may be ambulance charges, hospital charges, physician's charges, x-ray technician charges, and other charges. It is important to get your claim in as quickly as possible to ensure that the provider you work for is reimbursed at 100% and not at 90%.

Additionally, be sure to indicate on the bill that services are due to an accident. On the CMS-1500 claim form this is box 10b and 10c. With the date of the accident indicated in box 14. (The CMS-1500 claim form will be explained in detail in the chapter titled CMS-1500.) If your office does not use the CMS-1500, be sure there is a place to indicate that this was an accident, or type it on the bottom of the bill. This data should also be noted in the patient chart so that when the Explanation of Benefits (EOB) is received from the insurance carrier, you can determine if the correct benefits were applied (i.e., the bill was paid at 100%).

Pre-admission Testing

In the past, a patient would enter the hospital the day before surgery for routine tests such as a chest x-ray and a blood test. The hospital would then admit the patient and watch over them to ensure that they had nothing to eat or drink in the 24 hours prior to surgery. Insurance carriers realized there would be a great cost savings if the patient were to visit the hospital for the tests, return home, and then return the next day for the surgery. This eliminated the charges for an overnight stay in the hospital.

To encourage this practice, some insurance companies began offering an extra incentive for **pre-admission testing**, or testing done before the patient enters the hospital for surgery. Some insurance carriers now cover these charges at 100% rather than at their normal coinsurance percentage.

Tests performed at the facility where the patient will be admitted, and performed within 24 hours of admittance, are usually allowed under this benefit. If it is appropriate for the patient's condition, consider scheduling this option, or at least making the patient aware of it.

Second Surgical Opinions

Some insurance carriers cover a second surgical opinion at 100%. This originally started out as a cost-cutting measure. The hope was that only those surgeries that were necessary would be confirmed, with some patients receiving alternative (and less expensive) treatments, or with treatment being considered completely unnecessary.

Second surgical opinions have become less popular among insurance carriers since the cost savings seems to be minimal, if any. Many doctors are reluctant to go against the word or prescribed treatments of another physician. They don't want to contradict their peers, and also don't want to open themselves up to a lawsuit by suggesting a less radical treatment which may eventually prove less effective. Therefore, in they will often simply confirm the diagnosis and prescribed treatment of the original physician.

If you are billing for second surgical opinion services, be sure to use one of the second surgical opinion or consultation CPT® codes. These codes will be explained in details in the chapter on Reference Books.

Outpatient Facility Charges

Some surgeries are simple or routine enough to be performed on an outpatient basis. This means that the patient enters the facility in the morning, has surgery, and, after a brief recovery period, returns home the same day. There are no overnight or room and board charges. To encourage outpatient surgery when and where possible, some insurance carriers will cover such charges at 100%.

Major Medical Benefits

This section of the contract lists the particular benefits and stipulations which a contract provides.

Deductible

The first item usually listed is the amount of the **deductible**. This is the amount which the patient must pay prior to the insurance paying their benefits. Deductibles are usually accumulated according to a calendar year. Thus, each January 1st, the amount the patient has paid toward their deductible returns to zero and the patient must start paying again.

The exception to this is in contracts which have a "**carry-over provision.**" A deductible carry-over provision means that any amounts which the patient pays toward their deductible in the last three months of the year will carry-over and will be applied toward the next year's deductible. Remember, the patient pays their deductible before the insurance is required to pay any benefits. Therefore, if the patient is still paying a deductible in the last three months of the year, the insurance carrier hasn't had to pay any major medical benefits on this patient up to that time.

If you are in the month of September and it is appropriate for the patient's condition, ask the patient if they would like to schedule services for after October 1. The deductible payments will then apply not only for this year, but for the following year as well, if their plan has a carry-over provision.

Family Deductible

Family deductibles work the same way individual deductibles do in that once a certain limit is reached, no more deductible is taken. There are two ways to accumulate a family deductible: aggregate and nonaggregate.

Aggregate means that any amounts paid toward the deductible by any member of the family will be added up to reach the deductible. For example, if the Barton Family is covered under the Winter Insurance contract, their family deductible is $200, aggregate. Therefore:

Family Member	Deductible Met
Billy	$25
Barry	$45
Bobby	$85
Betty	$0

Family Deductible Met Total to date <u>$155</u>

Betty now submits a claim for $500 in services. She need only pay $45 toward her deductible since, when added to the family total the $200 family deductible limit is met. Even though none of the family members have met their individual limit, the family limit has been satisfied. Therefore no more deductible will be taken on any member of this family.

In nonaggregate family deductible limits, the added sum of what each family member has paid is not important. Rather, a specified number of individuals in the family must meet their individual deductible limit in order for the family limit to be met. Nonaggregate family limits often require that the family pay more money toward the deductible. For example, if the Barton family were covered under the Ball Insurance Carrier contract, the family deductible limit would be two family members. Therefore if:

Family Member	Deductible Met
Billy	$25
Barry	$45
Bobby	$85
Betty	$0

Family Deductible Met Total to date <u>$155</u>

Betty now submits a claim for $500 in services. She must pay the full $125 toward her deductible. Even then, the family deductible has still not been satisfied.

If the next claim is for Billy for $75, the full $75 amount would be considered part of the deductible, thus bringing the amount Billy has paid toward his deductible to $100. However, the family deductible still has not been met since only one family member (Betty), not two, have reached their individual family limit.

Only when Billy, Barry or Bobby has paid $125 toward their deductible will the family deductible be considered to be met. At that time, no more deductible would be taken on any member of the family.

As a biller, try to be aware of where each member of a family stands in relation to their deductible payments. This can be done fairly simply by looking at the patient ledger for each family member. The patient with the most charges during the year has probably gone the farthest toward meeting their deductible. Also, if the insurance carrier has previously made several payments, the deductible has usually (though not always) been satisfied.

If more than one member of a family is being treated, consider submitting the bill for the member(s) with the highest payments on their deductible. Then submit the claims for the other family members at a later date.

Let's assume that the entire Barton family came down with an illness and had to come in for office visits. The whole family comes in and is treated on the same day. You check their charts and discover that they are covered by the Ball contract and:

Family Member	Deductible Met
Billy	$25
Barry	$45
Bobby	$85
Betty	$0

Family Deductible Met Total to date $155

As a biller, it would be best to submit the claims for Bobby and Barry first, and then submit the claims for the remaining family members about a week later. This would ensure that only an additional $120 in deductible ($40 on Bobby and $80 on Barry) would have to be covered by the family. If all the bills were submitted at once, the claims examiner may choose to process the claims for Betty and Billy first, thus taking a deductible of $225 ($125 on Betty and $100 on Billy).

Coinsurance

Coinsurance is an agreement to share expenses between the member and the insurance carrier. This is usually expressed in percentages (i.e., the insurance covers 80% of the approved amount of a bill, and the patient covers 20%).

It is important for the biller to know the coinsurance percentage on a patient's insurance in order to collect the proper payment from the patient at the time services are rendered. Let's say you are visited by a patient who is covered under the Ball Contract and has not yet met their deductible. If the services totaled $500, you should collect $200 from the patient. First collect the $125 deductible which the patient will be responsible for, then collect 20% of the remaining $375 ($75).

Collecting the patient's portion of the payment before the patient leaves the office is one way to ensure that most of the bill will be paid. If a medical biller overcharges the patient, the insurance carrier will pay benefits to the provider only up to the amount of their bill. If additional monies are due, the insurance carrier will reimburse the patient.

Coinsurance Limit or Out-of-Pocket Limit

Many insurance companies are very aware that the financial effects of a catastrophic illness can ruin a family financially. Since insurance carriers want to keep people enrolled, they must leave them with enough resources to consistently pay premiums. For this reason many insurance carriers have a coinsurance limit, also called an out-of-pocket limit. This limit stipulates that if the coinsurance portion of a patient's bills reaches a certain amount, all subsequent claims will be paid at 100% of the allowed amount. For example, the Ball Contract has a coinsurance limit of $400. Since the coinsurance amount is based upon 20% of the allowed amount (with the insurance covering 80% of the allowed amount), the patient must have bills with approved amounts totaling over $2,125 in a calendar year ($125 is applied toward deductible, $2,000 multiplied by 20% equals the $400 limit).

As a medical biller, if your patient has an illness which generates numerous claims totaling large amounts, you should attempt to schedule as many of the visits in the same year as possible. This will allow bills which are over the coinsurance limit to be paid at a higher percent than those under it, thus decreasing the burden on the family and allowing the doctor a greater possibility of collecting the full amount.

Mental/Nervous Expenses

Mental and Nervous expenses include claims submitted for psychiatric services, marriage and family counseling services, and drug and alcohol treatment. Often there are different limits and coinsurance percentages for mental and nervous expenses.

Many contracts have a calendar year maximum or a maximum number of visits for these types of services.

It is important for the biller to understand any limits on the number of treatments or amounts covered by insurance. Make the doctor aware of these limits so that the doctor can suggest or schedule treatments accordingly.

Lifetime Maximum

There is a **lifetime maximum** payment amount placed on most contracts. Once the patient reaches the lifetime maximum amount, the insurance carrier will not cover any additional expenses. Essentially this amount is the total dollar payments the insurance carrier will make toward the lifetime care of this patient. However, this amount is so high that it is seldom reached, except in extreme cases.

Billers should be aware of this maximum amount, especially for patients with high medical expenses or who have been with the same insurance carrier (and under the same policy) for an extended period of time.

If the patient is about to reach their lifetime maximum (or may reach it within the next year) suggest to the patient that they may want to consider switching their insurance coverage. This is especially relevant if the patient is covered under a policy provided by their employer. If the employer offers more than one plan, the employee may be able to switch plans during the open enrollment period when they are sure to get coverage. Proof of good health is not required during an open enrollment period.

Pre-existing Limitations

Many contracts will not cover conditions which existed prior to a patient being covered under a contract (called **pre-existing limitations**). This prevents a patient from not paying for insurance coverage, then discovering they have a serious illness and seeking insurance to cover that illness.

The term pre-existing has a different meaning for each contract. Most often it is defined as a condition for which the patient has sought treatment within a given time period before insurance coverage has begun. If the patient has sought treatment for such a condition, within this time period prior to coverage, benefits for treatment may not be covered or may be limited to a certain dollar amount. Usually, the restraints for benefits will cease once the patient has been covered under a contract for 12 months or longer. A few contracts allow coverage after six months.

Some contracts also have a "treatment free" period. With this provision, if the patient can go without treatment for a specified period of time (often 90 days), then the insurance carrier will no longer consider the condition to be pre-existing and will cover the illness or condition under the normal terms of the contract.

Remember that treatment includes any kind of contact in relationship with the illness, including the office visit or testing which were used to diagnose the illness. It also includes treatment of the condition, tests or office visits to monitor the condition, and filling of prescriptions relating to the condition.

If you become aware that a pre-existing situation may exist, discuss the options with the doctor. It may be possible to schedule treatments in such a way that benefits will not be cut too drastically. Also, be sure to note when coverage for the condition will begin, usually after the person has been covered by the contract for 12 months. This may allow for better scheduling of treatments near that date so that the procedures are covered.

HIPAA/Health Insurance Portability

On August 26, 1996, new laws regarding health insurance were signed into law by President Clinton. This was called the Health Insurance Portability and Accountability Act of 1996 (HIPAA). The most important changes include pre-existing limitations and prior coverage certification.

Under the new law, pre-existing exclusions are limited to six months, and credit must be given for prior coverage. Therefore, if a person is covered by insurance, and then transfers insurance coverage to a new company within 63 days of ceasing coverage at the old company, the new insurance carrier may not apply pre-existing limitations to treatment. If there was a break of more than 63 days between the termination of the old coverage and the available date of new coverage, pre-existing exclusions are limited to six months.

Pre-existing limitations are also not allowed for pregnancy or newborns. Therefore, if a woman transfers coverage while she is pregnant, the new insurance carrier must cover the costs associated with the pregnancy.

If a person declines coverage under a new plan because they are covered under a previously existing plan, and then they loose their benefits under the old plan, they may then enroll under the new plan without pre-existing limitations. Pre-existing limitations may not be applied to those who transfer from one plan to another during a company's open-enrollment period.

Companies are also now required to provide written certification of all prior coverage. They must provide this information upon termination of coverage, and for up to 24 months after termination if the employee requests it.

Employees are no longer allowed to continue COBRA coverage on a policy if they are covered under a new policy. In the past, many employees would continue coverage on an old policy until the pre-existing limitation had been satisfied on the new insurance. Since the new insurance is no longer allowed to apply pre-existing limitations, the need for this coverage has been eliminated. Many people may still elect to continue coverage on the old policy until they have satisfied any length of employment requirements (i.e., must be employed for 90 days). However, the waiting period is not considered a break in coverage for purposes of the 63 day break in coverage. Therefore, if an employee terminates at one company (and ceases coverage), and is hired at a second company within 63 days, they are considered continuously covered even if they must satisfy a 90-day waiting period before coverage begins with their new employer.

When hiring, employers are not allowed to discriminate against those with higher medical costs. This is true even though the higher costs will eventually show an increase in the company's insurance premiums.

For those who do not satisfy the continuous coverage requirements, pre-existing exclusions are limited to conditions where treatment was received within six months prior to coverage. Exclusions are only allowed to remain in effect for 12 months. Therefore, after 12 months the carrier must cover the condition, whether it was pre-existing or not. If a person did not enroll when they first became eligible, then pre-existing exclusions are allowed to continue for up to 18 months. This is because some people won't apply for coverage until they have a condition which they know is going to require extensive treatment. They will then attempt to get coverage on that condition.

A new insurance carrier may choose to enact the pre-existing limitations on certain items that were not included in previous medical coverage. This allowance is limited to coverage for mental health, substance abuse treatment, prescriptions, dental care, and vision care. For example, if a participant's old plan did not include coverage for mental health benefits, then the new plan may elect to enact a pre-existing limit only on the mental health benefits which it normally offers in the plan.

How This Impacts Medical Billers
When a patient transfers insurance, changes employers, or looses eligibility under their insurance (i.e., a child reaches maximum dependent age), they should be issued a certificate which details their previous coverage. Since this is a new situation, many patients may not be aware of the significance of this certificate.

Ask patients to provide the practice with a copy of this certificate and file this copy in the patient's file. If the patient then receives treatment for a condition which would be considered pre-existing, include a copy of the certificate with the patient's claim. This will help to prevent denial of the claim.

Exclusions

Every contract will have a list of **exclusions**. These are items which the insurance carrier does not cover. It is important to check the list of exclusions before scheduling surgery or other expensive treatments for a patient. If the procedures or treatments are not covered, the patient will be responsible for the entire amount of the bill. Many doctors who routinely perform procedures which are not covered (i.e., cosmetic surgeons) will often require payment in full prior to scheduling the surgery.

Allowed Amounts

Insurance carriers limit payment to a specified amount of the allowed amount. The **allowed amount** is what the insurance company considers to be a reasonable charge for the procedure performed, and is often less than the amount which the doctor bills.

A nationwide listing of allowable amounts is not really fair since it costs a lot more to do business in Los Angeles (higher nurse and secretary salaries, rents, costs of supplies, etc.) than it does in a rural medical clinic in Louisiana. Because of this, a system called Usual, Customary and Reasonable (UCR) was established.

Under **UCR**, each procedure which is performed has been given a number value (called a relative unit value) based on how difficult the procedure is to perform, the overhead involved, and the chance of incurring a malpractice lawsuit. For example, it takes a lot more skill, time and medical supplies to perform brain surgery than it does to clean a skinned knee and put a bandage on it. Therefore, brain surgery is given a much higher unit value than cleaning and bandaging a skinned knee.

Since each procedure has a different unit value, there are often several codes for the same type of procedure. For example, there are five different codes for an office visit of a new patient. The code used depends on how difficult the patient's condition is to treat and the skill level involved in this treatment. Because different unit values are assigned to each code, it is important that the biller code the procedures correctly.

This unit value is multiplied by a conversion factor. The **conversion factor** is determined by the first three digits of the zip code in which the services were performed and what type of services they were.

The type of service is broken out into four groups:

- Medical Services (office visits),
- Surgical Services (procedures which invade the body),
- X-ray and Laboratory Procedures (x-rays taken and lab tests performed), and
- Anesthesia Services.

While the unit value for a procedure would remain the same no matter where in the nation it was performed, the conversion factor would change depending on the cost of doing business in a given area. Thus, the factors for Louisiana would be far less than those for Los Angeles.

By multiplying the conversion factor by the unit value, you get the **allowed amount**. This is the amount used to determine how much of the deductible has been met and how much of the charges will be covered. For example, if the claim is for $125 but the allowed amount of the procedure(s) is $75, the insurance carrier will only apply that $75 toward the deductible. Thus, even though the patient is paying $125 for the services, only $75 of their deductible limit has been met. The patient would still need another $50 (under the Ball Insurance Carriers contract) of allowed charges to meet their deductible.

Likewise, if the claim is for $500 and the allowed amount is $350, the patient could be responsible for quite a large a bill. Under the Ball Contract the $125 deductible would be subtracted from the allowed amount, leaving $225. This would then be multiplied by the 80% coinsurance rate and the insurance carrier would send a check for $180. The patient would be responsible for the remaining $320!

Not all insurance carriers use the same list of relative value units. Therefore, the allowed amount for one insurance carrier will be different from the allowed amount of a different insurance carrier.

Additionally, the insurance carrier will never consider more than the billed amount. Therefore, if the allowed amount for a bill is $200, but the doctor only charged $150, the insurance carrier will consider the billed amount to be the allowed amount of $150. The carrier will then subtract any remaining deductible to be paid, and multiply the remainder by the coinsurance percent.

As a biller, if you notice that the doctor's charges for a particular procedure are always the same as the allowed amount; it may mean that the doctor is charging less than what the insurance carriers consider to be reasonable for that procedure. Discuss this with the doctor and consider raising the billed amount for this procedure.

Likewise, if the allowed amount is always significantly lower than the billed amount, you may wish to discuss lowering the fee with the doctor. Be aware that allowed amounts are nearly always lower than billed amounts, so lowering of fees should not be done without serious consideration.

Pre-certification of Inpatient Admissions

To **pre-certify** means to get pre-approval for admission on elective, non-emergency hospitalization. Contact is made either with the plan administrator or another entity sanctioned to determine the necessity of the admission. Most often, these entities are composed of a specialized group of nurses working under the direction of a physician. The nurses deal directly with the physician's office and the facility to determine whether the admission is necessary and whether the number of days of care is medically necessary. If the patient stays longer than the approved number of days, the additional days of care may not be paid for or the usual payment may be reduced by a percentage specified by the plan. The objective in this program is to prevent unnecessary admissions and to get the patient out of the hospital as soon as is medically appropriate.

For these reasons it is important that all medical billers check the terms of the contract, if possible. Often information on pre-certification is included directly on the patient's insurance card. This information will say something to the effect of:

All voluntary inpatient admissions must be pre-certified 48 hours prior to admission. In case of emergency admission, please contact the carrier within 24 hours of admission or benefits may be reduced or services not covered.

Some programs provide for pre-certification only prior to or on the day of hospitalization. Other programs provide for a complete approach to managing the care, which entails a utilization review program. Utilization review is discussed in a later chapter.

As part of HIPAA, the Federal Government has mandated that no pre-certification can be required on maternity confinements. The law stipulates a confinement for a normal delivery cannot be limited to less than 48 hours (two days) or in the case of a cesarean section 96 hours (four days). The law, however, does not state that a concurrent review could not be done. Therefore, if the patient stays hospital confined beyond the two days for a normal delivery or a day for a C-section and the plan has concurrent review and extended stay provisions, applicable penalties can be imposed on those extra days.

Utilization Review

As previously indicated, **pre-certification** or a prospective review determines the need and appropriateness of the recommended care. A complete **Utilization Review (UR)** program contains the following three components:

1. Pre-certification (prior to) or prospective review.
2. Concurrent review (during the confinement).
3. Retrospective review (after termination of confinement).

Concurrent review determines whether the estimated length of time and scope of the inpatient stay is justified by the diagnosis and symptoms. This review is conducted periodically during the

projected length of time the patient is in the hospital. If the length of stay exceeds the criteria or if there is a change in treatment, the matter is referred to the medical consultant for review.

At no time does the consultant dictate the method of treatment or the length of stay. These decisions are left entirely to the patient and the attending physician. However, the consultant is entitled to inform the patient, physician, and facility that the continued stay exceeds the approved number of days and may not be covered by the plan as medically necessary. It is then the patient's responsibility to decide what course to take.

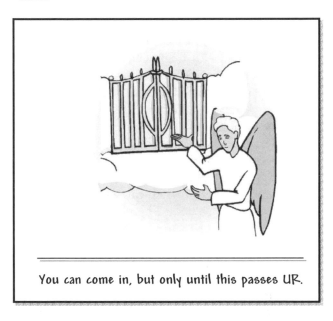

You can come in, but only until this passes UR.

Retrospective review is used to determine after discharge whether the hospitalization and treatment were medically necessary and covered by the terms of the benefit program. This type of review may be used as a substitute for admission and concurrent reviews when the failure to notify the UR program of an admission prevents the regular review procedures. However, the main drawback to the retrospective review is that the patient and providers are not notified about the services that will not be covered until after they have been provided. The best programs always work most effectively when the patient is notified beforehand that he or she will be primarily responsible for payment of services. This approach deters the member from incurring unnecessary expenses.

Second Surgical Opinion Consultations

Surgical claims represent the second highest categorical cost to carriers (hospitalization ranks first). The United States has the world's highest rate of surgical treatment because neither the physician nor the patient has much financial incentive to consider less expensive alternatives.

About 80% of all surgeries can be considered "elective." That is, they are not required because of a life-threatening situation. The objective of a **Second Surgical Opinion Consultation (SSO)** is to eliminate elective surgical procedures that are classified as unnecessary.

Unnecessary surgery is that which is recommended as an elective procedure when an alternative method of treatment may be preferable for a number of reasons, including:

- The surgery itself may be premature, taking into consideration all pathologic indications.
- The risk to the patient may not justify the benefits of surgery.
- An alternative medical treatment may be superior for both medical and cost-effective reasons.
- A less severe surgical procedure may be preferable under the circumstances. Or, no medical or surgical procedure may be necessary at all.

In this program, the patient consults an independent specialist to determine whether the recommended elective surgical procedure is advisable. This process is not intended to interfere with the patient-physician relationship or to prevent the patient from receiving necessary elective operations.

This program may be administered in one of two ways:

1. A **mandatory program** requires the patient to obtain an SSO for special procedures, or there is an automatic reduction or denial of benefits. For an example of this type of program, see the Rover Insurers, Inc contract.
2. A **voluntary program** encourages participants to have an SSO, but there is no automatic reduction of benefits if the patient does not comply. In both approaches, the SSO and related tests are usually paid at 100% so that the patient will not have any out-of-pocket expenses for conforming to the program.

The SSO program has met with much criticism because it has not effectively reduced the number of elective surgeries. One of the main reasons for this ineffectiveness is that physicians may be reluctant to tell a patient that a surgery is not necessary. This attitude stems from the growing number of malpractice lawsuits. For example, if a physician states that a patient does not need surgery and a sudden emergency situation arises that is related to the original need for surgery, the physician may be held liable under a malpractice suit. Consequently, many plans are abandoning the SSO plan provision.

Summary

It is vital that medical billers understand how to properly interpret the basic benefits of a contract. It will take practice to accurately understand the coverages provided under contracts and to suggest treatment options which will provide the greatest benefits.

Additionally, billers must understand items in a contract such as pre-authorization and pre-certification which can impact payment on a patient's claim.

Assignments

Complete the Questions for Review.
Complete Exercises 6 – 1 through 6 – 5.

Go through the following three contracts and be sure that you understand what coverages are provided.

Questions for Review

Directions: Answer the following questions without looking back into the material just covered. Write your answers in the space provided.

1. What is eligibility? _____
   _____

2. Basic benefits are usually paid at 100% and are _____

3. Define accident. _____
   _____

4. What is pre-admission testing? _____
   _____

5. What is outpatient surgery? _____
   _____

6. What is a deductible? _____
   _____

7. Define aggregate family deductible. _____
   _____

8. What is coinsurance? _____
   _____

9. What happens when a patient reaches their coinsurance limit? _____
   _____

10. What are mental/nervous expenses? _____
    _____

11. What happens when a patient reaches their lifetime maximum? _____

12. What is a pre-existing condition? _____
    _____

13. What is an exclusion? _____

14. What is an allowed amount? _____
    _____

15. How do you get the allowed amount? _____

If you were unable to answer any of the questions, refer back to that section, and then fill in the answers.

Exercise 6 – 1

Directions: Study the contracts on the following pages and complete the following questions. Write your answers in the space provided.

1. What are the eligibility requirements for:

   Winter _____

   _____

   _____

   Rover _____

   _____

   _____

   Ball _____

   _____

   _____

2. What is the individual and family deductible amount for:

   Winter _____

   Rover _____

   Ball _____

3. What basic benefits does each contract have?

   Winter _____

   _____

   Rover _____

   _____

   Ball _____

   _____

4. What are the terms of the accident benefit for:

   Winter _____

   _____

   Rover _____

   _____

   Ball _____

   _____

5. What is the coinsurance limit for:

   Winter _____

   Rover _____

   Ball _____

Exercise 6 – 2

Directions: Read each scenario below and determine whether or not the certificate of prior insurance should be included with the claim, and why or why not.

1. Jennifer received treatment for a chronic ulcer on 7/1/04 and again on 8/1/04. On 10/1/04 she quit her old job and began working for a new employer two weeks later, on 10/15/04. She immediately signed up for insurance and her coverage became effective after a 30-day waiting period, on 11/15/04. On 1/15/05 she was seen by a doctor for additional ulcer treatment. Should you send in a copy of her coverage certificate with the 1/15/05 claim?

2. Mary received treatment for diabetes on 7/1/03 and again on 8/1/03. On 10/1/03 she quit her old job and began working for a new employer two weeks later, on 10/15/03. She immediately signed up for insurance and her coverage became effective after a 90 day waiting period, on 1/15/03. On 10/15/04 she was seen by a doctor for additional diabetes treatment. Should you send in a copy of her coverage certificate with the 10/15/04 claim?

3. Tom received treatment for kidney disease 2/1/03 and again on 3/1/03. On 10/1/04 he quit his old job and began working for a new employer two weeks later, on 10/15/04. He immediately signed up for insurance and his coverage became effective after a 30 day waiting period, on 11/15/03. On 12/15/03 he was seen by a doctor for additional kidney disease treatment. Should you send in a copy of his coverage certificate with the 11/15/03 claim?

4. Betty received a routine visit for pregnancy on 7/1/04 and again on 8/1/04. On 10/1/04 she began working for a new employer. She immediately signed up for insurance and her coverage became effective after a 30-day waiting period, on 12/15/04. She did not have prior coverage. On 1/15/05 she was seen by a doctor for an additional routine visit. Should you send in a copy of her coverage certificate with the 1/15/05 claim?

5. Jessie received treatment for anorexia on 7/1/04 and again on 8/1/04. On 10/1/04 she quit her old job and chose not to continue coverage under COBRA rules. On 12/15/04 she began working for a new employer. She immediately signed up for insurance and her coverage became effective after a 30 day waiting period, on 1/15/04. On 10/25/04 she was seen by a doctor for additional anorexia treatment. Should you send in a copy of her coverage certificate with the 10/25/04 claim?

Exercise 6 – 3

Directions: Calculate the amount of deductible which will be taken and answer the following questions.

The Apple family is covered under the Winter Contract. Their previous deductible payments are as follows:

	Annie	**Adam**	**April**	**August**	**Ashley**
Carryover paid	0.00	5.00	10.00	55.00	0.00
Deductible paid	10.00	0.00	5.00	5.00	0.00

1. What is the individual deductible limit on this contract?   1. _____

2. What is the family deductible limit on this contract?   2. _____

3. Is the family limit aggregate or non-aggregate?   3. _____

4. How much has been paid toward the family deductible?   4. _____

5. Annie incurs allowed charges of $35. How much will be applied to the
   deductible?   5. _____

6. How much has Annie now met on her deductible?   6. _____

7. How much has now been paid toward the family deductible?   7. _____

8. August incurs allowed charges of $55. How much will be applied to the
   deductible?   8. _____

9. How much has August now met on his deductible?   9. _____

10. How much has now been paid toward the family deductible?   10. _____

11. April incurs allowed charges of $55. How much will be applied to the
    deductible?   11. _____

12. How much has April now met on her deductible?   12. _____

13. How much has now been paid toward the family deductible for?   13. _____

14. Adam incurs allowed charges of $60. How much will be applied to the
    deductible?   14. _____

15. How much has Adam now met on his deductible?   15. _____

16. How much has now been paid toward the family deductible?   16. _____

17. Annie incurs allowed charges of $35. How much will be applied to the
    deductible?   17. _____

18. How much has Annie now met on her deductible?   18. _____

19. How much has now been paid toward the family deductible?   19. _____

Exercise 6 – 4

Directions: Calculate the amount of deductible which will be taken and answer the following questions.

The Bear family is covered under the Rover Contract. Their previous deductible payments are as follows:

	Brad	**Bonnie**	**Barbra**	**Brian**
Carryover paid	0.00	5.00	10.00	55.00
Deductible paid	10.00	0.00	5.00	5.00

1. What is the individual deductible limit on this contract? 1. _____

2. What is the family deductible limit on this contract? 2. _____

3. Is the family limit aggregate or non-aggregate? 3. _____

4. How many people are needed to meet the family deductible for this year? 4. _____

5. Bonnie incurs allowed charges of $55. How much will be applied to the deductible? 5. _____

6. How much has Bonnie now met on her deductible? 6. _____

7. How many people are now needed to meet the family deductible? 7. _____

8. Brian incurs allowed charges of $85. How much will be applied to the deductible? 8. _____

9. How much has Brian now met on his deductible? 9. _____

10. How many people are now needed to meet the family deductible? 10. _____

11. Barbra incurs allowed charges of $105. How much will be applied to the deductible? 11. _____

12. How much has Barbra now met on her deductible? 12. _____

13. How many people are now needed to meet the family deductible? 13. _____

14. Brad incurs allowed charges of $60. How much will be applied to the deductible? 14. _____

15. How much has Brad now met on his deductible? 15. _____

16. How many people are now needed to meet the family deductible? 16. _____

17. Bonnie incurs allowed charges of $35. How much will be applied to the deductible? 17. _____

18. How much has Bonnie now met on her deductible? 18. _____

19. How many people are now needed to meet the family deductible? 19. _____

20. Brian incurs allowed charges of $35. How much will be applied to the deductible? 20. _____

21. How much has Brian now met on his deductible? 21. _____

22. How many people are now needed to meet the family deductible? 22. _____

23. Barbra incurs allowed charges of $55. How much will be applied to the deductible? 23. _____

24. How much has Barbra now met on her deductible?   24. _____

25. How many people are now needed to meet the family deductible?   25. _____

26. Brad incurs allowed charges of $60. How much will be applied to the
    deductible?   26. _____

27. How much has Brad now met on his deductible?   27. _____

28. How many people are now needed to meet the family deductible?   28. _____

29. Bonnie incurs allowed charges of $35. How much will be applied to the
    deductible?   29. _____

30. How much has Bonnie now met on her deductible?   30. _____

31. How many people are now needed to meet the family deductible?   31. _____

Exercise 6 – 5

Directions: Calculate the amount of deductible which will be taken and answer the following questions.

The Carpenter family is covered under the Ball Contract. Their previous deductible payments are as follows:

	Carry	Connie	Cathy	Chris
Carryover paid	0.00	5.00	10.00	55.00
Deductible paid	10.00	0.00	5.00	5.00

1. What is the individual deductible limit on this contract?   1. _____

2. What is the family deductible limit on this contract?   2. _____

3. Is the family limit aggregate or non-aggregate?   3. _____

4. How many people are needed to meet the family deductible?   4. _____

5. Connie incurs allowed charges of $35. How much will be applied to the
   deductible?   5. _____

6. How much has Connie now met on her deductible?   6. _____

7. How many people are now needed to meet the family deductible?   7. _____

8. Carry incurs allowed charges of $55. How much will be applied to the
   deductible?   8. _____

9. How much has Carry now met on her deductible?   9. _____

10. How many people are now needed to meet the family deductible?   10. _____

11. Chris incurs allowed charges of $60. How much will be applied to the
    deductible?   11. _____

12. How much has Chris now met on his deductible?   12. _____

13. How many people are now needed to meet the family deductible?   13. _____

14. Chris incurs allowed charges of $35. How much will be applied to the
    deductible?   14. _____

15. How much has Chris now met on his deductible?   15. _____

16. How many people are now needed to meet the family deductible?

16. _____

17. Connie incurs allowed charges of $95. How much will be applied to the deductible?

17. _____

18. How much has Connie now met on her deductible?

18. _____

19. How many people are now needed to meet the family deductible?

19. _____

20. Carry incurs allowed charges of $45. How much will be applied to the deductible?

20. _____

21. How much has Carry now met on her deductible?

21. _____

22. How many people are now needed to meet the family deductible?

22. _____

23. Cathy incurs allowed charges of $105. How much will be applied to the deductible?

23. _____

24. How much has Cathy now met on her deductible?

24. _____

25. How many people are now needed to meet the family deductible?

25. _____

26. Carry incurs allowed charges of $85. How much will be applied to the deductible?

26. _____

27. How much has Carry now met on her deductible?

27. _____

28. How many people are now needed to meet the family deductible?

28. _____

29. Chris incurs allowed charges of $85. How much will be applied to the deductible?

29. _____

30. How much has Chris now met on his deductible?

30. _____

31. How many people are now needed to meet the family deductible?

31. _____

32. Cathy incurs allowed charges of $90. How much will be applied to the deductible?

32. _____

33. How much has Cathy now met on her deductible?

33. _____

34. How many people are now needed to meet the family deductible?

34. _____

Honors Certification™

The certification challenge for this chapter will be a written test of the information contained in this chapter. Each incorrect answer will result in a deduction of up to 5% from your grade. You must achieve a score of 85% or higher to pass this test. If you fail the test on your first attempt you may retake the test one additional time. The items included in the second test may be different from those in the first test.

BALL INSURANCE CARRIERS *(800) 555-5432*
3895 Bubble Blvd. Ste. 283, Boxwood, CO 85926 (970) 555-5432

PLAN: **Blue Corporation**   Effective 09/1/93

ELIGIBILITY EMPLOYEE: Must work a minimum of 30 hours per week. Is eligible for coverage the first of the month following three consecutive months of continuous employment.
DEPENDENTS: Are eligible for coverage from birth to age 19, or to age 23 if a full-time student or handicapped prior to age 19/23 (proof of disability must be furnished within 31 days after dependent reaches limiting age). Not eligible as a dependent if eligible as an employee. Unmarried natural children, legally adopted and foster children are included (includes legal guardianship). If both parents are covered by the plan, children may be covered by one employee only.

EFFECTIVE DATE EMPLOYEE: If written application is made prior to eligibility date, coverage becomes effective the first of the month following three months of continuous employment.
DEPENDENTS: The date acquired by the covered employee becomes the effective date if written application is made within 31 days of eligibility date. If confined in a hospital on date of eligibility, coverage will not start until the first of the month following the date the confinement ends. Newborns are automatically covered for the first 30 days following birth. Coverage will be terminated after 30 days unless written application for coverage is submitted by the employee within 31 days of birth.

TERMINATION OF COVERAGE EMPLOYEE: Coverage terminates the last day of the month following termination of employment, or when the employee ceases to qualify as an eligible employee, or following request for termination of coverage.
DEPENDENTS: Coverage terminates the date the employee's coverage terminates or the last day of the month during which the dependent no longer qualifies as an eligible dependent.

BASIC BENEFITS

PRE-ADMISSION TESTING - Out-patient diagnostic tests performed prior to inpatient admissions; paid at 100% of UCR.
SUPPLEMENTAL ACCIDENT EXPENSE - 100% of the first $300 for services incurred within 90 days of accident.
INPATIENT HOSPITAL EXPENSE
    DEDUCTIBLE: $50.
    ROOM AND BOARD: Up to semi-private room charge. ICU up to $600 per day.
    MISCELLANEOUS FEES: Unlimited.
    MAXIMUM PERIOD: 10 days per period of disability.
SURGERY
    CONVERSION FACTOR: $8.50.
    CALENDAR YEAR MAXIMUM: $1,600 per person.
    REMARKS: Voluntary sterilizations covered.
ASSISTANT SURGERY
    CONVERSION FACTOR: $8.50.
    CALENDAR YEAR MAXIMUM ALLOWANCE: $320 per person. Maximum of 20% of surgeon's allowance or billed charge, whichever is less.
    REMARKS: Voluntary sterilizations covered for women only.
IN-HOSPITAL PHYSICIANS
    DAILY MAXIMUM: $21 for the first day; $8.00 per day thereafter.
    MAXIMUM PERIOD: Ten days per period of disability.
    REMARKS: Only one doctor can be paid per day.
ANESTHESIA
    CONVERSION FACTOR: $7.50.
    CALENDAR YEAR MAXIMUM: $300 per person.
    REMARKS: Voluntary sterilizations covered.
OUTPATIENT PHYSICIANS VISITS
    CONVERSION FACTOR: $7.50.
    CALENDAR YEAR MAXIMUM: $300 per person.
    REMARKS: Chiropractors, M.D.s, D.O.s and acupuncturists allowed. Mental and Nervous treatment not covered.

X-RAY AND LABORATORY
CONVERSION FACTOR: $7.
CALENDAR YEAR MAXIMUM: $200 per person.
REMARKS: Professional component charges covered at 40% of UCR allowance for procedure. Routine procedures are not covered.

MAJOR MEDICAL EXPENSES

INDIVIDUAL CALENDAR YEAR DEDUCTIBLE: $125; three month carryover provision.
FAMILY MAXIMUM DEDUCTIBLE: Two family members must satisfy their individual calendar year deductible in order to satisfy the family deductible.
STANDARD COINSURANCE: 80%.
COINSURANCE LIMIT: $400 out-of-pocket per individual; $800 out-of-pocket per family (not to include deductible, mental and nervous expenses); aggregate.
APPLICATION OF COINSURANCE LIMIT: Coinsurance limit applies in the calendar year in which the limit is met and the following calendar year.
OUTPATIENT MENTAL/NERVOUS EXPENSE: 50% coinsurance while not a hospital inpatient. $500 calendar year maximum per person.
LIFETIME MAXIMUM: $1,000,000 per person.
ROOM LIMIT: Semi-private room rate.
HOSPITAL DEDUCTIBLE: Not covered.
HOME HEALTH CARE: 120 visits per calendar year. Prior hospital confinement required.
PRE-EXISTING LIMITATION: If treatment received within six months prior to effective date, $2,000 maximum payment until patient has been covered continuously under the plan for 12 months.

MEDICARE
TYPE: Coordination of Benefits.
REMARKS: Assume all Medicare benefits whether or not individual actually enrolled. Subject to all other plan provisions.

EXCLUSIONS
1. Expenses resulting from self-inflicted injuries;
2. Work-related injuries or illnesses;
3. Services for which there is no charge in the absence of insurance;
4. Charges or services in excess of UCR or not medically necessary;
5. Charges for completion of claim forms and failure to keep appointments;
6. Routine or preventative or experimental services;
7. Eye refractions; contacts or glasses; orthotics (eye exercises); radial keratotomy, laser surgery or other procedures for surgical correction of refractive errors;
8. Custodial care;
9. Cosmetic surgery unless for repair of an injury or surgery incurred while covered or result of mastectomy;
10. Dental care of teeth, gums or alveolar process (TMJ) except: a) reduction of fractures of the jaw or facial bones; b) surgical correction of harelip, cleft palate or prognathism; c) removal of salivary duct stones; d) removal of bony cysts of jaw, torus palatinus, leukoplakia or malignant tissues;
11. Reversal of voluntary sterilization;
12. Diagnosis or treatment of infertility including artificial insemination, in vitro fertilization, etc.;
13. Contraceptive materials or devices;
14. Non-therapeutic abortions except where the life of the mother is endangered;
15. Expenses for obesity, weight reduction or diet control unless at least 100 lbs. overweight;
16. Vitamins, food supplements and/or protein supplements;
17. Sex-altering treatments or surgeries or related studies;
18. Orthopedic shoes or other devices for support or treatment of feet except as medically necessary following foot surgery;
19. Bio-feedback related services or treatment;
20. Experimental transplants;
21. EDTA Chelation therapy.

ROVER INSURERS INC.
5931 ROLLING ROAD
RONSON, CO 81369
(970) 555-1369

PLAN: RED ENTERPRISES, 7677 ROYAL ROAD, COLTER, CO 81293   Effective 01/01/96

ELIGIBILITY EMPLOYEES must work a minimum of 30 hours per week. They are eligible for coverage the first of the month following one consecutive month of continuous employment. DEPENDENTS are eligible for coverage from birth to age 19, or to age 25 if a full-time student or handicapped prior to age 19/25. Is not eligible as a dependent if eligible as an employee. Unmarried natural children, legally adopted children, foster children, and legal guardianship children are included. If both parents are covered by the plan, children may be covered by one parent only.

EFFECTIVE DATE - EMPLOYEE becomes effective, if written application is made prior to eligibility date, on the first of the month following 30 days of continuous employment. If employee is absent from work due to disability on the date of eligibility, coverage will not start until the first of the month following the date of return to active work.

DEPENDENTS become effective on the date the covered employee becomes effective, if written application is made within 31 days of eligibility date. If confined in a hospital on the date of eligibility, coverage will not start until the first of the month following the date the confinement ends. Newborns are automatically covered for the first 14 days following birth. Coverage terminates after 14 days unless written application for coverage is submitted by the employee within 31 days of birth.

TERMINATION OF COVERAGE - EMPLOYEE'S coverage terminates the last day of the month following termination of employment or when the employee ceases to qualify as an eligible employee, or following request for termination of coverage. DEPENDENTS' coverage terminates the date the employee's coverage terminates, or the last day of the month during which the dependent no longer qualifies as an eligible dependent.

EXTENSION OF BENEFITS - If covered under the plan when disabled, may continue coverage in accordance with COBRA. No other extension available.

COMPREHENSIVE MEDICAL BENEFITS

PRE-ADMISSION TESTING - Outpatient diagnostic tests performed prior to inpatient admissions are paid at 100% whether through a network provider or not.

PRE-CERTIFICATION - Voluntary, non-emergency inpatient admissions must be approved at least five days prior to admission. Emergency admissions must be pre-certified within 48 hrs. of admission. Benefits are cut to 50% if not done as required.

SECOND SURGICAL OPINION (SSO) - The SSO is paid at 100% of UCR. It is required for the following: bunionectomy, cataract extraction, chemonucleolysis, cholecystectomy, coronary bypass, hemorrhoidectomy, hysterectomy, inguinal herniorrhaphy, laparotomy, laminectomy, mastectomy, meniscectomy, oophorectomy, prostatectomy, salpingectomy, submucous resection, total joint replacement (hip or knee), tenotomy, varicose veins (all procedures). **IF SSO NOT PERFORMED, ALL RELATED EXPENSES PAYABLE AT 50%**

SUPPLEMENTAL ACCIDENT EXPENSE - 100% is paid on the first $500 for services incurred within 90 days of the date of accident. Subject to $20 copayment. After $500, payments are subject to calendar year deductible. Provider does not have to be a network member to receive 100% benefit. Common accident provision applies.

OUTPATIENT FACILITY CHARGES PAYABLE AT 100% - Network outpatient facility expenses for following procedures paid 100%. Does not include professional charges: arthroscopy, breast biopsy, cataract removal, bronchoscopy, deviated nasal septum, pilonidal cyst, myringotomy w/tubes, esophagoscopy, colonoscopy, herniorrhaphy (umbilical, to five years old), skin and subsequent lesions, benign and malignant (2cms+).

INDIVIDUAL CALENDAR YEAR - $150; three month carryover provision.
DEDUCTIBLE - All plan services subject to deductible unless otherwise indicated.
FAMILY MAXIMUM DEDUCTIBLE - $300, non-aggregate. Two family members must meet individual deductible limit.
STANDARD COINSURANCE - 80% Network; 70% Non-network.
COINSURANCE LIMIT - $1,250 out-of-pocket per individual; $2,500 out-of-pocket per family. Two individuals must meet their individual out of pocket limit to satisfy family limit. Limits not to include deductible, mental/nervous expenses, or surgery expenses reduced because SSO not done. 100% of allowed amount paid thereafter for network providers; 90% for non-network providers.
LIFETIME MAXIMUM - $1,000,000 per person.
IN/OUTPATIENT MENTAL/NERVOUS – maximum 25 visits allowed per year (includes substance abuse and alcoholism treatment).

PRE-EXISTING LIMITATION - If treatment is received within 90 days prior to effective date, no coverage on that condition for six months from the effective date (continuously covered for six consecutive months) unless treatment free for three consecutive months which ends after the effective date of coverage.

INPATIENT HOSPITAL EXPENSE IF NO PRE-CERTIFICATION, ADMISSION PAID AT 50%
DEDUCTIBLE - $200.00, waived for network facilities, applies to non-network. Inpatient hospital expenses not subject to regular Major Medical deductible.
ROOM AND BOARD - Network: 80% of semi-private/ICU; Non-network: 70% of semi-private/ICU.
MISCELLANEOUS FEES - Network: 80%; Non-network: 70%.
EXCLUSIONS - Well baby care. Automatic coverage for first seven days if baby is ill. Otherwise, no coverage.
MENTAL/NERVOUS/PSYCHONEUROTIC - Includes substance abuse and alcoholism. Exclusions: psychological testing, hyperkinetic syndrome, learning disabilities, behavior problems or autistic disease of childhood.
>OUTPATIENT MENTAL AND NERVOUS TREATMENT
>PAYABLE - $60 per visit for first 5 visits; $30 per visit for next 21 visits.
>COINSURANCE - 80% for first five visits (maximum payable: $60 per visit) 50% per visit for next 21 visits (maximum payable: $30 per visit).
>CALENDAR YEAR MAXIMUM - 26 visits.
>INPATIENT MENTAL AND NERVOUS TREATMENT
>PHYSICIAN SERVICES - 70% applies to network and non-network providers.
>HOSPITAL SERVICES - 70% applies to network and non-network providers.
>PARTIAL /DAY PROGRAM - Each day in a partial/day program: equals half day in an acute setting.
>PROVIDERS - Psychiatrists and clinical psychologists only.

MAMMOGRAMS
COINSURANCE - 80% Network; 70% Non-network.
REQUIREMENTS - Baseline mammogram for women ages 35-39; for ages 40-49, one allowed every two years; for ages 50+, one allowed every year.
X-RAY AND LABORATORY - PROFESSIONAL COMPONENTS - Professional charges paid at 25% of UCR.
DURABLE MEDICAL EQUIPMENT
COINSURANCE - 50%.
REQUIREMENTS - Prescribed by M.D.; must not be primarily necessary for exercise, environmental control, convenience, comfort or hygiene. Must be an article only useful for the prescribed patient. Covered up to purchase price only.
MEDICARE
TYPE - Maintenance of benefits.
REMARKS - Assume all Medicare benefits whether or not individual actually enrolled. Subject to all other plan provisions.

EXCLUSIONS
1. Expenses resulting from self-inflicted injuries;
2. Work-related injuries or illnesses;
3. Services for which there is no charge in the absence of insurance;
4. Charges or services in excess of UCR or not medically necessary;
5. Pre-existing conditions;
6. Charges for completion of claim forms and failure to keep appointments;
7. Routine or preventative or experimental services;
8. Eye refractions; contacts or glasses; orthotics (eye exercises); radial keratotomy, laser surgery or other procedures for surgical correction of refractive errors;
9. Custodial care;
10. Cosmetic surgery unless for repair of an injury or surgery incurred while covered or result of mastectomy;
11. Dental care of teeth, gums or alveolar process (TMJ) except: a) reduction of fractures of the jaw or facial bones; b) surgical correction of harelip, cleft palate or prognathism; c) removal of salivary duct stones; d) removal of bony cysts of jaw, torus palatinus, leukoplakia or malignant tissues;
12. Reversal of voluntary sterilization;
13. Diagnosis or treatment of infertility including artificial insemination, in vitro fertilization, etc.;
14. Contraceptive materials or devices;
15. Pregnancy; pregnancy-related expenses of dependent children for the delivery including Caesarian section. Related illnesses may be covered such as pre-eclampsia, vaginal bleeding, etc.;
16. Non-therapeutic abortions except where the life of the mother is endangered.

WINTER INSURANCE CO, 9763 WESTERN WAY, WHITTIER, CO 82963, (970) 555-2963
COMPANY: WHITE CORPORATION, POLICY **NAME: WHITE**, EFFECTIVE **DATE: 06/01/90**

ELIGIBILITY

EMPLOYEE: Must work a minimum of 35 hours per week. Is eligible for coverage the first of the month following 60 consecutive days of continuous employment.
DEPENDENTS: Are eligible for coverage from birth to age 19, or to age 24 if a full-time student or handicapped prior to age 19/24 (proof of disability must be furnished within 31 days after dependent reaches limiting age). Dependent is not eligible as a dependent if eligible as an employee. Unmarried natural children, legally adopted and foster children are included (also includes legal guardianship). If both parents are covered by the plan, children may be covered by one employee only.

EFFECTIVE DATE

EMPLOYEE: If written application is made prior to the eligibility date, coverage becomes effective the first of the month following 60 days of employment.
DEPENDENTS: The date acquired by the covered employee becomes the effective date if written application is made within 31 days of the eligibility date. Newborns are automatically covered for the first seven days following birth. Coverage will terminate after seven days unless written application for coverage is submitted by the employee within 31 days of birth.

TERMINATION OF COVERAGE

EMPLOYEE: Coverage terminates the last day of the month following termination of employment or when the employee ceases to qualify as an eligible employee, or following request for termination of coverage.
DEPENDENTS: Coverage terminates the date the employee's coverage terminates, or the last day of the month during which the dependent no longer qualifies as an eligible dependent.

EXTENSION OF BENEFITS - If covered under the plan when disabled, employee may continue coverage for 12 months following the date of termination or until no longer disabled, whichever is less.

COMPREHENSIVE MEDICAL BENEFITS

SUPPLEMENTAL ACCIDENT EXPENSE - 100% of first $300 for services incurred within 120 days of date of accident. Not subject to deductible.

PLAN BENEFITS
INDIVIDUAL CALENDAR YEAR DEDUCTIBLE: $100; three month carry-over provision.
FAMILY MAXIMUM DEDUCTIBLE: $200, aggregate.
STANDARD COINSURANCE: 90% except 100% of hospital room and board expenses for 365 days per lifetime.
COINSURANCE LIMIT: $750 out-of-pocket per individual; $1,500 out-of-pocket per family. Two separate members must satisfy the individual limit, not to include deductible, mental or nervous expenses. Applies only in the calendar year in which the limit is met.
LIFETIME MAXIMUM: $300,000 per person.
PRE-EXISTING LIMITATION: On 6/1/90 no restriction. After 6/1/90, if treatment received within 90 days prior to effective date, no coverage for that condition for 12 months from the effective date (continuously covered for 12 months) unless treatment free for three consecutive months ending after the effective date of coverage.

X-RAY AND LABORATORY
REMARKS: Professional component charges covered at 40% of UCR allowance for procedure. Routine procedures are not covered.

INPATIENT HOSPITAL EXPENSE
Room and board payable at 100% of semi-private room rate. Miscellaneous expenses covered at 90%. Non-medically necessary, well baby care and cosmetic services excluded. Personal comfort items not covered.

MENTAL/NERVOUS/PSYCHONEUROTIC
INCLUDES SUBSTANCE ABUSE AND ALCOHOLISM. Exclusions: psychological testing.

OUTPATIENT MENTAL AND NERVOUS TREATMENT
COINSURANCE: 50% while not hospital confined.
CALENDAR YEAR MAXIMUM: None.

INPATIENT MENTAL AND NERVOUS TREATMENT
PHYSICIAN SERVICES: Covered at 90%.
HOSPITAL SERVICES: Covered at 90%.
ALLOWED PROVIDERS: Psychiatrists and clinical psychologists. Marriage and Family Child Counselor and Licensed Clinical Social Worker allowed with referral from M.D.

EXTENDED CARE FACILITY
LIFETIME MAXIMUM: 60 days.
HOSPITAL SERVICES: 80% of billed room and board charge.
REQUIREMENTS: Stay must begin within 14 days of acute hospital stay of at least 3 days. Extended care must be due to same disability that caused hospitalization and continued hospital care would otherwise be required.

DURABLE MEDICAL EQUIPMENT
COINSURANCE: Covered at 90%.
REQUIREMENTS: Must be prescribed by M.D. Must not be primarily necessary for exercise, environmental control, convenience, comfort or hygiene. Must only be use for the prescribed patient. Covered up to purchase price only.

REMARKS
Covered expenses include charges for the initial set of contact lenses which are necessary due to cataract surgery. Handicapped children are limited to a $15,000 lifetime maximum after attainment of age 19. Coordination of Benefits according to National Association of Insurance Carriers (NAIC) guidelines. Subject to Third Party Liability and subrogation.

MEDICARE INTEGRATION
TYPE: Non-duplication of benefits applies.
REMARKS: Assume all Medicare benefits whether or not individual actually enrolled.

EXCLUSIONS
1. Expenses resulting from self-inflicted injuries, work related injuries or illnesses;
2. Charges or services: in excess of UCR, not medically necessary, for completion of claim forms, for failure to keep appointments; for routine, preventative or experimental services;
3. Eye refractions; contacts or glasses; orthotics (eye exercises); radial keratotomy, laser surgery or other procedures for surgical correction of refractive errors;
4. Custodial care and/or convalescent facility coverage;
5. Cosmetic surgery unless for repair of an injury or surgery incurred while covered or result of mastectomy;
6. Diagnosis or treatment of infertility including artificial insemination, in vitro fertilization, etc., contraceptive materials or devices, non-therapeutic abortions except where the life of the mother is endangered, reversal of voluntary sterilization;
7. Pregnancy-related expenses for dependent children.
8. Expenses for obesity, weight reduction, or diet control unless at least 100 lbs. overweight;
9. Vitamins, food supplements and/or protein supplements;
10. Sex altering treatments or surgeries or related studies;
11. Orthopedic shoes or other devices for support or treatment of feet except as medically necessary following foot surgery;
12. Bio-feedback related services or treatment, EDTA chelation therapy.

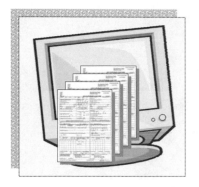

7

Medicare

After completion of this chapter you will be able to:

- Explain the impact of TEFRA and DEFRA on health insurance plans.
- State the eligibility requirements for Medicare.
- Describe the two types of Medicare coverage and the benefits for each.
- List the types of nonparticipating facilities that Medicare will not cover.
- List the types of service that require a UPIN in box 17A of the CMS-1500.
- List the differences on a CMS-1500 between billing for Medicare and billing other insurance carriers.
- State the exceptions when a patient may submit a bill themselves.
- List the guidelines for billing Medicare.
- State the guidelines for collecting the patient portion of a Medicare claim.
- Describe what "Acceptance of Assignment" is and how it affects billing.
- List the claims that require acceptance of assignment.
- Describe how to post Medicare payments.
- Describe "assignment of benefits" and how it can affect the amount collected on a Medicare claim.
- Properly "balance bill" a Medicare claim using a given scenario.

- State the most common reasons for a "not medically necessary" denial and describe how this affects the amount collected from the patient.
- Describe how to submit claims when Medicare is coordinated with other insurance.
- Show how a DRG benefit is calculated with a given scenario.
- Properly complete a Medicare advance notice and describe when it would be used.
- Describe the six levels in the Medicare appeals process.
- Describe the different levels of sanctions and penalties Medicare may impose.
- Describe what a Medicare Risk HMO is and how it works.
- State the requirements for a retiree to enroll in a Medicare Risk HMO.
- Describe the two types of Medicare HMOs.
- Describe the purpose of the Medicare Notice of Non-coverage.
- Properly complete a Medicare timeliness report.

Key words and concepts you will learn in this chapter:

Deficit Reduction Act of 1984 (DEFRA) – An act that amended TEFRA so that spouses age 65 years and older, of active employees who are under age

65 can elect their primary coverage, either Medicare or the private group plan.

Downcoding – When an insurance carrier changes a code to a similar code that has a lower level of service.

End-stage Renal Disease (ESRD) – A condition that occurs when a person's kidneys fail to function.

Explanation of Medicare Benefits (EOMB) – A document that lists all the claims which were paid for the specified time period.

Medicare – The Federal Health Insurance Benefit Plan for the Aged and Disabled.

Medi-Medi – A patient who is eligible for both Medicare and Medicaid.

Part A – Medicare's basic plan or hospital insurance.

Part B – Medicare's medical (supplementary, voluntary) insurance that covers physician services, outpatient hospital services, home health care, outpatient speech and physical therapy, and durable medical equipment.

Tax Equity and Fiscal Responsibility Act of 1982 (TEFRA) – An act which redirected the financial responsibility for medical coverage of active employees age 65 years and older and their spouses age 65 years and older.

Unique Physician Identification Number (UPIN) – A number for identifying the physician ordering or referring services.

Medicare is the Federal Health Insurance Benefit Plan for the Aged and Disabled, Title XVIII of Public Law 89-97 of the Social Security Act. This program is for persons 65 years of age or older and certain persons who are totally disabled.

Social Security Administration offices throughout the United States take applications for Medicare, determine eligibility, and provide general information about the program. The actual processing of the claims is administered by many different insurance companies, usually one or two within each state. Consequently, there may be diversity in the application or denial of benefits and in the Explanation of Medicare Benefit (EOMB) forms.

TEFRA/DEFRA

When the TEFRA/DEFRA federal program was first introduced, it was determined that Medicare would be the primary payor for individuals as of their 65th birthday, regardless of employment status. The **Tax Equity and Fiscal Responsibility Act of 1982 (TEFRA)** (and amendments to it) has redirected the financial responsibility for medical coverage of active employees age 65 years and older and their spouses age 65 years and older.

Initially, TEFRA regulations did not apply to spouses over age 65 of active employees who were under age 65. The **Deficit Reduction Act of 1984 (DEFRA)**, effective January 1, 1985, amended TEFRA so that now spouses, age 65 years and older, of active employees who are under the age of 65 can elect their primary coverage, either Medicare or the private group plan. These regulations apply only to those employees who become eligible for coverage after their 65th birthday, not those who are covered and then reach age 65 (i.e., ESRD).

The employers affected by these Acts are those who regularly employ 20 or more employees for each working day in at least 20 weeks of the current or preceding calendar year. Employees of such employers must be offered coverage under the group plan on the same basis as other employees. An election form choosing the primary plan must be completed and signed by each employee who is or becomes affected.

If coverage is chosen under the employer's group plan, the group plan will be the primary payor on all medical services. Medicare will provide the secondary coverage. If coverage under the group plan is rejected and thus Medicare is chosen, the employee or spouse, by law, can be covered only by Medicare. The group plan will not pay secondary.

Obviously, employers with fewer than 20 employees are exempt from the TEFRA/DEFRA regulations and Medicare is the primary carrier for their active employees and spouses 65 years of age or older. Medicare is also primary on all retired employees and on active employees and their spouses under age 65 who are totally disabled with conditions other than end-stage renal disease. (see Medicare Eligibility section.)

After it has been determined that the group plan is subject to TEFRA/DEFRA, it becomes necessary to determine the person's eligibility for Medicare.

Medicare Eligibility

Following are some of the guidelines governing Medicare eligibility.

Based on Age

An individual is eligible for Medicare coverage on the first day of the month in which she reaches age 65. Persons born on the first day of the month are eligible on the first day of the month preceding their birth date.

Example:
Birthday: June 25, eligible for Medicare June 1
Birthday: June 1, eligible for Medicare May 1

Based on Disability

Medicare coverage for totally disabled persons begins on the first day of the 25th month from the date approved for Social Security Disability or Railroad Retirement benefits. Those covered include disabled workers of any age, disabled widows between the ages of 50 and 65, disabled beneficiaries age 18 and over who receive Social Security benefits because of disability prior to age 22, the blind, and Railroad Retirement annuitants.

Based on ESRD

End-stage renal disease (ESRD) occurs when a person's kidneys fail to function. As a result, the patient must begin dialysis treatments. Because of the multiple problems associated with this disease, patients are considered to be totally disabled, even though some individuals with this disease continue to work. As a result, the following special rules apply to ESRD patients.

The employer's group health plan is the primary payor for the first 18 months after a patient (under age 65) with ESRD becomes eligible for Medicare. This 18-month period begins based on the earlier of (1) the month in which a regular course of renal dialysis is initiated, or (2) the month the patient is hospitalized for a kidney transplant.

Medicare is the secondary payor during this 18-month period but will revert to the primary status beginning with the 19th month. As a general rule, all services under a dialysis program are Medicare-assigned (defined later in this section).

Providers of Service

Providers of services and medical equipment suppliers under Medicare must meet all licensing requirements of the state in which they are located. To be a participating provider under the Medicare program, providers must meet additional Medicare requirements before payments can be made for their services. Medicare will not pay for the following types of care received in nonparticipating facilities:

- Hospital care,
- Skilled nursing facility,
- Home health agency,
- Hospice,
- Outpatient rehabilitation,
- Dialysis facilities,
- Ambulatory surgical centers,
- Independent physical therapists,
- Independent occupational therapists,
- Clinical laboratories,
- Portable x-ray suppliers, and
- Rural health clinics.

The Two Parts of Medicare

There are two parts to the Medicare program: Parts A and B. The services covered under the two parts of Medicare are as follows:

1. **Part A** is considered the basic plan or hospital insurance. This part covers facility charges for acute inpatient hospital care, skilled nursing, home health care, and hospice care.
2. **Part B** is the medical (supplementary, voluntary) insurance that covers physician services, outpatient hospital services, home health care, outpatient speech and physical therapy, and durable medical equipment.

Part A

The two parts have different eligibility requirements. Part A is automatic upon enrollment for the following individuals:

- All persons age 65 and over, if entitled to (a) monthly Social Security benefits, or (b) pensions under the Railroad Retirement Act,
- All persons who reached age 65 prior to 1968, whether or not under the Social Security or Railroad Retirement Programs, and
- Workers who reach 65 in 1975 or after, need 20 quarters of Social Security work

credits if female, or 24 quarters of Social Security work credits if male, to be fully insured.

Effective July 1, 1973, all persons age 65 years and over who are not otherwise eligible for Part A may enroll by paying the full cost of such coverage, provided they also enroll in Part B.

Those who are members of subversive organizations and aliens who have not been permanent United States residents for five years may be excluded from coverage in the Medicare program.

Benefits
Part A is the hospital insurance portion of Medicare. There is a deductible amount that is taken from the first inpatient hospital admission. If the patient is out of the hospital for at least 60 consecutive days (including the day of discharge), a new benefit period begins and another inpatient deductible would be taken if the patient is readmitted. (This is known as the period of renewal.) For 2005, the Part A deductible is $912.00.

If a member remains in the hospital for an extended period of time, additional copayments are required. Medicare deducts the copay amount from the billed amount and then pays the amount in excess of the copay.

The 2005 inpatient hospital copayments are as follows:
- 1st day--60th day = Deductible only, no additional copayment,
- 61st day--90th day = $228/day, and
- 91st day--150th day = $465. These days are known as the 60-day Lifetime Reserve. These copayments are not renewable. Once used, they are gone.

For skilled nursing facilities (SNF), there is a separate copayment schedule and requirement. To be eligible for this benefit, a doctor must certify the necessity of skilled nursing and rehabilitative care on a daily basis. Custodial care is not covered nor is occasional rehabilitative care. In addition, the Medicare intermediary approves the stay.

The 2005 SNF copayments are as follows:
- 1st day--20th day = No copayment. Since admission is usually from an acute care facility, during which time the deductible

was met, 100% of the allowable is generally paid by Medicare, and
- 21st day--100th day = $114 coinsurance/copay per day.

Multiple admissions can occur during a calendar year. However, the maximum number of allowable days is 100 per benefit period.

These deductibles and copayments are adjusted upward each calendar year, based on inflation.

Psychiatric inpatient hospital care is covered the same as regular hospital inpatient care. However, the facility must be a participating Medicare provider in order to be covered.

Foreign facilities are generally not covered. However, some qualified Canadian or Mexican hospitals may be covered during emergency situations. All such bills should be submitted to Medicare for consideration.

Part-time home health care may be covered under the following four circumstances:
1. The care needed includes intermittent skilled nursing care, physical therapy or speech therapy.
2. The patient is confined to the home.
3. A doctor prescribes the care and sets up a home health plan.
4. The home health agency is a participating provider.

Medicare will not cover the following services:
- Full-time nursing care in the home,
- Drugs and biologicals,
- Meals delivered to the home,
- Homemaker services, and
- Blood transfusions.

Hospice care may be covered under the following three circumstances:
1. A doctor certifies that the patient is terminal.
2. The patient chooses to receive care from a hospice instead of receiving standard Medicare benefits (inpatient).
3. Care is provided by a Medicare certified hospice program.

Special benefit periods and payments apply to this benefit. If additional clarification is required, refer to a Medicare handbook.

Part A does not cover the following services:
- The replacement fees for the first three pints of blood,

- Personal convenience items,
- Private duty nurses (while inpatient), and
- Private room difference, unless it is determined to be medically necessary.

Part B

Part B is the supplementary medical insurance, which covers physician and outpatient hospital services. It is considered a supplemental plan because each participant must pay a stipulated amount each month for the benefits. The monthly premium is adjusted each year based on inflation.

The rules, limits, and maximums under this coverage are subject to change every year. In addition, certain types of services are covered under some circumstances but not under others. Therefore, it is less confusing to have a general idea of the most common benefits without becoming overly concerned with the details. Normally, claims examiners will not be concerned with Medicare unless it is the primary payor. In such circumstances, you will need the EOMB to process the claim. The following briefly summarizes some of the more common benefits. For more particulars, refer to a Medicare booklet or carrier.

Benefits

The 2005 yearly deductible is $110, which has a 3-month carry-over provision. After the deductible has been satisfied, generally 80% of the approved charge will be paid.

Beginning January 1, 2006, the Medicare Part B deductible will be indexed to the increase in the average cost of Part B services for Medicare beneficiaries. In other words, the amount charged for the Part B deductible will depend on the amount spent by Medicare for payments for services.

The following services are covered by Part B:

- Manual manipulation of the spine for subluxation demonstrated by x-rays,
- Non-routine podiatric care,
- Dental care for surgery of the jaw-related structures and fractures of facial bones,
- Some non-routine optometry services,
- Outpatient hospital services,
- Outpatient physical/speech therapy-- maximums apply,
- Independent clinical laboratory/x-ray services,
- Ambulance transportation,

- Some durable medical and prosthetic equipment,
- Outpatient treatment of mental illness, and
- Home health care.

The following physician services are not covered by Part B:

- Routine physical examinations and related DXL (diagnostic x-ray and laboratory),
- Routine foot care,
- Eye or hearing examinations for eyeglasses or hearing aids,
- Immunizations (exceptions some pneumo-coccal and hepatitis B), and
- Cosmetic surgery (some exceptions).

Approved or Reasonable Charges

Medicare payments are based on what the law defines as "reasonable charges," which are the amounts approved by the Medicare carrier based on what is considered reasonable for the geographic area in which the doctor practices. Because of the way the approved amounts are determined and because of high rates of inflation in medical care prices, the approved amounts are often significantly less than the actual charges billed by providers. The charge approved by the carrier will be the lowest of either the charge billed by the provider or the prevailing charge (based on all the customary charges in the locality for each type of service) as determined by Medicare. Participating providers must write off the amounts in excess of the approved amount.

Billing Medicare Services

When billing for a patient who is a Medicare recipient, always request the patient's health insurance card. This card indicates whether the patient has both Part A (hospital) and Part B (medical) and when each became effective. A copy of this card should be made for your files.

The card also has a letter code indicating the recipient's status. The letter codes are as follows:

A--Wage earner
B--Husband's number
C--Disabled child
D--Widow

HDA--Disabled adult

J, K1, or J1--Special monthly benefits, never worked under Social Security

T--Uninsured and entitled only to health insurance benefits

Railroad retirees are indicated by the following letters preceding the patient's Social Security number:

MA	without any additional digits
A	with six additional digits
WA	with six additional digits
A	with nine additional digits
WA	with nine additional digits

The CMS-1500 should be used to bill for Medicare recipients' services. Instructions on completing the CMS-1500 are covered in a later chapter.

Unique Physician Identification Number

Medicare has established a **Unique Physician Identification Number (UPIN)** for identifying the physician ordering or referring services. This is a national number used to identify the physician. The following list of services requires the UPIN in box 17a of the CMS-1500 and the name of the ordering or referring physician in box 17 of the CMS-1500:

- Laboratory,
- Consultation,
- Diagnostic tests,
- Renal,
- Ambulance,
- Ultrasound,
- Radiology,
- Durable medical equipment,
- Parenteral nutrition,
- Magnetic resonance imaging,
- Computerized axial tomography (CT/CAT) scan,
- Prosthetics and orthotics,
- Physical therapy, and
- Chiropractic services.

If a physician is self-referring, his or her own individual UPIN should be entered on the claim.

Billing Guidelines

When billing Medicare, the provider must complete the appropriate billing forms. Most Medicare charges are billed on the CMS-1500 form. Items are completed the same as for any other type of claim except:

- Item 1a should contain the Medicare number, complete with any prefixes and suffixes,
- Items 4 and 7 should list the primary insurance policyholder's name and address,
- Item 9 - 9d should list the Medigap or supplemental policy information,
- Item 11 - 11d should list the primary insurance carrier, and
- Item 13 must be signed by the patient if the Medigap payment is to go to the provider.

Federal law demands that providers submit claims for Medicare patients, and providers who accept assignment are not allowed to charge for the service of billing Medicare. The patient may not submit the claim for payment themselves, except in the following situations:

1. If the patient has other insurance which should pay as primary, the patient may submit the claim and attach a copy of the other carrier's EOB.
2. If the services are not covered by Medicare, but the patient wishes a formal coverage determination for their records.
3. If the provider refuses to submit the claim (which is a violation of law and the provider may be penalized for such actions).
4. If services are provided outside the United States.
5. When the patient has purchased durable medical equipment from a private source.

The following suggestions will help with properly completing the billing forms, and complying with Medicare guidelines:

1. It is important that the proper ICD-9-CM code be used to denote the diagnosis. All diagnoses must be coded to the highest digit possible. If a five-digit code exists, it should be used rather than a four-digit code. Additionally, an appropriate ICD-9 code should be listed for each diagnosis and indicated in item 24E of the CMS-1500.
2. Keep for reference a fee schedule, list of unbundled services, list of denied services, list of procedures with limits on the number of services, and a list of those procedures which require pre-authorization from the carrier. Having these items

readily available will assist the physician in making informed decisions regarding the care and treatment of the patient while still receiving the maximum possible reimbursement for services rendered.

3. If modifiers are used, be sure to include any necessary documentation which substantiates the services rendered.

4. If you have a claim that has numerous procedures or confusing information, send a cover letter which clarifies the services performed and the documentation for the necessity of services.

5. Document everything. If you have received information over the phone, document the full name, title and department of the person who gave you the information, as well as the date and time of the contact. Sending a follow up letter which thanks them for their help, puts in writing your understanding of the important points of the conversation, and is also a wise practice. At the bottom of the letter include a note as follows: "If I misunderstood the information, please contact me at the above number or address to clarify." This letter provides proof of the contact should you need it in an audit. If a contact is received stating that you misunderstood the information be sure to document it, then notate it on the original letter.

6. Read your Medicare bulletins. They provide the best source of information for changing rules and regulations.

7. Providers may collect any deductible and coinsurance from the patient at the time of service. However, it may be best to wait until after receiving the Medicare EOB. This prevents the medical office from having to return any amounts that were for services which Medicare deemed were not medically necessary, and allows a more accurate calculation of the amount the patient owes.

8. Medicare rules state that the carrier must pay claims within thirty days for those claims without questions or in need of additional investigation. Claims for non-participating physicians are not processed as quickly as those for participating physicians. Also, claims submitted electronically are processed faster than those submitted on paper and often contain fewer errors since reentry of the data is not required.

9. Be courteous and kind when dealing with Medicare representatives.

10. If a record is missing or destroyed, a report should be made as soon as the problem is discovered. This note should include the items that are missing or destroyed, how the destruction occurred or when the items were discovered missing, who discovered the destruction or omission, the date and time of the report, and the name and title of the person writing the report. This should be placed in the patient's file. If an audit is conducted, such a report can help prove that files were not maliciously destroyed or lost to prevent the carrier from discovering abuses.

11. If the amounts listed on the EOMB do not match your data regarding allowed amounts or benefits, contact the carrier for clarification.

12. If you receive a check from Medicare which contains an overpayment, first check the records to be sure the payment is incorrect. If an overpayment has occurred, deposit the check and write to Medicare regarding the overpayment. Include in your letter copies of the EOMB, the check and the claim, along with an explanation of the amount that is overpaid and why you feel this to be an overpayment. If an overpayment has occurred, Medicare will deduct the overpayment from the provider's next check.

The **Explanation of Medicare Benefits (EOMB)** is a document that lists all the claims which were paid for the specified time period. The EOMB will list the patient's name, the date services were rendered, the services that were rendered, the billed amount, and the Medicare approved amount. It also shows the part of the approved amount that was applied toward the patient's deductible, the patient's coinsurance amount, and the amount Medicare is paying.

By adding together the billed amount and the patient's coinsurance, assigned providers can determine the proper amount to "balance bill" the patient.

Collecting Amounts Due From the Patient

You must bill the patient for any amounts which Medicare lists as the patient's responsibility and honestly attempt to collect these amounts. This means billing the patient at least three times before writing off any portion of the patients' amount. Additionally, you must use the same collection attempts for Medicare patients as you do for non-Medicare patients.

If the patient's portion of the bill is written off, there should be documentation as to why. Hardship conditions should be fully documented, as are bankruptcies or other conditions. The patient should be asked to sign a statement verifying this information.

Two cases may be allowed for non-collection attempts: hardship of the patient, and amounts which are too minimal to be cost-effective for established collection procedures. Hardship will usually only be accepted if the medical office can show that patients' portions were waived in only a limited number of cases. In cases of cost-effectiveness, the provider should have a cost analysis done which determines all the costs involved in collecting on an account. Amounts below this amount can be considered not cost effective to collect. The cost analysis should be updated periodically and kept on record.

Failure to balance bill can result in fines and penalties, exclusion from the Medicare program, and possible criminal charges.

Claims Which Require Acceptance of Assignment

Providers may usually accept assignment or not. However, there are some services which require acceptance of assignment. These include:

- Clinical diagnostic laboratory services,
- Medicare patients who are also eligible for Medicaid,
- Ambulatory surgery centers,
- Method II home dialysis supplies and equipment, and
- Physician's assistant, nurse midwives, nurse specialists, non-physician anesthetists, clinical psychologists and clinical social workers services.

Being a non-participating physician can net a return of up to 9.25% higher than for participating physicians. This percentage lowers depending on the number of claims assignment is accepted on. Providers must weigh this against the ability of patient to cover the increased portion, and the ill will of patients who discover that their bill would be lower if the provider was participating (some carriers place a statement on each EOMB stating how much the patient would have saved had they gone to a participating provider).

Billing Deceased Patients

Since Medicare pays for health care for the aged, some patients will die. Since the patient is unable to sign the claim form, place the words "Patient died on (date)" in the signature box.

There are two ways of handling unpaid bills for such patients. If assignment is accepted, Medicare will process the form without the necessary signature. If assignment is not accepted, Medicare may wait until the patient's estate is settled before making payment.

If the family of the deceased pays the bill, they should complete form CMS-1660 showing that they have paid, and attach the receipt. Medicare will then send payment to the person who paid the bill.

Posting Medicare Payments

Payments received from Medicare may be lower than the physician's billed charge. If the provider accepts Medicare's assignment, it is important that the medical biller knows how to post payments to the patient's ledger and make adjustments.

Upon receipt of the EOMB, the patient(s) chart(s) indicated on the EOMB should be pulled. Post each payment individually to each patient ledger card and to the daily journal. Separate entries should be made for each patient on the daily journal (not in a lump sum).

If the Medicare allowed amount is less than the billed charge, an adjustment or write-off will need to be made on the ledger card. After the payment has been posted, the next entry on the ledger card should be the adjustment to the charges. Enter the difference between the billed amount and the Medicare approved amount. This amount will be entered on the ledger card in the adjustment column and will be subtracted from the remaining balance. This entry will ensure that Medicare recipients are not being billed for charges that exceed the Medicare approved amount.

Part B Claims Time Limit

Medicare has established time limits for filing claims covered under Medicare Part B. These time limits are established according to the date of service.

For services rendered between October 1 and September 30, claims must be submitted by December 31 of the following year. However, if documentation is submitted that shows that the delay was due to an administrative error on the part of the Social Security Administration or the Medicare carrier, the time limit may be waived. Even if the claim is filed within the filing deadline, a 10% reduction in payment may be assessed on claims received more than 12 months after the date of service.

Medi-Medi
When a patient is eligible for both Medicare and Medicaid, that patient is considered to be a Medi-Medi patient. If a patient is eligible for benefits to be paid under Medicaid, Medicare will automatically forward the claim to the appropriate department for coordination of benefits. Through the use of computer files, Medicare cross-references all claims to check for Medicaid eligibility. Medicaid will always be the secondary payor to Medicare.

Assignment of Benefits

The Medicare Assignment of Benefits has nothing to do with the provider to whom the claims examiner will make payment. To be a participating provider, the provider must agree to accept assignment on all Medicare claims. By doing this, the provider receives payment directly from Medicare, rather than the payment going to the member. In addition, the provider has agreed to accept the amount approved by the Medicare carrier for the covered services. The patient is not responsible for any amount in excess of the approved amount. In such a case, the secondary carrier is also not responsible for the amount in excess of the approved amount.

Physicians Who Accept Assignment
When a physician agrees to accept Medicare assignment for a bill, Medicare will pay the physician directly for that bill. The physician may bill the patient only for any deductibles or coinsurance that Medicare has deducted from the assigned bill. As a result, the total fee that physicians may receive from Medicare and from beneficiaries for an assigned bill is limited to what Medicare deems to be an appropriate fee for the particular service or procedure (the Medicare "allowance").

To encourage physicians to accept assignment, the Medicare allowance is higher for physicians who agree to accept assignment for all bills for Medicare-eligible persons. These physicians are called "participating physicians." Thus, participating physicians agree not to practice "balance billing," or charging patients for more than the Medicare allowed amount.

The phrase "participating physician" can be confusing since physicians who sign these agreements are not the only ones who treat Medicare patients. Physicians who treat Medicare-eligible individuals but who decide whether to accept assignment on a case-by-case basis are called "nonparticipating physicians." In exchange for the freedom to make this choice for each patient, these nonparticipating physicians receive only 95% of the reimbursement that participating physicians receive from Medicare. For example, if the Medicare allowance for a procedure is $100 for participating physicians, the allowance for nonparticipating physicians would be $95.

Therefore, assuming that the patient's deductible had been paid, a participating physician would receive $80 from Medicare (80% of $100) and a nonparticipating physician would receive $76 from Medicare (80% of $95). While the participating physician cannot charge the Medicare patient more than the $20 copayment, the nonparticipating physician has no such restriction. However, if the nonparticipating physician agrees to accept assignment for that bill, he can only bill the patient for $19 ($95--$76).

Elective Surgery Over $500
Specific requirements must be followed for non-participating providers who perform elective surgeries over $500. For surgeries that are elective (surgery that is scheduled in advance and is not an emergency, and where delay would not result in impairment or death), are not assigned, and for which a charge greater than $500 is expected, the provider must notify the patient of certain information in writing. This information includes the:

- Name and description of the procedure,
- Fact that the surgery is elective,
- Expected charge for the surgery,

- Approximate Medicare allowable,
- Amount by which the physician's charge exceeds the allowable, and
- Amount the patient is responsible for.

Failure to provide this information could result in penalties being assessed. Medicare carriers may contact providers and request a signed copy of the notification.

Restrictions on Balance Billing

Balance billing by nonparticipating physicians is strictly limited. Participating physicians are not affected since they are not allowed to balance bill Medicare patients for any services.

Balance billing is restricted to no more than 15% above what Medicare allows. Following are two examples of how this rule affects the payment of claims.

Example 1. Provider accepts assignment.

Billed Charge	Approved Amt	Medicare Pays	Member Pays
$42	$35	$35 to ded = 0 pd	$35
$90	$75	$20 to ded, $55 @80% = $44 pd	$20 + 20% of $55($11)= $31
$480	$400	$400 @80% = $320	20% of $400= $80

Example 2. Provider does not accept assignment.

Charge	Approved Amt	Medicare Pays	Member Pays
$42	$33.25	$33.25 to ded = 0	$38.24*
$90	$71.25	$20 to ded, $51.25 @ 80% = $41 pd	$20 + 20.94 = 40.94*
$480	$380	$380 @ 80% = $304.00	$133.00*

*115% of Medicare approved amount minus what Medicare paid.

Some providers routinely write off any amounts not covered by Medicare. This practice is prohibited by law, since it means that Medicare covers 100% of the bill. Thus, there is no monetary incentive to the patient not to overuse services.

Medical Necessity Denials

The most common reason for denial of claims by Medicare is for services that are considered not medically necessary. In Medicare claim processing, this phrase has a wide variety of meanings. The three most common situations that are given a "not medically necessary" denial are:

1. The diagnosis does not match the service. If no clear connection can be made between the diagnosis and the related services, additional information should be provided to justify the medical necessity of services.
2. Frequency of services is greater than allowed. Medicare has specific limits for the number of times a specific service can be performed. For example, a patient age 65 and over is allowed one mammography screening every two years. If the second mammogram is done prior to the two year limit, it will be denied as not medically necessary.
3. Level of service does not match diagnosis. This denial is most often used with office visit codes. For example, if the diagnosis for a patient is a simple fracture of the arm, a Level V office visit would be denied. Some Medicare agencies will down code the level to the appropriate Level II code, but others will simply deny the visit as not medically necessary. **Downcoding** is when an insurance carrier changes a code to a similar code that has a lower level of service.

Additionally, claims with incidental services may list that certain procedures are not medically necessary. In such cases, Medicare is not stating that the service is not medically necessary, but that the second procedure is incidental to or an integral part of the first procedure. For example, a laparoscopy is an integral part of removal of a lesion. The removal procedure would be allowed and paid, however the laparoscopy procedure would be denied. Therefore, the second procedure would be denied as not medically necessary. In essence this is a form of downcoding, but the use of the "not medically necessary" denial can lead to confusion and concerns among your patients. It is important to check the CPT® and HCPCS codes carefully in order to be sure that a single code does not cover both procedures.

If a claim is denied as not medically necessary, any amounts paid by the patient must be refunded within 30 days of the notification of denial. If you wish to appeal the denial, send in the claim and any related documentation to the Medicare carrier and request a formal review. Be sure to detail exactly which services you are appealing (instead of asking the carrier to review the entire claim), and include documentation to support the medical necessity of services. The information will be reviewed to make a new determination regarding medical necessity.

If the claim is denied, you may request that the Medicare carrier provide you with all the information they used to make the denial determination. The request must be made in writing and should list the patient's name, the date of services, the services which were denied, and the reasons Medicare indicated on the forms for the denial. You should also state that you are requesting the information under the Freedom of Information Act. Any information sent by the carrier should be studied and retained for further information.

Coordinating Medicare With Other Insurance

Medicare pays secondary to employer sponsored group insurance, individual policies carried by the employee, workers' compensation insurance, automobile and/or no-fault insurance and third party liability. Medicare pays primary to Medicare supplemental plans (Medigap insurance), Medicaid, and after 18 months of End Stage Renal Disease.

The patient should be questioned during their first visit to determine all insurance coverage(s) which could affect payment of a claim.

Certain diagnoses have been identified as being workers' compensation related. If the patient is diagnosed with one of these conditions, the Medicare carrier will probably request additional information, or deny the claim as covered by workers' compensation. This list can be obtained from the Department of Labor.

When submitting a claim for secondary payments to Medicare, a copy of the claim as originally submitted to the primary carrier should be submitted. The primary insurance EOB should be attached, along with any necessary evidence to support services. No changes should be made on the claim, including altering the "amount paid" and "amount now due" boxes to reflect the payment made by the primary carrier.

If a Medicare patient is covered by primary insurance and receives a payment from the primary insurance which is greater than the Medicare allowed amount, the provider cannot charge the patient for any amounts (including the 20% coinsurance normally collected). The full allowed amount has been collected from the primary insurance carrier. The provider is allowed to keep any amounts paid by the primary insurance which are over the Medicare allowed amount without violating his agreement with Medicare. If the patient's insurance pays less than the amount Medicare determines to be the patient's responsibility (deductible and coinsurance amounts), the provider is allowed to bill the patient for the difference between the amount collected from the primary insurance and the patient's responsibility as determined by Medicare.

If a third party is determined to be liable for expenses (i.e., auto or other accident), that carrier should be billed first. If the carrier denies payment, a copy of the EOB should be filed with the Medicare claim. If the patient later sues and is granted monetary compensation, Medicare will demand a repayment of the benefits they have paid. The patient may be asked to sign a form which states that they will inform Medicare of the court's decision or a settlement. If the patient receives payment without informing Medicare, they are responsible for repaying Medicare.

Estimating Medicare Coverage

Sometimes, a member is entitled to Medicare but has not enrolled. In these circumstances, some plans estimate what Medicare would have paid had the person been enrolled properly. Benefits may then be reduced by the estimated amount.

In this situation, the medical biller should contact the patient and inform him that a balance is due on their bill. The patient must then pay the balance due. The medical biller should suggest that the patient apply for Medicare coverage to prevent the situation from occurring in the future.

Diagnosis-Related Group Billing

Effective October 1, 1983, Medicare instituted **Diagnosis-Related Group (DRG)** payments for inpatient hospital claims.

Under DRG, a flat rate payment is made based on the patient's diagnosis instead of the hospital's itemized billing. If the hospital can treat the patient for less, it keeps the savings. If treatment costs more, the hospital must absorb the loss. Neither Medicare nor the patient is responsible for the excess amount.

Provisions have been made for cases atypically expensive (based on the diagnosis) because of complications or an abnormally long confinement. Known as Outliers, these cases will be reimbursed on an itemized or cost percentage basis instead of DRG. The bill from the hospital must indicate that it is an Outlier.

Excluded from DRG are long-term care, children's care, and psychiatric or rehabilitative hospitals. Also several states have obtained waivers from DRG.

DRG Benefit Payment Calculations

As shown in the following examples, the maximum liability under a plan includes only the expenses that are covered by the plan and that the insured is legally obligated to pay.

Example 1. Itemized hospital bill exceeds Medicare DRG allowance.

Hospital Bill	$8,700
DRG Allowance	$7,000
Medicare Payment	$6,088
(Medicare Payment = DRG allowance - $912 Medicare Part A Deductible)	
Patient's Responsibility	$ 912
Hospital Write-off	$1,700

Although the Medicare DRG allowance is less than the itemized hospital bill, the insured is legally obligated to pay only the $912 Part A deductible.

Example 2. Medicare DRG allowance exceeds itemized billed amount.

Hospital Bill	$ 8,700
DRG Allowance	$10,000
Medicare Payment	$ 9,088
Patient's Responsibility	$ 912

Even though the Medicare payment exceeds the itemized hospital bill, the insured is still legally obligated to pay the $912 Part A deductible.

Medicare Denials

Medicare may deny claims for numerous reasons. If a claim is denied, the reason for the denial will appear under the "Claim Remarks" section of the EOMB. This will often be a code which refers to an in-depth explanation which is included on the last page.

One of the most common denials is due to "incorrect" patient information. In actuality, the information may not be correct, it may just be different from what Medicare's computer has. For example, if a patient is listed on the Medicare records as Sam S. Smith, and you list him as Samuel S. Smith, or Sam Simpson Smith, or Sam Smith, the Medicare computer may reject the claim. To prevent this from happening, copy the patient's data exactly as it appears on the Medicare card. This is the information you should have in your records and in the computer data banks, even if Mr. Smith completes his Patient Information Sheet differently.

Another message commonly found on Medicare claims is the following:

We understand that you may not have known that Medicare would not pay for this service. If you believe this service should have been covered, or if you did not know or could not have been expected to know that Medicare would not pay for this service, or if you notified the beneficiary in writing in advance that Medicare would not pay for this service and he/she agreed to pay, ask us to review your claim.

This indicates that the physician has provided a service which Medicare considers "medically unnecessary." If the physician could not be expected to know that this service would be considered medically unnecessary (i.e., Medicare never informed the physician either on a previous EOMB or through a newsletter or personal letter), then Medicare is obligated to pay the physician if the claim is submitted for review. For this reason, you should submit all denied Medicare claims for review.

Medicare Advance Notice

If a provider performs a procedure which Medicare determines to be not medically reasonable and necessary, the doctor will not be reimbursed by Medicare for that procedure. Additionally, the provider must refund all monies received from the patient for that procedure. An exception to this rule is if the provider informs the patient prior to the procedure that Medicare may not cover it. If the patient signs a waiver agreeing to be financially responsible for the procedure, even if Medicare determines it to be not medically necessary, the patient may be billed for the procedure. However, Medicare rules state that the provider may not ask all patients to sign such a statement for procedures. If Medicare determines that the provider is having a large number of patients sign such documents, they will be considered null and void.

In order to use the document, the provider must have reasonable cause to believe the procedure will be denied as not medically necessary. Reasonable cause can include a procedure that is listed as not covered under Medicare guidelines (i.e., cosmetic surgery), and a procedure which has been previously denied under similar circumstances.

Medicare has set forth strict guidelines as to the content of the consent form. The form in **Figure 7 – 1**, when completed, meets all requirements.

To complete this form, enter the procedures and their charges on lines 1-5 which you feel may be denied. On the following lines, list the number (1-5) which corresponds to each procedure and the reason it would be denied. For example, if the procedure which may be denied is a second nursing home visit within one month, list the visit and its charge on line 1. Then on the line in front of "more than one nursing home visit per month", place the number 1. This allows different procedures to be given their own reason for denial. Be sure the patient reads the bottom portion of the form, and signs and dates it.

The Medicare Appeals Process

There are six levels to the Medicare appeals process:
1. Inquiry
2. Review
3. Hearing
4. Administrative Law Judge
5. Appeals Council Review
6. Federal District Court Hearing

You should go through each level before moving on to the next level. The goal is to improve your reimbursement at the lowest appeal level possible.

Level One – Inquiry
Start by determining if the denial was due to an error or an omission on your part. If so, re-submit the claim with the mistakes corrected. Send the claim to the same address you used for the original submission. You should re-submit only for those services which were denied. Do not re-submit for any services which were already paid or Medicare will reject the entire claim as already considered and processed.

If you need further clarification on why a claim was denied, telephone your Medicare carrier. If there was not an error on your part and/or you are not satisfied with the settlement of the claim, proceed to the second level.

Level Two – Review
You have the right to a review if you are dissatisfied with the settlement of a claim. You must request a review within six months from the date of the original claim determination (EOMB date). This request must be in writing. Simply submit a statement which explains why you are dissatisfied with the reimbursement on the claim.

When submitting a statement, be sure to include:
1. A copy of the original claim, including any reports or attachments,
2. A copy of the EOMB,
3. Any additional information to support your position or to justify the medical necessity of the services, and
4. If you are appealing an unassigned claim, you must have a written authorization from the beneficiary that you are acting on his or her behalf.

End the request with a thank you and have the provider sign it. Some Medicare carriers require submission of a specific form to request a review. If this is the case in your area, obtain a copy of the form and complete and submit it.

ON PROVIDER'S LETTERHEAD

MEDICARE LIMITATION

Date: _____

Dear _____ :

Medicare limits payment to those services which it determines to be "reasonable and necessary" under Medicare Law, section 1862(a). If Medicare determines that a particular service, although it would be otherwise covered, is not reasonable and necessary under Medicare program standards, Medicare will deny payment for that service.

I have reason to believe that Medicare may deny payment for the following procedures:

1. _____
2. _____
3. _____
4. _____
5. _____

For the following reasons: Medicare does not usually pay for:

_____   this many visits or treatments
_____   this service or this many services within this period of time
_____   this injection or this many injections
_____   this procedure because it is treatment that "has yet to be proven effective"
_____   this office visit unless it is considered an emergency
_____   similar services by more than one doctor during the same time period
_____   similar services by two doctors of the same specialty
_____   this equipment
_____   this laboratory test
_____   this visit since it is more than one visit per day
_____   such an extensive procedure
_____   more than one nursing home visit per month

_____   _____
           _____

Should Medicare determine that any of the above listed procedures are not deemed medically necessary for any of the above reasons, you agree that you have been informed before the service(s) was rendered and you agree to be responsible for payment of these services. It is the professional opinion of this provider that these procedures are necessary to render high-quality medical care to you.

Patient's Signature: _____   Date: _____

Guardian's Signature: _____   Date: _____

Patient Name: _____   Medicare #: _____

Figure 7 – 1: Medicare Advance Notice

Medicare should respond within 45 days. If you do not hear from the claims reviewer by this time, call and ask about the status of the review. If the claim was assigned, the provider can be informed of the results of the review. If the claim was unassigned, the patient will be informed.

When requesting a review, do not use previous payments as justification for why a payment should be made. Medicare may decide that all payments were in error and you owe them a refund.

Level Three – The Fair Hearing

If you are not satisfied with the results of the review, you can request a Fair Hearing. To proceed to this level, the amount in controversy must be at least $100 and the hearing must be requested within six months of the review determination. If a single claim is not above $100 you can combine several claims for the same patient together to reach the $100 limit.

The Fair Hearing request form **(see Figure 7 – 2)** is usually sent to a different office from that of the Review, and the people who process these requests are typically more experienced than those at the lower levels. There are three types of hearings:

1. **On the record** – which is based on the written material and data which you have already submitted to Medicare and any additional data you provide.
2. **Telephone Hearing** – which allows you to introduce new information over the telephone and speak directly with the reviewer. You may be required to substantiate your phone information with additional written records. The physician should always be available for the telephone hearing so she may answer any questions regarding treatment.
3. **In person** – where the patient, physician and other parties meet in person. The proceedings are typed or recorded and the tape or transcript is usually available upon request.

A decision should be made within 120 days unless there are extenuating circumstances. You should receive a written explanation of the findings from the hearing. You may receive further reimbursement, or you may again be denied.

Level Four – Administrative Law Judge (ALJ)

This request must be made within 60 days of the Fair Hearing decision and involve at least $500 in controversy. It can take up to 18 months to receive an ALJ assignment. To succeed at this level you must prove that yours is an unusual case and deserves special consideration. Disagreement with Medicare policies will not be addressed at this level.

Your file will be looked at again. It may be immediately reversed (and payment made) or it may be forwarded to a non-Medicare employee. At this point you will be contacted regarding details for proceeding with the ALJ Hearing.

The Medicare carrier will usually not have a representative present at the ALJ Hearing. An authorized representative from the provider's office will need to be present to answer questions. You may submit additional data which shows special complications or situations that made your case unusual.

Level Five – Appeals Council Review

This Council is part of the Office of Hearings and Appeals of the Social Security Administration. You must request an Appeals Council Review within 60 days of the ALJ decision, or the Council may, on its own, review the ALJ decision if there is a question that the ALJ decision was not made in accordance with the law.

Level Six – Federal District Court Hearing

At least $1,000 must be in controversy at this level and an attorney must represent your case. You must appeal within 60 days of the Appeals Council decision. The provider's attorney will handle the case. The provider may want to contact his medical society for attorneys experienced in this level of the appeals process.

Reviews or Hearings After the Deadline

A review or hearing request must be filed within six months. You may file after the six month deadline if you can show "good cause" for not doing so sooner. Attach a letter to the request for Review or Hearing explaining the "good cause." Medicare defines "good cause" as:

- There were circumstances beyond your control or significant communication difficulties,

DEPARTMENT OF HEALTH AND HUMAN SERVICES
CENTERS FOR MEDICARE & MEDICAID SERVICES

REQUEST FOR HEARING
PART B MEDICARE CLAIM
Medical Insurance Benefits - Social Security Act
NOTICE—Anyone who misrepresents or falsifies essential information requested by this form may upon conviction be subject to fine and imprisonment under Federal Law.

CARRIER'S NAME AND ADDRESS	**1** NAME OF PATIENT
	2 HEALTH INSURANCE CLAIM NUMBER

3 I disagree with the review determination on my claim, and request a hearing before a hearing officer of the insurance carrier named above.

MY REASONS ARE: (Attach a copy of the Review Notice. NOTE: If the review decision was made more than 6 months ago, include your reason for not making this request earlier.)

_____

_____

_____

_____

4 CHECK ONE OF THE FOLLOWING

☐ I have additional evidence to submit.
(Attach such evidence to this form or forward it to the carrier within 10 days.)

☐ I do not have additional evidence.

CHECK **ONLY ONE** OF THE STATEMENTS BELOW:

☐ I wish to appear in person before the Hearing Officer.

☐ I do not wish to appear and hereby request a decision on the evidence before the Hearing Officer.

5 EITHER THE CLAIMANT OR REPRESENTATIVE SHOULD SIGN IN THE APPROPRIATE SPACE BELOW

SIGNATURE OR NAME OF CLAIMANT'S REPRESENTATIVE	CLAIMANT'S SIGNATURE	
ADDRESS	ADDRESS	
CITY, STATE, AND ZIP CODE	CITY, STATE, AND ZIP CODE	
TELEPHONE NUMBER	DATE	TELEPHONE NUMBER	DATE

(Claimant should not write below this line)

ACKNOWLEDGMENT OF REQUEST FOR HEARING

Your request for a hearing was received on _____ . You will be notified of the time and place of the hearing at least 10 days before the date of the hearing.

SIGNED	DATE

Form CMS-1965 (05/03)

Figure 7 – 2: Request for Medicare Hearing Form

- The delay resulted from your efforts to obtain documentation, which you did not realize could have been provided after filing for the Review or Hearing, or
- Your records were destroyed or damaged, delaying the filing of the request.

It may be difficult to convince your carrier to provide an extension of time to request a review or hearing. You may need to consider if the benefits are worth the time and effort.

Medicare Fraud and Abuse

It is important to understand the rules and regulations regarding Medicare reimbursement. Penalties are assessed for not complying with these rules. For minor violations, if the provider accepts assignment, the claim may be returned for correction of the problem and may be subject to post-payment review by Medicare. If the provider does not accept Medicare assignment, the provider may be subject to a penalty of $2,000 per claim. Some violations, or repeated violations, can subject the provider to audits, stiff fines, dismissal from the Medicare program, and in some cases criminal penalties and jail sentences.

Many providers and billers have the mistaken notion that they will not be caught for abuse of the Medicare system, or that they must commit "indiscretions" in order to gain the "proper" reimbursement for services. There have even been numerous courses and seminars on how to get around Medicare rules and "maximize reimbursement" from the Medicare carrier. As long as the provider is not committing fraud or abuse of the system, there is nothing wrong with obtaining the maximum amount the provider is entitled to. However, not understanding the rules or flagrantly disobeying them can get the provider and the biller into trouble, or even into jail.

Medicare Fraud

Fraud is the intentional misrepresentation of information which could result in an unauthorized benefit. The regulations are very specific about the activities that are allowed and not allowed under the Medicare rules and regulations. Examples of fraudulent practices include:

- Billing for services or supplies not rendered, including billing patients for not showing up to an appointment (since the patient never showed, no services were actually rendered),
- Altering the diagnosis to justify services,
- Altering claim forms to misrepresent or falsify data,
- Duplicate billing,
- Billing Medicare and an additional insurance both as the primary payor,
- Soliciting, offering or receiving a bribe, kickback, rebate or finder's fee for any services. This includes fees offered for referring a patient to a specific facility for additional tests or services. It also includes automatically writing off that portion of the bill that is the patient's responsibility, since this is considered a kick-back or bribe to the patient to induce them to obtain services from one provider over another,
- Unbundling or exploding charges, or billing for multiple services when one procedure code adequately describes the services provided. Many Medicare carriers provide a list of codes which are often unbundled. The computer is set up to look for these codes and automatically pays only the major procedure, denying the additional procedures,
- Providers who complete certificates of medical necessity or write prescriptions for patients they have not actually seen,
- Altering amounts charged for services, dates of services, identity of patients, or misrepresenting the services provided to obtain reimbursement. This includes up coding of services (i.e., billing for a level IV visit when a level II visit was performed),
- Altering the code or description of non-covered services to identify them as covered services,
- Any collusion between the provider and an additional party (i.e., patient, lawyer, etc.) to misrepresent charges or services to obtain reimbursement,
- Altering claims history or medical records to substantiate services which were up coded or misrepresented,

- Using or allowing the use of an incorrect or additional person's Medicare card to obtain coverage for services,
- Billing inappropriately for "gang visits." For example, heading a group psychotherapy session, but billing for each patient as if they had an individual visit,
- Not disclosing or providing false data regarding physician ownership of a clinical laboratory, medical supplier, or other related entity. Physician's are not allowed to refer patients to a lab or medical supplier which they have a financial interest in,
- Split billing, or billing supplies and services as if they were provided over a series of dates rather than during a single visit,
- Collusion with an employee of the insurance carrier to generate false payments, and
- Repeated violations of Medicare regulations when warning and instruction has been provided.

Medicare Abuse

Unlike fraud, Medicare abuse does not require the proof of intent to defraud the Medicare system in order to be assessed. Abuse includes any item or procedure that is inconsistent with accepted norms or practices. This can include:

- Excessive charges for procedures or supplies, or billing over the limiting charge,
- Billing for services which are considered not medically necessary. This includes ordering more tests than necessary for diagnosis or ordering services which are of no great benefit to the patient,
- Billing at different rates for Medicare and for other insurance (unless a lower amount is charged to Medicare in order to comply with fee schedules or limiting charges). There are some exceptions to this rule regarding service fees set by a contractual agreement with a Health Maintenance Organization. This violation includes accepting another insurance carrier's payment as payment in full for services (thus waiving coinsurance amounts). Such a practice results in charging non-Medicare patients 20% less than Medicare patients,
- Improper billing of Medicare when another carrier should be billed, or billing

Medicare first when they should be the secondary payor,
- Violation of any of the provisions of the Medicare participation agreement, and
- Unintentional unbundling, up coding, or violations of rules. Medicare may accept "I didn't know" as an excuse for a single violation of any of the Medicare rules and regulations. However, repeated abuses, especially after a provider has been warned will result in the upgrading of a violation from an abuse to intentional fraud.

It is unwise to think that the Medicare carrier will not catch instances of provider fraud and abuse. Due to the capacity of the Medicare carrier's computer database, the carrier can detect alterations in the billing patterns of providers. Additionally, carriers extensively use post-payment review of claims wherein they pull a sampling of a provider's claims and audit them.

If the carrier identifies overpayments or abuses, they may contact the provider and request documentation to substantiate the claims, or will simply send a request for repayment of an overpaid amount. Do not ignore letters requesting a refund of overpayment. If the provider disagrees with the request, you should file additional documentation to substantiate the services and request a review. If the provider agrees with the overpayment, the Medicare carrier should be reimbursed as soon as possible, along with any fines levied by the carrier. Since a decline in service results in a lower allowed amount, often repayments must also be made to the patient for excessive payment of coinsurance amounts.

Medicare will often audit claims using a peer review system. This is a group of physicians who review documentation regarding the services provided. If they find medical or documentation errors, points will be counted against the provider. When a provider receives a certain number of points, he may be subject to forfeiture of his license. Because of this, it is important that proper care be rendered and all evidence supporting the care and the justification of services be fully documented.

Sanctions and Penalties

Different levels of penalties and sanctions have been included in the Medicare provisions. The most common sanctions include:

1. **Educational contact and/or warning.** If Medicare determines that you are improperly billing, you may be contacted and instructed of the proper procedures and the necessary steps to rectify the situation. Such a contact may or may not include a formal warning which is placed in the provider's file.

2. **Recoupment of overpayments.** A letter may be sent requesting repayment of any amounts they feel have been overpaid. If payment is not received (and no review is requested), the carrier may withhold future payments to recoup the losses.

3. **Fines.** Many penalties include the assessment of fines for failure to follow regulations. Fines can range from $2,000 per incident to $25,000 per incident. Penalties of up to twice the overpayment amount may also be levied. Additional fines may be levied for not repaying overpayments in a timely manner.

4. **Criminal prosecution.** Providers or billers may be criminally prosecuted for fraudulent actions against the Medicare system. Penalties include conviction of a misdemeanor or felony, and may include additional fines and even jail time.

5. **Suspension or dismissal from the Medicare program.** Repeated or severe abuses can cause a provider (or a biller) to be excluded from the Medicare program. This sanction may be imposed for a limited time (suspension, often for up to five years), or permanently (dismissal). In such a case, announcements are made to all patients and in the press that the provider is no longer allowed to accept Medicare patients. If a patient submits a claim after the provider has been dismissed, they will be informed that the provider is not allowed to provide Medicare services and no coverage exists. A provider who is excluded from participating in the Medicare program may also be excluded from participating in Medicaid, Maternal and Child Health Services (EPSDT program), and Social Service Block Grants.

6. **Referral to licensing agencies and professional societies.** Extremely severe cases, especially those involving fraud, mismanagement of patient care, improper or unprofessional conduct, or unethical practices may be referred to a state licensing agency or a professional society for possible revocation of licensure.

If the Medicare carrier determines that a penalty or sanction has not solved the problem, they may proceed to the next level of penalty or sanction. Since the provider is responsible for what happens in his office, he will be held responsible for abuses and fraudulent actions committed by his employees or an independent billing service contracted by him.

Medicare Supplement

Supplements are separate plans written exclusively for Medicare participants. A supplement plan may be written with any optional benefits the policyholder wants. Three common options are:

1. Physicians' services – Covers Part B deductible and 20% coinsurance for reasonable charges.
2. Hospital services – Covers Part A deductible and may or may not cover the various copays not covered by Medicare.
3. Nursing care, prescriptions, and the non-replaced fees on the first three pints of blood.

With the changes in Medicare, supplemental plans have become much more flexible. Therefore, the benefits can be very complex and comprehensive or very basic.

Medicare and Veterans

Veterans may possess benefits with the Veterans Administration (VA), and at the same time be eligible for Medicare coverage. In such a case, the patient is required to make a choice between being covered by VA benefits or by Medicare. They can not be covered by both.

Once a patient has chosen, and completed the proper enrollment forms, claims for services rendered should be sent to the appropriate office. If a patient is covered by Medicare, some providers think that they must first send the claim to the Veteran's Administration and wait for a denial before submitting the claim to Medicare. This is erroneous and causes payment delays and unnecessary processing of claims by the VA.

Medicare and Managed Care

In 1985, Medicare began looking at the managed care market as a way to save costs. Medicare began in 1936 as a way to provide health care coverage for Americans aged 65 or older or those who are totally disabled.

Medicare Risk HMOs

A new trend has emerged lately, **Medicare risk HMOs**. These HMOs are set up exclusively to provide care to Medicare recipients who use about four times the amount of health care services as those under 65. Medicare risk HMOs must provide a minimum of the same basic benefits that Medicare would cover without the Medicare copayments and deductibles, but many HMOs provide more benefits.

A decade ago, in an effort to curb the ever increasing cost of treating those over age 65, Medicare began looking at alternatives. One of those alternatives was to have larger insurance companies set up HMOs for Medicare recipients. In return, the Health Care Finance Administration (HCFA), which oversees Medicare, determines the amount that is usually spent in treating an average Medicare recipient in a given area. HCFA then contracts with Medicare risk HMOs to provide benefits for those over age 65 at a cost lower than they would normally spend. This amount is usually 95% of the cost Medicare would normally pay in a given county, adjusted by the age and sex of the individual over age 65.

In exchange, the HMO assumes all the risk for treating that patient. In high cost areas like South Florida, New York and California, Medicare HMOs can be paid $500 to $600 per month for each patient.

Since many HMOs can drastically reduce the cost of treating these patients, the HMO can offer its benefits at no cost or a very low cost to them. Some HMOs offer a zero monthly premium, and some offer increased benefits to induce retirees to sign up.

The benefit for the retirees includes less paperwork to fill out and the ability to budget their health care costs. With the exception of the nominal copayment fee, all costs are covered by the monthly premium. The monthly premium costs for some HMOs are similar to premium costs for other insurance plans. However, with an HMO the more the retiree utilizes the provider's services, the greater the savings becomes since they are paying only the nominal copayment rather than a deductible and a portion of each service.

Because the HMOs have much lower costs, they are able to offer more benefits to the retiree, such as unlimited prescription drugs, 100% of hospitalization costs and 100% of physicians' visits. Currently, Medicare charges a deductible for hospital benefits along with a patient copay amount for over 60 days in the hospital and pays 80% of the approved fee for physician visits after payment of a $100 deductible.

Also, many HMOs offer a low-option package and a high-option package. The low-option package usually includes the basic options offered by Medicare with the high-option package offering greater benefits.

The disadvantages to the retiree are the same as with any HMO: limitations on choice of providers and increased rules on gaining pre-authorization for services or visits to specialists. Additionally, for those retirees who enjoy travel, or who spend a portion of the year in two separate places (i.e., summers in Maine, winters in Florida) the Medicare HMO may not have providers in both areas, or may not be licensed to practice in both areas. Emergency visits for retirees who are traveling may also require pre-approval, adding stress and paperwork in an already difficult time.

Medicare risks HMOs are also targeting employers whose retiree benefit plans include medical coverage. Traditional medical insurance coverage for a person over 65 can run up to $1,500 or more per year. By offering a Medicare risk HMO plan, employers can cover the entire premium and still save hundreds of dollars a year. Especially since most Medicare risk HMOs charge between zero and $40 per month for coverage.

By mid 1996, about 3.2 million retirees received benefits through Medicare HMOs. That's nearly 9% of the total 36 million Medicare population, and the market has just begun to explode. In December of 1994 there were 154

Medicare risk HMOs. Fourteen months later 194 had signed contracts with Medicare and 45 applications were pending. However, most Medicare risk HMOs operate only in high medical cost areas. In more rural settings, where an HMO has fewer providers and members and, thus, higher costs, Medicare risks HMOs are virtually non-existent.

There are some eligibility requirements that must be meet in order to enroll in a Medicare risk HMO:

1. The retiree must be eligible for and enrolled in both Part A and Part B of Medicare.
2. The retiree may only join an HMO that has a contract set up with Medicare.
3. An HMO is contracted for only a certain geographic area, and the retiree must live within that area. If the retiree resides outside a certain area for a specified number of consecutive days during the year, they may not be eligible for enrollment.
4. The retiree can only be enrolled during the open enrollment period. However open enrollment periods can last from a minimum of 30 days to all year.
5. Special requirements apply and the retiree may be denied admittance to a Medicare risk HMO if they qualify for Medicare due to ESRD or they are receiving hospice benefits.
6. If the retiree is dissatisfied with the HMO, he or she can discontinue coverage and return to the regular Medicare program.
7. If the retiree wishes to drop the HMO program, they must do so on a prescribed form. The form must be received by the HMO by the tenth of a month in order for coverage to be dropped by the first of the following month. At times the paperwork may take up to 60 days to complete the transfer process. The retiree is considered covered by the HMO until they receive a letter clearly stating that the retiree is reinstated in Medicare.

Medicare also has certain requirements which are usually higher than the requirements that states impose for licensing of an HMO. These include:

1. The retiree cannot be denied enrollment due to their health (unless they qualify for Medicare due to ESRD or are receiving hospice benefits). As a condition of enrollment, HMOs cannot require a retiree to have a physical examination or to provide proof of their health. However, the HMO may limit enrollment for some health conditions to the low-option package, denying the higher-option benefits. The low-option package must have at least the same basic benefits which are provided by Medicare.
2. The retiree cannot have their membership revoked due to poor health or a change in their health. Membership also cannot be revoked due to the costs of treating a retiree.
3. Emergency facilities must be available 24 hours a day, 7 days a week. All other Medicare-covered services must be available with reasonable promptness when needed.
4. The HMO must give 60 days notice to all its Medicare enrollees if they are ending their contract with Medicare and dropping coverage for all Medicare beneficiaries.
5. A retiree may be dropped from the HMO only if they move out of the service area which the HMO is licensed for, or if the HMO can prove that the retiree has been "grossly uncooperative" with administrative rules. Grossly uncooperative includes such items as allowing others to use a membership and/or identification card, and not paying monthly premiums.

The Two Types of Medicare HMOs

There are actually two types of Medicare HMOs: wrap-around policies and all-in-one (or total care) HMOs. There are basic differences, and not knowing these differences could cost retirees a large amount of money.

HMO/Medicare Wrap Around

A wrap-around HMO policy is actually a Medicare supplement plan, similar to many indemnity Medicare supplements. They are designed to provide protection for items that Medicare does not cover (i.e., deductibles and copayments). Often these types of plans are available to individuals who are in an employer sponsored HMO plan and then turn 65.

The employee's standard Medicare policy remains in force, but the retiree can save the costs of deductibles and coinsurance by going to the HMO provider. In essence, the HMO premium (added to any amounts Medicare pays) will cover the entire cost of a visit.

However, if the retiree chooses to visit a provider who is outside the HMO, standard Medicare benefits of 80% (after payment of a deductible) would be paid. Additionally, if the doctor did not accept Medicare assignment, there might be additional amounts that are "balance billed" to the retiree (the difference between what Medicare allowed and what the doctor charged, with limitations).

Medicare supplements may have fewer benefits than all-in-one HMO Medicare plans. For example, a Medicare supplement HMO may not cover or may have severe limitations on prescriptions, psychiatric treatment and nursing care.

Retirees must be careful to determine what is and isn't covered, the limitations that exist, what out-of-area treatments may be covered, what the HMO considers emergency or urgent care, and what the reimbursement is for going outside the HMO for care.

All-In-One Medicare HMOs

All-in-one Medicare plans (also known as competitive medical plans or CMPs) have recently appeared on the scene. These plans actually combine the retiree's Medicare and supplemental plan in one package. In essence, Medicare pays a capitated amount based upon the average costs for care in the HMOs area (adjusted for the age and sex of the member). In exchange, the HMO offers a complete package of benefits which covers at least as much as Medicare, and usually more.

The main difference is the "lock-in" provision. With the all-in-one plan, the HMO takes over the normal Medicare plan. Therefore, the retiree is limited to the benefits of the plan. If the retiree goes to the HMO providers, all benefits are covered. If the retiree goes to a non-HMO provider, the visit is not covered. Since the retiree is enrolled in this plan and is no longer enrolled in traditional Medicare, the normal 80% copayment provided by Medicare does not apply. The retiree is responsible for 100% of the visit.

If a specialist or a certain type of care is medically required by the member, but not provided by the plan, the plan should refer the retiree and cover the costs.

Once again, many plans will cover emergency visits if the retiree is out of the HMOs service area, but if the visit is declared a non-emergency there is no coverage.

If a retiree becomes dissatisfied with the plan, they are allowed to disenroll, then to re-enroll in Medicare. In theory, the member files for disenrollment, this becomes effective on the first day of the month following the application for disenrollment. However, there have been reports of delays in paperwork, perhaps leaving a member without coverage where they have been disenrolled from the HMO plan but not yet re-enrolled in Medicare.

There is one additional advantage with all-in-one Medicare HMOs. Because Medicare pays some (if not all) of the cost of coverage, if the plan generates excess funds (too much profit) it must either use the funds to provide additional benefits, or lower premiums for members.

Medicare Preferred Provider Organizations - PPOs

Medicare PPOs work much the same as Medicare HMOs, but with more freedom of choice. In such instances, the retiree is free to choose any provider for any visit. However, there are financial incentives for choosing a network provider (a provider who has signed contracts with the PPO and is on their approved list). Higher deductibles and copayment amounts will usually be required for visits to a non-network provider.

Many PPOs have fewer benefits than HMOs, but they often provide more benefits than standard Medicare coverage. The requirements for Medicare PPOs are somewhat less stringent than those for Medicare HMOs. They receive a contracted amount from Medicare for each retiree enrolled and the amount is based upon the local cost of treating Medicare patients. Usually, the higher the cost area the PPO is doing business in, the higher their payments and, thus, the lower their premiums (if any) and the more benefits they provide.

Medicare Notice of Non-Coverage

A **Notice of Non-Coverage** must be provided to all Medicare HMO members at the time of discharge from an inpatient facility. This is a letter, advising them of their right to an immediate professional review on a proposed discharge. This allows patients who feel they are being discharged too early to appeal the decision.

Additionally, all providers and groups must provide Medicare members with a copy of "An Important Message From Medicare" at the time of admission to any inpatient facility. This letter informs patients of their rights in regards to treatment. Inpatient facilities include hospitals, skilled nursing facilities, convalescent hospitals, psychiatric hospitals and any other facility where the patient will be staying overnight and/or receiving 24-hour care.

When filling in the variable fields on the letter, make sure the entries are easily understood. The notice should be hand delivered to the member and the member's signature should be obtained acknowledging receipt of the notice. A copy of the notice, signed by the member, must be placed in the patient chart.

If a Medicare member disagrees with a plan for discharge from an inpatient medical facility, he/she has the right to request an immediate review of the proposed discharge. If the review is requested by noon of the day following receipt of the notice, the member is not financially liable for the inpatient services until they receive notification that the review board has agreed with the discharge. If the patient does not file the request for review within the specified time period, they may still request a review. However, they will be financially responsible for treatment after the proposed discharge date if their request is denied.

In all instances, the member is responsible for convenience services and items not covered by Medicare or the plan.

Medicare Timeliness Reports

Each medical provider or group who contracts with an HMO to provide Medicare services must complete a Medicare "Monthly Report of Claims Processing Timeliness" each month **(see Figure 7-3)**.

Medicare designates that claims for Medicare services must be paid within a specified time period (usually 30 days on clean claims). When HMOs contract with groups or facilities that administer their own claims (i.e., have delegated claims processing to the provider or group or facility), HMOs are required by law to insure that those payors meet HCFA requirements.

The HMO monitors the timeliness of Medicare claim payments by use of the Monthly Report of Claims Processing Timeliness.

The claims to be monitored and reported include all Medicare risk claims that may be processed for allocation of risk pool (capitation) dollars. NOTE: The beginning of the 30 or 60 day period is the earliest date stamp on the claims you cannot prove are not yours or anyone contracted with the HMO to process. The end of the period is the date on which the payment or denial notice was mailed, not the examiner's release or adjudication date.

When filling out the Monthly Report of Claims Processing Timeliness, it is important to remember two things:

1. Medicare risk includes treatment for any patient for which the HMO, not the provider or group, receives a monthly capitation amount from the Federal Government. Any claims that are received are the responsibility of the HMO. There is no additional reimbursement from Medicare, regardless of the type or amount of services provided to the patient. The alternative to Risk is "Cost" or "Fee-For-Service" where claims are adjudicated by Medicare intermediaries or carriers that reimburse providers directly based on cost or fee schedules.

2. A denied claim is considered to be a claim where (a) one or more services will not be paid by the HMO (including its contracted groups/IPAs, hospitals, or facilities, and (b) payment is the responsibility of the patient. This does NOT include claims:

   ▪ For patients who remain enrolled with the same HMO, but who have transferred from one IPA to another and you are forwarding the claim,

   ▪ For which payment responsibility belongs to another contracting entity (health plan, hospital, IPA) and you are forwarding the claim,

   ▪ That are duplicates,

   ▪ That are encounter only/capitated claims and no patient liability is involved, and

MONTHLY REPORT OF CLAIMS PROCESSING TIMILINESS

Report as of _____/_____/_____   Note: *Report due within 7 calendar days of status date.*   _____/_____/_____
_{Status Date (Last working day of month)}   _{Date Report Prepared}

Names of management company/claims processing agent (if any) _____

Provider Name _____

Name and title of individual submitting report _____

Phone Number _____   Signature _____

1. At least 95% of **"clean" Medicare Risk*,** claims from **unaffiliated* (non-contracted), providers** to be paid or denied within 30 calendar days of receipt:

    Paid (+) Denied (=) Total

    A. Number of those claims processed during this reporting month   _____ + _____ = _____

    B. Total number of those claims processed in 30 days or less   _____

    C. Percent <u>meeting</u> 30-day standard (1B divided by 1A = %)   _____%

2. All other Medicare risk claims, which are to be paid or denied within 60 calendar days of receipt:

    Note: 2A should <u>not</u> include the claims reported in part 1A.   **Paid (+) Denied (=) Total**

    A. Number of Medicare Risk claims processed during this reporting month other than those reported in Part 1.   _____ + _____ = _____

    B. Total number of those claims processed in 60 days or less   _____

    C. Percent <u>meeting</u> 60-day standard (2B divided by 2A = %)   _____%

3. Reason for non-compliance or volume variation from prior month and corrective action plan/comments.

    _____

    _____

    _____

Please submit this report to: Medicare
                                   P.O. Box 123456
                                   Anywhere, AB 01234

Figure 7 – 3: Monthly Report of Claims Processing Timeliness

> ▪ That involves reduced payments due to contract terms or Medicare fee schedules (allowed amounts).

Summary

Medicare billing guidelines are changed several times a year. The medical biller must keep abreast of all the changes that occur.

Medicare intermediaries send out bulletins on a regular basis. The medical biller should read through these bulletins as soon as possible to become familiar with any updates or changes in the billing procedures.

Assignments

Complete the Questions for Review.
Complete Exercise 7 – 1.

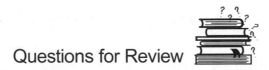

Questions for Review

Directions: Answer the following questions without looking back into the material just covered. Write your answers in the space provided.

1. What is Medicare? _____

_____

2. What three criteria is Medicare eligibility based on? _____

_____

3. Medicare _____ is considered the basic plan or hospital insurance and Medicare _____ is the medical insurance which covers physicians' services.

4. Briefly explain how to file an appeal on a Medicare claim. _____

_____

_____

5. What does it mean if a provider accepts assignment of benefits in regards to Medicare? _____

_____

_____

If you were unable to answer any of the questions, refer back to that section, and then fill in the answers.

Exercise 7 – 1

BALANCE BILLING

Directions: Calculate the adjustment and the amount which you may bill the patient in the following examples. Assume in all cases that the patient has fully met their deductible for the year and that the provider is a non-participating provider.

	Billed Amount	Medicare Approved	Medicare Paid	Collectible Amount	Adjustment	Balance Due From Patient
1.	175.00	115.40	92.32	_____	_____	_____
2.	35.00	3.00	2.40	_____	_____	_____
3.	375.00	323.60	258.88	_____	_____	_____
4.	45.00	40.00	32.00	_____	_____	_____
5.	1,500.00	1225.60	980.48	_____	_____	_____
6.	950.00	138.05	110.44	_____	_____	_____
7.	20.00	4.72	3.78	_____	_____	_____
8.	95.00	86.86	69.49	_____	_____	_____
9.	175.00	135.70	108.56	_____	_____	_____
10.	75.00	50.30	40.24	_____	_____	_____
11.	260.00	250.00	200.00	_____	_____	_____
12.	545.00	295.95	236.76	_____	_____	_____
13.	1,200.00	968.53	774.82	_____	_____	_____
14.	450.00	445.00	356.00	_____	_____	_____
15.	750.00	560.15	448.12	_____	_____	_____

Honors Certification™

The certification challenge for this chapter will be a written test of the information contained in this chapter. Each incorrect answer will result in a deduction of up to 5% from your grade. You must achieve a score of 85% or higher to pass this test. If you fail the test on your first attempt you may retake the test one additional time. The items included in the second test may be different from those in the first test.

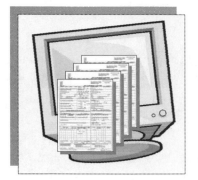

8

Medicaid

After completion of this chapter you will be able to:

- Describe the purpose of the Medicaid program.
- Explain how to verify a patient's eligibility for Medicaid coverage.
- List the benefits covered under the Medicaid program.
- Define and describe the EPSDT program.
- State the rule for time limits for Medicaid claims and the exceptions to this rule.
- List the services that require a Treatment Authorization Request.
- Properly complete a Treatment Authorization Request.
- Describe how providers are reimbursed for Medicaid services.
- State the guidelines for submitting Medicaid claims.

Key words and concepts you will learn in this chapter:

Categorically Needy – People who usually make less than the poverty level every month.

Early and Periodic Screening, Diagnosis and Treatment (EPSDT) – A preventive screening program designed for the early detection and treatment of medical problems in welfare children.

Eligibility Card – A card that shows that a recipient may be eligible for Medicaid.

Medicaid – A health care program established under Title XIX of the Social Security Act to provide the needy with access to medical care.

Medically Needy – Those whose high medical expenses and inadequate health care coverage (often due to catastrophic illnesses); have left them at risk of being indigent.

Provider Service Network (PSN) System – A system that requires the provider to maintain a machine that will read the magnetic strip on the back of the eligibility card.

Medicaid is not a health insurance program. The Federal Medicaid program was established under Title XIX of the Social Security Act of 1965. The purpose of this program is to provide the needy with access to medical care.

Medicaid Eligibility

The regulations governing eligibility under this program are extremely complex. Individuals may be entitled to coverage due to medical, family or financial situations. The fact that the individual has private insurance does not preclude him from being eligible for Medicaid benefits.

Most Medicaid recipients belong to one of two classes, the categorically needy and the medically needy. **Categorically needy** recipients usually make less than the poverty level every month. They may or may not be working, and may or may not have other health insurance. Coverage for some programs may be limited to pregnant women or their children.

Medically needy recipients are those whose high medical expenses and inadequate health care coverage (often due to catastrophic illnesses); have left them at risk of being indigent. Many disabled and elderly persons fall into this category.

For a claimant's services to be covered under Medicaid the claimant must be a Medicaid beneficiary and the provider must be an approved Medicaid provider. To be an approved provider, the provider of services must agree to accept Medicaid's determination of approved amounts as binding. That is, similar to Medicare's approved amount on assigned claims, the provider is not allowed to bill the patient for any amount not approved by Medicaid. In recent years, many providers have dropped out of the Medicaid program because their allowances and payments are extremely low, even lower than those provided by Medicare.

Medicaid Billing Procedures

Medicaid eligibility is determined monthly through the county welfare office. When billing for services for Medicaid recipients, you must have a copy of the Medicaid eligibility card for the month the services are rendered. If the eligibility card has adhesive stickers, one of the stickers must be attached to the billing form for payment. The following services are covered benefits under Medicaid:

- Inpatient hospital care,
- Outpatient hospital services,
- Physician services,
- Laboratory and x-ray services,
- Screening, diagnosis, and treatment of children under age 21,
- Immunizations,
- Home health care services,
- Family planning services,
- Outpatient hospital services, and
- EPSDT services.

Early and Periodic Screening, Diagnosis and Treatment (EPSDT) services is a preventive screening program designed for the early detection and treatment of medical problems in welfare children (known in California as the Child Health and Disability Prevention (CHDP) program).

The EPSDT program includes such things as medical histories and physical examinations of children, immunizations, developmental assessments, and screening for dental problems, hearing loss, vision problems, anemia, tuberculosis, sickle cell disease (and the sickle cell trait), bacteriuria, and lead poisoning. If problems are found, states may be required to provide services and treatment.

Additional benefits may be offered in various states. These can include items such as:

- Ambulance charges,
- Emergency room care,
- Podiatry services,
- Psychiatric services,
- Dental services,
- Chiropractic services,
- Private duty nursing,
- Optometric services (eye care),
- Eyeglasses and eye refractions,
- Intermediate care,
- Care in a clinic setting,
- Prosthetic devices,
- Diagnostic and screening services,
- Preventive and rehabilitative services (i.e., physical therapy),
- Treatment for allergies,
- Dermatologic treatments,
- Some medical cosmetic procedures (often reconstructive), and
- Prescription drugs.

To determine those services covered by your state, obtain further information from your state's Medicaid agency.

Medicaid recipients will have an **eligibility card** to show that they may be eligible for Medicaid. This card can be either plastic or paper. The paper eligibility card has adhesive stickers. These stickers are used for payment when claims are billed to the Medicaid office. Medicaid eligibility is determined on a monthly basis. The paper eligibility cards are issued monthly. You must have a copy of the card for the month when services are rendered to receive payment. The plastic cards are issued once and are to last throughout the participant's eligibility on Medicaid. Verification of coverage must be obtained for each month services are rendered. Most states have a telephone verification eligibility system that requires you to respond to various questions asked by a computer by pressing numbers or symbols on the headset.

The eligibility of the member on the card can be determined through a **Provider Service Network (PSN) system**. The system requires the provider to maintain a machine that will read the magnetic strip on the back of the eligibility card. The machine resembles a credit card machine. The card is swiped through the PSN, and the computer network will verify the eligibility of the person seeking services. The PSN system is able to indicate what benefits are available to the recipient, any restrictions, any third party coverage, or Medicare coverage.

Some Medicaid covered services require the Medicaid beneficiary to pay a small fee for services, called a copayment. The services that require copayments vary from state to state.

Medicaid claims must be submitted within 60 days of the end of the month for which services were rendered. There are six exceptions to this rule (these services must be billed within one year of the date of service):

1. Dental bills.
2. Obstetric care.
3. Treatment plan completion.
4. When the patient has other insurance coverage.
5. Retroactive eligibility.
6. In the event that the patient did not inform the provider that there was Medicaid coverage.

Treatment Authorization Request

In many cases, prior authorization is required before services are rendered. A Treatment Authorization Request (TAR) form is completed to obtain authorization for specific services **(see Figure 8 – 1)**. This form must be completed and sent to the appropriate agency for authorization to be given, prior to services being rendered. Please check with your state's Medicaid fiscal intermediary for prior treatment authorization guidelines. Some of the services that require TARs are:

- Inpatient hospital services,
- Home health agency services,
- Hearing aids,

- Chronic hemodialysis services, and
- Some surgical procedures.

Instructions for Completing the TAR

Each state Medicaid agency will have a form for requesting authorization for treatment of Medicaid patients. This form must be completed prior to the rendering of services. An explanation of how to complete the sample form is given below.

Verbal Control Number – This number is given when there is insufficient time to request a Treatment Authorization Number for the services provided. Once a Verbal Control Number is given, you must complete and submit a TAR immediately.

Type of Service Requested--Place an "X" in the appropriate box.

Request is Retroactive--Place an "X" in the appropriate box.

Is Patient Medicare Eligible?--Place an "X" in the appropriate box.

Provider Phone Number--Enter the area code and phone number for the provider.

Patient's Authorized Representative (If Any) Enter Name and Address – If the patient has an authorized representative enter the name and address of that representative here.

Provider Name and Address – Enter the name and address of the provider.

Provider Number – Enter the provider's Medicaid assigned number.

For State Use – Leave this area blank. This is where the Medicaid consultant will indicate if the services requested are approved, approved but modified, denied or deferred. If the TAR is approved but modified, denied or deferred, the consultant will give an explanation in the Comments/ Explanation section. The reviewing consultant must sign and date the TAR or it is not valid.

Name and Address of Patient – Enter the patient's last name, first name and middle initial. Enter the patient's address and telephone number on the following lines.

Medicaid Identification Number – Enter the patient's Medicaid identification number as it appears on the eligibility label or ID card.

Sex – Enter "M" for male or "F" for female.

Age – Enter the age of the patient.

Date of Birth – Enter the patient's date of birth in a six digit format (i.e., 01/01/2000).

Patient Status – Place an "X" in the appropriate box.

Treatment Authorization Request [TAR]

Verbal Control No.	Type of Service Requested ☐ ☐ Drug Other	Request is Retroactive? ☐ ☐ YES NO	Is Patient Medicare Eligible? ☐ ☐ YES NO	Provider Phone No.	Patient's Authorized Representative (IF ANY) Enter name and address:

Provider Name and Address | **Provider Number** | **FOR STATE USE** Provider your request is:

☐ Approved As Requested

☐ Approved as Modified (items marked below as authorized may be claimed

Name and Address of Patient
Patient Name (Last, First, MI) | Medicaid Identification Number

☐ Denied

☐ Deferred

Street Address | Sex   Age | Date of Birth | |

City, State, Zip Code | **Patient Status** ☐ Home   ☐ Board & Care

By: _____
Medi-Cal Consultant

Phone Number | ☐ SNF/ICF   ☐ Acute

Comments/Explanation

Diagnosis Description | ICD-9 CM Diagnosis Code

Medical Justification

Line No.	Authorized Yes | No	Approved Units	Specific Services Requested	Units of Service	NDC/UPC or Procedure Code	Quantity	Charges
1	☐ ☐						
2	☐ ☐						
3	☐ ☐						
4	☐ ☐						
5	☐ ☐						
6	☐ ☐						

To the best of my knowledge, the above information is true, accurate and complete and the requested services are medically indicated and necessary to the health of the patient.

Authorization is valid for services provided
From   Date   To   Date
  | | | |

_____ _____ _____
Signature of Physician or Provider   Title   Date

Office | **Sequence Number**

Figure 8 – 1: Example of Treatment Authorization Request Form

Diagnosis Description – Enter the description of the diagnosis.

ICD-9 CM Diagnosis Code – Enter the ICD-9 Diagnosis code for these services. Diagnosis descriptions and codes must relate to the services requested in the section below.

Medical Justification – Enter the medical justification (attach consultation report or other medical documentation if necessary) for the Medical Consultant to determine medical necessity. Enter the hospital name and address on the first line on the Medical Justification section. If the patient is inpatient in a SNF/ICF, enter the name and address of the facility in the Medical Justification section.

Authorized Yes/No – Leave blank. These boxes will be checked by the Medicaid consultant if some services are approved, but others are denied.

Approved Units – Leave blank. The Medicaid consultant will enter the approved number of units.

Specific Services Requested – Enter the name of the procedure or service requested. Up to six services may be requested on each TAR.

Units of Service – Enter the means for determining units of service (i.e., 15-minutes for treatments that are calculated per 15-minute blocks).

NDC/UPC or Procedure Code – Enter the procedure (CPT) code or the drug code for the procedure or drug you are requesting authorization for. The code on the claim submitted and the TAR must be the same.

Quantity – Enter the number of times the service or procedure is to be performed.

Charges – Enter the usual and customary fee for the requested services.

Signature of Physician or Provider – Signature of the provider of services or authorized representative must appear in this space. Enter the title of the person signing the TAR and the date.

Authorization is Valid for Services Provided – This section will be completed by the state agency reviewing the TAR. The authorized services must be completed within the dates specified. If the TAR is for a hospitalization, the claim submitted cannot have a date of service earlier than the "from Date" on the TAR.

Sequence Number – The TAR control number is preprinted on the form at the time of production. The consultant may add additional numbers or letters. This number must be entered as the TAR control number on the claim when submitted to Medicaid.

Reimbursement from Medicaid

By law, Medicaid is always secondary to private group health care plans. Therefore, if the patient has other coverage through their employer or through any other insurance carrier, that carrier should be billed first. Once payment has been received, Medicaid should be billed, and a copy of the EOB from the other carrier attached to the claim.

If Medicaid inadvertently pays primary, it will exercise its right of recovery and seek reimbursement from the private plan. The private plan is required to process Medicaid's request for reimbursement and pay Medicaid back the monies it paid the provider of services.

The Medicaid program does not process its own claims. Medicaid contracts with an organization to act as the fiscal intermediary, similar to Medicare. The intermediary processes the claims according to specifications set forth by the Medicaid program.

The rates under this program are based on the results of reimbursement studies conducted by the Department of Health Services. Reimbursement for hospital inpatient services are based on each facility's "reasonable cost" of services as determined from audit cost reports and annual limitations on reimbursable increases in cost.

Providers are not allowed to bill or submit a claim to the Medicaid beneficiary for any service included in the program's scope of benefits except to collect money from a patient's private health care coverage prior to billing Medicaid or to collect the patient's "share of cost."

Some Medicaid systems collect a small share of cost payment from the patient. This amount will not be printed on the Medicaid recipient's eligibility card. You should always ask about any share of cost when you contact Medicaid to verify the patient's eligibility

Medi-Medi

Patients who have both Medicare and Medicaid coverage are called medi-medi or crossover patients. Medicare should always be billed first on these patients. Medicaid may provide reimbursement for services which are not covered by Medicare or for the Medicare deductible and coinsurance.

Posting Medicaid Payments

As with Medicare, Medicaid payment will probably be lower than the actual billed charges. Because Medicaid recipients are not financially responsible for the balance, an adjustment to the patient's account will have to be made. When the explanation of benefits is received from Medicaid, each patient ledger will need to be pulled and the payments recorded. The adjustments should be made on the next corresponding entry line on the ledger card. The payment amount should be subtracted from the billed amount and the difference should be written off. If the patient's eligibility for Medicaid is terminated at the time services are rendered, the patient becomes financially responsible for the charges. At that time the patient should be billed directly.

Appeals

If a Medicaid claim payment is not satisfactory to the provider of services, the provider has the option to file an appeal. An appeal must be made to the fiscal intermediary within 90 days of the action causing the grievance. The appeal must be submitted in writing. Copies of the appeal letter, claim, and any additional documentation should be included with the submission.

The Medicaid Claim Form

Medicaid Claim Forms are required to be filled out when submitting claims to Medicaid. Many states now use the CMS-1500 form for billing; however, a few states may have a form specifically for their Medicaid recipients. Much of the information on these forms will be the same as those for the CMS-1500. Additional information on completing the CMS-1500 is covered in a later chapter.

General Guidelines

The following guidelines should be followed for the completion of Medicaid Claim Forms:

1. If possible, type the claim rather write it.
2. Use capital letters only when typing claims.
3. Do not strike over to correct errors.
4. Do not use N/A; leave space blank.
5. Be as complete and accurate as possible.
6. Code accurately and to the greatest possible number of digits, using the ICD-9 and CPT®.
7. Use all appropriate modifiers and list them in order of importance.
8. Be sure diagnosis codes substantiate the services provided.
9. If a claim is unusual, it may be better to send it manually rather than electronically. Electronic claims do not allow for the addition of medical reports or additional data to substantiate services.
10. Since Medicaid pays secondary to Medicare, claims for patients who are eligible for both programs should first be billed to Medicare. If the provider accepts assignment, the claim will automatically be forwarded to the Medicaid carrier after payment by Medicare. If the provider does not accept assignment, a copy of the EOMB must be obtained from the patient and attached to the Medicaid claim. Often Medicare pays more than the Medicaid allowed amount and no payment will be forthcoming, unless the patient has a deductible which has not been met.
11. If the patient is over age 65, but is not eligible for Medicare, this should be indicated on the claim in the Remarks section, along with the reason. For example, if the patient is an alien, "over 65 and not eligible for Medicare--ALIEN".

Many state's Medicaid forms are read by computer, so it is important to complete it correctly. It is important to use the proper Medicaid billing form for your state in order to receive reimbursement from Medicaid. Without it, Medicaid may refuse to pay.

Summary

Medicaid was established under Title XIX of the Social Security Act of 1965 to provide the needy with access to medical care. Medicaid eligibility is determined monthly. The information contained on this card must be used when billing for Medicaid services.

It is important to remember that providers who accept Medicaid patients are not allowed to bill the patient for any amounts that Medicaid does not cover. If the patient is covered by other insurance, the other insurance carrier is primary to Medicaid and should be billed first.

Each state's Medicaid program dictates the appropriate form to use for billing. The correct form must be used or Medicaid may not accept the claim for payment.

Complete the Questions for Review.

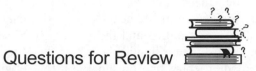

Questions for Review

Directions: Answer the following questions without looking back into the material just covered. Write your answers in the space provided.

1. What is the purpose of the Medicaid program? _____
   _____

2. (True or False?) By law, Medicaid is always primary to private group health insurance plans. _____

3. In what situation are providers allowed to bill or submit a claim to the Medicaid beneficiary? _____
   _____

4. Once Medicaid pays, is the doctor allowed to balance bill the patient for any amount Medicaid did not
   cover? _____

5. In order for a claimant's services to be covered under Medicaid, the claimant must be a _____
   _____ and the provider must be an _____.

If you were unable to answer any of the questions, refer back to that section, and then fill in the answers.

Honors Certification™

The certification challenge for this chapter will be a written test of the information contained in this chapter. Each incorrect answer will result in a deduction of up to 5% from your grade. You must achieve a score of 85% or higher to pass this test. If you fail the test on your first attempt you may retake the test one additional time. The items included in the second test may be different from those in the first test.

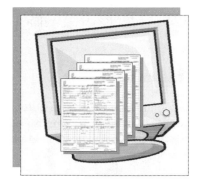

9

Workers' Compensation

After completion of this chapter you will be able to:

- Describe the eligibility and basic benefits of workers' compensation.
- List situations or places that would be covered by workers' compensation if an accident were to occur.
- List the types of claims workers' compensation provides coverage for.
- Describe the three disability levels for workers' compensation claims.
- Describe the benefits provided by workers' compensation coverage.
- List the types of issues that most of the new workers' compensation laws deal with.
- Describe what a medical service order is and what it is for.
- Describe how to handle patient records for workers' compensation cases.
- Describe the Doctor's First Report and how it is used.
- State the information that should be included in a Doctor's First Report and Subsequent Progress Reports.
- List the factors that may delay the close of a workers' compensation case.
- State the guidelines for billing for workers' compensation related services.
- Explain how to handle delinquent claims.
- List signs to look for that may indicate fraud or abuse of a workers' compensation case.
- Describe how third party liability on a workers' compensation case can affect the medical biller.
- Properly complete lien documents.
- Explain how to handle a claim that is reversed or denied by the workers' compensation board.

Key words and concepts you will learn in this chapter:

First Report of Injury – A form containing information on the doctor's findings.

Lien – A legal document that expresses claim on the property of another for payment of a debt.

Medical Service Order – A form which states that the patient is being referred to the provider in regards to a work-related injury and that the employer is responsible for coverage of services.

Non-disability – Minor injuries that will not require the patient to be kept from his job.

Temporary Disability – A situation where the patient is not able to perform his or her job requirements until he or she recovers from the injury involved.

Workers' Compensation (WC) – A separate medical and disability reimbursement program which provides 100% coverage for job-related injuries, illnesses and/or conditions arising out of and in the course of employment.

Workers' Compensation (WC) is a separate medical and disability reimbursement program which provides 100% coverage for job-related injuries, illnesses and/or conditions arising out of and in the course of employment. The employer, by law, is responsible for the benefits due an employee for work-related injuries and illnesses. WC insurance includes benefits for medical care expenses, disability income and death benefits.

When a patient first enters the office for treatment of an accident, it is important to obtain a statement of exactly what happened so that you can determine if a claim is covered by WC or by the patient's regular insurance. Job related injuries include any injuries which happen during the performance of work-related duties, whether they are in or out of the office. Occupational illnesses are considered to be any disorders, illnesses or conditions which arise at work or from exposure to factors at work. Occupational illnesses may be caused by inhaling, directly contacting, absorbing or ingesting the hazardous agent. Some occupational illnesses may take years to develop, or remain latent for a number of years before flaring up. For this reason, some states have WC laws which cover workers for years after they cease active employment in a field. For example, construction workers who dealt repeatedly with asbestos may develop asbestosis years after exposure.

Federal WC programs cover Washington DC workers, Federal workers, coal miners (black lung program), longshoremen and harbor workers. State WC laws cover everyone else. States set up their own guidelines, with the Federal government mandating a minimum level of benefits.

Each state's WC Appeals Board has the sole authority to oversee the rights and benefits of an injured or ill worker. It is through this Appeals Board that an applicant (employee) will file their WC application.

As a general limitation, most insurance plans specify that the claimant will not be entitled to payment for "bodily injury or disease resulting from and arising out of any employment or occupation for compensation or profit."

Most insurance plans will investigate and then provide benefits for medical care if they suspect that a claim(s) is work-related. Because the resolution of a WC case usually takes one to two years, private plans are obligated to pay the benefits for which the member is entitled and then file a lien with the member and the WC Board to recover their losses when the case is settled.

Once the WC carrier has accepted liability for the claim(s), the plan will discontinue providing benefits for medical care. At that point, the claim would be denied on the basis that it is work-related.

Employee Activities

The following section contains some general guidelines as to what constitutes an injury or illness as recognized by a WC Board in most states based on the type of activity, not injury.

Company Activities
Company activities can be defined as the following:
1. An injury sustained while attending an activity sponsored by an employer for the purpose of obtaining some business gain (i.e., company party for morale purposes; sporting activity for which the employee is provided transportation and/or the company gains advertisement by virtue of having the employee wear a company "athletic shirt").
2. An injury sustained by an employee for which the company provides remuneration.
3. An injury sustained while in the course of a person's occupation.

Use of Company Vehicles
Most WC laws provide coverage for an injury sustained while driving or as an authorized passenger in a company vehicle. This is true whether the injury is incurred in the course of the person's occupation, or if the vehicle is provided as a part of the employee's benefits to use to and from work.

The law's interpretation of "in the course of employment" is very different from most laymen's interpretation. For instance, someone injured while eating lunch at a company-sponsored event may be considered covered by WC. Therefore, always do investigations and let the Board handle the final determination.

Business Trips
Most WC laws provide 24-hour coverage for a person who is on a business trip. This coverage is applicable to the entire trip, so long as the person is performing routine activities. Of course, there are always exceptions to this rule.

Company Parking Lot

Most WC laws provide that if an employee is injured in a parking lot which is owned or maintained by his employer and furnished to the employee free of charge, he may be covered under WC. In addition, coverage would extend, in some instances, to an injury sustained by the employee while on neutral ground between the parking lot and the place of employment. An exception would be if such incidents were specifically excluded in the WC law, or if the injuries were sustained from willful or negligent actions on the part of the employee.

Usually, WC is not liable for injuries sustained in a parking lot which is owned by the employer and for which a rental fee is charged for the parking space. In such instances, the employee has a free choice to park elsewhere which would relieve the employer of any and all responsibility.

Occupational Disease

Most of the time, coverage will extend to employees who contract a disease which develops by working within a certain industry. For instance, most states provide compensation for individuals working with asbestos material over a period of years who then develop asbestosis or silicosis. Likewise, individuals can develop dermatitis from working with certain chemicals, such as in the exterminating industry.

Sometimes, a claimant may have an occupational illness which is submitted to the WC Board, and a concurrent non-occupational illness for which he may be reimbursed under the plan. In such instances, a separate billing should be completed by the provider indicating those charges which were solely for the treatment of the non-occupational disability.

Time Limits

Employees must report their injury or illness to their employer within a reasonable period of time. What is considered reasonable will often vary from state to state. However, many states require that the employee report an injury within 24 hours.

If a patient indicates that they are being treated for a work related injury, be sure they have notified the employer of the injury. If they have not, encourage them to do so immediately. Let them know that their WC benefits may be cut if they do not report the injury within a specified period of time. Also, let them know that many states will refuse to pay anything for claims if the injury is not reported in a timely manner.

Types of Claims

WC provides benefits for:
1. Medical expenses, including medical services, hospital treatment, surgery, medications and prosthetics or appliances, and durable medical equipment.
2. Temporary disability, allowing payments to continue to the employee even though they are not currently working. Payments are based upon the employee's salary and the length of the disability. Payments are usually not taxable as income.
3. Permanent disability, either in the form of weekly or monthly payments, or as a lump sum distribution.
4. Death, to compensate spouses and dependents for the loss of an employee. Some states also provide for a burial benefit to help cover the cost of funeral services.
5. Rehabilitation, to cover rehabilitation services or vocational retraining for permanently disabled workers who are unable to continue in their present position.

There are three types of WC claims. They are non-disability claims, temporary disability claims and permanent disability claims.

Non-disability Claims

Non-disability claims are for minor injuries that will not require the patient to be kept from his job. The patient is able to continue working throughout the extent of the injury. Upon the first visit to the physician the physician should complete a "Doctor's First Report of Occupational Injury or Illness (First Report)." This form and a copy of the bill should be submitted to the WC carrier.

Temporary Disability Claims

Temporary disability claims are when the patient is not able to perform his or her job requirements until he or she recovers from the injury involved. When a physician sees a patient in this situation a

First Report will be submitted and ongoing reports will be issued every two to three weeks until the patient is discharged to return to work.

Each state has a waiting period before temporary disability becomes effective, usually three to seven days (except in the Virgin Islands where the waiting period is one day). During temporary disability the employee is paid a portion of their salary as a tax free benefit. Temporary disability ends when the patient is able to return to work, even with limitations or to a different department, or when the patient's condition ceases to improve and the patient is left with a permanent disability.

Permanent Disability Claims

Permanent disability usually commences after temporary disability when it is determined that the patient will not be able to return to work. The physician will prepare a discharge report stating that the patient is "permanent and stationary." This means that nothing more can be done and the patient will have the disability for the rest of his or her life. The case will be reviewed by the WC Board and if determined to be permanent, a compromise and release will be issued. This is a settlement from the insurance carrier for a payment to the injured party.

The amount of the settlement is based upon the age of the disabled worker, the amount of money they were making at the time of the injury and the severity of the injury. The older an employer is, the higher the disability rating. This is due to the idea that a younger patient has a better chance of finding other employment or of being retrained for another job than an older worker would. Additionally, death benefits and rehabilitation benefits may be provided.

Death Benefits

Death Benefits compensate the family of a deceased employee for the loss of income which the employee would have provided to the family. Some states also provide a burial benefit to assist with the funeral and burial expenses for the employee.

Rehabilitation Benefits

If an employee is found to have a permanent disability, some states allow for a **rehabilitation benefit**. This benefit can be provided to retrain the employee in a physical ability which will help them to seek future employment (i.e., proper use of a wheelchair, use of the left hand when a person looses their right).

Some states participate in a "work hardening" program, wherein an employee is assigned therapy similar to their work in an attempt to strengthen them and build up their endurance toward a full days work. Often, employees in such a program will be returned to work on a limited or restricted basis. Physicians, therapists, employers, insurance carriers and all others concerned with the employee's case must keep in constant communication to ensure that the patient is not returned to work either sooner or later than possible, and that the employee will continue to receive adequate benefits that do not encourage them to cease work.

Many states also allow for vocational rehabilitation or retraining in a different job field when the employee is unable to return to their former position. This can include courses in colleges and vocational schools, or on-the-job training programs. Often employees are paid a weekly allowance (as in the case of temporary disability) while they are attending school and for a limited time after graduation. The time after graduation is to allow them time to locate a job. The employee is then considered to be off temporary disability and having returned to work. Vocational rehabilitation can also include job guidance, resume preparation and placement services.

Insurance carriers will often attempt to get the employee retrained and back to work as soon as possible, especially since the longer a person is off work, the higher the likelihood that they may never return to full-time employment.

Vocational rehabilitation has been an area of high abuse in the past. Often, employees have gone through a lengthy training program only to announce that they are unable to find a job in that field. In fact, some refuse to accept employment that is offered. Some employees and vocational schools will state that an employee needs additional training to bring their skills up to a minimum level, thus increasing the length of the program and the compensation to both the school and the employee.

Due to abuse of the system, many states have instituted reform to limit the amount of training an employee may receive and the amount of time an employee may receive compensation after retraining.

Benefits of Workers' Compensation

Before WC, employees were responsible for their own care, regardless of whether they were hurt on the job or at home. Employees would have to seek and pay for their own medical care, and then attempt to collect from their employer if they felt the company was at least partially responsible for their injury. Many times, the only way to collect was by bringing a lawsuit against the employer, thus creating hard feelings between the employer and the employee.

If the employer accepted the blame for the accident and agreed to cover medical expenses, they would often choose the medical provider based on price rather than quality of service.

Additionally, employers were not encouraged to stress safety in the workplace since the damages awarded in an accident often had more to do with the employee's injury than with the amount of negligence on the part of the employer.

With the implementation of WC and the inclusion of the WC insurer, both the employer and the employee have a third party to address grievances to and to assist with the rehabilitation of the employee. WC has the following benefits:

1. It allows employees to seek the best available care without irritating their employer, since the WC insurance carrier will be covering the bills.
2. It allows employees and employers to understand the rights and responsibilities of employees injured on the job. This eliminates many of the lawsuits and the animosity they entail. It also allows the employee to be reimbursed quickly, without waiting for the lawsuit to settle, and to gain a higher portion of the award since there are no attorney's fees and court costs involved.
3. It allows the injured worker to continue to receive income during their disability.
4. It relieves the employer of liability for workplace injuries, except in cases of gross negligence.
5. It relieves hospitals, providers and public charities of the obligation to cover the costs of those employees who are unable to pay for services, especially in the case of an accident which causes permanent disability.
6. It allows for compilation of reports which allow studies of workplace accidents. This provides additional information for reducing preventable accidents and for assisting employers with upgrading workplace safety.
7. It allows special provisions for coverage of minors under age 18 (or age 21 in some states). In some states WC laws allow for double compensation or additional penalties.
8. It allows coverage for all employees, regardless of the wealth of the employer or the business engaged in. Most states require WC for all businesses with one or more employees; however, a few states require a minimum of three to five employees.

Workers' Compensation Reform

Billions are spent on WC care each year. The system had numerous abusive and fraudulent claims. Even claims for legitimate work-related injuries were getting out of hand. Due to this, many states began restructuring their WC laws. Most new laws deal with:

- Limiting benefits,
- Increasing penalties for fraud and increasing prosecution of employees, physicians and lawyers who abuse the system,
- Not allowing a physician to refer a patient for further treatment to a lab or facility in which they have a financial interest,
- Requiring higher proof of medical necessity for treatment and proof of disability,
- Pre-authorization for expensive procedures,
- Encouraging companies to transfer workers to a different position in the company, allowing them to continue working while recovering,
- Limiting benefits for vocational rehabilitation,
- Increasing safety in the workplace,

- Limiting payment amounts to medical providers by the use of fees schedules or allowed amounts,
- Tighter review of records to catch duplicate charges, payments and billings, and
- Requiring or using mediators to settle disputes.

Medical Service Order

The first indication that a patient is being treated for a work-related injury is usually when the employee enters the provider's office for treatment with a medical service order. Many employers have a standard **medical service order** which states that the patient is being referred to the provider in regards to a work-related injury and that the employer is responsible for coverage of services. A copy of a medical service order is shown below.

ON LETTERHEAD

To Dr./Hospital/Clinic _____
Address _____

We are requesting treatment for _____(name)_____,
in accordance with the workers' compensation statutes for the state of XX. Please submit any necessary reports to the State Compensation Insurance Fund as soon as possible. Compensation cannot be paid without the completion of the proper reports.

Thank you,

Employer Representative _____
Title _____

If the employee is unable to return to work immediately, please so indicate by signing and dating this form below. If the employee is able to return to work with limitations or restrictions, please describe any limitations on the reverse of this form. This form should be returned to the employee for forwarding to the employer.

Dr. _____
Signature _____
Date/Time _____

If the patient does not arrive with a medical service order, the biller should contact the company immediately and request that one be faxed over. If the employer does not have a medical service order, the provider should fax one to the employer, and ask the company representative to complete it and fax it back immediately. This form can assist with the collection of a claim in cases of dispute, and a copy should be attached to any claims when they are sent in for processing.

In order to preserve the original signatures for your records, a photocopy should be made of the medical service order prior to its completion by the doctor. The original should be kept for your records. The copy should be signed by the doctor, if necessary, and a photocopy made of the front and back for the records. The copy which was signed by the doctor should then be returned to the patient.

If the patient must be referred to an additional facility for testing or treatment, authorization should be obtained from the employer prior to transferring the patient. The medical biller should call the employer and give the reason for the transfer or referral, the name and address of the facility the patient is being transferred to, and the treatment needed at the facility. Ask the employer to fax an authorization for transfer or referral. If verbal authorization is given, be sure to record the date and time, and the name and title of the person giving the authorization. The authorization (whether by faxed copy or the verbal information) should be placed directly on or attached to the transfer or referral order and a copy retained for your records.

Medical billers should be aware that some employers may attempt to cover the costs of a work-related injury themselves. This prevents them from reporting the injury to the state. Since premiums are often based on the past history of the employer, the more injuries reported, the higher the premium for the employer. Non-reporting of a work-related injury is illegal. The provider is in violation of the law if they know an illness or injury is work-related and do not file the appropriate forms.

Since this form constitutes an agreement for the company to cover the medical expenses, a contract exists between the employer and the physician, not the patient and the physician. Thus, all privacy guidelines that would normally apply between the patient and the physician now apply between the employer and the physician. If anyone, including the patient, requests information from the medical records, permission must first be obtained from the employer. Likewise, the employer has the right to examine the medical records if they choose.

If a patient refuses to see the physician recommended by the employer, the patient then becomes responsible for payment of the bill, and confidentiality guidelines would apply between the patient and the physician.

Patient Records

If a patient is being treated for a work-related injury, all records relating to the injury and treatment should be kept separate from the patient's regular medical records. Since employers are covering the costs of treatment, privacy guidelines are somewhat different than the normal privacy agreement between patient and provider. In WC cases, the agreement is actually between the provider and the employer, not the employee. The employer may request to see records regarding the injury, and these records may be subpoenaed. No information pertaining to the employee's non-work related treatment should be made a part of this file, so that confidentiality between the provider and the patient is not breached for non-work related treatments and conditions.

Many providers place work-related injury records in a colored file so it can be clearly identified as different from the patient's normal file.

If the physician finds a non-work-related condition during their injury-related examination (i.e., during the exam the physician discovers the patient has a heart condition), the WC agreement would be in force for all treatment relating to the injury, and the patient and his normal insurance carrier would be responsible for treatment of the non-work-related condition. It is important to clarify this with the patient and, if possible, treat the two conditions at separate times. At no time should the doctor bill twice for the same examination, both to the WC insurance carrier and to the patient. The examination should be charged according to the main activity of treatment (i.e., was most treatment related to the work-related injury or the non-work-related injury).

Doctor's First Report

Regardless of the type of claim or benefits, the doctor must file a **First Report of Injury (see Figure 9 – 1)**. This form contains information on the doctor's findings. It may have a different name, depending on the state; however, nearly all states require the completion of a similar form.

Physicians must make a report of injury, disability or death within a specified time period. This varies from immediately upon knowledge of the incident to within 30 days. Different states set different time limits and different requirements for reporting. There may also be different limits for different levels of injury (i.e., injury, disability, death).

This report is considered a legal document and it should be signed in ink by the provider. All information should be typed or printed clearly. The original should be submitted to the WC agency and a copy of the form sent to the insurance carrier. One copy is retained in the patient's records, and many providers also send a copy to the employer.

If the provider chooses to send a narrative report along with the standard report, the following information should be included:

- A history of the accident, injury or illness,
- Diagnosis,
- Any connection between the primary injury and any subsequent injuries, especially if the interrelating factors between the primary and secondary injuries are not immediately discernable, and
- Subjective and objective findings.

Subjective findings are those that cannot be discerned by anyone other than the patient (i.e., pain, discomfort). The physician should give an opinion as to the extent of pain, description of activities that produce pain and any other findings.

The original form should be submitted to the WC agency and a copy of the form sent to the insurance carrier. One copy is retained in the patient's records, and many providers also send a copy to the employer.

It is important to include all available information since most WC insurance carriers make an estimate of the total costs that will be associated with each case. Money is then set aside to cover the costs of treatment, disability benefits and, if necessary, rehabilitation or permanent disability benefits.

In describing the patient's pain or discomfort: severe pain limits ability and movement, moderate pain handicaps the patient in the performance of an activity, slight pain would cause a mild handicap in the performance of an activity, minimal or mild pain would be an annoyance, but would not preclude performing the activity.

DOCTOR'S FIRST REPORT OF OCCUPATIONAL INJURY OR ILLNESS

Within 5 days of your initial examination, for every occupational injury or illness, send tow copies of this report to the employer's workers' compensation insurance carrier or the insured employer. Failure to file a timely doctor's report may result in assessment of a civil penalty. In the case of diagnosed or suspected pesticide poisoning, send a copy of the report to Division of Labor Statistics and Research, P.O. Box 420603, San Francisco, CA 94142-0603, and notify your local health officer by telephone within 24 hours.

	PLEASE DO NOT USE THIS COLUMN
1. INSURER NAME AND ADDRESS	
2. EMPLOYER NAME	Case No.
3. Address No. and Street City Zip	Industry
4. Nature of business (e.g., food manufacturing, building construction, retailer of women's clothes.)	County
5. PATIENT NAME (first name, middle initial, last name) 6. Sex ☐ Male ☐ Female 7. Date of Mo. Day Yr. Birth	Age
8. Address: No. and Street City Zip 9. Telephone number ( )	Hazard
10. Occupation (Specific job title) 11. Social Security Number - -	Disease
12. Injured at: No. and Street City County	Hospitalization
13. Date and hour of injury or onset of illness Mo. Day Yr. Hour ____ a.m. ____ p.m. 14. Date last worked Mo. Day Yr.	Occupation
15. Date and hour of first examination or treatment Mo. Day Yr. Hour ____ a.m. ____ p.m. 16. Have you (or your office) previously treated patient? ☐ Yes ☐ No	Return Date/Code

Patient please complete this portion, if able to do so. Otherwise, doctor please complete immediately, inability or failure of a patient to complete this portion shall not affect his/her rights to workers' compensation under the California Labor Code.

17. DESCRIBE HOW THE ACCIDENT OR EXPOSURE HAPPENED. (Give specific object, machinery or chemical. Use reverse side if more space is required.)

18. SUBJECTIVE COMPLAINTS (Describe fully. Use reverse side if more space is required.)

19. OBJECTIVE FINDINGS (Use reverse side if more space is required.)
   A. Physical examination

   B. X-ray and laboratory results (State if non or pending.)

20. DIAGNOSIS (if occupational illness specify etiologic agent and duration of exposure.) Chemical or toxic compounds involved?   ☐ Yes   ☐ No
   ICD-9 Code __ __ __ - __ __

21. Are your findings and diagnosis consistent with patient's account of injury or onset of illness? ☐ Yes   ☐ No   If "no", please explain.

22. Is there any other current condition that will impede or delay patient's recovery? ☐ Yes   ☐ No   If "yes", please explain.

23. TREATMENT RENDERED (Use reverse side if more space is required.)

24. If further treatment required, specify treatment plan/estimated duration.

25. If hospitalized as inpatient, give hospital name and location   Date admitted   Mo.   Day   Yr.   Estimated stay

26. WORK STATUS -- Is patient able to perform usual work?   ☐ Yes   ☐ No
   If "no", date when patient can return to: Regular work ___/___/___
                                               Modified work ___/___/___   Specify restrictions _____

Doctor's Signature _____   CA License Number _____

Doctor Name and Degree (please type) _____   IRS Number _____

Address _____   Telephone Number (___) _____

FORM 5021 (Rev. 4)
1992

Any person who makes or causes to be made any knowingly false or fraudulent material statement or material representation for the purpose of obtaining or denying workers' compensation benefits or payments is guilty of a felony.

Figure 9 – 1: Example of a Doctor's First Report

Many First Report forms have a space for the occupation of the patient. It is important to list the patient's actual job, so the insurance carrier can determine if the employee was engaged in a normal work activity. This also allows the carrier to insure that the employer listed job titles and normal work activities accurately. Some employers attempt to list workers in less hazardous jobs (i.e., office worker rather than cutting machine operator) since insurance premiums are based upon the hazards the employee may encounter in the job.

If the First Report requests the time the patient was examined, it is important to list the date and time of the examination, as well as the date and time of the injury. This allows the insurance carrier to know how much time elapsed between the injury and the patient seeking treatment for the injury.

Be sure to indicate the provider's complete address and telephone number on the bottom of the form. This is the address payment will be sent to. The provider's title (i.e., M.D., D.C.) should be included, as well as their complete license number.

Copy the required number of forms prior to signing, and then have the physician sign each copy in ink. Stamped signatures are not acceptable. Additionally, the preparer should place their initials in the lower left-hand corner.

Subsequent Progress Reports

Following the First Report, the physician should follow up with subsequent progress reports (sometimes called supplemental reports) every two or three weeks. Many states have forms for subsequent progress reports; however, they may also allow a narrative report to be filed, rather than the completion of the specified form. Retain a copy for the files and provide the insurance carrier with their required number of copies (usually three or four). Subsequent reports should also be sent at the end of a hospitalization, even if the patient is expected to be readmitted later. This report serves as both a report on the patient's condition, and as a bill.

If the physician chooses to send in a narrative report, the following information should be included:

- Complete identification of the patient, including WC Case, Number, name and address of the patient,
- Date and description of all examinations and treatment procedures performed since the last report was submitted,
- Progress of the condition since the last report,
- Any proposed changes in the treatment plan,
- Any lab tests, function tests or other items which show any change in the patient's condition, and
- The status of the patient's disability, including an estimated time the patient can return to work, or any estimated permanent disability. If this changes from the doctor's report of first injury it should be brought to the attention of the insurance carrier so it may adjust funding to cover the new situation.

If the patient's condition changes significantly, a Re-examination Report, or a detailed progress report, should be filed with the insurance carrier.

Physician's Final Report

The WC carrier will often wait until the physician indicates that the patient's condition is permanent and stationary before finalizing a claim. The physician should then notify the WC carrier that no further treatment is needed (or that no further treatment will significantly alter the patient's condition) and that the patient has been discharged. This is called the **Physician's Final Report**. Some states require the final report be submitted on a specified form, and some states use the same form for both subsequent and final reports. The Physician's Final Report should indicate that the patient has been discharged, the level of the patient's permanent disability, if any, and the balance due on the patient's account (usually provided as a patient's statement showing services, dates of service, charges, and any payments rendered). Once this information is received, the WC carrier will establish the level of permanent disability, if any, medical and other expenses will be paid, and the case will be closed.

Delay of Adjudication

When a patient is released to work, all benefits have been paid, and the case is closed, the claim is said to have been adjudicated. Often adjudication occurs within two to eight weeks after the physician submits the report stating that the patient has been discharged and is able to return to work.

If the patient suffers a permanent disability, adjudication can take much longer, especially if the amount of permanent disability is protested and a lawsuit ensues. Additional factors which may delay the close of a case include:

1. Confusion or questions on any of the reports submitted by the employer, employee, or physician. This can include conflicting information from one or more parties, or vague or ambiguous terminology (especially by the physician) or illegible items.
2. Omitted information on a report, including incomplete forms, boxes not filled in, or signatures not included.
3. Incorrect billing or questions on the billing provided by the physician.
4. Insufficient progress reports to update the insurance carrier on the status of the patient.

Billing for
Workers' Compensation Services

When billing WC claims, it is important to follow all guidelines and regulations provided by the state WC agency. Using incorrect forms or not following procedures can cause delays in claims, or difficulty in collecting for procedures performed. Following are general guidelines regarding billing WC cases:

1. As mentioned previously, services rendered in a WC case are the responsibility of the employer, not the injured employee.
2. Some states pay WC cases according to a fee schedule, while others may use the amounts based on Medicare's allowed amounts. A fee schedule limits the amount providers can charge for services. Each service is given a different allowed amount based upon the difficulty of the procedure, the time involved, the risk to the patient, and other factors. Fee schedules prevent doctors from overcharging for services. The amount paid under a fee schedule is considered payment in full for the services and the biller should write off any amounts not covered. If possible, the biller should obtain a copy of the fee schedule for their state, and should charge for services according to this schedule.
3. If there are unusual factors which affect the amount the physician has charged, documentation should be sent with the claim to substantiate the increased fees charged. The insurance carrier will then determine if the fees are warranted.
4. If any procedures are listed as By Report (BR) on the fee schedule, a complete report of the procedure, initialed by the doctor, should accompany the claim. This report will allow the insurance carrier to determine the appropriate payment for the procedure. Be sure to attach any lab reports, x-rays or other data which supports either the excess fees, or the BR procedure.
5. As a biller, always remember to ask if a case is work-related when a patient first visits for treatment of an injury, illness or condition. This prevents billing the wrong party and having to go through costly adjustments and reimbursements. If the case is work-related, the patient should be instructed to provide the doctor's office with the Case Number as soon as they obtain it.
6. Since WC cases often go before a jury, every contact with the patient, his employer, his attorney, or anyone else related with the case should be documented and placed in the file. This includes contacts in person, by phone, or through a third party. Be sure to include the date and time of the contact, the full name of the person contacted, who initiated the contact (i.e., patient called, carrier called), and the details of the contact.
7. Be sure to use the proper CPT and ICD-9 codes and to complete all boxes on all forms. Incomplete information is one of the main causes of delay in closing a case.
8. In WC cases, all materials and drugs should be itemized in detail and charged at cost.
9. If a patient is injured in one state and then seeks treatment in a different state, the

laws of the state where the claim occurred would cover the employee. This situation occurs most often in cities which straddle a state line, or in rural areas where the nearest hospital is in a neighboring state.

When treating such patients, be sure to obtain a fee schedule and all pertinent information from the WC insurance carrier in the state with jurisdiction. The WC carrier should be contacted prior to treatment, if possible, since some states have restrictions on treatment. If treatment is approved, be sure to get a written authorization, preferably by fax for speed, then a hard copy for permanent records. Be sure to ask the state to fax or send all necessary forms for physician's first report of illness, progress reports, physician's final reports, and any other reports needed since these forms often vary from state to state. Also ask about billing requirements. Some states insist on a CMS-1500 or other form and some will accept an itemized patient statement or superbill.

10. Be sure to file claims for workers' compensation services as soon as possible. Many states have time limits on when you can submit a claim to the insurance carrier (i.e., six months after treatment). If you are past the time limit, some WC carriers will cut the benefit payment and others may refuse to pay it completely.

If you have questions regarding the payment of a particular claim, call the WC insurance carrier and ask to speak with the adjuster in charge of the case. General questions regarding the state WC benefits, rules and legislation information can be obtained from your state's WC appeals board. Information regarding WC coverage for those covered under one of the three Federal programs can be obtained from the Department of Labor Employment Standards Administration in Washington, DC.

Delinquent Claims

If payment is not received within 45 days of billing the WC insurance carrier, the biller should contact the adjuster in charge of the case and ask the reason for the delay. Often the proper forms have not been received from one party or another. If such is the case, ask which form is missing and who is responsible for sending it. If the form is required by another person (i.e., the employer) contact that person and request that the form be completed as soon as possible so you may receive payment.

If the employer or other party has not completed the necessary item within 30 days of your contacting them, send a letter to the WC Board or Industrial Accidents Commission in your state. The letter should state that you are requesting their help in securing the necessary items from the party. Be sure to include the case number, the name, address and phone number of the party who should provide the item, the patient's name and address, the date of the injury, and the name and address of the insurance carrier or other person the item should be sent to. Also list the patient's balance due.

Fraud and Abuse

Unfortunately, fraud and abuse occurs frequently in the WC system. Many employees, employers, providers and insurance carriers find it easy to defraud the system and reap significant financial rewards.

In the past there has been little deterrent to abusing the system. It was frequently possible to find a doctor who was willing to testify that injuries were more serious than was first thought. Likewise, numerous lawyers stepped in and set up relationships with doctors to produce claims where no actual injury or illness existed. This is especially true when work-related stress became a popular diagnosis for any one of a number of ailments. Many of these lawyers would locate people in the unemployment office and convince them they could get better reimbursement through WC than they could through unemployment.

It is important for the medical biller to realize that committing fraud or abuse of the WC system is a felony in most states. Additionally, not reporting suspected or known cases of fraud or abuse is also illegal in many states. While most claims are legitimate, the medical biller should recognize what constitutes fraud. Following are some signs of fraud or abuse to look out for.

An injured employee who:
- Cannot clearly describe the pain or injury, or whose description changes each time details of the incident are related,
- Is overly dramatic regarding their injury,
- Complains of an injury which cannot be substantiated by medical evidence. This may include soft tissue injuries which cannot be seen on an x-ray, or a patient who insists there is a serious injury, even when there is medical evidence to the contrary,
- Delays the reporting of an injury, especially an injury that is reported on a Monday when the employee claims it happened on Friday,
- Reports the injury to an attorney or regulatory agency prior to reporting the injury to their employer,
- Changes physicians frequently, or shows up for a first treatment, but seems unhappy with the diagnosis and changes physicians. Patient may be seeking a physician who will grant additional time off work or will testify to a greater degree of injury,
- Is a short term worker, or who was scheduled to terminate employment just after the injury occurred,
- Has a history of curious or an excessive amount of WC claims, or
- Complains of a severe injury and an inability to perform certain tasks, but is seen having used the injured limb or body part while in the waiting room.

An employer who:
- Refuses to accept that an injury occurred on the job when there is evidence to the contrary, or
- Refuses to complete the necessary paperwork and instead attempts to pay for medical services through the company.

A medical provider who:
- Orders or performs unnecessary procedures or tests,
- Inflates the severity of the injury to qualify for higher reimbursement (i.e., lists a fracture as open rather than closed, bills for a high complexity exam rather than a moderate complexity exam),
- Charges for services that were never performed, or adds additional procedures onto existing claims,

- Makes multiple referrals to a lab, clinic or hospital and receives a referral fee from these organizations,
- States that an injury exists and needs treatment when no injury is actually present,
- Sends in duplicate billings with information changed (i.e., dates) to make it appear services were performed more than once,
- Files many claims with subjective injuries (i.e., pain, strain, emotional disturbance, inability to perform certain functions), or
- Files claims for several employees of the same company which show similar injuries (i.e., injuries for which reports or x-rays may be duplicated).

An attorney who:
- Pressures a provider to provide additional treatment or to increase the severity of the diagnosis,
- Encourages a provider to charge for services not rendered, stating that the insurance carrier will cover it, or
- Refers numerous clients to a specific provider, which suggests they may be in collusion with each other.

The above instances suggest signs a medical biller should look for. If a biller suspects fraud, it should be reported to the appropriate authority immediately. If a biller becomes aware of fraud by the provider they work for, they should seek the help of an attorney. A biller can be considered guilty of fraud if they knew of the fraud and did nothing to prevent it. This is true even if the biller receives no money from the fraud.

Third Party Liability

It is possible to have third party liability in a WC case. For example, George works at a restaurant and is taking trash out to the trash bin behind the building. A plumber had been visiting the restaurant. Upon leaving, he backed up without looking and ran over George's leg.

Since George was clearly injured in the normal performance of his duties, the accident would be covered by WC. The WC insurance carrier would be required to pay all benefits George is entitled to. However, since the accident was clearly the plumbers fault, the insurance carrier may encourage George to sue for damages. If George wins the case against the plumber, the insurance carrier has a right to collect all monies it has paid out for George's benefits. Anything left over, would go to George.

This situation often does not affect the way the medical provider is paid since it usually takes an extended time period for a lawsuit to be resolved. By this time the WC insurance carrier has covered the medical expenses.

However, in such cases the doctor may be called upon to testify for either party. The doctor would be considered an expert witness, and compensation would be allowed for time spent preparing records, waiting to testify (if the doctor had to cancel appointments), giving a deposition, and for the testimony. A deposition is when a person answers questions under oath, but not in open court. Depositions are often tape recorded or are transcribed word for word.

When the biller is preparing a claim for these services, all items should be broken out and the time indicated for each item separately. Often each item carries a different amount of reimbursement. The actual amounts paid for these services should be worked out between the provider and the WC insurance carrier prior to rendering of services. All items are billed by description; however, the CPT® code 99075 is also given for Medical Testimony.

Liens

In permanent disability a compromise and release will be issued by the insurance carrier for the injuries to the patient. If the physician has been seeing the patient and there are unpaid medical expenses, a lien should be filed for payment of services rendered. A **lien** is a legal document that expresses claim on the property of another for payment of a debt **(see Figure 9 – 2)**. A lien is completed and submitted to the attorney representing the injured party to be paid upon monetary settlement of the WC claim.

A lien should be sent along with the bill for the initial visit. Whenever additional services are rendered, a copy of the bill should be submitted to the attorney so that all concurrent care will be included in the lien. All services must be for the care of the injury covered under the WC claim.

Many states have a special lien form for WC purposes. These forms can be obtained through the local Division of Industrial Accidents. (A sample copy of a lien is shown in **Figure 9 – 3**.) Complete the lien form and send copies to the WC appeals board, the patient's employer, the patient, and the WC insurance carrier. A copy should also be kept for the files.

If a lien is not filed, all monies recovered at the close of the case officially belong to the patient. It is then the patient's responsibility to cover the medical expenses. If any liens are filed, the patient must first pay the liens, and then pay any other resultant expenses. Therefore, if the lawyer files a lien and his fees exhaust most of the money, there will be little or none left for other expenses. If at all possible, patients should be persuaded to pay for medical services prior to settlement of the claim.

If a lien is filed, the biller should have their copy of the lien letter signed by the patient and the patient's attorney. This makes the attorney responsible for payment of the physician's bills. If the attorney does not remit the necessary funds from the patient's settlement, the attorney must cover the medical expenses.

A lien should have a specified time limit on it, often a period of one year. If settlement has not been reached by that time, or there are ongoing charges on the patient's account relating to the WC injury, an amended lien should be filed. The subsequent lien should state the balance of the patient's account, and should have the word AMENDED stamped across the top or below the Appeals Board Case Number.

The biller should place all files with liens in a special section and hold them until the cases have been settled. It is illegal to continually bill or harass the patient when a lien agreement has been signed.

In effect, the lien acknowledges the provider's agreement to wait for reimbursement until the case has been settled. The biller should contact the patient's attorney at least once every quarter for an update on the case and to determine when settlement is expected to occur. The attorney should also be contacted within two weeks after the date settlement is expected to find out the results of the case and ask when payment can be expected.

In some states, the law allows the provider to be paid prior to the attorney or patient collecting any monies from the settlement. Statutes in your state should be checked to protect you. If your state has such a provision, attorneys may not collect their fee and then state that insufficient funds were recovered to cover your total bill. Some states also allow the physician to bill the patient for any funds which were not received from the settlement. Once again, check with the laws of your state to determine if patients can be billed or if any amounts not collected should be written off.

Liens are an inexpensive way of insuring that the physician will be reimbursed for their services. The cost is much less than suing the patient and assures that payment will be received when the dispute between the patient and the WC insurance carrier is settled. A lien is a legal document that will be recognized by the court and will provide protection in the event of litigation.

Reversals

Occasionally, an accident which was thought to be WC will turn out not to be. This can happen when a patient hides or omits facts regarding when and how the accident occurred. It can also be found that there is a non-industrial, underlying condition which caused the accident. For example, a patient may have epilepsy and suffer a seizure at work. Any injuries directly received on the job site could be considered WC; however, the treatment of the underlying epileptic condition would not be WC.

In some cases the employee may be found to be negligent in their actions, or willfully not abiding by established workplace rules. In such cases, injuries sustained as the result of negligence of the employee may not be considered industrial accidents. For example, if the employee is told they must refrain from wearing hoop earrings, but they chose to anyway, they may be considered liable if the earrings are caught on machinery and ripped from the ear.

In such cases, the WC board would deny payment on the claim. All claims for treatment should then be sent to the patient's regular insurance carrier with the denial notice from the WC Board. A letter should also be sent to the employee notifying them that their claim was denied and their regular insurance is being billed for the charges.

Summary

WC insurance is a separate medical insurance program which covers work-related injuries, disabilities and death. A wide range of activities may be covered under WC laws.

Assignments

Complete the Questions for Review.
Complete Exercise 9 – 1.

TO: Attorney _____

_____

_____, California

RE: Medical Reports and Insurance Carrier Lien

FOR_____

I do hereby authorize the above insurance carrier to furnish you, my attorney, with a full report of any records and resultant payments of myself in regard to the accident in which I was involved.

I hereby authorize and direct you, my attorney, to pay directly to said insurance carrier such sums as may be due and owed for payment of medical services rendered me or the provider of services both by reason of this accident and by reason of any other bills that are due, and to withhold such sums from any settlement, judgment or verdict as may be necessary to adequately protect said insurance carrier. And I hereby further give a lien on my case to said insurance carrier against any and all proceeds of any settlement, judgment or verdict which may be paid to you, my attorney, or myself as the result of the injuries for which I have been treated or injuries in connection therewith.

I fully understand that I am directly and fully responsible for reimbursement of any payments for all medical bills submitted for services rendered and that this agreement is made solely for said insurance carriers additional protection and in consideration of its awaiting payment. And I further understand that such payment is not contingent on any settlement, judgment or verdict by which I may eventually recover said fee.

Dated: _____   Patient's Signature: _____

The undersigned being attorney of record for the above patient does hereby agree to observe all the terms of the above and agrees to withhold such sums from any settlement, judgment or verdict as may be necessary to adequately protect said insurance carrier named above.

Dated: _____   Attorney's Signature: _____

Mr. Attorney: Please sign, date, and return one copy to our office at once.

Keep one copy for your records.

Figure 9 – 2: Sample Copy of a Lien Letter

WORKERS' COMPENSATION APPEALS BOARD

STATE OF CONFUSION

CASE NO. _____

NOTICE AND REQUEST FOR ALLOWANCE OF LIEN

_____
LIEN CLAIMANT   ADDRESS
VS.

_____
EMPLOYEE   ADDRESS

_____
EMPLOYER   ADDRESS

_____
INSURANCE CARRIER   ADDRESS

The undersigned hereby requests the Workers' Compensation Appeals Board to determine and allow as a lien the sum of

_____ dollars ($_____) against

any amount now due or which may hereafter become payable as compensation to _____
                                                                             EMPLOYEE

on account of injury sustained by him/ her on _____.
                                              DATE

This request and claim for lien is for: (Mark appropriate box)
- ❑ The reasonable expense incurred by or on behalf of said employee for medical treatment to cure or relieve from the effects of said injury; or
- ❑ The reasonable medical expense incurred to prove a contested claim; or
- ❑ The reasonable value of living expenses of said employee or of his dependents, subsequent to the injury, or
- ❑ The reasonable living expenses of the wife or minor children, or both, of said employee, subsequent to the date of injury, where such employee has deserted or is neglecting his family; or
- ❑ The reasonable fee for interpreter's services performed on _____.
                                                                DATE

NOTE: ITEMIZED STATEMENTS MUST BE ATTACHED
The undersigned declares that he delivered or mailed a copy of this lien claim to each of the above-named parties on

_____
ATTORNEY FOR LIEN CLAIMANT   DATE

_____
ADDRESS OF ATTORNEY FOR LIEN CLAIMANT   LIEN CLAIMANT

EMPLOYEE'S CONSENT TO ALLOWANCE OF LIEN

I consent to the requested allowance of a lien against my compensation.

_____
ATTORNEY FOR EMPLOYEE   EMPLOYEE

DEPARTMENT OF INDUSTRIAL RELATIONS
DIVISION OF INDUSTRIAL ACCIDENTS

Figure 9 – 3: Sample Copy of a State Lien Form

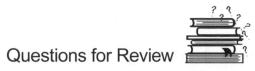

Questions for Review

Directions: Answer the following questions without looking back into the material just covered. Write your answer in the space provided.

1. What is workers' compensation?_____
   _____

2. What items are likely to cause a delay in adjudication of a case?_____
   _____
   _____

3. What do you do if a patient states this is a WC injury but he has nothing from the employer to prove it?
   _____
   _____

4. What is a lien? _____
   _____

5. Why should you file a lien?_____

6. What signatures should you get on a lien?_____

7. Define Temporary Disability?_____
   _____

8. Define Permanent Disability?_____
   _____

9. What is a non-disability claim?_____
   _____

10. If an employee is injured while at a company-sponsored game, is it considered a WC case?_____

If you were unable to answer any of the questions, refer back to that section, and then fill in the answers.

Exercise 9 – 1

Directions: Complete a Doctor's First Report for the following case.

Patient:	Joel Johnson 1234 Jerome Way Jersey City, NJ 11111 (111) 123-4567	**Insurance Carrier:**	Just Workers Insurance 1234 Jingle Road Jersey City, NJ 11112 (111) 987-6543
DOB:	10/01/63		
SSN:	123-45-6789		
		Physician:	Joanne Jones, M.D. 1029 Jonathan Lane Jersey City, NJ 11121
Job Title:	Waiter/Hostess		(111) 123-0987
Employer:	Jerry's Cafe	**License #:**	A1234567
	5678 Joseph Lane	**EIN:**	11-0987654
	Jersey City, NJ 11113		
	(111) 567-8901		

Incident: Patient states that at 5:10 pm on 10/16/XX, he was carrying a dessert tray. He slipped on some soda that was spilled on the floor and landed on his back, striking his head on the floor. The dessert tray turned upside down and landed on him. The patient is complaining of headache and difficulty in breathing through nose.

Injuries: Concussion (no fracture, no apparent brain damage), foreign matter (chocolate mouse) in both eyes, foreign body (cherry) lodged in nose.

Procedures Performed: Physical examination and history, new patient, moderate complexity ($70.00), x-ray of the skull, 2 views (negative for fracture $45.00), removal of foreign body from nose ($85.00), irrigation of eyes ($18.00).

Treatment Plan: Bed rest for two days, wake patient every hour during first 24 hours to insure no LOC, limited activity for two weeks, re-check in ten days. Patient estimated able to return to work 10/30/XX.

Signed: Joanne Jones, M.D.,   10/166/XX 6:05 pm

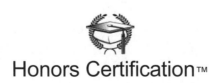

Honors Certification™

The certification challenge for this chapter will be a written test of the information contained in this chapter. Each incorrect answer will result in a deduction of up to 5% from your grade. You must achieve a score of 85% or higher to pass this test. If you fail the test on your first attempt you may retake the test one additional time. The items included in the second test may be different from those in the first test.

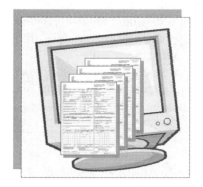

10

Managed Care

After completion of this chapter you will be able to:

- List the reasons for rising health care costs.
- Describe ways that insurance carriers decrease costs.
- Describe the main types of managed care organizations and their function.
- List the common HMO benefits.
- Describe the various types of Preferred Provider Organizations and their function.
- Explain the purpose of the membership card and eligibility rosters.
- Explain the difference between reporting patient encounters on a CMS-1500 and billing on a CMS-1500.
- Describe how risk for expenses is shared between groups/IPAs and the HMO.
- Explain how providers are reimbursed in a capitation agreement.
- Describe how a medical management incentive program works.
- Describe the purpose and reason for supplemental capitation and how to request it.
- Describe the purpose and reason for additional capitation and how to request it.
- Describe the proper handling of the patient's medical record.
- Appropriately schedule appointments using a given scenario.
- Appropriately handle a missed appointment using a given scenario.
- Properly handle authorizations, referrals and second opinion referrals using a given scenario.
- List the steps in the second opinion process.
- List the information that must be included on member appeals of denied HMO claims.
- List the steps to be taken in the case of a member grievance or complaint.
- Properly complete a grievance log.
- Describe PCP transfer procedures.
- State the reasons why a member may be disenrolled and the information that must be documented in a disenrollment.
- Describe the standard provisions for continuing care when a provider terminates their agreement with an HMO.
- Properly complete a patient population record.
- Properly generate a payment to an outside provider using a given scenario.
- Properly complete a denial notice.
- Describe stoploss and the procedures for obtaining stoploss reimbursement from the HMO.

Key words and concepts you will learn in this chapter:

Capitation – A monthly payment made to a provider in exchange for providing the health care needs of a member.

Clean Claim – A claim that can be paid as soon as it is received because it is complete in all aspects.

Complaints – Verbal expressions of dissatisfaction with a provider or services.

Copayment – An amount which the member pays at each visit.

Disenrollment – When a patient transfers their care from a provider.

Eligibility Roster – A list of patients who have chosen the provider as their Primary Care Provider.

Exclusive Provider Organization (EPO) – A plan where the patient must select a Primary Care Provider and can use only physicians who are part of the network or who are referred by the PCP.

Gatekeeper PPO – A plan where patients must choose a regular provider. Those who wish to consult a specialist or receive additional tests or procedures must get prior approval from their regular provider.

Grievances – Written complaints made by a member regarding dissatisfaction with a provider or services.

Health Maintenance Organizations (HMOs) – Organizations or companies that provide both the coverage for care, and the care itself. Members pay a set amount every month and the HMO agrees to provide all their care, or to pay for the covered care they cannot provide.

Independent Practice Associations (IPAs) – A group of medical organizations and providers who have banded together to form their own HMO.

Managed Care – An attempt by insurers to control health care costs using a number of different methods.

Management Service Organization (MSO) – A separate corporation set up to provide management services to a medical group for a fee.

Physician Hospital Organization (PHO) – An organization of physicians and hospitals that bands together for the purpose of obtaining contracts from payor organizations.

Preferred Provider Organizations (PPOs) – A plan where the insurance carrier contracts with providers to join their "network." These providers agree to provide services at a reduced amount in exchange for the referrals from the carrier, and the carrier agrees to reimburse network providers at a higher percentage than providers outside the network.

Primary Care Provider (PCP) – The provider a patient has chosen for their primary medical care.

Self-Insurance – A plan where employers place monthly premium amounts into an escrow account and pays all medical claims from this account.

Stoploss – An attempt to limit payments by an insured person, or a group/IPA in the case of a catastrophic illness or injury to a member.

Utilization Review – A process whereby insurance carriers review the treatment of a patient and determine whether or not the costs will be covered.

Health care costs in the American economy have escalated out of control. Higher prices for services and insurance have American consumers demanding some type of reform. Managed care contracts were created in an attempt to bring health care costs under control by having providers share some of the financial risks of health care with the patient and the insurance carrier.

Rising Health Care Costs

There are numerous reasons for the rising cost of health care in America. Some of the most common include:

1. The higher costs of doing business, including rising rents, employee salaries, etc.
2. The rising costs of education for medical professionals. Doctors who incur tremendous debt gaining their education expect to be able to pay off these debts and still make a healthy profit.
3. Little or no competition among providers. It is not customary for doctors to advertise their prices. Additionally, the American consumer often does little comparison shopping on the basis of cost when trying to find a physician, especially when insurance carriers cover most of the cost of services.
4. Little or no control by traditional indemnity plans on the utilization of care. These plans normally paid on claims with little or no restrictions. Only lately have these companies begun trying to regulate health care costs by tightening controls, requiring pre-authorizations for treatment and by reviewing the treatment provided to determine the necessity of services.

5. Greater number of lawsuits, causing ever increasing malpractice insurance premiums. Additionally, doctors are ordering more tests and trying more treatments in order to protect themselves against possible lawsuits. This "over care" not only costs more money, but can be harmful to the patient, putting them at risk for increased medical problems. For example, if a doctor orders surgery when a less invasive treatment would work as well, the patient is at risk from infection, adverse reaction to anesthesia or other drugs, or complications of surgery.

6. Higher utilization of medical services. As late as the beginning of this century, many people didn't go to a doctor for minor illnesses or injuries. They relied on home remedies and time to take care of medical problems. Now many people see a doctor for even the most insignificant reason.

7. The cost of new medical technology. Patients like to see doctors who have the latest technology and equipment. Unfortunately, this equipment costs a tremendous amount of money. Some medical equipment can cost as much as $500,000.

8. More people are living longer, and those over 65 use more of the medical services than any other age group. This will be especially true in another 12 to 15 years when the baby boomer generation begins reaching retirement age.

9. Over 37 million people have no insurance. These people utilize services and then are unable to pay, or pay on a delayed timetable. The costs associated with treating the uninsured are often passed on to those patients with insurance.

10. There are more catastrophic illnesses in the world today, including the AIDS epidemic.

Decreasing Costs

Now that we know why the problems exist, what can be done about increased health care costs?

Numerous ideas have been put forward regarding health care reform. Everything from health maintenance organizations to a national, federally run health insurance program have been proposed or tried, with varying degrees of success.

More often than not the issue is not whether to cut costs, but how. The ideas most often proposed include limiting unnecessary services and restricting access to providers who have not agreed to cut costs.

Each idea seems to have its good and bad points. Often the idea itself is not at issue, but rather where to draw the line.

Cutting Unnecessary Costs

Cutting unnecessary costs is often the first idea proposed when considering how to trim the health care budget. But what is unnecessary to one person may be considered vital to another. For example, if costs are trimmed among administrative personnel, causing delays in service and/or delays in payments for services, many patients may complain. In America we have grown used to the idea of having health care on demand. When we are injured or don't feel well, we want attention and a remedy immediately. Patients who have to wait a week or more for services often express dissatisfaction regarding their health care. Additionally, some patients will refuse to wait, instead seeking care in a hospital emergency room, thus creating higher costs.

What about cutting out procedures which aren't necessary? Currently, the health care system is run on a fee for service basis; that is, providers are paid according to the number of services they provide. This type of system encourages providers to order tests or procedures that may be of limited value in diagnosing or treating the patient. However, the more tests the provider requests, the higher he is paid. Additionally, many patients are uncomfortable with providers who don't prescribe a battery of tests or procedures. They want to be sure the health care provided to them is the best they can get. In the patient's mind, this often means that the more testing provided, the better their overall care must be.

When these factors are added to the threat of malpractice, providers are often reluctant to consider a test or procedure unnecessary if there is any chance that it may benefit the patient.

But at what point does a test become unnecessary? Currently doctors may prescribe an MRI (magnetic resonance imaging) scan of the head for patients who are showing signs of stupor or confusion which indicate a blood clot or other life threatening condition. But they may also often prescribe an MRI for a patient complaining of headaches and dizziness. In only one of every 2,000 cases does this MRI reveal a blood clot or life threatening condition, at a cost of two million dollars per life saved. Whether the cost is justified often depends on whether or not that one life that was or wasn't saved is someone you know.

At what point do you draw the line? If a test or procedure results in a life saved for every $100 of testing done, it is easy to make a determination. But what if the costs were $2,000 or $10,000 for every life saved? At what point does that one life become not worth the cost of testing patients with similar symptoms?

Restricting Access to Providers

Many plans are experimenting with limiting patients to those doctors who have agreed to limit or curb their costs. Some plans pay nothing for a patient who sees a doctor outside the limits set by the plan. Others pay a smaller portion of costs than they normally would (i.e., 70% rather than the 80% they would pay to a provider on their list for the same services).

These types of arrangements (most common in HMOs and PPOs) force a patient to see a specified doctor, perhaps giving up the trusted physician they have seen for years. This has become less of an issue since so many patients have less allegiance to their family physician (due perhaps to frequent moves to a new area or more frequent job changes than in past history). Additionally, many physicians understand that managed care is here to stay and are signing up with HMO and PPO organizations. This creates a situation where patients may not need to change providers even though they change insurance carriers.

But what about the patient that desperately feels they need a second opinion or a referral to a specialist? Are they forced to pay the costs for this care if the original provider is unable to see them, gives them a diagnosis they disagree with, or refuses to refer them to a specialist?

Managed Care

Managed care is the wave of the future. It is touted by experts as one of the ways of gaining control over spiraling health care costs. But what is managed care and how does it work?

Managed care is simply an attempt by insurers to control health care costs using a number of different methods.

Due to the dilemmas listed above, there are many different types of managed care organizations, including Health Maintenance Organizations, Preferred Provider Organizations, Gatekeeper PPOs, Exclusive Provider Organizations, Physician Hospital Organizations, and Management Service Organizations, just to mention a few.

Health Maintenance Organizations

Health Maintenance Organizations (HMOs) are one of the most common managed care trends. Many other managed care models may start with an HMO base and modify it based upon the needs of the members. HMOs are organizations or companies that provide both the coverage for care, and the care itself.

Under an HMO policy, members pay a set amount every month and the HMO agrees to provide all their care, or to pay for the covered care they cannot provide. The HMO hires physicians and sets up hospitals (or contracts with existing physicians and hospitals). The member chooses a specific provider for their care (called a primary care provider or primary care physician (PCP)). This provider is paid a set amount every month to take care of you.

HMOs (and independent providers) are based on the principal that in any given month most of its members will not need treatment. The premium payments these members make will be offset by the treatment the other portion of the membership incurs. Often capitation amounts paid to a physician for a single member are far less than the cost for a single office visit. However, if a physician has 500 members who have chosen him as a PCP, the payments for the 500 people will offset the costs of treating the 50 or so people who seek treatment during any given month.

Members can sign up for HMO coverage through their employer or with an individual policy.

Many HMOs require a copayment amount from the member for each visit, usually a nominal fee of $3 to $20. This is the entire amount the patient must pay. Additionally, members often receive benefits that are not usually covered under regular indemnity service such as yearly physicals, mammograms and pap smears. Another benefit is the lack of paperwork for the patient since the provider completes any paperwork for reimbursement for treatment.

In return, the member is locked into visiting one physician or provider. If the member wishes to see a provider other than their normal provider, they must seek pre-approval from the HMO or must cover the costs themselves. One complaint that many members often have of HMOs is the lack of freedom of choice in choosing providers. Many find the location of HMO facilities inconvenient. Some members also feel there is a reluctance by their providers to give referrals as often as the member feels they should. This is an attempt by the HMO to cut costs by eliminating visits to specialists which they feel are medically unnecessary.

Health Maintenance Organizations are so named because of their initial belief that health care costs could be cut by providing services that maintained and encouraged the health of its members. By adding benefits such as low cost physician visits and yearly check-ups, they felt members would be encouraged to seek medical attention for minor medical problems before they became serious medical emergencies.

Since the provider is paid a set amount according to the number of participants enrolled in his office, it forces the provider to live within a budget. This is far different from the traditional plan whereby providers were paid for each service performed, encouraging them to perform as many tests or procedures as the patient's condition could justify. Traditional insurance has placed limits on how much will be reimbursed (or allowed) for each service performed, however the provider who wished to increase his income simply performed more procedures rather than charged more for the ones he did. Thus, health care costs kept increasing year after year.

With the HMO philosophy, the provider is rewarded for keeping testing and procedures to a minimum while ensuring the health of the patient.

There are several different types of HMO organizations. The most common include:

Staff Model
This is the original concept of HMO services. A physician or provider is hired to work at the HMOs' own facility. They are usually paid a salary and may receive additional bonuses. The provider works only for the HMO and sees no outside patients.

Group Model
The HMO contracts with providers or provider groups to make services available. These practitioners agree to see only HMO members, but they do so at their own facilities.

In the group practice model care is often provided at a centrally located facility. The HMO may have several facilities in the region they service, or just a few, depending on the size and diversity of the population they serve.

The HMO will also own one or more hospitals which provide the inpatient services which members need. These hospitals are owned and run by the HMO and all physicians and other personnel are on staff and paid a salary by the HMO. Any specialists needed to treat the patients are brought in by the HMO.

Some HMOs are contracting with hospitals to take over a specified number of beds, or a wing of an existing hospital, rather than build their own facilities. This is due to the increased costs associated with building a new hospital and the decreased utilization of hospitals. With HMO providers being encouraged to shorten the length of stays at hospitals, some hospitals have only 40% to 50% of their beds filled at any given time. Sharing a facility can be a good way to provide an HMO the resources and treatment options needed while at the same time increasing the revenues of the hospital. HMO personnel are usually used to care for patients at these facilities.

Approximately 85% to 90% of all HMO enrollees are members of a group practice model; however, the enrollment in IPAs is growing.

Independent Practice Associations (IPAs)
Independent Practice Associations (sometimes called Individual Practice Organizations or IPOs) came about in the 1950s in Central California. Concerned by the amount of business the Kaiser-Permanente plan was gaining, several county medical organizations banded together to form their own HMO.

There are two arms to this type of organization. The HMO arm acts as an insurer, oversees the program, enrolls members, collects premiums and handles the claims. The medical groups organize physicians and contract with the HMO for discounted rates on services. The medical group as a whole is paid a capitation amount for each member, and the group oversees the care of the members and attempts to control costs.

The individual physicians (who are members of the medical groups) agree to see patients in their own offices along with their regular fee-for-service clients. The providers were able to easily gather a large number of patients by joining the HMO, and at the same time they retained their autonomy and freedom, unlike the traditional HMO providers who were hired by the HMO and placed on salary.

This type of arrangement allows the HMO to add numerous providers which allows patients a wider freedom of choice. Since providers are paid a capitation amount according to the number of members they see, there is no additional cost to the HMO for adding numerous additional providers.

The providers agree to offer discounted fees to the medical group for their services, and the medical group covers the fees from the capitation amount. In addition to the discounted fees, the individual physicians will usually have a small amount deducted from each claim which is placed into a general fund. This is placed in an escrow account to cover any unexpected fees the medical group or HMO might run into. Any excess money in the escrow fund at the end of the year would be reimbursed to the physicians as a bonus.

The medical groups create their own cost-control measures and some are more successful than others. For those who pay their physicians a capitation amount, the physicians seem to do very well at managing their own costs. However, some still pay the physicians on a discounted fee-for service basis. These providers still gain higher rewards by performing more services with less chance to limit costs.

With the fee-for-service type physician, HMOs reacts by performing utilization reviews that attempt to limit unnecessary treatment. Pre-authorization, or prior approval, for hospital stays may also be required. However, these measures alone do not limit costs since providers still receive a fee for each treatment or test performed. Providers are now making sure to substantiate the reasons for each test or treatment, but are continuing to utilize more services than in group HMO practices. Because of these increased costs, some IPA-type HMOs often have higher premiums than group practice HMOs.

Network Model

In this instance the HMO contracts with several providers in a given area, allowing some overlap in a geographic region This allows more of a choice for subscribers and allows an HMO to increase its subscriber base without worrying about unduly overloading a single provider. In the network model, providers see not only the HMO members, but continue to see their regular fee-paying patients as well.

There are two payment types within HMOs, those that utilize capitation, and those that pay according to services provided. **Capitation** is the practice of paying a provider a set amount per month for the treatment of a patient. The provider is paid each month, regardless of whether or not the patient visits the provider. The savings of being paid for those that don't visit is usually offset by those people who require more treatment than the average member.

HMO Coverage

Most HMOs offer a higher level of coverage than traditional indemnity plans. For example, not only do HMOs cover physician visits and necessary testing, but treatment by a specialist (when the patient is referred by their PCP) is also often covered. HMOs also tend to cover prenatal care, emergency care, home health care, skilled nursing care, drug and alcohol abuse treatment, physical therapy, allergy treatment and inhalation therapy, often to a higher degree than coverage provided by indemnity plans. Most physician visits require a small copayment from the member, usually between $3 and $20.

Hospitalization is covered in full by many plans. However, many plans require a copayment. A $100 per day copayment for the first five days is not uncommon. If a patient is seen in the emergency room there is often a $25 to $30 copayment.

Additionally, HMOs often cover preventive services. Preventive coverage includes items such as an annual physical, cancer screening (pap smears, mammograms, etc.), flu shots, immunizations, and well-baby care. Many also cover health education, cessation of smoking classes, nutrition counseling (especially for diabetics and those needing weight control) or exercise classes. Traditional indemnity plans either limit or restrict coverage of such services.

Eye exams for both children and adults are covered by most HMOs; however, additional vision services (glasses, contacts, etc) may not be.

For those plans that cover prescription drugs there is often a small copayment required from the member ($3 to $5) for each prescription. Prescriptions are often limited to a 30-day supply, but many HMOs have no limit to the number of prescriptions which may be filled in a month.

Mental health treatments often requires a higher copayment than physician visits ($15 to $25) and are often limited to short-term care. There are also limits on the number of visits (often 20 a year).

Physical therapy is often covered only for a brief period of time (six to ten weeks) and only if significant improvement is expected for the patient.

Controversial or experimental procedures (i.e., temporomandibular joint (TMJ) surgery, laser surgery, and gastric stapling) are often not covered. Cosmetic procedures are virtually never covered.

Likewise, coverage is generally not provided for nontraditional treatments. These can include treatments provided by chiropractors, homeopaths, naturopaths and reflexologists. Some states mandate coverage for certain providers (i.e., California law mandates that chiropractic care be covered). In such instances such care will usually be covered (if deemed medically necessary). However, the HMO may not have such practitioners on staff and the patient may need to be referred to an outside provider.

Treatments provided by non-licensed or certified practitioners are usually not covered.

Those HMOs which are federally qualified must provide the following minimum benefits:
1. Preventive care.
2. All hospital inpatient services with no limits on costs or days.
3. Hospital outpatient diagnosis and treatment services, including rehabilitative services, with some limitations.
4. Skilled nursing home and home health care services.
5. Short-term detoxification treatment for drug and alcohol abuse.
6. Medical treatment and referral for substance abuse.

Preferred Provider Organizations

Preferred provider organizations (PPOs) are the second most common managed care alternative with HMOs. They are, in essence, a hybrid mix of HMO and indemnity plan philosophies.

The insurance carrier contracts with providers to join their "network." These providers agree to provide services at a reduced amount in exchange for the referrals from the carrier. Additionally, the carrier agrees to reimburse providers in their network at a higher percentage than providers outside their network.

In a PPO, the insurance carrier will contract with a group of hospitals and/or physicians to provide services at a set fee for each service. Some services may be covered by a capitation amount (like the HMOs). Those fees that are not covered by the capitation amount will be billed on a discounted basis to the carrier.

Many services will be covered by the insurance carrier in full. Other services will have a standard coinsurance percentage (i.e., 80%).

However, this option allows patients more freedom of choice. Patients can choose to go to a provider who has not contracted with the insurance carrier (a non-network provider), but they must pay more. Usually, the patient is responsible for a higher coinsurance amount (i.e., the insurance pays only 70% instead of the normal 100% or 80%) and there may be additional deductibles or other amounts the patient is responsible for. Additionally, when a patient sees a provider within the group, claims forms are usually taken care of between the provider and the insurance carrier. When a patient sees an outside practitioner they may be required to handle and submit their own paperwork to the insurance carrier.

Gatekeeper PPOs

A **gatekeeper PPO** works much the same as a regular PPO. However, patients must choose a regular provider. Those who wish to consult a specialist or receive additional tests or procedures must get prior approval from their regular provider. Their regular provider acts as a "gatekeeper" and determines whether a referral to a specialist is necessary. If a patient chooses to go to a specialist or requests services that have not been approved by their regular provider, they must pay for the cost of these services themselves.

When a referral is approved or given, the specialist may or may not be in the same network group as the regular physician.

Exclusive Provider Organization

In the Exclusive Provider Organization (EPO), the patient must select a PCP and can use only physicians who are part of the network or who are referred by the PCP. EPO providers are paid as services are rendered.

Physician Hospital Organization

A Physician Hospital Organization (PHO) is an organization of physicians and hospitals that bands together for the purpose of obtaining contracts from payor organizations. The PHO bargains as an entity for preferred provider status with various payors. The organization also refers clients to each other.

Management Service Organization

A Management Service Organization (MSO) is a separate corporation set up to provide management services to a medical group for a fee. Individual physicians and providers contract with the MSO for services. An MSO may be owned by a single hospital, several hospitals, or investors.

Self-Insurance

Many employers are turning to a concept called self-insurance. Instead of paying monthly premiums to an insurance carrier, they place the money in an escrow account. When an employee receives medical attention they submit the claim to their employer and are reimbursed according to the terms of the employer's contract.

This idea works well for employers with large numbers of employees, but not for those with fewer employees. For example, a company with only ten employees who is paying $1,000 a month in health care premiums would have $12,000 in their account for use each year. One employee with a catastrophic illness could wipe out this account with only a few weeks of treatment.

However, if the employer has 1000 employees, with premiums of $100,000 a month, the account would receive a total of $1,200,000 during the year, which is more than enough to handle most cases.

Additionally, these plans are not regulated by the insurance industry. Therefore, a company can change the terms of the policy with little or no warning, and there is little or no recourse for employees who disagree with the payment of a claim.

These companies, in essence, create their own little insurance company. They must hire employees to oversee the collection of premiums from employees (if any), the accounting of the department, the processing of claims, and all other aspects an insurance company covers with perhaps the exception of a marketing department. These additional employees generate additional costs.

To sidestep these costs, some companies hire Administrative Services Only (ASO) companies or Third Party Administrators (TPAs) to handle the processing of claims. The employee sends any claims directly to the ASO, and may not even know that the plan is self-funded by their employer. This often happens in the cases of large insurance carriers which have an ASO arm, such as Blue Cross/Blue Shield. The ASO handles the paperwork, processes the claims, and pays benefits out of the escrow account.

Companies who choose to go with a self-insurance plan run the risk that their employees may utilize more care than the premiums they would have paid. They could then loose money. However, by tightening controls or altering benefits, they can keep costs under control.

They can also help save costs by offering "wellness incentives." These include stop-smoking programs, diet and nutrition education, and exercise programs. They can also judge the efficiency of these programs.

One reason this strategy works is that employees tend to be healthier, as a whole, than the general population. There are no elderly, and most of the people are well enough to show up to work on a regular basis.

Many self-insurance plans also buy the services of a "reinsurance" company. This is basically an insurance policy which protects the company against catastrophic medical costs levied against their plan, either by a single employee or by all employees as a whole. This protects the employer in cases of a company disaster (i.e., plant collapsing and injuring numerous workers, fire, chemical poisoning, etc.), a non-work related disaster (i.e., earthquake, flood, tornado, with numerous injuries to employees and their families), or in a generally unhealthy year.

Billing Managed Care

Providers who treat patients covered by nearly all types of PPOs and self-insurance plans create the same bills they would for any other insured patient.

The main difference is in pre-approvals and in the patient's choice of providers.

Billing HMOs

HMOs however, have specific rules and regulations which must be followed regarding the keeping of patient charts, determining member eligibility and all other pertinent data. These rules will be set forth in a Policies and Procedures manual which will be given to each provider/group/IPA upon the signing of a contract with the HMO. It is important that all office staff understand the rules and regulations contained within this manual in order to abide by the contractual obligations of the HMO.

Disobeying any of the rules could result in substantial loss of revenue to the provider, or in termination of their contract with the HMO.

The Membership Card

Upon enrollment, each HMO member is issued a membership card. This card shows the member's name and will contain a record number or other means of identifying the patient. Often there will be a magnetic strip on the back of the card which will have additional information encoded on it.

The membership card may also list a plan number or type which will indicate the benefits covered for this individual.

The reverse of the card contains the magnetic strip and may show contact numbers for authorization of emergency treatment.

If an HMO member transfers from one medical group to another, or changes their benefits, the HMO may issue a new membership card.

Whenever a member seeks treatment, the provider should check the identification card to verify eligibility and to insure that the correct patient chart has been pulled. If necessary, the provider may request an additional piece of identification to insure that the person using the card is actually the member to whom it was assigned.

Eligibility Rosters

Since the membership card is retained by the patient and remains unchanged from month to month, most HMOs will issue an **eligibility roster** to assist the provider in determining who is eligible for treatment. These rosters list those patients who have chosen the provider as their PCP. There will often be several different rosters.

The active member roster lists those whose coverage has continued into the next month. This usually means the insured or their employer has paid the monthly premium to continue coverage for another month.

The new member roster shows those patients who have signed up for HMO coverage and have chosen the provider as their PCP. In addition to members who have just begun coverage, the new member roster shows those existing patients who have recently chosen this provider as their PCP.

The terminated member roster shows those members whose coverage has been terminated or who have chosen to terminate this provider as their PCP. For those whose eligibility has terminated, this list is most accurate for those whose coverage is handled by their employer. In such a case, the employer will notify the HMO that the employee is no longer with the company and that their benefits are being terminated.

There may be those clients who do not show up on any of the rosters. This may be because they have not formally terminated their coverage; however, they did not pay their monthly premium prior to the time the rosters were created. If a patient does not show up on any of the lists, and is seeking treatment, contact the HMO to verify that they are still eligible for coverage prior to providing services. If they are still eligible for coverage, see the following guidelines under SUPPLEMENTAL CAPITATION to insure that the provider receives the capitation amount for these patients.

Be sure to verify that the member is eligible for service for the month and that they have chosen this provider as their PCP, the amount of their copayment, and the correct group or plan number they are covered under. The group or plan number will determine which services are covered by the capitation amount and which services should be billed to the HMO.

The roster may also contain information in addition to the patient's name. This may include identifying information such as social security number, date of birth, gender, insurance information such as covered benefits, the employer group number, the plan effective date, and other data.

Member rosters are the primary means of identifying eligibility for a patient. The medical group should verify the member's eligibility every time they seek treatment. If the medical group provides services without verifying eligibility, the medical group is at financial risk for the services it provides and may not receive reimbursement from the HMO.

Copayment Amounts

HMOs do not have deductibles which must be satisfied each year. Instead, they have **copayment** amounts which the member pays at each visit.

The eligibility roster, or the group designation chart, will identify the services covered by the capitation amount. It will also identify the copayment amount which should be collected from the patient for each visit. This copayment is per provider visit. Therefore, if a patient sees one provider in a medical group and is referred to a different provider within that group, the group should collect the copayment twice, once for each visit with each provider. If this money is not collected at the time of the visit, the provider must absorb the loss of this amount.

Copayment amounts may be different for different services. For example, the member may have a $10 copayment for outpatient visits, and a $20 copayment for inpatient visits. For this reason it is important to check the contract for each of the services performed.

For purposes of copayments, services are often broken into the following five categories:

- Outpatient services, including physician office visits, outpatient lab and radiology, outpatient surgery, durable medical equipment, home health services, etc.,
- Inpatient services, including facility charges, drugs, anesthesia, inpatient laboratory and radiology, emergency services, etc.,
- Pharmacy and prescription services,
- Vision care services, and
- Dental care services.

Some contracts may not cover some of these services (i.e., vision and dental care), and some contracts may not cover items which are listed under a specific type of service (i.e., durable medical equipment).

Occasionally, there may be two designated copayment amounts due to the different types of services performed in a single visit. In such a case, only one copayment should be collected from the member. Most groups/IPAs will collect the higher of the two amounts.

HMO System:

PATIENTS
- Choose an HMO and contract with that HMO to provide all medical care for a set monthly premium,
- Choose a provider who has contracted with the HMO as their primary care physician, and
- Visit the chosen primary care physician for all medical needs unless an emergency situation exists, and pay a copayment for each medical visit.

HMOS
- Collects premiums from patients,
- Contracts with providers to provide certain services,
- Oversees quality of care, and
- Authorizes and pays for services not covered by the doctor's capitation plan.

PROVIDERS
- Provide all capitated care for patients,
- Refer patients to specialists when needed,
- If specialist services are not covered by capitation, obtains authorization for referral from HMO, and
- If specialist services are covered by capitation, provides reimbursement (payment) to the specialist from their capitation amount.

GROUPS/IPA
- Contract with providers to join a group so they have greater bargaining power with the HMOs, and
- Contract with the HMOs to provide care for HMO patients in a specified region.

SPECIALISTS
- Treat patients referred by provider and authorized by provider or HMO, and
- Bill provider or HMO for services, and may sign a contract with the provider or HMO to limit his charges for services to managed care patients.

Patient Encounter Forms

The group/IPA must report all patient encounters (i.e., visits) to the HMO. This is true regardless of whether the visit occurs at the group/IPA, or at one of its contracted providers. This reporting is often done using an encounter form. If the group/IPA does not have data regarding an encounter (which may happen if they are not contractually obligated to cover the services), but they receive information regarding the encounter, they should report what they know of the encounter to the HMO.

The HMO may specify the use of a designated form for reporting encounters, or they may use the CMS-1500.

Encounters for consultation, second opinions and other outside visits should be reported prior to adjudication and/or payment of the claim.

Some HMOs have their providers or group/IPAs report patient encounters on a CMS-1500. When this is done, the only difference between this and a normal CMS-1500 is in item 24F, the charges. If the charges are covered by a capitation amount, then there is no charge for these services. Therefore, the indicated charges will be $0. The total charges and the balance due will, likewise, be $0.

If there are services which a provider renders which are not covered by the normal capitation amount, the amount for these charges should be placed in item 24F. Some HMOs may have providers or group/IPAs submit charges that are the HMO's responsibility on a separate claim form from those that are covered under capitation. Thus, two claim forms for the same provider, patient and dates of service may be necessary.

Groups/IPAs

Medical groups are a group of physicians who are signed under or work for the same company. **Independent Physician Associations (IPAs)** are groups of providers who have banded together for the sole purpose of signing a contract with an HMO.

Most HMOs require the group or IPA to have a certain number of physicians in varying specialties. For example, they must often have a general practitioner or internist, a pediatrician, an obstetrician/gynecologist, a cardiologist, etc. This allows the group to treat all aspects of the patient's care and to provide appropriate services to all members who choose that group/IPA as their PCP.

HMO to Group/IPA Risk
HMOs often use existing providers to deliver care to their patients by signing the providers to contracts. They introduce a mechanism for financial risk-sharing by providing cost incentives to providers in order to contain their expenditures (i.e., the provider is paid a set amount, regardless of the services they provide to the patient).

In many HMO situations, the risk for patient services is shared between the group/IPA and the HMO. The contract between the HMO and the group/IPA will outline who is responsible for what services and any conditions or limitations that apply to those services.

Risk determinations are usually considered to be:

- No risk contracts for which the HMO collects and keeps the monthly capitation amount, and merely pays providers on a fee-for-service basis for the treatment rendered to members. This is similar to a regular insurance carrier set-up, except that the member pays only the copay amount, no deductibles or copayment percentage. This arrangement is almost never seen.
- Partial risk--the HMO is responsible for most services; however, the capitation covers basic services.
- Shared risk--the HMO and the group/IPA share the responsibility for services. A contract will designate which services or treatments are covered by the HMO and which are covered by the provider.
- Full risk--the group/IPA is responsible for most, if not all of the services. The HMO is just in the business of selling policies and writing contracts with groups/IPAs.

Most HMO contracts with providers are on a shared-risk basis. The HMO will provide a list to the group/IPA of all possible services (often indicated by CPT® codes and descriptions, and an indication of who is responsible for those services **(see Figure 10 – 1).** A letter code will often designate who is responsible for payment for that service (i.e., G = Group/IPA responsibility, H = HMO responsibility, etc.).

If an HMO offers numerous different types of policies (i.e., group coverage, individual coverage, Medicare HMO coverage, etc.), then each of these plans may be listed on the same sheet. It is important for the biller to be sure they are looking at the correct procedure code and the correct plan to determine who is financially responsible for a service.

This document will also list any services which are denied and the appropriate copayment amount for many of these services. It is important to note that if the plan is a Medicare HMO, any services which are normally covered by Medicare should be covered services under the HMO contract (regardless of whether the group or the HMO has financial responsibility). Therefore, if Medicare determines that they will begin covering a specific type of treatment, then the HMO Medicare contract must also begin covering that type of treatment.

Group/IPA to Physician Risk

In addition to the HMO transferring all or part of the risk to the group/IPA, the group/IPA may transfer some or all of their risk to an individual capitated provider as well. The levels of risk transferred to the capitated provider include:

- No risk--The group/IPA keeps the entire capitation payment and providers are paid on a fee-for-service basis. There are usually no withholds or bonuses as part of the provider's contract. However, there will often be a fee schedule incorporated as part of the contract agreement, so the amount the provider receives for services will be determined by the fee schedule.

- No referral risk transferred--This means that all or part of the payment to the provider involves risk, but that the risk is not tied to referrals. Only the capitation amount, bonuses and withholds are at risk (i.e., the provider may perform more services than the capitation, withholds and bonuses cover). Under this arrangement, referral means any service not provided for by the provider. Essentially, it is expected that the capitation, withholds and bonuses are the only payments for any and all care which the provider renders to the member. The provider is not responsible for paying for referrals, and the amount of money paid to the provider is not affected by the decision of the provider to make referrals to other providers.

- Referral risk is transferred, but is not substantial--This means that part of the payment to the provider is dependent on the decisions the provider makes to refer patients to other providers. However, that part of the payment is not substantial (i.e., is under 25%). Therefore, if this type of provider makes too many patient referrals

to other providers, up to 25% of his or her capitation amount may be withheld.

- Substantial risk for referrals is transferred, but stop-loss protection is in place--If more than 25% of total payments to the provider are at risk for referrals, the medical group/IPA must have aggregate or per-patient stoploss protection in place. **Stoploss** protection means that if the costs to the provider exceed a specified amount, the provider will be reimbursed by the group/ IPA for at least 90% of expenditures over that amount.

In general, the higher the risk that is transferred to the provider, the higher the capitation amount. If less risk is transferred to the provider, the group/IPA keeps a higher percentage of the capitation amount to cover its expenses.

Capitation Payments

Capitation refers to a monthly payment made to a provider. When a contract is signed between an HMO and a provider, an agreement is made regarding a capitated fee. This fee is often dependent upon the type of plan the patient is covered under. Varying factors such as the gender and age of the patient and their overall health may also be considered. The provider and HMO will also agree which services are covered by the capitation amount.

Often, capitation amounts pay for all the basic treatment the patient needs during the month. If the patient does not see the physician that month, the physician keeps the fee. If the patient becomes ill and requires treatment, the physician is expected to provide the necessary services without additional compensation by the HMO. Usually, the amount saved and the extra amount spent balances out.

The capitation amount for each provider is determined by those who are included on either the active or new member roster. The PCP usually receives capitation payments for the prior month. The amount of the capitation payment will vary according to the coverages or plans which have been selected. Additional amounts may be provided for patients who have entered a hospice or skilled nursing care facility, as well as those who have been diagnosed with specific diseases (i.e., HIV or ESRD) (see the Additional Capitation Section).

The HMO may withhold a portion of the monthly capitation amount to protect the HMO from inadequate patient care or financial management by the PCP. They may also withhold a portion to insure the quality of care given to patients and promptness of payments to outside providers. This amount is outlined in the contract signed by the group and the HMO.

For example: The 123 HMO withholds 3% of the capitation amount to cover financial insolvency and unpaid claims by the group/IPA. If all obligations have been met, this amount will be returned when the group terminates its contract with the HMO. Additionally, the 123 HMO will withhold 5% of the capitation for its Medical Management Incentive Program. This program stipulates that the 5% will be reimbursed to the group/IPA if the following guidelines are met:

- 25% of the withheld amount will be reimbursed if the group/IPA has submitted less than their budgeted amount of hospital expenses which are covered by the HMO.
- 10% of the amount will be reimbursed for customer satisfaction. The HMO will randomly survey patients to determine their satisfaction with the provider and the services rendered. If the provider is above the average in customer satisfaction, he or she will receive this amount.
- 10% of the withheld amount will be reimbursed for low disenrollment. If the provider/group maintains less than 2% disenrollment (those terminating HMO coverage or transferring to another provider), then they will receive this amount.
- 40% of the withheld amount will be reimbursed for quality of care. This will be determined by a review of medical records by the HMO. If the Medical Review Panel agrees with the treatment given at least 80% of the time, the provider will receive this amount.
- 15% of the withheld amount will be reimbursed for protocol compliance. This is calculated as follows:

- o 5% for compliance with all facility requirements as determined by an audit of the facility.
- o 5% for timeliness of claim payments.
- o 5% for timeliness in submission of all contractually required statements to the HMO.

If the provider meets all the stipulations outlined, they will keep the 5% quality care amount.

You can see how the things you do as a biller may affect the amount the provider receives in his or her monthly capitation check. If you are rude to a patient and a complaint is made, or a member chooses to transfer to another provider, it could cost the group/IPA. If you do not process claim payments promptly, submit statements to the HMO on time, or let the providers in the group know that they are near the limit on their hospital costs, there will be additional amounts withheld. It is important that the biller understand all factors that can cause withholding from the provider's capitation amounts and do their best to see that the goals are met for compliance with HMO guidelines.

Supplemental Capitation

On occasion, an eligible member will not appear on the eligibility rosters. The biller should keep a list of all eligible patients seen by the provider. If at any time a patient does not show up on an eligibility roster, the biller should contact the HMO to find out why.

There may be a legitimate reason (i.e., the patient has transferred to another PCP, but you have not yet received the transfer paperwork), or the patient may have been inadvertently left off the list.

If you discover a patient who should have been on the list and was not included, contact the HMO to determine the correct procedure for having the patient put on the list. Additionally, ask what paperwork needs to be filed by the provider to receive the capitation amount for this patient. Since the capitation amount is only paid for those patients on the eligibility roster, the provider has not received capitation amounts for anyone who is not on the rosters.

Covered Services	MEDICARE		COMMERCIAL						
	Standard	Medi-Medi	AMG	Rocky	CAT	MIPC	CAIT	SBA	RICE
Abortion - Elective (CPT 59840 - 59841) Note: Refer to Super Panel contracts for financial responsibility for specific procedures	G/P[1]	G/P[2]	G/P[2]	G/P[1]	G/P[2]	G/P[2,3]	G/P[4]	G/P[4]	G/P[4]
Abortion - Therapeutic (CPT 59812 - 59857) If the life of the mother could be endangered if the fetus is carried to term, or in cases of fetal genetic defect.	-	G	G	G	G	G	G	G	G
Acupuncture	-	-	-	-	-	-	-	-	G
Acute Care									
• Facility Component	G	G	G	G	G	G	G	G	G
• Hospital Based Physicians, including clinical and anatomical pathologist (CPT 80002 - 83999), radiologist (CPT 70010 - 76499), anesthesiologist (CPT 00100 - 01999, 99100 - 99140)	P	P	P	P	P	P	P	P	P
• Professional Component, including consultations and follow up care visits (CPT 99217 - 99239, 99251 - 99275)	G	G	G	G	G	G	G	G	G
• Closed panel physicians under contract with a hospital for test reading (e.g. EKG)[5]	P	P	P	P	P	P	P	P	P
• Special services and reports, miscellaneous (CPT 99000 - 99090, 99175 - 99199)	G	G	G	G	G	G	G	G	G

[1]Not covered except in cases of rape or incest, or when the life of the mother would be endangered if the fetus were brought to term.
[2]Covered for the first thirteen (13) weeks of pregnancy only.
[3]Copay for HIPC is the same as for in-patient hospitalization.
[4]Covered through the second trimester (24 weeks) of pregnancy only.
[5]Plan to confirm closed panel status.

Legend: G = Medical Group Responsibility; P = Plan/HMO Responsibility; G/P = Shared Responsibility; -- = Not Covered

This chart shows a sampling of CPT codes and the party that bears responsibility for covering costs for each procedure under numerous different plans. It is important to check the correct column for the plan being processed to determine if services are covered or not.

Figure 10 – 1: Distribution of Responsibility

Often the HMO will require you to fill out a Supplemental Capitation Request form. An example of this form is included in **Figure 10 – 2.** The form is rather simple, requesting only the member's name, their type of coverage and their membership number.

The patient list should be compared with the eligibility roster as soon as the eligibility roster is received from the HMO. Many HMOs have very strict deadlines as to when the forms must be submitted in order to receive capitation amounts for someone left off the list.

The procedures for filing these forms should also be followed in the case of a patient who comes in for treatment and is not on the eligibility roster. The provider has not received the monthly capitation payment for these patients.

Additionally, there will be many patients who sign up for HMO coverage, but do not immediately choose a PCP. These people may not choose a PCP until they feel the need for treatment. At that time they will choose a provider and will be added to that provider's new member roster.

The billing office should contact the new members as soon as possible to determine how long they have been a member and what precipitated their decision to choose this provider as their PCP. If they have been an HMO member for a while, but simply had not requested a specific provider, the HMO has been keeping the capitation amounts for that patient and not assigning them to a specific provider. The contract between the provider and the HMO, or the HMO and the member, may stipulate that the HMO will assign a PCP to any enrollee who does not choose one within a specified time. If this is not being done, the physician/group should be notified that they may want to contact the HMO regarding the matter. They may be due additional patients (and capitation amounts), from new members who should be assigned to a PCP.

Additional Capitation Amounts

Many HMOs will pay an amount in addition to the regular capitation amount for those patients who have been diagnosed with certain illnesses or whose illness or condition has required them to enter a hospice or skilled nursing facility.

It is the responsibility of the provider to inform the HMO of changes in the patient's status in order to receive the additional reimbursement. The biller should consult the HMO's Policy and Procedure Manual to determine which conditions allow for additional reimbursement and which form to file to obtain this reimbursement. The biller should then make a list of those conditions which qualify for additional reimbursement and the time limits and other conditions for applying for the reimbursement.

As with supplemental capitation, there are usually specific forms and deadlines which must be met in order for a provider to receive the additional capitation. For example, if the deadline for submitting the paperwork is not met, the HMO may refuse to add the additional capitation amount until the following month and the provider forfeits the additional capitation for the current and preceding months.

Billing for Services

While the monthly capitation amount covers most services, some services will be reimbursed on a fee for service basis. This means that the provider will bill the HMO for these services when they are performed. Most agreements between a provider and an HMO will have a list of those services which are covered by the capitation amount, and/or those which are considered to be on a fee-for-service basis. Fee-for-service procedures are billed on a CMS-1500 or superbill the same as non-HMO services.

The medical biller should familiarize themselves with those services which are covered and those which are billed prior to treating a patient. They should also collect the copayment amount from the patient prior to treatment being rendered by the provider.

Patient Charts

Patient charts for HMO covered patients are the property of the HMO, not the provider. As such, the HMO will dictate the specific order and types of forms which can be used in the patient chart.

When the HMO requires specific forms, they will often provide copies of these forms to the provider. The billing department needs to be aware of the difference between these charts and the charts which are for their regular patients. The HMO forms should not be used for patient charts of non-HMO members.

The Patient's Medical Record

The patient's medical record is a legal document. However, unlike regular insurance patients, the medical record of an HMO patient belongs to the HMO, not to the physician. This allows the record to be transferred between physicians when the patient transfers their care. When a member disenrolls from the HMO, the patient's record must be returned to the HMO.

Because of the transient nature of the medical record, it is more important than ever that all services, contacts or information be documented in the patient's chart.

The HMO may require the provider to use specific forms and/or to keep the information in the chart in a specific order. All rules given by the HMO should be followed.

If the physician feels a need to maintain a copy of the patient chart for his or her own files, a second copy should be made for this purpose. The original document remains the property of the HMO. It is suggested that when a patient transfers their care or disenrolls, the biller should make a complete copy of the patient chart for the practice's files. This chart should be clearly labeled as a copy of the medical record. It should also note that this patient was disenrolled or transferred, the date of the disenrollment or transfer, where the original of the chart was sent, and the date the copies were made. No changes should be made to this chart after this date without those changes being clearly labeled as changes, a notation of when the changes were made, and the initials of the person making those changes.

No loose papers or self-stick notes should be placed in the patient file. All data should be clearly written on forms and attached in the chart using fasteners.

A patient's medical record may be considered inactive when the patient has not been seen for a period of two years.

If a member has disenrolled from a practice or transferred to another practice (as shown by the eligibility rosters), the biller should contact the HMO and request what to do with the patient's chart.

HMO Appointment Scheduling

The HMO will usually dictate the maximum amount of time a patient must wait for an appointment (i.e., the appointment must be scheduled within four weeks of the patient's request for an appointment). Different time frames may be given for routine appointments and for urgent care appointments.

Many HMOs require that there be a certain number of appointments set aside for emergencies. This allows a patient to be seen within 24 hours if an emergency situation arises. All decisions as to whether a patient should be seen immediately are the responsibility of the patient and the provider. At no time should a medical biller attempt to determine the emergent nature of the patient's condition. All triage and assessment, including over the phone, should be performed only by a licensed medical provider.

It is important that these time frames be met. Failure to do so could result in sanctions against the provider. Numerous sanctions could result in the provider losing their contract with the HMO.

If the provider is unable to meet the patients request for an appointment within the allotted time, the provider should refer the patient to another appropriate provider who can see the patient within the allotted time. The charges for this appointment will be the responsibility of the provider.

If you are scheduling elective surgery, whether inpatient or outpatient, you should avoid the ending and the beginning of the month so that eligibility may be cleared. Additionally, many HMOs will insist that the surgical procedure be done on the first day of admission. Any necessary pre-admit testing should be done on an outpatient basis the day before surgery. If this is not possible, the documentation to substantiate the need for an overnight stay prior to surgery should be attached to the Treatment Authorization Request (TAR).

Missed Appointments

Each time a patient misses an appointment; the provider must review the patient's chart and determine the appropriate follow-up activity. This decision should be documented in the patient chart and initialed by the provider. The following are appropriate follow-up activities:

- No follow-up needed. Wait for patient to call for a new appointment.
- Send a letter to the patient advising them that they should call to reschedule an appointment.
- Telephone the patient to reschedule the appointment

Supplemental Capitation Request

TO: _____   FROM: _____
    Provider Network Manager   Medical Group Name and Number

Date Submitted: _____   For Eligibility Month/Year: _____

Member Name	Plan Type	Member Number	DRG/Diagnosis

Figure 10 – 2: Supplemental Capitation Request Form

All follow-up activities must be documented in the patient chart.

If the appropriate follow-up was a letter, the letter should contain the member's name, the date and time of the missed appointment, the reason for the appointment, the provider's name and address, and a phone number where the patient can call to reschedule their appointment.

If the appropriate follow-up is a phone call to reschedule the appointment, record any phone calls or attempts to contact the member in the patient record. This should include the date and time of the call, name and title of the person making the call, and the outcome of the call (i.e., new appointment scheduled, left message, no answer, etc.).

If the physician notes that the patient should be seen as soon as possible, the biller should attempt to contact the member the same day as the missed appointment. The member should then be scheduled for the first available emergency appointment.

If there is no telephone number, or if there has been no contact after three attempts, a letter should be sent to the member requesting that they call the office to reschedule their appointment. A copy of this letter should be placed in the patient chart.

If any correspondence to the patient is returned by the postal service as undeliverable, it should be date stamped and filed in the patient's chart. The doctor should be informed, and a notation of his or her decision of follow-up placed in the patient's chart.

Authorizations, Referrals and Second Opinions

It is important that the medical biller familiarize themselves with the agreement between the HMO and the provider. Often the HMO will require a second surgical opinion (SSO) or a pre-authorization for treatment. If the patient is to be admitted to the hospital, a pre-certification may be required. These items will often have timeliness limits on when they are to be performed. For example, pre-certification must often take place at least five days before a scheduled inpatient admission and emergency treatments require notification to the HMO within 48 hours of admission.

With pre-certification and pre-authorization, the HMO will evaluate the proposed treatment and inform the provider and patient as to whether or not they will cover the services. If the HMO decides that the services are not necessary, they will deny payment. The provider and patient must then decide whether they will abandon the treatment, seek authorization for an alternate treatment, or if they will go ahead with the treatment with the understanding that the patient is completely responsible for the charges.

Pre-authorization

It is important to obtain pre-authorization for services which are the responsibility of the HMO. If these services are performed without pre-authorization, the group/IPA may be responsible for payment of services. Each HMO may have their own specific Treatment Authorization Request (TAR) form.

Often a TAR approval will be valid for a limited time, usually 30 days. If services are not performed within that time you will need to complete an additional TAR and obtain another pre-authorization. In the case of ongoing treatments (i.e., chemotherapy, dialysis), you will often need to obtain monthly authorizations of services covered by the HMO.

If you have not received the authorization back from the HMO within 10 to 15 days, you should contact the HMO. If they never received the TAR, you may need to reschedule the patient and resubmit a new TAR. For this reason it is best to choose a date which is several weeks in the future. However, you should also attempt to avoid the beginning and ending of the month since the patient's eligibility may be changing and the HMO will often insist that all routine follow-up care and/or hospital stays be included in the one authorization.

TARs are often three or four part forms. If not, be sure to make a copy of the TAR for your records before sending it in to the HMO. If you feel additional documentation is necessary to substantiate the need for services, this should be included with the TAR, and firmly attached to it.

If it is not possible to reschedule the patient's surgery due to the nature of the treatment, many HMOs have an emergency request procedure which allows faxing of the TAR and overnight approval. If the patient cannot wait for this approval they should be instructed to go to the emergency room and the hospital will call the HMO and request approval for an emergency admit.

If you list a specific date of surgery on the TAR, surgery must be performed on that date. TARs may not be valid for any dates other than the date listed. In such a case, the group/IPA may be responsible for payment of services, not the HMO.

The HMO will also indicate the number of days allowed for the patient to remain in the hospital (if it is an inpatient admission). If it becomes necessary for the patient to remain in the hospital for a longer period (i.e., due to complications), then the group/IPA should submit a request to the HMO as soon as possible with the documentation to substantiate the need for additional inpatient days.

Different rules may apply for inpatient admission for psychiatric care or chemical dependency.

Utilization Review

Utilization review (UR) is a process whereby insurance carriers review the treatment of a patient and determine whether or not the costs will be covered. Many insurance carriers began creating utilization review departments in an effort to control costs and avoid unnecessary procedures. While this process was started with traditional insurance carriers, managed care carriers have taken the concept a step further, creating complete UR departments and reviewing every outside procedure which may require additional costs and every referral to a specialist.

Many providers dislike the utilization review process. They feel the UR committee cannot always make an effective decision based on the data provided in the medical report. They dislike being second guessed by a committee that is not familiar with the patient and their problems. Many providers have found a need to hire an additional office person just to review medical information over the phone with the insurance companies in order to get their procedures approved.

However, insurance carriers insist that the process has prevented numerous unnecessary surgeries and helped providers to consider alternate forms of treatment which may be as much or more beneficial to the patient.

Additionally, UR committees are becoming more selective in the items and providers they choose to review. Those procedures which are nearly always allowed, such as a cystourethroscopy, are being automatically allowed while more questionable procedures such as MRIs on the knees are being reviewed. Additionally, some insurers are tracking the records of providers. Those that are known for ordering tests or procedures that are nearly always necessary are less closely watched than those who have a history of ordering questionable procedures.

Specialist Referrals

If a member requests to see a specialist, the provider must discuss the request with the member. If the request is denied, the procedures for denial of services must be followed, including the sending of a denial letter to the member.

If the provider agrees with the member's request, or recommends the member to see a specialist, an appropriate referral form should be completed and approved by the medical group/IPA. The decision to refer or not to refer a member is a medical judgment which should be made by the provider and the group/IPA.

The group/IPA must provide a written notice of its decision to the member. If the request is approved, the notice must advise the member of the name, address and phone number of the consultant and either state an appointment time, or inform the member how to schedule an appointment.

The group/IPA is required to have contracts with its specialists. They must maintain contracts with a sufficient number of specialists so that members are not inconvenienced by excessive appointment waiting times. The provider's office should also keep a log of all patients referred to a specialist. This log should include:

- The name of the member or patient,
- The request date,
- The appointment date,
- The referring physician,
- The consulting physician or specialist,
- The problem or reason for the referral,
- The date the report was received from the specialist, and
- Any comments.

This log can help the practice keep track of patients who have been seen by a specialist and whether or not the results of that referral have been received from the specialist.

Denial of Services to Members

If a member requests a specific treatment and the group/IPA feels this treatment or service is not medically necessary, would be detrimental to the patient, or would provide no medical benefit to the patient, they may deny the service (i.e., refuse to perform the treatment). The provider should discuss with the member why they feel these services would not be beneficial to the patient. If the patient wishes to pursue the request, they can ask for a second opinion, or ask the provider to reconsider the treatment.

Second Opinions

Many HMOs have a second opinion policy designed to resolve differences of opinion regarding proposed treatment among providers, members, consultants, and/or the HMO. Second opinions are often provided in the following instances:

- At the request of the member before a surgical or other invasive procedure,
- If the provider's opinion is contrary to the member's expressed expectations, even after the physician has counseled the member,
- If the opinion of the provider differs substantially from the recommended treatment plan of the specialist on the case, or
- At the request of the HMO.

There are several steps to the second opinion process:

1. A request is made by the provider, member, consultant or HMO for a second opinion. This request may be either verbal or in writing.
2. The patient's chart is documented with the request.
3. An internal review is done. This is a second opinion performed by another physician affiliated with the same group/IPA as the provider.
4. If the member is still dissatisfied, or if the two opinions differ substantially, an external review may be performed. This is an opinion provided by a physician who is not a member of the group/IPA to which the member belongs. If the member is still dissatisfied, they should contact the HMO to request the external review. The HMO reviews the records and, if they deem it necessary to have an external review, they will inform the provider and the member. The HMO may send the member to a physician of their choosing.

5. All records are forwarded to the HMO's Chief Medical Officer who makes a determination of the proper course of treatment. The provider will then be informed of the decision and it is their responsibility to carry out the proposed treatment plan. This may mean treating the patient themselves, or referring the member to a specialist for treatment.

Financial responsibility for second opinions is usually split among the group/IPA and the HMO as follows:

1. The group/IPA is responsible for the internal review.
2. The HMO is responsible for the external review unless the group/IPA failed to document the internal review, did not properly complete a TAR and obtain authorization before sending the member for an external review, and/or if the opinion of the external review physician differs substantially from the group/IPA decision.

All activities regarding the second opinion process must be thoroughly documented in the patient's record. Any time the HMO must bear financial responsibility for any services, including the external review, a TAR must be completed and the treatment pre-authorized.

Because of substantial delays in receiving authorizations and/or referrals, and member complaints, some HMOs are now allowing members to refer themselves for a second opinion. However, they are limited to obtaining a second opinion from another provider who is affiliated with the same HMO, and the number of times they may refer themselves for a second opinion is limited (i.e., once every six months).

Denials of Service after a Second Opinion

Once the member has exhausted the second opinion process, or chooses not to proceed with the process (i.e., accepts the decision of the internal review), the group/IPA must send a denial letter to the member. A copy of this letter must also be sent to the HMO with any supporting documentation.

This letter must state the patient's name, the date services were requested, the services that were requested, and the reason for the denial of services.

The HMO will often keep a log of these denials. If they feel a group/IPA is denying too many treatments, they may ask for a review of the record to monitor the quality of care given to the patients.

Member Appeals of Denied Services

Members may appeal any decision which involves the denial of services which they believe should have been performed or covered. This includes the right to appeal decisions both before and after the service has been performed. It also applies to the proposed termination of treatment which the patient is currently receiving (i.e., termination of a hospital stay or continued plan of treatment).

To file an appeal, the member must contact the HMO, usually in writing, and include the following items:

- Patient name,
- Member name (if different from patient),
- Member identification number,
- Member address,
- Phone number,
- Name of medical group/IPA,
- Name of provider,
- Date service was rendered if previously done,
- Complete description of the problem and/or why they feel services should not have been denied, and
- Member signature.

If the member delivers this appeal to the group/IPA, they should be told to mail it to the HMO, or the group/IPA may be required to accept the appeal and mail it to the HMO themselves.

The HMO will review the appeal and all appropriate supporting evidence. They will also look up the denial and supporting evidence that was filed by the group/IPA. This is why it is so important that the group/IPA file their notices of denial in a timely manner and with all necessary supporting documentation.

Within a specified time limit (usually 30 days) the HMO will make a decision regarding the denial of services. If they determine that the services should have been covered or performed, they will instruct the group/IPA to do so. If they uphold the decision of the group/IPA that the services were correctly denied, they will inform the member by letter. A copy of this letter will also be forwarded to the group/IPA and should be placed in the patient's record.

For services that have not yet been performed, some HMOs have an expedited appeal process in which the HMO is required to make a decision within a few days. This expedited appeal process is required to be available to Medicare members, but may also be available to other members.

Member Grievances and Complaints

Grievances are written complaints made by a member regarding quality of services, access to care, interpersonal communication, or any other aspect of their care or relationship with their provider. **Complaints** are verbal expressions regarding the above dissatisfactions. Members may file a grievance or complaint with the provider, the group/IPA or the HMO.

If the member files the grievance or complaint with the provider or the group/IPA, the following steps should be taken:

1. The provider or group/IPA should attempt to resolve the issue through patient counseling, whether in person or over the phone.
2. If the provider or group/IPA is unable to resolve the grievance or complaint, or it is outside his or her scope of responsibility (i.e., the member is dissatisfied with their HMO contract), the provider must refer the grievance to the HMO. There is usually a time limit associated with this procedure. Often the provider must refer the grievance within one working day of receiving it if they are unable to resolve it. For this reason it is imperative that all members of the group/IPA and their staff take complaints from member very seriously.
3. If the grievance or complaint has been resolved at the provider level, the group/IPA must send a letter confirming the resolution of the issue to the member. A copy of this correspondence and any supporting documentation must also be mailed to the HMO.
4. If the provider is unable to resolve the complaint within a specified time limit (i.e., 30 days), they must give the member the opportunity to file a written complaint with the HMO.

5. If the grievance or complaint concerns any aspect of medical care, it must be reviewed by the group/IPA medical director.

Grievance Logs

Often group/IPAs are required to keep a log of all grievances in addition to documenting all grievances in the patient chart. Some HMOs require that a copy of this log be forwarded to them at set intervals (i.e., every 30 days). If a copy of the log is required, but no grievances or complaints have been received, the group/IPA must submit a log with the words "NO GRIEVANCES" printed on it.

The following items are often required on a grievance log:

1. Member name,
2. Member identification number,
3. Date of grievance or complaint,
4. Type of grievance or what the grievance was about, and
5. Date of resolution letter or date referred to HMO.

If numerous grievances or complaints are received the HMO may withhold a portion of the monthly capitation amount, or may terminate their relationship with the group/IPA.

Transfers

A member may transfer from one provider to another at any time. Often, the HMO will require the patient to complete a request for transfer. There will then be a waiting period while the HMO verifies that the member is eligible for coverage and has chosen a provider who is contracted under the member's plan. The transfer will then become effective at the beginning of the next month. Since capitation amounts are paid month to month, this eliminates the need to split a capitation amount between two or more providers.

Usually, if one member of a family chooses to transfer to another medical group as a provider, then all members of the family must transfer to the same medical group. However, each family member may see a different provider within that medical group. This is often the reason that a medical group will be required to have providers of different specialties within their group (i.e., general practitioner, pediatrician, cardiologist, etc.).

Any member requesting a transfer must complete a transfer request form. This form must also be completed if a patient chooses to transfer from one provider to another within the same medical group. Upon receipt of the transfer form, the medical group must forward a copy of the patient's medical records to the HMO. The HMO will then forward them to the new provider. If there is no chart available (i.e., the patient has never visited the provider), then the original provider must inform the HMO that there is no chart on this patient.

If the provider feels a need to have a copy of the patient chart, a copy should be made prior to sending the chart to the HMO. This copy should be notated that the patient has been transferred to XXX facility and the date, and then the entire file should be placed in an "inactive" file. If the biller for a medical group receives a notice that a patient is transferring into their medical group, it is their responsibility to be sure that they have received a copy of the patient's medical record before treating that patient.

Disenrollment

When a patient transfers their care from a provider, they are considered to have "**disenrolled**" from that provider. A patient may disenroll from a provider at any time by requesting a transfer to another provider. A patient may also disenroll from the HMO program by stopping the payment of their premiums or by seeking other insurance coverage.

Because an HMO is responsible for all care given to a patient, there is often no secondary insurance coverage under an HMO. Many HMOs will include a provision in their contract with the patient that states that if the patient enrolls in another HMO or obtains other insurance coverage, their policy with the HMO will be immediately terminated.

HMO Initiated Disenrollment

The HMO may disenroll a member for various reasons. These reasons must have been previously stated in the contract with the member, and verified by documentation by the provider and/or the HMO.

The reasons for disenrollment can include, but are not limited to:

1. The member disregards the enrollment agreement by habitually seeking covered services, other than emergency care, from a provider who is not a contracted provider.
2. The patient/physician relationship has broken down. This can be evidenced by a pattern of broken appointments, refusal to follow physician advice or orders. The HMO may require that the member be referred for psychiatric evaluation prior to initiating this type of disenrollment to insure that the patient can be held mentally competent and legally responsible for their actions.
3. Physical or verbal abuse of the provider or his or her staff. This must often be documented and a police report filed. The HMO may also require these members to be sent for psychiatric evaluation prior to initiating disenrollment.
4. The member moves out of the service area covered by the HMO. By law, HMOs are only allowed to provide service within a designated area. Additionally, they must have the required number of physicians within the designated area to ensure that each patient can receive proper care without excessive travel or undue hardship (i.e., waiting incessantly for appointments).
5. Failure to pay the required monthly premium.

Each pattern of missed appointment, abusive behavior, or failure to follow medical advice must be carefully documented by the provider and made a part of the patient's record.

Once a provider has documented a habitual problem, they may request disenrollment of the patient. This is often accomplished by filing a request for disenrollment form. These forms vary from one HMO to another but usually contain only basic patient information. The request must then be substantiated with documentation. This documentation should include the following:

1. Documentation in the patient record or progress notes showing dates of visits or missed appointments, or a listing of these. There should be a sufficient pattern shown to document the "habitual" nature of the offense.
2. Documentation in the patient record or progress notes or in a grievance log showing the date, time and subject of any counseling the member received from the group/physician's staff in an effort to prevent or repair the breakdown in the relationship.
3. Explanation of why the problem cannot be resolved.
4. If appropriate, a discussion of why a change to another provider is not appropriate or has not been done.
5. Copies of any correspondence sent to the member in an effort to resolve the situation, or to assist the member in understanding the plan procedures (i.e., when to use the emergency room, need for prior authorization, importance of keeping medical appointments, etc.).
6. Evidence the member has demonstrated a total lack of cooperation with the plan, has continued to misuse services, or has been physically or verbally abusive after receipt of the correspondence or other written attempts to correct the problem. In many cases a police report will meet this requirement.
7. Evidence that the non-compliant or abusive member has been referred to a psychiatrist, or reason why this action was not appropriate.

The provider will be required to continue treating the patient until they are officially notified by the HMO that the member has been disenrolled.

The Health Care Financing Administration (HCFA) oversees all Medicare HMOs, and HCFA approval must be obtained before the HMO may disenroll a Medicare patient.

Continuing Care

There are times when a provider or group chooses to terminate their contractual obligation with the HMO. If a physician terminates their contract with the HMO or with the group, the remaining members of that group continue to be responsible for the treatment for that patient. Members are assigned to a group, as well as to a physician within that group, and that relationship will continue regardless of whether one provider removes himself from the group or not.

However, if an entire group/IPA terminates their contract with the HMO, there may be a need for continuation of coverage for some members who were being treated by the terminating group. Continuation of coverage exists when a specified treatment was begun by the terminating group/IPA, and must be continued by the newly assigned provider or group/IPA. For continuing care coverage to exist, the following rules often apply:

- The patient must be involved in a specific treatment plan which has been previously authorized by the medical director of the terminating group/IPA.
- The treatment has a clearly identifiable termination (ongoing treatments for a condition which has no cure (i.e., diabetes) would not be reimbursable under continuing care rules).
- Medical care was terminated due to the group/IPA situation, rather than through any fault of the member.
- If the patient is pregnant, specific rules may apply regarding the length of the gestation and time left to the termination of treatment.

In such cases, the newly assigned group may be allowed additional compensation for the continuing care treatment which is provided to these patients. For example, the provider may be reimbursed by the HMO for each treatment which he provides in relation to the continuing care at the normally contracted rate. The regular capitation amount will apply for all treatments which are provided for a reason other than the continuing care.

Specific rules must be followed to obtain the proper reimbursement, and the Policies and Procedures manual should be checked prior to the rendering of services. For example, in order to qualify for an additional reimbursement under continuing care rules, the provider may need to seek pre-authorization for all treatments.

It is often the responsibility of the group/IPA which receives the member to identify the need for continuing care coverage. These people should be identified as quickly as possible so that proper rules and reimbursement can be applied.

Miscellaneous Services

Certain rules can apply to select types of services under an HMO agreement. These services can include outpatient surgery, emergency room services, durable medical equipment, and prescriptions.

Outpatient Surgery

Some HMOs will provide a list of surgeries that must be performed in an outpatient setting. This is most often done in a shared risk contract when the group/IPA is financially responsible for outpatient services and the HMO is responsible for inpatient services.

It is important to know which surgeries must be performed on an outpatient basis. If these guidelines are not followed, the group/IPA may be financially responsible for all inpatient costs in relation to the surgery.

The biller should be aware of this list and keep it handy. If he or she receives a TAR for services that should be performed on an outpatient basis, but the provider is requesting inpatient authorization, inform the provider immediately. If the provider feels the surgery should be done inpatient due to complications or other circumstances, the documentation for these circumstances should accompany the TAR.

Emergency Room Services

If the group/IPA is considered financially responsible for emergency room services, then they are responsible for managing the member's utilization of ER services and for paying for the cost of these services. The group must provide written information to its members on how to access these services. The group/IPA must have procedures for the authorization of these services. Payment may not be denied based on lack of notification or lack of authorization for these services.

If the member seeks emergency room services from a non-contracted provider, the group/IPA usually has 30 minutes to respond from the time of the non-contracted provider's first call. Lack of response means that the emergency room may provide whatever services it deems necessary to treat the emergency situation and the group/IPA is obligated to pay for _all_ charges.

Therefore, if a biller receives a call requesting authorization for emergency services, it is important that he or she transfer the call to the appropriate person immediately, or get any necessary information so that the provider may return the call as quickly as possible. The biller should not authorize or deny services. The authorization or denial of services should be done only by a licensed medical professional.

Durable Medical Equipment

All durable medical equipment (DME) must be ordered and prescribed by the physician for the patient use. If the financial responsibility for durable medical equipment rests with the group/IPA or HMO, it is imperative that authorization be obtained as soon as possible. Requests and prescriptions for durable medical equipment must include a specified time period. Often HMOs will only authorize the rental of DME for a month at a time. Thus, the authorization must be requested each and every month for patients with chronic conditions (i.e., a glucometer for a diabetic). Also, each request for DME must be on a separate prescription or authorization request form. Thus, it is possible for one patient to have several outstanding DME authorizations (i.e., for oxygen, bed, wheelchair). Each specific DME request will be assessed based upon member eligibility and medical necessity. Therefore, it may be necessary to include a copy of the documentation with each DME request.

Prescription Coverage

When an HMO offers prescription coverage to a member, there are often limitations:

1. The member must purchase the drugs from an HMO contracted facility. If they obtain prescriptions from a non-contracted pharmacy, the member will bear the cost of the pharmacy services. There may be exceptions to this rule for emergency situations, or situations where the patient is outside the service area, or the prescription is not available from a contracted pharmacy.
2. They may limit drugs and medications to a 30-day supply.
3. They will only cover prescription drugs. Over the counter medications are not covered.
4. They may only include oral and topical drugs. Injectable drugs are often not covered under the pharmacy benefit. They

may, however, be covered under the medical benefit. This is especially true for injectable medications which the patient needs for survival (i.e., insulin for a diabetic).
5. They may also insist that the generic equivalent of a drug be prescribed if it is available. If there is no generic equivalent, the HMO will often cover the brand name at the standard copayment amount. However, if there is a generic equivalent, the HMO may only cover the cost of the generic equivalent. Thus, the member will be charged the standard copay, plus the difference between the generic and the brand name medication.

Some generic drugs are not the same as their brand name counterparts. They may have a similar, but different active ingredient, or they may be in a different dosage amount from the brand name drug. In such a case they are not considered to be therapeutically equivalent. For these drugs, the HMO may require the physician to prescribe the generic drug, or they may allow the full benefit for the brand name drug.

Facility Requirements

At any given time a group/IPA must be able to provide information about its patient population, the types of health plans accepted and the percentage of patients covered under Medicare, Medicaid, commercial plans, cash patients and HMO covered patients. This information may be required by the HMO at any time, so it is imperative that medical record keepers determine these amounts every month.

This is most easily done by keeping a log of all patients who transfer into and out of a practice during the month (see Figure 10 – 3). Monthly figures can then be updated using the previous month's figures. A simple chart such as the following can help a practice to maintain these records.

While these records must be maintained, it is important that there be no discrimination between patients with various types of coverage. All patients must be treated equally and allowed access to the same rooms, treatments, facilities, etc.

PATIENT POPULATION RECORD

Month _____

Provider: _____

Type of coverage (i.e., HMO, commercial insurance, Medicare, Medicaid, cash patient, etc.) _____

New patients (Name and Member Number): _____

_____

_____

_____

_____

Patients who have left the practice (Name and Member Number): _____

_____

_____

_____

_____

Number of this type of patient last month _____

Plus number of new patients _____

Minus number of patients who have left the practice _____

Total patients of this type this month _____

Total number of patients this month _____

Divide type of patients by total patients _____ %

Figure 10 – 3: Patient Population Record

Medical billers represent the practice. Therefore, they should be familiar with the forms and procedures regarding each of the following issues:

- Grievances,
- Informed consent policies,
- Referrals,
- Telephone advice,
- Emergency procedures,
- Appointment scheduling,
- Preventative services (i.e., pap smears, mammograms, etc.), and
- Handling and disposing of infectious waste.

All HMO records (and all patient records) should be stored in a lockable area. This area should be kept locked so that no one outside the staff has access to these records. Any time a patient chart is removed from the storage area, a retrieval card should be kept in its place. This retrieval card indicates the chart number being taken, the name of the person taking the chart, where the chart is, the date the chart was taken, and the expected date of its return.

The facility will be audited on a regular basis and the auditor may question the staff regarding these procedures and policies.

Sanctions

If a group fails to meet the quality standards, reporting requirements or any other provisions of its contract with the HMO, the HMO may impose sanctions on the group/IPA or the individual provider. These sanctions usually include the withholding of specified amounts (i.e., $1,000 or 5%) of the group/IPA's monthly capitation and/or not allowing any new members to be enrolled to that group/IPA (members may not choose them as a provider).

It is not uncommon for sanctions to escalate for additional offenses. Therefore, an HMO may impose a $1,000 (or 5% of capitation) sanction for the first offence, $3000 (or 10% of capitation) for the second offense and $10,000 (or 15% of capitation) for the third offence. If there are additional offenses, the group/IPA or the individual provider may be terminated.

Because of these sanctions, it is important that all reports, forms or claim payments be properly completed in a timely manner and all rules be expressly followed.

Additionally, if the HMO receives any fines or penalties from a government agency as a result of any action by a provider or group/IPA, the HMO can impose sanctions, fines, penalties or any other type of sanction imposed by the regulatory agency or governing body on the HMO or group/IPA.

Claim Payments

If a provider is deemed to be responsible for payment of services, then the provider/group/IPA must either provide these services, or pay for the providing of these services. Often groups/IPAs will attempt to sign a wide variety of providers to their group/IPA so that they do not need to refer patients to outside providers. This often means that they will enter into a contractual agreement with a specific provider (i.e., a chiropractor) in their area to provide services for their patients at a specified rate. This specified rate may be on a fee-for-service basis or on a capitation basis.

Clean Claims

Claims from providers outside the group/IPA must be paid from group/IPA funds if the group/IPA is contractually obligated to cover or provide these services. There are usually time limits on how long a provider may take to pay a clean claim.

A claim is considered "clean" if all information to process the claim is within the plan or group/IPA. A **clean claim** is defined as one that can be paid as soon as it is received because it is complete in all aspects, including patient information, coverage information, coding, itemization, dates of services, and billed amounts.

If a claim is submitted without a piece of information which is included in the group/IPA patient chart, omission of this information alone will not make it an unclean claim. For example: if pre-authorization was required, the leaving off of an authorization number alone should not make the claim unclean. The group/IPA should have this information available in the patient chart.

Additionally, the need for medical review of a claim to determine appropriateness of services does not make it an unclean claim.

When a claim is unclean (it does not have the necessary information to be processed), the group/IPA must send a written notice to the provider advising the provider of the information needed to process the claim. Many providers have a standard form letter for this purpose.

If you do not receive a response within 30 days, send a denial notice stating that the services were denied. A copy of a denial notice is shown in **Figure 10 – 4.**

Group/IPA Payment Responsibility

When a claim is received from a provider outside the group, or is paid on a fee-for-service basis, the following steps need to be done:

1. Date stamp the claim and any supporting documents. This will help to prove the timeliness of your claim payments. There are state and federal laws governing how soon you should pay a claim (usually within 30 days). Additionally, the HMO may require that the claim be paid within a specified time period or the provider may forfeit a portion of his capitation amount (see Capitation Payments).
2. Notify the provider in writing if the claim is incomplete, improperly completed, or if additional reports or documentation need to be attached. A copy of this notification should be attached to the claim.
3. Complete eligibility verifications and any internal review (i.e., were treatments authorized or allowed, or did the member choose to see the provider on their own?).
4. Prepare a proper remittance advice or denial notice in the case of denied claims.
5. Determine the proper payment amount.
6. Prepare and mail a check. For timeliness guidelines, a claim is usually considered paid when the check is placed in the mail.

Additionally, the group/IPA is required to provide an Explanation of Benefits to any fee-for-service provider showing the patient information, service rendered, date of service, amount billed, disposition of copayment (if any), amount group/IPA is paying, and a reason code for any denied services or amounts.

If the provider is paid on a capitated basis, the group/IPA must provide a count of members listed by plan, a payment amount for each plan, and copies of the member rosters. In essence, the same type of document which the group/IPA receives from the HMO when they are paid their monthly capitation amounts must be provided.

Determining the Proper Payment Amount

If there is no contract in place between the provider and the group/IPA prior to the rendering of services, the group/IPA has no legal basis for discounting payment to a provider. They must pay the full amount of the bill, minus any copayment amounts which should have been collected from the patient.

Legally, if a member has met their contractual obligations (i.e., seeking pre-authorization or emergency authorization for treatment), they have no responsibility for payment for services other than the copayment amount stipulated in their contract. Therefore, the group/IPA must pay a provider's billed amount, minus any copay. A statement should accompany payment to the provider stating that the copayment is the only amount which may be collected from the patient.

If there is a contracted amount for services, the terms in the contract should be adhered to. Usually, a fee schedule will accompany contracted terms. This fee schedule may be different for each provider which the group/IPA contracts with. The proper contract should be pulled and the correct allowed amount determined. The member's copayment amount should then be subtracted from this amount, and the remainder paid to the provider. A notice should accompany the EOB stating that this is the contracted amount for this service and no amounts other than the copayment may be collected from the member.

It is the responsibility of the group/IPA to insure that neither the member nor the HMO incurs any financial responsibility for claims which are contractually deemed to be the responsibility of the group/IPA.

For services rendered to seniors who are covered by Medicare HMOs, the fee schedule may indicate that fees are limited to the Medicare fee schedule. Under this arrangement, Medicare participating providers are limited to the allowed amount as determined by the most recent Medicare Fee Schedule. Non-participating providers would be paid the non-participating fee amount. The non-participating fee equals 95% of the participating fee amount. The maximum amount a non-participating physician or supplier will receive is the Medicare limiting charge, which is equal to 115% of the non-participating provider amount.

In either case, if the fee is being limited by contractual agreement with the provider, a copy of the contract and the accompanying fee schedule should be attached to the claim when it is filed.

Claim Files

Claims are usually filed in a separate claim file, along with all documentation submitted by the provider, and a copy of the explanation of benefits (fee for service providers) or member rosters and capitation amounts (capitated providers).

Additionally, a copy of the claim or some documentation showing the services rendered should be placed in the patient chart. If any of the documentation supporting the claim payment is pertinent to further treatment of the patient, this information should also be copied and filed in the patient chart. At no time should any information regarding capitation payments be placed in the patient chart. This information is a part of the contract between the provider and the group/IPA and should be considered privileged information.

Denial of a Claim or Service

If a claim or service is denied, a denial letter must be included with the EOB indicating the reason for the denial. The denial notice must also include a statement that the provider has the right to appeal the denial within 60 days, and the address of where to file an appeal.

If the claim is for emergency services, the member or provider is requested to notify the HMO within 48 hours of the initiation of care. However, some HMOs may limit the ability of a group/IPA to deny claims based upon the lack of notification within this 48 hour period.

If it is believed that these services were not medically necessary, or were not true emergency services, then the claim must be sent through a medical review process. The medical review should use the presenting diagnosis rather than the discharge diagnosis as the basis for their decision making, and must consider the member's understanding of the medical circumstances which led to the emergency service.

Date:

Member Name
Address
City, State Zip

File # _____

Dear:

We have received your request for the specific service or referral described below.

Service/Referral Requested: _____
_____

This Service/Referral request is being denied for the reason(s) shown below:
_____   Services are not a covered benefit with your plan.
_____   You have exhausted the benefit for this particular service.
_____   Service/Referral request denied because _____
_____
_____
_____

If you believe this determination is not correct, you have the right to request a reconsideration. You must file the request in writing within 60 days of the date of this notice. File the appeal with: Your HMO, Attn: Member Services, Address, City, State, Zip.

In addition to the complaint process described above, you may also contact the Department of Corporations (DOC). The DOC is responsible for regulating health care service plans in this state. The DOC has a toll-free number (1-800-XXX-XXXX) to receive complaints regarding health plans. If you have a grievance against the health plan, you should contact the plan and use the plan's grievance process. If you need the DOC's help with a complaint involving an emergency grievance or with a grievance that has not been satisfactorily resolved by the plan, you may call the DOC's toll free number.

Please include your name and date of birth on all correspondence. If you have any questions about this notice, please call YOUR HMO at 1-800-XXX-XXXX.

Sincerely,

Name of Medical Group/IPA

cc: Member Services
    Quality Assessment
    Primary Care Provider

Figure 10 – 4: Denial Notice

If this medical review determines that the services were not medically necessary or were not true emergency services, then a specific denial letter is required for these claims. This denial letter must meet federal requirements. The HMO will often provide a copy of an appropriate denial letter in their Policies and Procedures Manual. In such a case, this letter should be used verbatim, and the wording left unaltered.

All denial notices must contain an explicit reason, in layman's terms, of why the service(s) are being denied. If the HMO provides a list of denial reasons, then the appropriate denial reason should be written on the denial letter. You may not use a code unless you indicate the meaning of that code in the denial letter. Additionally, all denial letters must meet the following criteria:

1. The decision to deny must be correct and based upon approved medical practices.
2. The denial reason must be clear to the member and must use HCFA-approved denial reasons.
3. The denial letter must include mandated appeals language and the correct health plan address.
4. The denial letter must be sent to the appropriate parties (the provider, the member, or both).
5. The denial notice must be issued within required time frames.

There are additional guidelines which mandate that certain items be included and that the type font be of an appropriate size to be read by most members. The HMO should furnish all providers with copies of appropriate denial letters, and these should be used by the provider.

If the member is not covered by the group/IPA, then certain steps must be taken before the claim can be denied. First, call the HMO to determine if the member was covered at the time services were rendered, and who the assigned provider was at that time. If the member was not covered at all, then the claim may be denied for that reason. If the member was not eligible under the group/IPA, but was a covered member under the HMO, then the claim must be forwarded to the HMO. You are not allowed to simply deny the claim and return it to the provider.

Additionally, any claims which have been denied by the group/IPA must be sent to the HMO with a copy of any contact or denial letters to the member or provider. Many HMOs also require the use of a denied claim log which includes the following information:

- Current month and year,
- Group name,
- Contact person,
- Phone number,
- Member name,
- File/member number,
- Provider name,
- Whether the provider was contracted or non-contracted,
- Date of service,
- Reason for the denial,
- Date the claim was received,
- Date the notice was sent to the member, and
- Date the notice was sent to the provider.

A copy of this log should be forwarded to the HMO on a regular basis. If there are no denials for the month, a copy of the log should still be forwarded to the HMO with the words NO DENIALS on the first line of the log.

Appeals

Any member or provider has the right to appeal a denied claim. All denial letters, by law, must include a statement saying that the receiver has the right to appeal the decision and whom to contact to begin the appeal process.

If a member or provider appeals a denied claim, the HMO will review the claim and make a determination of whether to uphold or reverse the denial. If the HMO determines that the services should have been covered, it will inform the group/IPA of its decision and will instruct the group/IPA to pay the claim.

The payment should be generated immediately and a copy of the proof of payment (EOB and copy of the check) sent to the HMO. If the HMO does not receive proof of payment in a timely fashion, it has the right to pay the claim and deduct the payment from the group/IPA's capitation amount. The HMO may have a fund set up under the provider's name in which it has withheld a portion of the group/IPA's monthly capitation amount (i.e., 3%). If so, the claim will be paid from this fund.

If the HMO processes the claim and makes payment to the provider, it not only goes against the provider's record, but the HMO has the right to charge an administrative fee for processing the claim. This fee can be as much as $100 or more.

Medical billers should be aware of the appeals process and should routinely appeal all claims in which services performed by their provider were denied. If possible, additional information substantiating the need for the services or the urgent nature of the services should be included with the appeal.

HMO/Plan Responsibility

If the group/IPA determines that the HMO is responsible for payment of a claim, they must forward the claim to the HMO. The following steps should be completed:

1. Determine which services, if any, are the responsibility of the group/IPA and process these claims according to the guidelines given above.
2. Indicate on the EOB or write a letter stating which services are the responsibility of the HMO, and indicate that the claim is being forwarded to the HMO for payment.
3. There is usually a transmittal form which must be sent with any claims. A copy of this form is shown in **Figure 10 – 5.**

Reinsurance/Stoploss

Stoploss is an attempt to limit payments by an insured person, or a group/IPA in the case of a catastrophic illness or injury to a member.

Many HMO contracts have a stoploss or reinsurance clause included in them. This clause states that the group/IPA will be financially responsible for the first set amount (i.e., $7,000) in expenses for each member in a contract year. After those expenses have been paid, the HMO will reimburse the group/IPA for verified expenses which exceed the set amount.

If the provider's contract has a stoploss clause, it is important that the medical biller be aware of the set amount. They will need to file a claim with the HMO for any services which exceed that set amount. The biller should also be familiar with that portion of the provider's contract with the HMO, since there are often limits put on the billing. For example, the HMO may require that claims be submitted within a specified time period, or that pre-authorization be obtained before the services are rendered. Some contracts may also stipulate that the year runs from July 1, to June 30. If the biller is unfamiliar with the terms required to achieve stoploss reimbursement, the provider could stand to lose a substantial sum of money.

Often the HMO will require that a claim for reimbursement be submitted on specific forms. An example of this form is shown in **Figure 10 – 6**.

Incorrect Denials

If a group/IPA arranges, refers, or renders services or equipment that are not covered under a plan, the group/IPA must inform the member ahead of time that the services or equipment are not covered by the plan and the member is liable for coverage. The group/IPA should have a form for the member to sign stating that they understand that such services are not a covered expense. If the member is not informed of the non-coverage and financial liability in advance, the member cannot be held liable for the cost of the services or equipment.

If the HMO has a Medicare HMO plan, they must agree to cover at least the minimum of services which are covered under Medicare. Therefore, it is important that providers and their billers understand what items are covered under Medicare so these items are not denied.

Many HMO plans have a limit on the number of visits or units which a member may utilize during a year (i.e., 20 chiropractic visits). When the member has exhausted their benefits under such an arrangement, it is important to notify the member that they have reached their limit and any additional treatments will not be covered by the plan. Failure to do so could cause the group/IPA to be liable for the services.

It is important that billers note in a patient's file if they are covered under an HMO plan. If a member receives services that should have been pre-authorized, and the provider is a contracted member with a plan, the provider forfeits their fee for those services.

For Example: Sarah James is seen by Dr. Dorman. She indicates that she is covered by Medicare when she is actually covered by a Medicare HMO. Dr. Dorman is contracted with the Medicare HMO which Ms. James is a member of. Thinking that Ms. James is covered by Medicare, he renders services that need pre-authorization by the HMO. Because the provider did not inform Ms. James in advance that the services were not pre-authorized or were not covered by the HMO, the services will be denied. Because he is a contracted provider with the HMO, Dr. Dorman is not allowed to bill the patient for these services. Therefore, the provider forfeits his fee.

To prevent this from happening, it is important to verify insurance coverage prior to the first visit, and also to ask each patient if their insurance coverage has changed since their last visit on subsequent visits.

Provider Network Services
CLAIMS TRANSMITTAL FORM

Date: _____

To: Claims Services

From: _____, Administrator for _____

The attached claims are the responsibility of [the HMO].

Authorization Number _____

___ Inpatient Hospital (IP) Charges

___ Outpatient Surgery (OPS) Facility Charges

___ Anesthesia for approved IP or OPS

___ Radiology for approved IP, OPS or SNF

___ Pathology for approved IP, OPS or SNF

___ Emergency services which resulted in admission to Inpatient status

___ Ambulance

___ Durable Medical Equipment

___ Dialysis Facility Charges

___ Radiation Therapy

___ Member not on roster for date of service. Include relevant roster page(s).

NOTE: Use a separate form for each type of Plan expense. Multiple providers may be grouped if the authorization number is the same.

[The HMO] will not send denial notices for services which are the responsibility of the Group/IPA.

Refer to the Medical Services Agreement for questions of coverage and financial responsibility.

Figure 10 – 5: Transmittal Form

Excess Risk Limit Cost Summary

I.   Group Name: _____   Enrollee Name: _____   II.

      Address: _____   Enrollee PF#: _____

      _____   Date of Eligibility: _____

      Contact Person: _____   Contract Year: _____

      Phone Number: _____   For HIV/AIDS cases, list qualifying hospital stays:

      Date Submitted: _____

      _____   _____   _____

      _____   _____   _____

Type of Submission

___ Original   ___ Medicare
___ Supplemental   ___ Commercial
___ Resubmittal   ___ OO Care
___ AIDS/HIV   ___ CCC

III.

Provider of Service / Provider #	Date of Service	CPT4, RVS, or SMA code	Units	Billed Amount	Amount Paid	For HMO use only
				TOTAL THIS PAGE:		

Figure 10 – 6: Excess Risk (Stoploss) Form

Summary

Health care costs in the American economy have escalated out of control. Higher prices for services and insurance have American consumers demanding for some type of reform. Managed care contracts were created in an attempt to bring health care costs under control by having providers share some of the financial risks of health care with the patient and the insurance carrier.

There are numerous types of managed care organizations, including HMOs, PPOs, Gatekeeper PPOs, EPOs, PHOs, and MSOs, to mention a few.

HMOs are one of the most common managed care trends. HMOs pay providers a set capitation amount each month for the patients on their eligibility roster, and in return the provider is expected to cover many of the services that member needs. A written contract will dictate those services which the provider will cover and those which the HMO will cover. There are also numerous forms which the provider must complete to keep the HMO informed of services rendered and the daily operations of the practice.

Assignments

Complete the Questions for Review.

Questions for Review

Directions: Answer the following questions without looking back into the material just covered. Write your answers in the space provided.

1. What is a PPO? _____

   _____

   _____

2. In a _____ the insurance carrier will contract with a group of facilities and/or providers to provide services at a set fee per month.

3. What should a biller do if a patient requests treatment and they are not included on the provider's eligibility roster?

   _____

   _____

   _____

4. What is a TAR and what is its purpose? _____

   _____

   _____

5. What is a gatekeeper PPO? _____

   _____

   _____

If you were unable to answer any of the questions, refer back to that section, and then fill in the answers.

Honors Certification™

The certification challenge for this chapter will be a written test of the information contained in this chapter. Each incorrect answer will result in a deduction of up to 5% from your grade. You must achieve a score of 85% or higher to pass this test. If you fail the test on your first attempt you may retake the test one additional time. The items included in the second test may be different from those in the first test.

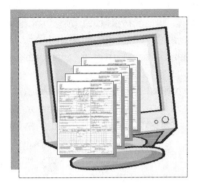

11

Miscellaneous Billing Procedures

After completion of this chapter you will be able to:

- Describe the use of the charge slip and the information it contains.
- List procedures or situations when delayed billing is appropriate.
- Describe items that may affect the billing amount of a service or procedure.
- State the most common billing forms used and their applicability.
- List the guidelines that can facilitate the quickest possible payment of a claim.
- Describe how follow-up days, maternity bundling, unbundling, diagnosis related groups, and ambulatory patient groups can affect the procedures and amounts billed.
- List the tips that will help you obtain maximum reimbursement on a claim.
- Properly calculate the patient's portion of a bill using a given scenario.
- Describe the purpose of the patient claim form and list the information it contains.
- Properly define the terms used in coordination of benefits.
- Use the OBD rules to determine the proper primary, secondary and tertiary payor on a given claim.
- Discuss how benefits are coordinated with an HMO.
- Describe the most common TRICARE programs and how a biller would bill for these services.

Key words and concepts you will learn in this chapter:

Allowable Expense – Any necessary, reasonable, and customary item of medical or dental expense, at least partly covered under at least one of the plans covering the patient.

Explanation of Benefits (EOB) – A letter from a payor indicating how a member's benefits have been applied in response to the submission of a claim.

Group Plan – A group insurance plan is a plan under which members of a structured group insure themselves against potential losses in the event of death, disability and the need for medical treatments that may occur. This form of coverage allows coordination of benefits.

Order of Benefit Determinations (OBD) – The 13 rules determining the order of insurance benefit payment.

Overinsurance – A situation that occurs when a person is covered under two or more policies and is eligible to collect an accumulation of benefits that will actually exceed the amount charged by the provider.

Primary Plan – The plan that determines and pays its benefits first without regard to the existence of any other coverage.
Secondary Plan – The plan that pays after the primary plan has paid its benefits.
Self-funded Plan – A company that insures itself and its own workers.
TRICARE – The Department of Defense's health care program for members of the uniformed services and their families and survivors, and retired members and their families.

In this chapter we will discuss general billing guidelines as well as several types of claims that will require special handling when they are encountered in the medical office. We will also discuss coordination of benefits and TRICARE.

Billing for Services

After the patient has seen the doctor, the doctor will complete a charge slip or fee ticket. The **charge slip** is a form used by the provider to indicate the services rendered, the diagnosis for the visit, and whether a return visit is required **(see Figure 11 – 1)**. This form usually has a list of service descriptions along with the corresponding numeric billing codes and a list of diagnoses and diagnoses codes.

The charge slip is given to the patient after the visit is complete. The patient will in turn give the charge slip to the receptionist for payment to be made and a return visit to be scheduled, if required. At that time, the receptionist should collect any amounts that the patient owes. For cash patients (those without insurance or responsibility by a third party payor), the entire amount is often collected or a payment plan is set up. For many patients covered by insurance, a small payment will be required. The receptionist should issue a receipt for any monies collected and list the amount received and the form of payment (cash or check) on the charge slip.

If the services rendered are complicated, the medical biller may need to refer to the medical record for a report to substantiate the amount charged for the services. The physician is required to dictate a report if this information is necessary for billing.

When billing the carrier, double-check to make sure the CPT®, ICD-9, and DRG codes are accurate (coding will be discussed further in later chapters). Improper coding is the most common error made on billing forms, and it can result in improperly paid as well as delayed claim payments. Since codes can frequently change, it is important that the most up-to-date information and reference books are available.

Also, make sure that all the necessary information has been filled in on a claim form prior to submitting it to the carrier. Medical billers and front office personnel have many tasks and responsibilities. Without proper organization it is very easy to forget valuable information on a form or forget to call for pre-authorization of services. Therefore, organize your office in such a way that the opportunity for these mistakes is at a minimum. Also, take the time to do things correctly. It prevents having to correct it later.

When the above information has been used and the claim form is complete, the claim form is then mailed to the insurance carrier. The patient is also sent a copy of the billing information. If the charge slip or superbill has carbon copies, one of these may be used as a bill for the patient.

Delayed Billing
If a procedure is expected to take an extended period of time (i.e., pregnancy, multiple surgeries), billing for the procedure should be delayed until the entire process is complete. The appropriate CPT® code usually covers all services. Waiting until the completion of services insures that the correct billing will be done. For example, in the case of a pregnancy, all prenatal visits for nine months prior to the delivery are included under CPT® code 59400, as well as the delivery of the baby and the post-partum care. If the provider were to bill prior to the delivery, several scenarios could cause an error in billing. The patient could be rushed to the hospital in advanced labor and the baby delivered by another doctor, or a complication could occur which requires the baby to be taken by cesarean section.

It is impossible to determine exactly what procedures a doctor will perform until they are actually done, so billing should be postponed until all related services have been performed. Also, billing for procedures which have not been performed (even if you expect to perform them in the future) is considered fraud.

Determining the Proper Billing Amount

Providers may have different charges for the same service, depending upon the situation. For example, if the patient is covered by Medicare, there are limits to the amount which Medicare will cover, and to the amount which may be collected on the overall bill.

Medicare Limitations

Medicare limits the amount which may be charged by providers. While this limit may not always show up on the initial bill, the amount which can be balance billed to the patient is limited.

Network Provider limits

If the provider has signed a contract with a PPO carrier, there may be limits to the amounts which the provider may charge for services.

The provider must limit balance billing to the patient so that the total amount collected for the service does not exceed the contracted amount.

Providers sign PPO agreements because they often receive more patients under a PPO contract than they might otherwise receive. Patients will often seek treatment from PPO providers because the carrier will often pay a higher amount for these providers (those who have signed contracts – network providers) than for non-network providers (those who have not signed contracts).

Before calculating any payments it is important to determine the amount which the patient should be billed, and the total amount which may be collected. This prevents overbilling the patient and having to make a refund at a later date.

If the provider has signed a contract which limits payments, there should be a comprehensive listing of the procedures which have limits, and the amounts which may be charged for those procedures. Billers must first look up the appropriate CPT® or HCPCS code for the services that were rendered. This description of service and code is then compared to the amount listed in the PPO contract. If there is a limit to the charge, it will be listed under the appropriate CPT® or HCPCS code.

Sample chart

CPT® Code	Description	Approved Charge
99211	Office Visit, minimal	$65
99212	Office Visit, problem-focused	$75
99213	Office Visit, low complexity	$85

Billing Forms

Billing forms usually come in three types: the superbill, the CMS-1500, and the UB-92. These forms are covered briefly in the next sections. The CMS-1500 and the UB-92 will be covered in depth in later chapters.

The medical biller will be required to use several types of billing forms, depending on the type of services rendered and to whom the bill is being submitted for payment.

Superbill

Superbills are billing forms used by many providers of service and suppliers. The superbill serves as a charging slip to expedite the process of medical insurance reimbursement. The standard superbill has four copies: one copy for the office, one for insurance filing, one for the patient, and a fourth for the patient's record. As long as a superbill contains the required information, many insurers will accept it for payment; however, Medicare will not.

A superbill is an invoice and, as such, is subject to the same accountability requirements as other standard billing forms.

The superbill is different depending on the provider of service and the form he chooses to use; therefore, we will not discuss the completion of these forms. However, the type of information required by payors is generally the same as those found on the following medical billing forms.

CMS-1500

The Centers for Medicare and Medicaid Services (CMS) 1500 is the basic form for billing services from physicians and suppliers. The medical biller uses the CMS-1500 when billing for payment from insurance carriers and Medicare programs. The medical biller can extract the necessary information to properly complete the form from the patient's record or operative report. When billing Medicare, the most current version of the CMS-1500 should be used.

UB-92

The Uniform Billing-92 (UB-92) is used for billing hospital services. Information for completing the UB-92 can be taken from the hospital medical records or from Triage Reports. Triage Reports are generated in the emergency rooms of hospitals or at the scene of an accident.

Charge Slip

Date of Service: _____ Account Number: _____

Name (Last, First, Middle): _____

X	Code	Description	Fee	X	Code	Description	Fee	X	Code	Description	Fee
Initial				**Established**				**Special Procedures**			
	99204	Extended Exam	100.00		99211	Minimal Exam	35.00				
	99205	Comprehensive Exam	110.00		99212	Brief Exam	40.00				
					99213	Limited Exam	45.00				
					99214	Intermediate Exam	60.00				
					99215	Comprehensive Exam	90.00				
Consultations				**Laboratory**				**Prescriptions**			
	99244	Comprehensive	150.00		36415	Venipuncture	15.00				
					81000	Urinalysis	10.00				
					82948	Glucose Fingerstick	18.00				

X	Code	Diagnosis	X	Code	Diagnosis	X	Code	Diagnosis
	466	Bronchitis, Acute		401	Hypertension		460	Upper Resp Tract Infection
	428	Congestive Heart Failure		414	Ischemic Heart Disease		599.0	Urinary Tract Infection
	431	CVA		724.2	Low Back Syndrome		616	Vaginitis
	250.0	Diabetes Mellitus		278.0	Obesity		**ICD-9**	**Other Diagnosis**
	625.3	Dysmenorrhea		715	Osteoarthritis			
	345	Epilepsy		462	Pharyngitis. Acute			
	0009.0	Gastroenteritis		714	Rheumatoid Arthritis			
	784.0	Headache		477	Rhinitis, Allergic			
	573.3	Hepatitis		471	Sinusitis. Acute			

Remarks/Special Instructions	New Appointment	Statement of Account	
		Old Balance	
		Today's Fee	
Referring Physician	Recall	Payment	
		New Balance	

Figure 11 – 1: Charge Slip

Additional Suggestions

The following are four additional suggestions for the medical biller.

1. Give the patient a copy of the bill when she leaves the medical office. This can be a superbill, a copy (not the original) of the CMS-1500, or a listing of the charges incurred during this visit.
2. If an Assignment of Benefits Form is not on file or if the patient's insurance carrier requires it, have the patient sign the Assignment of Benefits box on the claim form before leaving the office.
3. Batch Medicare, Medicaid, HMO, and PPO forms in separate groups before sending them to the computer center. This way each of these types of forms will be processed at one time and you will have a separate batch total for each type.
4. Make sure that the forms that the medical office or the computer service generates are compatible with the required submission format for the insurance carrier. If your office is considering a new form, send a copy to all the insurance carriers you submit claims to and ask for a written approval of the form. Requesting the approval in writing can solve problems later. It may take six weeks or more to get approval, so check with your supervisor before switching to a new form or system.

There are a number of things to keep in mind when dealing with patients. Of course, customer service should always be your first and foremost concern, but at the same time you need to have regard for the medical office. It is important to obtain all necessary information from the patient. Remember that the primary objective of the medical biller is to minimize the amount of time between the physician's service and the complete payment of the bill. The information that can facilitate this process may include the following:

1. Ask the patient to fill out all the forms required for the patient file. Give the patient sufficient time to fill out the forms and check that they have been filled out completely before accepting them. Many offices mail the forms to the patient prior to their visit to ensure their completeness.
2. Be sure you understand the policies of the office you work for regarding the completion of forms and payment for bills. This way you can explain it accurately to the patient.
3. Use the office forms consistently and accurately so that the tracking of information proceeds smoothly, regardless of who enters the information.
4. Secure all the details of the insurance information. If the patient or insured has a card, make a copy of it for the patient file. Make sure the information contains the subscriber's name, the policy number, the effective date, the company that holds the policy or the name of the policy, and the insurance carrier's address.
5. Make sure the patient understands the provider's policy regarding any amounts that the insurance carrier does not pay or does not cover.
6. Complete all insurance forms accurately and completely. This is the most important paper to ensure the prompt payment of claims by the insurance carrier. Also, use the forms preferred by the insurance carrier. Use of other forms can result in a delay in the processing of the claim.
7. Make sure the claims and all necessary papers have been signed by the physician, nurse, and any other necessary persons.
8. Maintain a copy of all paperwork and claims submitted to the insurance carrier. Also keep a log of the date of submission of the claim.

Billing Tips/Issues

There are a number of situations which can affect billing for patient services. The most common of these include the following:

Follow-up Days

When billing for surgical services, the total surgical care is included in the charge for the surgery. Total surgical care includes the initial visit with the patient before surgery, the surgical procedure, and the routine follow-up care. If visits are related to a prior surgical episode, you cannot bill separately for them. For further information on this issue, see the chapter on CPT® Coding.

Maternity Bundling

All maternity procedures are usually bundled together. This includes one visit per month in the months leading up to the delivery, and the actual delivery service itself. Additionally, some carriers consider certain tests to be included in the overall maternity care, such as urinalysis tests and ultrasounds.

Be sure to determine the exact services that are considered part of maternity care. Any procedures which are not routinely part of this care may be billed separately.

Unbundling

Codes for individual lab tests include the taking of a specimen for each test. If a single blood specimen is collected and a number of lab tests run from that single specimen, a panel test code should be chosen to report the procedure. Panel test codes report multiple tests run from a single specimen.

If you are billing for several laboratory tests together, make sure you use the appropriate code and charge for the combined test.

Unbundling is discussed more fully in the chapter on CPT® Coding.

Diagnosis Related Groups

Some diseases or conditions are covered under a Diagnosis Related Group (DRG) billing. DRG billings lump all charges for hospital treatment of a specific diagnosis under one payment. For example, if a hospital treats a patient for one of these conditions, they will be paid a lump sum charge which will cover all treatment. If the hospital's charges are higher than the amount provided in the lump sum payment, they must write off any charges above the payment. They are not allowed to balance bill the patient for this amount. However, if the hospital's charges are less than the lump sum payment, they are still paid the same amount. The hospital may keep the extra money. DRGs are only for hospital treatment.

Ambulatory Patient Groups

An Ambulatory Patient Group is similar to a Diagnosis Related Group, except that it is for outpatient treatment (treatment outside a hospital setting). The same rules apply regarding the lump sum payment.

Special Services

Physicians may bill charges other than medical services. Some medical offices charge for completing insurance or claim forms, late charges on past due amounts, charges for missed appointments, and charges for phones calls by or from patients. These services are usually not covered by insurance carriers and are the sole responsibility of the patient.

A Professional Courtesy is when a doctor renders medical services to another professional, such as a doctor, pharmacist, or nurse, or to a relative. Billing procedures vary from not charging the patient, to a percentage of the physician's usual charges for these services. You should familiarize yourself with the provider's billing procedures prior to billing for these services.

Maximum Reimbursement Tips

Following are a few rules that will allow you to receive the maximum reimbursement possible on each claim.

1. Be sure the claim form is filled out completely and accurately.
2. Be sure that each procedure is linked to its appropriate diagnosis and that the diagnosis substantiates the need for the procedure.
3. Check the contract provisions (or contact the insurance carrier to request information regarding contract provisions). Follow all provisions carefully, including pre-certifying procedures, pre-authorization of hospitalizations, need for second surgical opinions, etc.
4. Be sure that any benefits which are reimbursed at a higher benefit amount are clearly indicated. This can include outpatient surgery being paid at a higher percent than inpatient surgery; pre-admit testing paid at a higher percent, accident provisions, etc.
5. If a common accident provision applies, send in the claim for the patient who has previously paid the most toward their deductible first.
6. Make a notation at the top of the file copy of the claim regarding the benefit level you expect this claim to be paid and why (i.e.,

100% accident benefit). When the claim is paid, double-check the EOB to insure that the claim was paid at the expected benefit level. If not, contact the insurance carrier for an explanation.

7. Double-check all EOBs to insure that all procedures were paid or accounted for. In cases of paper claims, it is easy for a single procedure to be omitted.

8. Appeal all decisions that you do not agree with, especially in cases of downcoding or denials due to medical necessity. Be sure to include appropriate information as to why the services should be allowed at the level indicated. Simply adding a modifier is not enough. Provide lab tests, operative reports, or other written data which substantiates your point of view.

Collecting the Patient Portion

Many medical offices will collect the estimated amount due from the patient at the time services are rendered. This estimated amount is based upon the patient's portion of the coinsurance amount and any deductible which has not yet been satisfied. This practice requires that medical billers contact the patient's insurance company prior to treatment being rendered (usually within 24 hours of the scheduled appointment). The biller should confirm that the patient is covered by the insurance, determine the correct coinsurance amount, any special circumstances which may apply to the treatment, and any deductible which has not yet been met by the patient.

Once this information has been obtained, the biller should determine the estimated amount which is the patient's responsibility. Let's look at the following example.

Barney Bumpkiss is scheduled for a high complexity office visit for the treatment of diabetes ($130). The doctor is expected to perform a glucose monitoring of the patient ($30), and a CBC ($30).

Upon calling the insurance carrier, you determine that Barney is currently covered by insurance which has a $125 deductible. Barney has received prior treatment, satisfying $75 of his deductible. The remaining services are covered at 80% for medical services and 70% for laboratory services.

The patient's estimated amount should be determined as follows:

Charges

Office visit	$130
Glucose monitoring	$30
CBC	$30
Total	$190

Deductible to Be Satisfied

Amount of deductible	125
Deductible paid	75
Deductible Remaining	50

Office visit ($130) - deductible remaining ($50) = $80
$80 x 20% (patient's coinsurance) = $16
Lab charges ($60) x 30% (patient's coinsurance) = $18
Total patient portion ($16 + $18) = $34
+ unmet deductible of $50 = $84 Estimated patient payment due.

Be sure to inform the patient that this is an estimated amount based upon your charges. The insurance carrier may allow a smaller amount, which may result in a higher amount being due from the patient.

If the patient is enrolled in the Medicare program, it is important not to over collect on the patient's portion of the payment. Since Medicare limits the amount a provider can collect to the Medicare allowed amount, it is important to determine the appropriate Medicare allowed amount prior to calculating the patient's portion of the payment.

Many medical offices will have a list of their most commonly rendered services and the Medicare allowed amount for these services. It may be necessary to either contact the Medicare carrier and ask what the allowed amount is, or to go back through past Medicare payments (especially those for this patient if this treatment is for an ongoing condition) to determine the allowed amount for the estimated procedures.

If an office does not have a listing of approved amounts, the Medicare carrier may have a list they can distribute. If not, the biller should consider creating a list and adding in the Medicare approved amount from each Explanation of Medicare Benefits (EOMB) which it receives.

Additionally, if Medicare determines that the services are not medically necessary, you must refund all monies paid to the patient, even if you are appealing the decision and are waiting for a final determination.

Remember that any amount collected which is more than the Medicare allowed amount for the procedure will need to be refunded to the patient. This can cause ill feelings on the part of the patient, especially Medicare patients who are on a fixed income.

Patient Claim Form

In addition to the billing forms, a medical biller may occasionally receive a Patient Claim Form **(see Figure 11 – 2).** This form is provided by self-funded plans. A **self-funded** plan is a company that insures itself and its own workers.

Some companies are so large that it is less expensive to insure themselves. Rather than pay insurance premiums to an insurance carrier every month, they instead put funds in a specific company bank account. When patients seek services, the claims are paid out of this fund. If a company has several thousand employees, it can be a lot less expensive for them to pay for all medical services themselves, rather than pay the insurance premiums for that many people.

If the patient is a member of a self-funded plan, the plan may have a specific form for the provider to use when billing for services.

The information contained on this form is self-explanatory. The member should complete the information entitled "To Be Completed by Member" and the provider of services should complete the information entitled "To Be Completed by Physician."

Coordination of Benefits

Coordination of Benefits (COB) is a process that occurs when two or more group plans provide coverage on the same person (see definition in next section). Coordination between the two plans is necessary to allow for payment of 100% of the allowable expenses but no more.

This process was developed in response to a growing problem of overinsurance. **Overinsurance** occurs when a person is covered under two or more policies and is eligible to collect an accumulation of benefits that will actually exceed the amount charged by the provider. The purpose of COB is to allow coverage and usually payment of 100% of allowable expenses without allowing the covered member(s) to make money over and above the total costs for care.

In response to the diversity of handling procedures used by various carriers and administrators in coordinating coverages, the National Association of Insurance Commissioners (NAIC) developed a standardized model for COB administration. The majority of benefit plans follow this model, but it is not mandatory.

Definitions
Words commonly found in COB provisions are defined as follows:

Allowable Expense – Any necessary, reasonable, and customary item of medical or dental expense, at least partly covered under at least one of the plans covering the patient. Items excluded by the secondary plan, such as dental services and vision care services, would not be considered allowable. Conversely, amounts limited under the secondary plan would be considered allowable (the entire charge). For example:

1. Each plan provides a limit of $35 per visit for outpatient psychiatric care. The psychiatrist charges $50 per visit. As long as the $50 is within the UCR guidelines of one of the two plans, the entire $50 would be considered an allowable expense under COB.
2. Based on the primary plan's UCR guidelines, the amount allowed for a surgery is $1,200. The secondary plan's UCR for the same surgery is $1,000. When coordinating benefits, the secondary plan would allow the greatest amount allowed by at least one of the plans. Therefore, the allowable amount when coordinating would be $1,200.

Claim Determination Period – Usually, means a calendar year. It does not include any part of a year before the effective date of duplicate coverage under the secondary plan.

Explanation of Benefits (EOB) – A letter from a payor indicating how a member's benefits have been applied in response to the submission of a claim. The EOB indicates deductibles, coinsurance amounts, non-allowed amounts, UCR limitations, and other variable items. An EOB is required by law to be generated on each claim submission showing the disposition of the claim (how it was paid, denied, or pended for additional information).

Patient Claim Form

Information must be printed or typewritten. Claim form must be completed and returned to us at the indicated address.

Medicare Patients: Submit this claim to Medicare FIRST! A copy of the Medicare Explanation of Benefits must be submitted with this claim form.

TO BE COMPLETED BY MEMBER

1. Information Pertaining To Member				
Name: Last, First, M.I.	Sex:	Date Of Birth	Social Security Number	
Home Address: Street City	State Zip		Telephone Number	
Marital Status	Name Of Spouse	Spouse's Date Of Birth	Spouse's Social Security #	
Is Spouse Employed?	If Yes, Name And Address Of Employer	Employer Phone Number		

2. Information Pertaining To Patient				
Patient Name: Last, First, M.I.	Sex	Date Of Birth	Social Security Number	
Home Address: Street City	State Zip		Telephone Number	
Is Patient Employed? Full-Time Part Time No	Relationship To Employee?	If Dependent Child Over 19, Name Of School Where Full-time Student:		

3. Information Regarding Current Treatment				
Related To Illness?	Related To Pregnancy?	Related To Work?	Description Of Illness Or Injury	
Date Of Accident	Where Happened?	Describe Accident		

4. Information Regarding Insurance	
Are You, Spouse Or Dependent Children Covered By Any Other Insurance?	Name Of Insured
If Yes, Name And Address Of Insurance	Insurance Phone Number

Patient's Or Guardian's Signature

I certify that the above information is true and correct and I authorize the release of any medical information necessary to process this claim.

Signed: Date:

Assignment of Benefits:

I assign payment of benefits to the following provider:

Address: Street City	State Zip	Telephone Number

Figure 11 – 2: Patient Claim Form Side 1

TO BE COMPLETED BY PHYSICIAN

Patient's Name: Last, First, M.I.				

Home Address: Street	City	State	Zip	Telephone Number

Is Condition Due To Illness?	Injury?	Work Related?	Pregnancy?	If Yes, Date Of Last Menstrual Period

Diagnosis Or Nature Of Illness Or Injuries. Give Description And ICD-9 Code.

_____

_____

Date Of Service	Place Of Service	Description Of Medical Services Or Supplies Provided	CPT® Code	ICD-9 Code	Charge

Date Of First Symptoms	Date Of Accident	Date Patient First Seen		Total Charges	
Dates Patient Unable To Work From To:	If Still Disabled, Date Patient Should Return To Work			Amount Paid	
Patient Still Under Care For This Condition?	Date Of Same Or Similar Illness Or Condition		Does Patient Have Other Health Coverage?		

Under Section 6019 Of The Internal Revenue Code, Recipients Of Medical Payments Must Provide Identifying Numbers To Payors Who Must Report Such Payments To The Internal Revenue Service.   Taxpayer ID Number: _____ Social Security Number: _____

Physician's Name: _____   Signature: _____

_____

Street Address	City	State	Zip

INFORMATION REGARDING THIS CLAIM FORM

A Separate Claim Must Be Filed For Each Different Injury Or Illness.

A Claim Must Be Filed Within 90 Days of The Date Of Service Or Claim Benefits May Be Reduced.

If Patient Is Medicare Eligible, Claim Must First Be Submitted To Medicare For Payment. We Cannot Process Claim Without Information Regarding Medicare's Payment.

Figure 11 – 2: Patient Claim Form Side 2

Group Plan – A form of coverage with which coordination of benefits is allowed. A plan may include:

- Group, blanket, or franchise insurance policy or plan if not individually underwritten,
- Health maintenance organization or hospital or medical service prepayment policy available through an employer, union, or association,
- Trusteed policy or plan, union welfare policy or plan, multiple employer policy or plan, or employee benefit policy or plan,
- Governmental programs (Medicare) or policies or plans required by a statute, except Medicaid, or
- "No fault" auto policy or plan. (Applies to some plans only. The plan must specify whether or not this is applicable.)

Primary Plan – Benefit plan that determines and pays its benefits first without regard to the existence of any other coverage.

Secondary Plan – Plan that pays after the primary plan has paid its benefits. The benefits of the secondary plan take into consideration the benefits of the primary plan and may reduce its payment so that only 100% of allowable expenses are paid.

Order of Benefit Determination

Before standardized coordination rules were adopted by the benefits industry, a person covered under two policies could collect full benefits from both. Thus, the individual would make a profit by being sick.

Since each plan would prefer to pay as the secondary payor, it became necessary to develop rules to determine when a plan should pay as primary, secondary, or tertiary.

The 13 rules determining the order of benefit payment are referred to as the **Order of Benefit Determinations (OBD)** and are as follows:

1. The plan without a COB provision will be primary to a plan with a COB provision.
2. The plan that does not have these OBD rules and, as a result, the plans do not agree on the OBD, will determine the order of payment.
3. The plan that covers a person as an employee will be primary to a plan that covers that person as a dependent.
4. If the person is an employee under two plans, the primary plan is defined as the one that has been in effect the longest.
5. If an employee is an active employee under one plan and retired (or laid off) under another, the active plan will pay primary.

The parent birthday rule, explained in rules six and seven, affects the OBD for dependent children of parents who are living together and married (not divorced or legally separated).

6. The plan of the parent whose birthday (based on month and day only) occurs first in the calendar year is the primary plan.
7. When both parents' birthdays are the same (based on month and day), the benefits of the plan that covered one parent the longest is the primary plan.

For dependents of legally separated or divorced parents and those whose parents have remarried, the Order of Benefits Determination will be based on the following rules:

8. If there is a court-approved divorce decree, the plan of the parent specified as having legal responsibility for the health care expense of the child is the primary plan.

If there is no court decree:

9. The plan of the parent with custody is primary.
10. The plan of the step-parent with whom the child resides is secondary.
11. The plan of the natural parent without custody is tertiary.
12. The step-parent (if any) who does not reside with the child has no legal right to declare dependency of the child and, therefore, no coordination should be performed, since the child is (probably) not an eligible dependent under the plan.
13. For joint custody with no additional responsibility designation, the plan of the parent whose coverage has been in effect the longest would be the primary payor.

Right of Recovery

If the amount of the payments made by the plan is more than should have been paid under the COB provision, the plan may recover the excess from one or more of the following:

- The person(s) it has paid or the person(s) it has paid on behalf of,
- Other insurers/plans, or
- Other organizations.

The "amount of the payments made" includes the reasonable cash value of any benefits provided in the form of services.

When billing for patients who have dual coverage, determine the primary carrier to be billed first. After payment is received from the primary carrier, post the payment to the patient's ledger card to determine the balance. When billing the secondary carrier, always attach a copy of the primary carrier's explanation of benefits to the claim being submitted. The secondary carrier will not process the claim without this information. Upon receipt of the secondary carrier's payment, post the payment to the patient's ledger card. Any balance remaining after all adjustments should be billed to the patient.

COB With
Health Maintenance Organizations

A Health Maintenance Organization (HMO) is a type of prepayment plan in which providers agree to charge members for their services in accordance with a fixed schedule of rates. The HMO insured may pay a specified copayment at the time the service is rendered or may not be required to pay anything. The patient and the doctor are never involved in having to complete claim forms for submission to a payor. Instead, the HMO is billed directly or the HMO pays a monthly retainer fee to the physician for membership plus other specified fees.

If the required medical services are available through the HMO but the insured does not go to an HMO provider for the treatment, he may be held entirely responsible for all of the expenses.

Prepayment plans are included in the definition of the type of policies to which COB provisions apply. However, many HMOs do not have COB provisions, although more are now starting to incorporate this concept since the spiraling costs of medical care are affecting them, as well.

An example of an HMO is Kaiser Permanente. Kaiser provides a prepayment policy for hospital and professional medical services at no cost or at a small fee, as long as the member goes to a Kaiser facility. Subsequently, they provide the member with a "reasonable cost statement," which represents what would have been charged to a non-member. If the HMO does not have a COB provision, they would be considered the primary payor. To coordinate benefits, a request must be made for receipts or statements showing the actual out-of-pocket expense. The secondary plan would pay no more than the amount that would be considered the allowable expense. If the HMO does have a COB provision, the regular OBD determination rules should be applied.

TRICARE

TRICARE is the medical program for military personnel. There are several different health care programs under the TRICARE banner. The most commonly used include:

- **TRICARE Prime:** A managed care option similar to an HMO. All active duty personnel are required to be enrolled in this option. Their spouses and dependents are also encouraged to enroll, though it is not mandatory for them.
- **TRICARE Extra:** A preferred Provider Organization. Patients who seek treatment from a network provider are covered at 85% of the allowed amount while those who seek treatment from a non-network provider are covered at 80% of the allowed amount.
- **TRICARE Standard:** This is the new name for what was formerly called the Civilian Health and Medical Program for the Uniformed Services (CHAMPUS). This option provides coverage on a fee for service basis.
- **TRICARE For Life and TRICARE Plus:** Medigap insurance which covers those who are 65 or over and covered by Medicare.

TRICARE provides a comprehensive program of health care benefits for active-duty and retired services personnel, their dependents, and the dependents of deceased military personnel. Persons eligible for TRICARE will be enrolled in the **Defense Enrollment Eligibility Reporting System (DEERS)**. This is a computer database used to verify TRICARE eligibility.

TRICARE is secondary to all other insurance or health policies except Medicaid and TRICARE supplemental insurance. However, most military personnel will be treated free of charge or at a minimal fee at veterans' administrative clinics and facilities. Because of this, many medical billers will never have to bill TRICARE.

When treating TRICARE patients, be sure to list the name, rank, station and ID number from the enrollment card onto the medical record. Also copy the card and place it in the medical record.

TRICARE claims can be submitted on a CMS-1500 or a UB-92. Complete the CMS-1500 and submit it to the fiscal intermediary for the state. Claims for TRICARE must be submitted no later than the last day of the calendar year following the year in which the services were rendered.

Summary

Properly handling the billing of claims is the prime responsibility of the medical biller. If the proper general guidelines and procedures are not main-tained, it can cause a delay in the reimbursement for services.

Two types of billing require special handling: TRICARE, and Coordination of Benefits. It is important for the medical biller to understand the basic benefits provided by TRICARE and to know how to coordinate benefits when there is more than one payor who may cover payment for a patient. This will allow the provider to recover the maximum amount possible from the various payors, leaving less of a balance for the patient to pay or for the physician to write off.

Assignments

Complete the Questions for Review.
Complete Exercise 11 – 1.

Questions for Review

Directions: Answer the following questions without looking back into the material just covered. Write your answers in the space provided.

1. What does COB stand for?_____

2. What is the purpose of COB?_____

_____

3. The _____is the benefit plan that determines and pays its benefits first without regard to the existence of any other coverage.

4. The _____is the plan that pays after the primary plan has paid its benefits.

5. What is TRICARE?_____

_____

If you were unable to answer any of the questions, refer back to that section, and then fill in the answers.

Exercise 11 – 1

Directions: Determine the correct amount to be collected from the patient prior to the rendering of services.

Yellow Insurance covers 90% of all procedures except anesthesia, which is covered at 80%. They have a $125 annual deductible.

1. Yvonne Yang is scheduled to receive drainage of a cyst in the mouth ($340), an x-ray of the mouth and throat ($85) and an esophagotomy ($624). She has met none of her deductible.

    Amount to be collected: _____

2. Yasmin Yarrow is scheduled to receive a straightforward office visit, new patient ($100). She has met $10 of her deductible.

    Amount to be collected: _____

Brown Insurance covers patients at 80% for medical services. The carrier requires a deductible of $150 annually.

3. Betty Boston is scheduled to have a straightforward office visit ($85) to have a skin lesion looked at. She has met all of her deductible.

    Amount to be collected: _____

4. Betsy Bryman is scheduled to receive the removal of a 2.1 cm lesion on her arm ($560). She has met $30.50 of her deductible.

    Amount to be collected: _____

5. Barry Barker is scheduled to receive a moderate complexity office visit ($110) and an x-ray of his arm ($65). He has met $5 of his deductible.

    Amount to be collected: _____

Honors Certification™

The certification challenge for this chapter will be a written test of the information contained in this chapter. Each incorrect answer will result in a deduction of up to 5% from your grade. You must achieve a score of 85% or higher to pass this test. If you fail the test on your first attempt you may retake the test one additional time. The items included in the second test may be different from those in the first test.

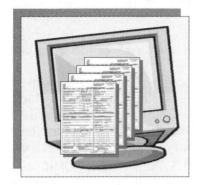

12

Patient Accounting

After completion of this chapter you will be able to:

- Explain and use the ledger card and patient statements.
- Properly post payments to the patient account.
- Properly create a payment plan.
- Properly handle a collections call using various given scenarios.

Key words and concepts you will learn in this chapter:

Accounts Receivable – Money being received by a business.

Accounts Payable – Money paid out, usually for goods or services.

Adjustments – Changes which can either increase or decrease the remaining balance.

Balance Billing – Sending an additional bill to another party for payment of any remaining amounts on a claim.

Bankruptcy – The act whereby a debtor announces they no longer have the ability to pay creditors and asks relief from the federal courts.

Defendant – The person being sued.

Dunning Notice – A statement or sentence reminding the recipient to make a payment on their account.

Explanation of Benefits (EOB) – A form from the insurance carrier which shows the patient, the date of the service, the service performed, the amount which was allowed for the procedure, the percentage covered by insurance and the amount which the insurance carrier is paying.

Insurance Tracer – A form or letter sent to the insurance carrier to inquire about the disposition of a previously submitted claim.

Ledger Card – A card used to indicate a chronologic record of all services rendered to a patient.

Patient Statement – An individual summary (either by patient or by family) that lists all the services, charges, payments, adjustments, and balance due that occurred during the month.

Pended – Held for further information.

Post – To list items such as payments or charges in a log.

Skip – A person who has received services without payment and has moved and left no forwarding address.

Statute of Limitations – The maximum time that a debt can be collected from the time it has been incurred.

Billing is not the only function of the medical biller. Once a bill has been sent out, it is the biller's responsibility to collect on that bill and to make sure the patient's account is properly credited.

Often the biller begins by submitting a claim to the patient's insurance carrier. When payment is received from the carrier it is credited against the patient's account. The patient, or a secondary insurance carrier if there is one, is then billed for any remaining amount left unpaid on the claim.

If payment is not received from the insurance carrier in a timely manner, an insurance tracer is sent on the claim. If payment is not received from the patient in a timely manner, the medical biller is responsible for handling collections on the account. If necessary, the account may be sent to small claims court in an effort to collect.

Let's look at each step of this process in more detail.

Accounts Payable/Receivable

The main function and purpose of any bookkeeping system is to provide a way to keep an accurate account of money being received and paid out. Most accounting systems are set up on a principle of accounts payable and accounts receivable. In simple terms, money being received is considered **accounts receivable** and money paid out is referred to as **accounts payable**. In any business, the objective is to have more money coming in (accounts receivable) than there is going out (accounts payable).

Since the medical office provides a service and also functions as a business, one of the responsibilities of the medical biller includes the continued updating of financial records.

In the medical office, the biller is often responsible for collecting payments from services to patients. This amounts to most, if not all of the accounts receivable which a medical practice may have. Therefore it is important for the medical biller to insure that all accounts are paid in a timely manner.

Due to this, billers must keep highly accurate records of patients and the services they receive, bill for those services promptly, record payments, do balance billing in a timely manner, and institute collections procedures when necessary.

Often the practice will have a second person (if not the doctor themselves) who is responsible for handling all accounts payable. However, it is important that the medical biller be aware of any major purchases which the practice may need, and have a general idea how much the office expenses are each month. This does not need to be a detailed understanding of how much each person is paid or how much the expenses are. However, if the medical biller is aware that the practice has approximately $10,000 in expenses each month they will know what they need to collect to cover those expenses.

Several bookkeeping systems may be used in the medical office to keep track of incoming and outgoing finances.

There are two main ways of keeping patient accounts: computerized and manually. Most computerized billing systems also allow you to handle patient accounting. Thus, they not only generate the claim, but they record all charges and payments into the system.

If you are using a computerized system, the accounting system is automatically set up when you enter patient information into a record. When a claim is created it is automatically posted to the patient's account. To **post** means to list items such as payments or charges in a log.

When payments are received the information is recorded on a payment screen, and the amount paid is automatically deducted from the patient's account.

The pegboard system is one of the most frequently used manual systems because it is the simplest to use. Ledger cards, charge slips, and daily journal sheets all are used in the pegboard system. This system uses NCR (no carbon required) material on its forms to allow information written on one form to be recorded on all the rest.

The Ledger Card

When you are using a manual system for patient accounting, the patient's account is often kept on a Ledger Card **(see Figure 12 – 1).** The **ledger card** is used to indicate a chronologic record of all services rendered to a patient, and record all payments and adjustments made on their account.

Each service, payment or adjustment should have its own line or column on a ledger card. Any services provided are added to the remaining balance (if there is one), and any payments received are subtracted from the remaining balance. **Adjustments** are changes which can either increase or decrease the remaining balance.

Items should be entered in chronological order. Thus, the charges for services performed would be entered before any payments for those services. The remaining balance shown on the last line of the ledger card is the amount that is still owed on the patient's account.

Ledger Card

RESPONSIBLE PARTY: _____

ADDRESS: _____

TELEPHONE #: _____

PATIENT NAME: _____ PATIENT #: _____

SPECIAL NOTES: _____

Date	Description of Service	Charge	Payments	Adjustments	Remaining Balance

Figure 12 – 1: Ledger Card

To post items to a ledger card, complete the items below.

Responsible Party: Enter the name of the person ultimately responsible for payment of this bill. This is often the patient, or the parent or guardian of a minor patient.

Address: Enter the address of the person ultimately responsible for payment of this bill.

Telephone #: Enter the telephone number of the person ultimately responsible for payment of this bill.

Patient Name: Enter the name of the patient. Each patient should have their own, separate ledger card. Never place more than one patient's account information on a card.

Patient Number: Enter the patient's account number.

Special Notes: This is where you may enter any special circumstances regarding this patient and their account.

Date: Enter the date of the transaction. This is the date services were rendered in the case of most charges, or the date a payment was received for payments.

Description of Service: Enter a description of the reason this account is being changed. If you are recording charges, indicate the services that were performed. If you are recording a payment, indicate that it is a payment, and who is making the payment (i.e., Green Insurance Carrier Payment, check #1234). If you are recording an adjustment, indicate the reason for the adjustment (i.e., adjustment to Medicare allowed amount).

Charge: Indicate the charge for any services that were performed. If you are recording a payment, leave this space blank.

Payments: Enter the amount of the payment. If there is no payment, leave this space blank.

Adjustments: Enter the amount of the adjustment. If there is no adjustment, leave this space blank.

Remaining Balance: Add the amount of any charges to the prior amount in this field. Subtract the amount of any payments from the prior amount in this column. Adjustments can be either increases or decreases to the patient's accounts.

It is important to always keep the patient's ledger card updated. Any changes to the patient's account should be promptly noted. This can prevent numerous problems with the patient's account, including interest charges or late charges being assessed.

Insurance Payments

The insurance carrier is often the first entity to make a payment on a claim. Once the insurance carrier has processed the claim, they will send an Explanation of Benefits with the check (if applicable) to the party designated as the payee. If benefits are assigned, this would be the provider. If benefits are not assigned, this would be the patient. If the patient is designated as the payee, the provider will not receive any contact from the insurance carrier. It is the biller's responsibility to collect the full amount due for services from the patient.

Understanding an EOB

When benefits are assigned to the provider, the insurance carrier will create an **Explanation of Benefits (EOB)** for the claim and send payment directly to the provider. This EOB will list the patient, the date of the service and the service performed. It will also list the amount which was allowed for the procedure, the percentage covered by insurance and the amount which the insurance carrier is paying.

If benefits are not assigned to the provider, the EOB will be sent to the patient, along with payment amount. The full amount should be collected from the patient, regardless of what was paid by the insurance carrier (unless Medicare or Medicaid is involved).

It is important to check the EOB carefully against the patient's account. Be sure that the codes which were paid were the ones that were billed. Errors can often occur in the inputting of codes, thus causing improper calculation of the benefits.

There are many different EOB styles and formats. EOBs may list one patient or they may list several on the same page. If several are listed together, be sure that you are crediting the payment to the proper patient. Some providers will choose to list each procedure separately on their records and record the amount received for each service. Others will combine all the services provided on the same date and apply the payment to that total.

If the EOB combines payments for several dates of service, be sure that you separate the amount of the payment according to the proper dates. Some EOBs do not contain information that is detailed enough to do this. In such a case, add together the amounts billed on the claim and apply the total amount against this.

December 15, 20XX
Claim for Joann Johnson
Claim number: 478-78-4

Dear Ms. Johnson:

We received a claim for you. The following details the benefits which were paid on this claim. Please save this form for your tax records. If you have any questions, please contact the customer service office.

DATE OF SERVICE	PROCEDURE	BILLED AMOUNT	ALLOWED AMOUNT	% OF PAYMENT	PAYMENT AMOUNT	DENIED AMOUNT	REASON CODE
11/06/04	HOSP CONSULT	$200.00	$140.00	90%	$ 36.00* *	$ 60.00	55
11/07-08/04	HOSP VISIT	$150.00	$100.00	90%	$ 90.00	$ 50.00	55
11/09/04	HOSP D/C	$100.00	$ 75.00	90%	$ 67.50	$ 25.00	55
TOTAL		$450.00	$315.00		$193.50	$135.00	

55   Denied amount exceeds the amount covered under your plan.
** $100 applied to deductible.

Figure 12 – 2: Sample EOB

See the sample EOB in **Figure 12 – 2**. On this EOB, Joann Johnson received a hospital consultation, two hospital visits and a hospital discharge. All charges were allowed (though not at the billed amount), and were paid at 90%. However, the patient had not yet met $100 of her deductible, so this amount was taken from the $126 that otherwise would have been paid on the first line item.

On this claim, the billed amount was $450. Since the insurance only paid $193.50, the patient (or any additional insurance if the patient is covered by more than one policy) should be balance billed for the remaining $256.50.

Posting Payments

When payment on the claim is received, you will need to post the payment to the patient's account. This can be done on a computerized system, or with a manual system.

Be sure to record all the pertinent information regarding a payment. This should include not only the name of the person or entity making the payment, but the type of payment (i.e., cash, check, money order), and the number of the check or money order.

Post each of the appropriate amounts from the EOB onto the patient's account. In the case of a Medicare or Medicaid EOB, be sure to write off any amounts that were not allowed. Next, determine the amount which is still owed on the claim.

Balance Billing

If there are any remaining amounts owed, you will need to balance bill. **Balance billing** is sending an additional bill to another party for payment of any remaining amounts on a claim. If the patient has more than one insurance carrier, a second copy of the claim should be sent to the secondary carrier to coordinate benefits between the two carriers. Be sure to attach a copy of the primary carrier's EOB so that the secondary payor may see how much was paid by the primary payor. Do not alter any of the information on the form. You should send an exact copy of the form to the secondary insurance carrier. Many CMS-1500 forms have several carbon copies for this purpose.

If there is no second insurance carrier, the patient should be balance billed for any remaining amounts. Patients are usually billed using a patient statement. Most insurance carriers will send a copy of the EOB to the patient at the same time they send one to the provider. However, some providers prefer to include a copy of the EOB to allow the patient to view how the payment was credited to the account.

Patient Statements

A **patient statement** is an individual summary (either by patient or by family) that lists all the services, charges, payments, adjustments, and balances due that occurred during the month. This statement is sent to the patient every month. It acts as both a statement of his or her account and as a bill.

Often these statements contain a **dunning notice**, which is a statement or sentence reminding the recipient to make a payment on their account. There are certain days which are more appropriate for sending out patient statements. These dates are usually between the 8th and the 12th of the month and between the 20th and the 27th of the month. Sending out patient statements on these dates receives a higher response, since most people receive their paychecks on the 15th and the 30th or 31st of the month.

Follow-Ups

A claim may be denied or **pended** (held for further information) by the insurance carrier if there are omissions or errors on the form. The most common reasons why claims are denied include missing or incomplete diagnoses, diagnoses not corresponding with services rendered, incorrect dates, charges not itemized, incorrect patient insurance information, incorrect procedure codes, and documentation not submitted to substantiate services rendered.

If the claim was denied or pended for these or any other reasons, complete or correct the information and resubmit the claim.

If the payment was denied on all or part of a claim and you feel the denial is incorrect, write to the insurance carrier and ask for a review or appeal of the claim. Every insurance carrier has an appeals process and will give you the required directions and information or forms to use.

Make sure that you have a good system set up to remind you when to follow up on a claim. If you have not heard from the carrier six weeks after you have filed a claim, it is definitely time to follow up.

When a Claim is Rejected

An insurance carrier may reject all or part of a claim. Before billing the patient for the remaining balance, be sure you determine why the claim was rejected. Many claims are rejected due to minor errors which can be fixed easily. These can include things such as the following:

1. The patient is not listed as covered under the mentioned policy. Many insurance carriers (and their computer systems) track patients according to policy numbers, group numbers and/or social security numbers. If any of these numbers is incorrect, the claim may be rejected because the patient and the policy numbers do not match up.

2. Office visits are rejected because they fall within the follow-up days for a surgical procedure. If the office visit was for a reason (diagnosis) other than as a follow-up to the surgery, be sure this is clearly indicated on the claim. Box 24e of the CMS-1500 should reference the additional diagnosis. Modifier -24 can also be used to indicate unrelated E/M services by the physician during a post-operative period. Some providers (including Medicare) may require additional documentation proving that the visit was unrelated to the surgical procedure.

3. The claim (or some services) is rejected as not being medically necessary. If procedures seem unrelated to the listed diagnoses, those procedures may be rejected. Be sure that each procedure has an appropriate diagnosis listed for it. If you need additional room for more diagnoses, list procedures on two separate CMS-1500s, according to their related diagnoses.

4. Item 12, release of information, was not completed. After ensuring that the signature is on file, type the words "Signature on File" in the box. Some insurance carriers require that the patient's name or the name of the person who signed the release appear in this field, and will reject claims with "Signature on File."

5. The patient was not covered at the time the treatment was begun. If special conditions exist which negate the pre-existing provisions, be sure to attach this information. These special conditions can be the meeting of certain requirements such as the patient being treatment free for a specified period of time, or the patient's

medical insurance transferred when the patient moved from one job to another.

6. The claim is rejected because the facility or doctor is incorrect for the type of procedure being performed. For example, if ear surgery is being performed by an obstetrician it would probably be rejected. Be sure that the procedure codes listed are correct for those procedures that were performed.

7. The claim is rejected because the patient's gender or age is incorrect for the type of procedure being performed. For example, a male is not treated for gynecological procedures. If the gender is listed incorrectly on the patient's form, the claim could be resubmitted.

Carriers are required to provide the reason why the claim or procedure was denied. If you do not understand the wording or why the claim was denied, contact the person (or department) listed on the EOB to inquire.

If the error is a minor one, fix the error and resubmit the claim. If more explanation is needed (i.e., an operative report to justify services performed), include the additional information, and resubmit the claim.

If everything on the claim is correct and you disagree with the claims examiner's judgment on the claim, contact the claims examiner and discuss the situation. If you cannot come to an agreement on the claim, ask what the appeals process is for such a situation. All companies have an appeal or claim review process.

Insurance Tracer

If you have not received payment from an insurance carrier within six weeks of sending in the claim, you should submit an insurance tracer. An **insurance tracer** is a form or letter sent to the insurance carrier to inquire about the disposition of a previously submitted claim. Be sure to include the patient's name, their social security number or insurance number, their policy name and number, and the patient's address. You should also include the date of services, the diagnosis, and information regarding their employer.

Many medical offices have a form letter for this purpose. A sample form letter follows:

ON PROVIDER'S LETTERHEAD

INSURANCE TRACER

Date: _____

Dear Insurance Carrier:

    We sent a claim to you over six weeks ago and have not heard back from you.
Patient:
Insured:
Address:
SSN/Birth Date:
Group Number:
Claim Amount:
Date Billed:
Date of Services:
Date of Illness or Injury:
Diagnosis:
Employer:
Address:

    Please supply the following information on the above named claim within ten days. Payment on this claim is overdue and we would like to avoid involving the patient and the state insurance commissioner in a reimbursement complaint.

Claim pending because:_____
_____

Payment in progress. Check will be mailed on:
_____

Payment previously made. Date: _____
To whom:_____
Check #: _____ Payment Amount: _____
Claim denied. Reason: _____
_____

Patient notified: Yes   No
Remarks: _____
_____
_____

Thank you for your assistance.

Completed by: _____

Payments from insurance carriers should normally be received within four to six weeks. When the payment is received, the amount of payment should be compared with the actual claim originally sent. The payment should then be posted to the patient's account.

Collections

The patient is always financially responsible for payment of services rendered, regardless of whether or not he is covered by insurance. The following are two exceptions: (1) if the patient is a minor, in which case the financial responsibility lies with the parent(s) or legal guardian; or (2) if the patient was injured on the job and the services rendered are related to this injury. In this case (2), the company's workers' compensation carrier would be responsible for payment.

After the claim is paid by the insurance carrier and the payment is posted to the patient's account, any remaining balance is billed to the patient. If no payment has been received within 30 days, a follow-up reminder should be sent.

If payment is not received within 15 days of the second notice, send a courteous collection notice reminding the patient that payment is now seriously delinquent, followed by a courtesy call ten days later. Keep accurate records of when each contact was made and the outcome of that contact. Also record the date you should follow-up if you have not received payment.

The longer an account ages, the less likely you will be to recover the money due. This can be as much as 40% or more if the bill is overdue by six months or more.

Often, providers are wary of becoming "bill collectors" because the image is not consistent with that of a healer. However, if revenues are not collected in a timely manner, it can be difficult for the provider to meet the cost of their overhead and other obligations.

Therefore, a balance must be achieved that allows for the collection of revenues without tarnishing the provider's image. The best way to achieve this is to set reasonable credit limits and to stress to patients that they are responsible for payment of the bill. Create a credit agreement, and then ask each patient to sign and date it. Also make sure that the patient understands that by signing the credit agreement, she agrees to abide by its terms.

Do not make your credit policy too stringent. You do not want to lose patients because they cannot afford your terms. If you need to put a little pressure on clients without alienating them, try blaming a third party (i.e., your accountant).

When collections are being made by telephone, there are also laws to be followed under the Fair Debt Collection Practices Act. Harassing, frightening, or abusive calls are a violation of this act, along with calling during odd hours, or calling friends or neighbors.

A **statute of limitations** is the maximum time that a debt can be collected from the time it was incurred and/or became due. The statute of limitations varies from state to state, so check with your state legislation.

When all other methods of collection are exhausted, a collection agency may be retained to collect delinquent accounts. Most collection agencies charge a percentage of the account once the debt is collected. Therefore, usually only large amounts are sent to a collection agency.

Many companies use a standard collection letter. A sample of a collection letter is shown below.

COLLECTION LETTER

Dear Sir/Madam:

We are currently showing a past due amount on your account. According to our records your payment of $____ was due on/by _____. As of this date, payment has not been received.

Please remit payment as soon as possible. If you have recently sent payment, please disregard this notice.

Sincerely,

Collections Representative

If the standard collection notice does not gain a response within 30 days, a delinquent notice should be sent.

DELINQUENT NOTICE

Dear Sir/Madam:

Your account is seriously delinquent. According to our records we have not yet received your payment of $_____. This payment was due by _____ and reflects services which were rendered on _____.

If payment is not received by _____ we may be forced to send your bill to collections. Doing so may damage your credit rating.

If you are unable to pay the full amount, please contact our office immediately to set up a payment plan.

Sincerely,

Collections Representative

Collections Procedures

The medical biller often needs to work as a bill collector in order to obtain reimbursement for amounts not covered by insurance or other sources. Usually, these amounts need to be collected from the patient. Occasionally, due to an error on a previous claim payment, it may become necessary for a medical biller to recover monies that were paid in error. For these reasons, we will cover the basic laws and regulations regarding collections.

Although the specific laws and regulations vary from state to state, you should become familiar with several general guidelines. These include:

1. You are never allowed to make frightening or abusive calls. This includes making any threats to the person, calling names, or making derogatory statements. Racial or ethnic statements should never be made.
2. It is illegal to call people at odd times of the day. In most states, this means any time between 8 p.m. and 8 a.m. In some states, it is also illegal to contact people at their place of employment.
3. It is illegal to request collection through another party, including friends or neighbors. This means that you are not allowed to leave a message with anyone

other than the debtor concerning details of the collection attempt. This includes, but is not limited to, the amount you are trying to collect, any payment amounts or details that may have been worked out, and the nature of the bill. If you call the debtor and reach a family member or roommate, you are allowed to leave a message giving your name, company and phone number, and a request that the person you are trying to contact return your call.

4. You are not allowed to harass the person from whom you are trying to collect. The legal definition of harassment varies from state to state; however, it is illegal to do things such as call and speak to the debtor several times a day or even several times a week. For this reason, it is important that you remind them of the debt and then ask when you can expect to receive payment. If they are unable to pay in full and if your company allows payment plans, try to work out a payment plan for the amount owed. Make detailed notes of the conversation in the patient file. You should not contact the person again until after the date payment is expected.

Payment Plans

If the patient cannot pay the entire bill when contacted and your company allows it, payment arrangements should be made. If a payment plan was worked out – whether over the phone or in person – it is advisable to write down the terms of the agreement and have it signed by both parties (the debtor and a representative of the company to which the money is owed).

If the payment requires more than four installments, the federal Truth in Lending Act will apply. Regulation Z of the Truth in Lending Act requires that a written disclosure be made. When the installment plan is being discussed, the following important points should be covered:

- The amount of the debt,
- The amount of the down payment,
- The estimated date of final payment,
- The amount of each installment, and
- The date each payment is due.

A statute of limitations is the maximum time a debt can be collected from the time it is incurred and/or became due. Remember that the statute of limitations varies from state to state, so check with your state legislature. You should always be aware of the statute of limitations within your state since the entire debt must be paid off prior to this time or the physician will forfeit any amounts remaining unpaid.

Date:
Doctor:
Patient's Name:
Patient's Address:

Cash price (total fee):
Less cash down payment:
Unpaid balance of cash price:
Amount financed:
FINANCE CHARGE:
ANNUAL PERCENTAGE RATE:
Total of payments:
Deferred payment price:

Patient hereby agrees to pay to (provider's name) at the address shown above, the total payments shown above in _____ monthly installments of $_____, first installment being payable 20 _____, and all such installments on the same day of each consecutive month until paid in full.

Signature _____ Date_____

Truth in Lending Form

Many doctors have a pre-printed form for payment plans. This insures that they comply with all requirements of the Truth in Lending Act. The following form meets all requirements of this act if it is printed on the provider's letterhead. Please note that the words FINANCE CHARGE and ANNUAL PERCENTAGE RATE must appear in capital letters.

Payment Schedule Form

A Payment Schedule Form is designed to track the payment history of a patient making payments through an installment plan. Some providers prefer to use a payment schedule which may be placed on half of an 11 x 8.5 sheet of paper (with the Truth in Lending Form contained on the right-hand side of the paper), or with a payment schedule attached to or printed on the back of the Truth in Lending document.

A payment schedule lists the due date of each installment, the paid amount of the installment, the date the payment was received, and any follow-up notes (usually notes of a phone call if the payment was not received on time). Some practices will use the follow-up area to include the check number of the payment. This helps to track the payment if there are any questions.

Using a form such as this allows the biller to easily see how many payments have been received and if the patient is behind or ahead in their payments. It also helps to determine if a patient has missed a payment. Occasionally, a payment will be missed, and the patient will then pay subsequent payments on the due date. The patient may believe they are up to date on their payments when in fact they are a month behind. By using a Payment Schedule Form this information can be quickly accessed.

Tracing a Skip

A **skip** is defined as a person who has received services without payment and has moved and left no forwarding address. Skips are usually identified by mail being returned to the medical office by the post office and postmarked "return to sender" or "address unknown." In attempting to trace a skip, use the information on the patient information sheet. The person shown in the "person to contact in case of emergency" space should be contacted. Another source is the local Department of Motor Vehicles. If the patient owns a car, it must be registered. The motor vehicle department may be able to provide information regarding the patient's whereabouts. Under no circumstances should information regarding the patient's medical condition be given to the third party.

Tracing a skip is a very tedious and challenging task, which requires tact as well as patience. If the methods just mentioned prove to be futile, the account may be written off or turned over to a collection agency.

Bankruptcy

Bankruptcy laws allow protection for a debtor. By filing for **bankruptcy**, a debtor announces that he no longer has the ability to pay his creditors and requests relief for his debts from the bankruptcy court. A provider who is owed money by a patient is considered to be a creditor for that patient. There are several types of bankruptcy filings:

- Chapter 7 (straight bankruptcy). The debtor lists all those to whom he owes money. If the debtor has no assets, all debts are cancelled with no recourse to the creditor. If there are assets to be distributed, a claim must be filed by the creditor. The provider will usually be notified of the need to file a claim.

- Chapter 11 (company reorganization). This type of bankruptcy is for companies who wish to reorganize their business and attempt to pay off a portion of their debts. The court determines the amount which each creditor would receive if the company were to be completely liquidated. The company must then agree to pay at least this amount and have a valid plan, budget and repayment schedule. Chapter 11 allows a company to remain in business.

- Chapter 12 (farmer reorganization). Similar to Chapter 11, but for a farmer rather than a company.

- Chapter 13 (wage earner's bankruptcy). The debtor agrees to pay a certain amount (agreed to by the court) to a trust organization or court appointed trustee every month. The trust organization will distribute the available funds among the creditors. Providers should file a claim as soon as possible to insure at least partial payment of the patient's account. Often the amount paid is less than the actual claim against the debtor (i.e., creditors will get 25 cents for every dollar they are owed).

If the patient includes the outstanding provider's fees as part of a bankruptcy filing, the fees owed may be discharged by the court. This means the debtor does not need to repay the debt.

A claim should be filed on all bankruptcy proceedings, regardless of whether one is requested or not. This protects the provider in case he or she does not receive word that a claim is required. If a claim is not filed within a specified period of time (usually 90 days) the creditor relinquishes his claim on the debtor.

The proper claim forms can be obtained from the bankruptcy court, or standard forms are available in many stationery stores. Debts with collateral (secured debts) will be paid off first. Debts without collateral (unsecured debts) will be paid last. A provider's debt is considered an unsecured debt, since there is no property which has been pledged as collateral against the debt.

As soon as an office is informed that a patient has filed bankruptcy, you are no longer allowed to attempt collection on that account. This often includes not only the patient, but also accounts for all members of the patient's family. If the account was turned over to a collection agency, immediately notify the collection agency that the patient has filed bankruptcy. Many doctors will write-off the patient's debt when they are notified of the bankruptcy filing. This prevents statements from continuing to be sent out.

It is not necessary for a patient to notify their creditors in writing that they have filed for bankruptcy protection. A phone call is legally sufficient; however, many offices will request a copy of the bankruptcy filing.

Dear _____:

We are sorry to hear about your recent financial difficulties. Unfortunately, due to your situation, Dr. --- will no longer be able to treat you and your family. We will continue treatment for the next 30 days to allow you to find a new physician, however, during this period payment must be made in cash prior to services rendered. We will be happy to inform you of an estimate of the cost of services prior to an appointment to allow you to bring in the required funds.

When you have chosen a new physician, and upon your written request, we will be happy to provide copies of any medical reports or information on your treatment to the new physician.

Please sign and date one copy of this letter to acknowledge understanding, and return it to our offices in the enclosed envelope. Thank you very much.

Sincerely,

_____, M.D.

This letter should be sent certified mail. Even if the patient refuses to sign and return the letter, the provider is allowed to discontinue treatment of the patient 30 days after receipt of the letter and not be charged with patient abandonment.

Small Claims Court

At times, a patient who is able to pay his account will refuse to pay. In such cases it may be necessary to take the patient to small claims court and ask for a judgment against the person.

Attorneys are not allowed in small claims court, so each party represents themselves. Each side tells their side of the story and the judge renders a decision. There is a maximum limit of $5,000 per case in most areas. Your claim should ask for all money which the defendant owes you, plus any collection costs, court costs, and any other costs incurred in attempting to collect the debt.

Before filing a claim, you must show that you attempted to recover the money and that your efforts have not been successful. This means that you should bill the patient at least three times, and send collection letters demanding payment. If the patient makes no attempt to pay the bill, contact the Municipal Courthouse in your area and request a plaintiff claim form.

Complete the plaintiff claim form and send it to the court with any required filing fees. The **defendant** (the person you are suing), will be notified of the law suit and you will be given a court date.

On the scheduled date, show up in court and bring any and all available documentation to support your case. You should include copies of the pertinent portion of the medical record showing the services performed, the billing for those services, and any letters or copies of statements which show collection attempts.

The judge will take all the evidence into consideration and render a verdict. Often the verdict will come several weeks after the court date. If the decision is in your favor, the defendant will be ordered to pay you the money. If not, you are unable to collect the money requested.

Many states have a provision for the defendant to pay "through the court." In such a case, the court collects the money and reimburses you. There is usually a charge for this service, often based upon the amount of money being collected. However, this charge can be much less than trying to collect from a defendant who still refuses to pay, even though the court has ruled against him.

If you choose this option, be sure to discuss it with the clerk of the court prior to trial.

Summary

Keeping accurate patient accounts is one of the most important jobs of a medical biller. Patients must not only be billed for the services they receive, but insurance carriers must be billed, payments posted to accounts, and patient's balance billed for any remaining amounts on the claim.

If payment is not received from an insurance carrier in a timely manner, an insurance tracer must be completed.

Collections are also an important aspect of the job. Some patients will refuse to pay their bill and collection attempts must be made. At times this involves tracing a skipped patient or filing a claim in small claims court. If the patient files bankruptcy, all collections on the account must stop and the patient must be properly informed if the provider refuses to continue to treat the patient.

Assignments

Complete the Questions for Review.
Complete Exercise 12 – 1.

Questions for Review

Directions: Answer the following questions without looking back into the material just covered. Write your answers in the space provided.

1. What information is listed on a patient statement? _____

   _____

   _____

2. Under the Truth in Lending Act, what items must be included in a payment plan? _____

   _____

   _____

3. What is the purpose of the ledger card? _____

   _____

4. If you are attempting to collect on a bill, is it legal to call the person names or to make derogatory comments regarding them, their sex, race or ethnic background? _____

   _____

   _____

   _____

5. What information are you allowed to give if you call a debtor and speak instead with a roommate or other family member?_____

   _____

If you were unable to answer any of the questions, refer back to that section, and then fill in the answers.

Exercise 12 – 1

Directions: Make three copies of the ledger card shown in **Figure 12 – 1**. Complete a patient ledger card for each of the following patients.

1. The following services were billed for: Abby Addison   Date of Service 9/19/xx
      99204 – Moderate Complexity Exam ($140)
      82948 – Glucose Fingerstick ($18)
      81000 – Urinalysis (30)
   Patient made a cash payment of $60 on this visit.

2. The following services were billed for: Bobby Bumble   Date of Service 9/19/xx
      99205 – Comprehensive Exam ($160)
      81000 – Urinalysis ($30)
      36415 – Venipuncture (20)
   Patient made a payment by check of $75 on this visit.

3. The following services were billed for: Cathy Crenshaw   Date of Service 9/19/xx
      99204 – Moderate Complexity Exam ($140)
      81000 – Urinalysis ($30)
   Patient made a payment by check of $110 on this visit.

Honors Certification™

The certification challenge for this chapter will be a written test of the information contained in this chapter. Each incorrect answer will result in a deduction of up to 5% from your grade. You must achieve a score of 85% or higher to pass this test. If you fail the test on your first attempt you may retake the test one additional time. The items included in the second test may be different from those in the first test.

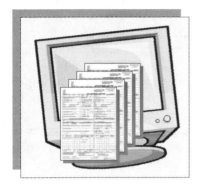

13

Office Accounting

After completion of this chapter you will be able to:

- Explain and use the daily journal.
- Properly balance petty cash money using a petty cash count slip and petty cash receipts.
- List the main reports a medical office may use and their purposes.

Key words and concepts you will learn in this chapter:

Accounting Control Summary – A weekly or monthly report form that shows each day's charges, payments, and adjustments for the period indicated.

Cumulative Trial Balance – A list that shows each patient alphabetically and shows any charges, payments, or adjustments to the patient's account.

Daily Journal – A daily balance sheet that shows the patient's name, the individual fee charged for the day, any payments made, and the current balance.

Deposit Slip – An overview and balance of monies being deposited.

Petty Cash Fund – A fund that is used for giving change to customers who are making cash payments and for buying miscellaneous small supplies.

Petty Cash Receipt – A form that is used whenever money is removed from the petty cash fund indicating how much money was removed and who received it.

As a medical biller, you are often responsible for keeping a petty cash drawer, for collecting payments from patients, and for reconciling the amount in petty cash. At the end of each day you will prepare a deposit slip indicating all payments received that day. You should recount the petty cash to insure that the same amount remains at the end of the day as there was at the beginning. Also be sure that the money in petty cash is sufficient for making change for customers.

When a patient makes a payment, place the check or cash into the petty cash drawer. If change is needed, remove the proper change from the petty cash drawer.

Petty Cash

Most offices have a **petty cash fund** to start the business day. This fund is used to make change for patients who are making cash payments and for purchasing miscellaneous small offices supplies. Keeping track of this fund on a daily basis is essential.

Petty Cash Count Slips

Most offices use a **petty cash count slip (see Figure 13 – 1)** to keep track of the amount of money kept in petty cash. The petty cash count slip has space to write the date and time at the top. The remainder of the slip shows various denominations of currency and coins.

To use the petty cash count slip, count the number of each denomination you have. Put the number of items on the first line. Then multiply the denomination by the number of items. This is the amount of money you have for that denomination.

Once you have counted all the money in the drawer, total the amount on the petty cash count slip. Most offices will also require the person making the count to sign the slip with their name or initials.

This count is often performed at the beginning of the day before any money is taken from or added to petty cash, and at the close of the day.

The morning's petty cash count slip is usually kept in the petty cash box for the day.

When closing at the end of the day, all monies added to the petty cash drawer should be taken out. These will be deposited in the bank. The remaining amount is counted using a second petty cash count slip. While the denominations of the currency or coin may change a bit, the total amount in petty cash should be the same at the end of the day as it was at the beginning, unless money was removed to purchase supplies or other items.

Petty Cash Receipts

At times the money in petty cash will be needed to pay for small office supplies or other items for the office (i.e., a cake to celebrate an employee's birthday).

There are usually only a few people who are allowed to take money from petty cash. Each time cash is removed, the medical biller should get the permission of a supervisor. This is usually documented using a **petty cash receipt (see Figure 13 – 2).**

Each person who takes money from petty cash should sign a petty cash receipt showing the date the money was taken, the amount, and what it is to be used for.

Petty cash receipts should be kept in the petty cash box until a purchase receipt and change are obtained. This allows all reimbursements and outgoing monies to be monitored and approved by a supervisor.

After purchases are made the receipt and any change left over should be returned to the petty cash drawer. Be sure that the amount of the receipt and the change total the amount that was originally taken from petty cash. Indicate on the petty cash receipt the amount of change returned. Then staple the purchase receipt to the petty cash receipt.

At times someone may purchase an office supply with their own money and need to be reimbursed with petty cash funds. A petty cash receipt should also be completed for these types of purchases. The exact amount should be returned to the person, and the purchase receipt stapled to the petty cash receipt.

Petty cash receipts should be kept in the petty cash drawer. When reconciling funds at the end of the day, petty cash vouchers should be counted as cash. This will help you to determine if your amounts have balanced.

All petty cash receipts should be consecutively numbered and treated as amounts paid out.

PETTY CASH COUNT

DATE _____

TIME _____

	QUANTITY	AMOUNT
CURRENCY		
$100	_____	_____
$50	_____	_____
$20	_____	_____
$10	_____	_____
$5	_____	_____
$1	_____	_____
TOTAL		_____
COINS		
$1	_____	_____
Half $	_____	_____
Quarters	_____	_____
Dimes	_____	_____
Nickels	_____	_____
Pennies	_____	_____
TOTAL		_____
RECEIPTS TOTAL +		_____
GRAND TOTAL		_____

Figure 13 – 1: Petty Cash Count Slip

```
┌─────────────────────────────────────────────────────────────┐
│                                                               │
│         RECEIVED OF PETTY CASH              01278             │
│                                                               │
│  NUMBER _____ DATE _____    │
│  AMOUNT _____ │
│  FOR _____ │
│  _____ │
│  _____ │
│  CHARGE TO ACCOUNT _____   │
│  _____  _____  │
│  APPROVED BY                        RECEIVED BY               │
│                                                               │
└─────────────────────────────────────────────────────────────┘
```

Figure 13 – 2: Petty Cash Receipt

The Daily Journal

At the end of the day, the daily journal will need to be balanced. The **daily journal** is used as a balance sheet. This form indicates the patient's name, the individual fee charged for the day, any payments made, and the current balance **(see Figure 13 – 3).** All receipts for the day and any insurance or other payments should equal the cash/check total collected on the daily journal.

The beginning line on the daily journal should be the petty cash total for the day. All entries should be made on the journal for insurance payments, cash payments, or any other miscellaneous payments or adjustments. To balance, make a total of the cash receipts for the day, any petty cash disbursements, and the petty cash on hand. A receipt should be made for all payments made in the office or by mail. Total all insurance payments received. Combine the receipts total and the insurance payments total. Total the payments column on the daily journal. This total is equal to the combined insurance payments, cash receipts, and petty cash totals.

If the daily journal does not balance, go back through the charge slips and ledger cards for the day. By comparing the amounts written, you should be able to find your error.

Deposit Slips

All checks should be stamped on the back with a bank deposit stamp and entered on a deposit slip **(see Figure 13 – 4).** A deposit slip is an overview and balance of monies being deposited.

Be sure to fill out the correct deposit slip. Several companies have more than one bank account. The deposit slip has space for coin, cash, and check deposits. Add up the amount of money you have in coins and enter it in the first box. Next, add up the amount of cash you have and list it in the second box.

Checks are listed individually. Fill in the bank number of the check. This is a four to six-digit number with a hyphen in the middle (i.e., 66-123). This number refers to the bank and the branch of the bank that the check is drawn on. Next to this number and below the previous amounts, list the amount of the check. If you run out of space for all of your checks, there is usually additional space on the back of the deposit slip.

When all amounts have been entered, total them and put the amount at the bottom. This will give you the total amount of your deposit.

Office Reports

There are numerous reports designed to help the office run smoothly and to keep track of the cash flow. These include the daily journal, accounting control summary, insurance request form, and patient statements.

Accounting Control Summary

The **accounting control summary** is a weekly or monthly report form that shows each day's charges,

Daily Journal

Mike Moriarty, M.D.
0123 Any Way
Anytown, USA 12345
(123) 555-6789

Date	Name	Description of Service	Charge	Payments	Adjustments	Remaining Balance

Figure 13 – 3: Daily Journal

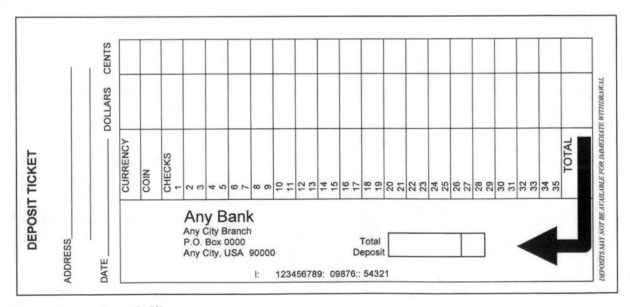

Figure 13 – 4: Deposit Slip

payments, and adjustments for the period indicated. The medical biller uses this form to double-check the figures against her records. This ensures that all information that is to be input reaches the computer properly and has been entered correctly. It also lists items that were not entered.

Items may not be entered or "held in suspense" for a variety of reasons, including wrong account numbers, incorrect spellings, missing code numbers, and no master record for the family.

Cumulative Trial Balance

The **cumulative trial balance** lists each patient alphabetically and shows any charges, payments, or adjustments to the patient's account. This allows the medical office to keep track of all accounts and the amounts that are owed and have been paid.

Summary

Keeping accurate patient accounts is one of the most important jobs of a medical biller. It is also important to balance bill patients for any amounts not received and to keep a daily journal of the office transactions. It is the medical biller's responsibility to reconcile petty cash and prepare a deposit slip of the day's receipts.

Collections are also an important aspect of the job, as well as maintaining numerous other reports.

Assignments

Complete the Questions for Review.

Questions for Review

Directions: Answer the following questions without looking back into the material just covered. Write your answers in the space provided.

1. What is the purpose of the petty cash count slip and how do you use it? _____

   _____

   _____

2. What is the purpose of the daily journal? _____

   _____

3. What is included on a daily journal? _____

   _____

   _____

4. What is the purpose of the petty cash receipt? _____

   _____

5. What are some of the most common accounting reports used in a medical office and what is their purpose? _____

   _____

   _____

   _____

If you were unable to answer any of the questions, refer back to that section, and then fill in the answers.

Honors Certification™

The certification challenge for this chapter will be a written test of the information contained in this chapter. Each incorrect answer will result in a deduction of up to 5% from your grade. You must achieve a score of 85% or higher to pass this test. If you fail the test on your first attempt you may retake the test one additional time. The items included in the second test may be different from those in the first test.

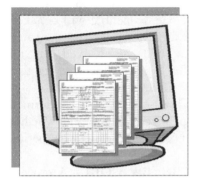

14

Terminology

After completion of this chapter you will be able to:

- Recognize and define insurance terms.
- Identify providers by their professional abbreviation to determine appropriateness of services rendered or benefits payable.
- Properly identify medical abbreviations and medical symbols.

Key words and concepts you will learn in this chapter:

Abbreviation – A shortened version of a word.
Acronym – An abbreviation formed of a set of words or title using the first letters of several related words.

It is impossible to bill or handle insurance claims properly without learning and understanding the industry terminology. Without terminology, coding of diagnoses and procedures is far less accurate. In addition, there is a higher percentage of error in the filling out and processing of forms. This leads to incorrectly paid benefits and payment delays.

As with learning anything new, the first step is to memorize the terms of what you are studying.

One of the easiest ways to accomplish this is by relating the term, whenever possible, to experiences in your own life. By internalizing the terms, it becomes easier to both remember the meaning and to incorporate the use of the terms in your vocabulary. Of course, the more you use the terms during your classroom experiences, the faster and better you will retain the meanings.

Insurance Terminology

The following terms will follow you in your medical billing career, regardless of the type of provider you work for. Therefore, it is absolutely essential that you learn to use and understand this terminology.

Accumulation Period – Period of time (normally January 1 through December 31) in which to satisfy the deductibles, accumulate COB credit reserves, reach maximums, and so on.

Actively at Work Requirement – The provision of a group plan that requires an otherwise eligible employee to be actively at work on the day he or she becomes covered. Furthermore, if the employee is not actively at work on the date that the coverage becomes effective, coverage will be delayed until the date he or she returns to active work. For an eligible dependent that is hospital-confined on the date that coverage was to become effective, the coverage will not become effective until after the dependent's release from the hospital.

Adjustment – A correction of the application of benefits or coding on a claim.

ASO – Administrative Services Only. The provision of services such as actuarial benefit plan design, claim processing, data recovery and analysis, employee benefits communications, financial advice, medical care conversions, preparation of data for reports to governmental units for a self-funded plan, or the like. ASO's are provided on a contract basis by an insurer or a Third Party Administrator.

Administrator, Third Party – See Third Party Administrator.

Assignment of Benefits – In health coverage, a method under which a claimant requests that his or her benefits under a claim be paid to a designated person or institution, usually a physician or hospital.

Audit, Claim – Checking the accuracy of claim payments in accordance with the contract provisions of the plan. The claimants and the providers eligibility is usually also verified.

Automatic Annual Reinstatement – A specified amount of money (credit) that may be added to the balance of available lifetime benefits. Usually, this is important only when a member has a catastrophic illness or injury and will be calculated only when lifetime benefits have been exhausted.

Basic Benefits – The portion of a plan of benefits that is not usually subject to a deductible and usually pays from the first dollars submitted by a provider. Generally, a maximum amount is allowed for payment for each basic benefit.

Beneficiary – The person designated or provided for by the policy terms to receive the proceeds from the policy upon the death of the insured.

Benefit – The amount payable by the plan to a claimant, assignee, or beneficiary under each coverage.

COBRA – Consolidated Omnibus Budget Reconciliation Act of 1985. This act provides for continuation of coverage for employees no longer considered eligible by a plan.

Coinsurance – The arrangement by which both the member and the plan share a specific ratio of the covered losses under a policy. For example, the plan may reimburse the provider or member 80% of covered expenses, and the member will be responsible for the remaining 20% of such expenses.

Common Accident Provision – An arrangement that only one deductible will be taken for all members of a family involved in the same accident. Deductibles will be waived on all remaining members for expenses incurred for that accident.

Concurrent Review – A review performed while a patient is hospitalized to determine whether the stay is medically necessary and for what period of time.

Coordination of Benefits (COB) – A process that occurs when two or more group plans provide coverage on the same person. Coordination between the plans is necessary to allow for payment of 100% of the allowable expenses, but no more.

Copay – The amount that the member/insured must pay "out-of-pocket." This would normally be the 20% not paid by the coinsurance. The plan copay amount may or may not include the major medical deductible. The policy will state this specifically. Also known as the out-of-pocket expense (OOP).

Covered Expenses – The amount of those expenses that are allowable under the plan.

Customary and Reasonable (C&R) – See UCR.

Deductible – The amount of covered expenses that must be paid by the insured/member before benefits become payable by the insurer/plan. Usually, this is a calendar year deductible (taken once each calendar year), but not always. The deductible is always taken out of the first eligible expenses submitted each year.

Individual Deductible – The amount of covered expenses that must be paid by the individual family member before benefits become payable by the plan.

Family Deductible – A specified number of family members must satisfy their deductibles. The deductible is then considered met for the remaining family members. There are two types of family deductibles: aggregate and non-aggregate.

Aggregate Deductible – All major medical deductibles applied for all family members that are added together to attain the family limit.

Nonaggregate – A specified number of individual deductibles must be satisfied before the family limit is met.

DEFRA – Deficit Reduction Act of 1984. Requires that employers with 20 or more employees offer the spouses, age 65+ of active employees the same coverage offered to younger spouses.

DXL – Diagnostic x-ray and laboratory tests.

EIN – Employer Identification Number. A number assigned by the IRS for tax purposes. This number is used by businesses in place of a social security number. (May also be called a taxpayer identification number (TIN).)

Eligibility Period – A specified length of time (usually 31 days) following the eligibility date, during which an individual member of a particular group will remain eligible to apply, without evidence of insurability, for coverage under a group life or health plan. A newborn child must be enrolled within 31 days of birth.

ERISA – Employee Retirement Income Security Act of 1974. This act governs every aspect of private pension and welfare plans and requires employers who sponsor plans to operate them in compliance with ERISA standards.

ESRD – End-stage renal disease is a complete or near complete failure of the kidneys to function to excrete wastes, concentrates urine, and regulates electrolytes.

Evidence of Insurability – A health questionnaire used to determine a person's physical and mental condition and/or other factual information affecting the acceptance of the applicant's application for health or life coverage. Normally, this is required only when the individual is attempting to obtain coverage after the period of eligibility has lapsed on a group plan. However, this is a common requirement to obtain coverage on an individual policy.

Exclusions – Specified conditions or types of services for which the policy does not provide benefits.

Experience Rating – The process of determining the premium rate for a group risk wholly or partially on the basis of that group's experience (dollars paid out in claims). This also takes into consideration administrative costs, inflation, and probability of the next year's costs.

Explanation of Benefits (EOB) – A statement generated by the claim payor, which indicates how the benefits were applied, paid, or denied on a particular claim. It would also show when and to whom the benefits, if any, were paid.

Explanation of Medicare Benefits (EOMB) – Issued by the Medicare claims payor to explain the application of benefits on claims submitted on behalf of Medicare participants.

Extended Benefits – The continued entitlement of a member, under certain circumstances, to receive benefits after the coverage has terminated until either the person is no longer totally disabled or until a specified period of time has elapsed. A doctor's certification of disability is required before benefits can be extended. Usually, such coverage will continue only for expenses incurred for the condition that caused the disability and for a maximum of 12 months following the date of disability or the date that the member is no longer totally disabled, whichever period of time is less.

Full-Time Student – A dependent who is attending a recognized educational facility on a full-time basis. The facility may include vocational schools, colleges, junior colleges, universities, high schools, or any other type of institution specified by the plan. The contract must specify the maximum age limit allowed under this provision and the student cannot be the subscriber, employee, or member.

Health Maintenance Organization (HMO) – An alternative form of health care delivery that refers all patients to a set location and provides a full range of health services. All patients must be enrolled in the plan.

Last Quarter Carry-Over – Amounts applied to the deductible in the last three months of the calendar year, which are carried over (applied) to the next year's deductible.

Major Medical Benefits (MM) – The portion of a health plan that pays benefits at a set percentage usually subject to a deductible.

Management Information System – A system that processes data and makes the resulting information available to those who request it.

Maximum(s) – The maximum amount payable by the plan. The maximum may refer to a calendar year or a lifetime maximum. In addition, it may apply only toward expenses paid under Basic or only toward expenses paid under MM or a combination of all payments, basic and Major Medical. The policy must specify what type.

Medical While Hospitalized (MWH) – Medical care while confined in a healthcare facility. This can include doctor's visits to a patient while the patient is hospitalized.

Order of Benefit Determination (OBD) – The process by which claim payors determine who is the primary, secondary, and tertiary payor on a patient covered under more than one plan.

Out-of-Pocket Expense (OOP) – Applies to expenses for which the insured is held responsible and must pay "out-of-his-or-her-own pocket," such as the deductible and coinsurance. Also known as Copay.

OOP Max – The yearly limit on the OOP that the insured is responsible for paying. (Most contracts have this.) When this limit or maximum is reached, the plan pays additional covered expenses at 100% instead of the usual percentage for the remainder of the calendar year.

Pre-Admit Testing (PAT) – Testing performed on an outpatient basis prior to admittance to an inpatient facility.

Peer Review – Independent review by a group of physicians to determine whether the services submitted by another physician are usual, customary, and reasonable for the condition being treated.

Plan Document – The legal document prepared by the fiduciaries of a self-funded/self-insured health and welfare fund. This outlines all the terms and conditions of the plan benefits. The plan document is essentially the same as a policy except that the term "policy" is usually associated with insured plans, whereas a "plan document" is associated with self-insured plans.

Policy – The legal document issued by the insurance company to the policyholder, which outlines the terms and conditions of the insurance.

Pre-existing Exclusion – When specified by the plan, a condition that is treated within a specified time period prior to the effective date of coverage. All charges related to the condition would not be covered at all for a stated period of time, or payment for the condition would be limited to a stated dollar amount.

Preferred Provider Organization (PPO) – A medical group of physicians who negotiate discounted fees and who does utilization review and quality assurance in exchange for a referral of a population of patients or monthly per capita payments. The arrangements under this heading vary widely within the industry.

Subrogation – Contract provision that provides a plan with the authority to recover money paid on claims that are covered by a third party, such as automobile carriers and lawsuit settlements. See also Third Party Liability Provision.

Summary Plan Description (SPD) – A summary of the plan document that is distributed to the members of a self-funded plan. A copy of the SPD is kept on file at the Department of Labor.

Tax Equity and Financial Responsibility Act of 1982 (TEFRA) – Requires employers with 20 or more employees to offer active employees age 65 and over and their spouses of the same age the same coverage under any group plan that is offered to younger workers. See the chapter on legal issue for details.

Taxpayer Identification Number (TIN) – A unique nine-digit identification number required by the IRS for a provider or business for tax purposes.

Terminal Liability – Benefits payable after the termination of a contract.

Third Party Administrator (TPA) – A firm that handles all functions related to the operation of a group insurance/self-funded plan. The kind and number of services provided vary, depending on the contract. As an administrator only, the client uses the money to pay for the health care coverage. The administrator provides the personnel and equipment to perform the services for the client.

Third Party Liability Provision – Provision by a plan that when an injury is covered by a third party (another coverage), reimbursement will be provided to the plan if recovery is made through that coverage. For example, in an automobile accident, a lawsuit is won and damages are recovered for medical services rendered. The member would have to pay back the plan the money that the plan paid out for coverage of the injury. See also Subrogation.

Three-Month Carry-Over Provision (C/O) – Eligible charges incurred in the last quarter of the calendar year (October, November, December) and applied toward the member's deductible. These amounts will apply toward satisfaction of the deductible for that member for the next calendar year. These monies normally are not applied toward the family limit.

Usual, Customary, and Reasonable (UCR) – Also known as U&C, R&C and C&R--The amount determined to be the maximum allowable by the plan, based on the contract provisions, procedure, date of service, and geographic location of the provider.

Provider Abbreviations

Many types of insurance benefits are based on the type of licensing of the provider and the type of service being provided. Therefore, in order to properly apply these types of benefits, billers and examiners must understand the various types of licensing available and the types of services which that particular type of provider is allowed to perform. The following is a list of the more common types of licensing that are covered under most contracts and the types of services they usually provide.

CA – Certified Acupuncturist. Usually required for other than an M.D. or D.O. Provider must have this certification to provide acupuncture treatments.

Clinical Psychologist – Licensed to perform psychological testing and therapy. Referral by an MD is usually not required.

CRNA – Certified Registered Nurse Anesthetist. Certified to administer anesthesia under the direction of an M.D.

DC – Doctor of Chiropractic. Performs manual manipulations of the spine and other musculoskeletal areas. Licensed for office visits, x-rays, nutritional supplements, manipulations, ultrasound and physical therapies. All other services should be questioned. Cannot draw blood or perform surgery.

DDS – Doctor of Dental Surgery. Licensed to perform all dental care including dental surgeries and surgeries to the face and jaw.

DMD – Doctor of Medical Dentistry. Licensed to perform dental care including dental surgeries and surgeries to the face and jaw. The only difference between a DDS and a DMD is the school attended; the training and licensing authorizations are the same.

DO – Doctor of Osteopathy. Licensed to perform any service that an M.D. can perform. Training is essentially the same as an M.D.

DPM – Doctor of Podiatry Medicine. Licensed for the care, treatment, and surgery of the feet.

DSC – Doctor of Surgical Chiropody. The same as a podiatrist; deals with foot surgeries. DSC is an old licensing designation that is seldom seen today.

EdD – Doctor of Education. An educational degree, not a licensing. The licensing needs to be obtained. Without appropriate licensing, services by this provider would not usually be covered.

EMT – Emergency Medical Technician. Licensed to administer emergency procedures such as CPR. Cannot perform tracheotomies. Usually works in an ambulance.

LCSW – Licensed Clinical Social Worker. Licensed to provide psychological counseling. Referral from an MD is usually required.

LPN – Licensed Practical Nurse. Equivalent to an LVN. LVNs are in California, whereas LPNs are from other states.

LVN – Licensed Vocational Nurse. Lower level (usually a two year program) nurse, not certified to perform IV-Push (injecting medications directly into a vein) and cannot be a charge nurse on a floor.

MD – Medical Doctor. Licensed to perform any and all medical care/procedures.

MFCC – Marriage, Family, Child Counselor. Licensed to provide psychological counseling and marriage and family counseling. Usually requires a referral from an M.D.

Midwife – Licensed as a registered nurse and certified as a nurse midwife. Usually handles routine maternity cases. Must be associated with an M.D. or a D.O. to handle emergency cases.

MSW – Master of Social Work. Licensed to provide family and psychological counseling. Referral from an MD is usually required.

MT – Medical Technologist. Usually works in a laboratory and can draw blood and perform lab testing. An MT also can administer injections and perform EKGs.

Myofunctionist – Licensed to perform myofunctional speech therapy. This involves the reeducation of the facial muscles needed to speak and breathe.

NA – Nurse's Aide. Licensed to assist patients not requiring skilled nursing care. Normally employed in skilled nursing facilities, nursing homes and home health agencies. (Also known as a CNA--Certified Nurse's Aide.)

NP – Nurse Practitioner. A nurse practitioner is a registered nurse (RN) who has completed advanced education and training in the diagnosis and management of common medical conditions. They provide some of the same care provided by physicians and maintain close working relationships with physicians.

OD – Doctor of Optometry. An optometrist. Not licensed to perform surgery. Most commonly performs eye refractions, dispenses glasses and contacts.

OT – Occupational Therapist. Licensed to perform occupational therapy. Occupational therapy is the retraining of muscles and nerves, usually in the hands and arms, necessary for the performance of routine daily movements (i.e., learning to feed oneself, brush hair, and other activities of daily living.)

PA – Physician Assistant. Physician Assistants are health care professionals licensed to practice medicine with physician supervision. PA responsibilities include conducting physical exams, diagnosing and treating illnesses, ordering and interpreting tests, counseling on preventive health care, assisting in surgery and writing prescriptions. PA-C stands for Physician Assistant-Certified; the person that holds the title has taken a national certification examination.

Paramedic – Licensed to administer emergency care. Has more extensive training than an EMT. Normally works in an ambulance or for a fire department.

PhD – An educational degree (doctorate) not a licensing. Services by this provider would be covered only when there is also appropriate licensing.

RN – Registered Nurse. Registered nurses provide direct patient care. This level of nursing is higher than an LVN/LPN.

RPT – Registered Physical Therapist. Licensed to perform physical (muscle) therapy when services are prescribed by an M.D. or D.O.

Medical Abbreviations

An **abbreviation** is a shortened version of a word (i.e., aglut for agglutination). An acronym is an abbreviation formed by using the first letters of several related words (i.e., AIDS for Acquired Immune Deficiency Syndrome).

The following listing shows some of the most common medical abbreviations and acronyms. It is not necessary to memorize the abbreviations listed here. However, this reference list should be reviewed and kept handy to understand items which may be listed in the text and/or the medical reports. Many medical practices will have a more comprehensive medical abbreviation listing, and many medical dictionaries also contain abbreviations and acronyms.

AA	Aortic aneurysm
ABD	Abdomen
ABG	Arterial blood gas
ACTH	Adrenocorticotropic hormone
ADI	American Drug Index
ADL	Activities of daily living
ADR	Adverse drug reaction
AFIB	Atrial fibrillation
AFO	Ankle-foot orthosis
AG	Antigen
AGGLUT	Agglutination
AGL	Acute granulocytic leukemia
AHS	Allied Health Services
AIDS	Acquired immunodeficiency syndrome
AK	Above knee
AKA	Above-knee amputation
AL	Aluminum
ALK	Alkaline
ALS	Amyotrophic lateral sclerosis
AMA	Against medical advice
AMI	Acute myocardial infarction
ANS	Autonomic nervous system
AODM	Adult-onset diabetes mellitus
APP	Application
AR	Accounts receivable
AROM	Active range of motion
ASBD	Arteriosclerotic brain disease
ASC	Ambulatory surgical center
ASCHD	Arteriosclerotic coronary heart disease
ASCVD	Arteriosclerotic cardiovascular disease
ASD	Atrial septal defect
ASHD	Arteriosclerotic heart disease
AVF	Arteriovenous fistula
AVR	Aortic valve replacement
AZT	Azidothymidine
BBB	Bundle branch block
BILI	Bilirubin
BK	Below knee
BKA	Below-knee amputation
BLS	Basic life support
BMR	Basal metabolic rate
BOM	Bilateral otitis media
BP	Blood pressure
BR	By report
BS	Blood sugar
BSO	Bilateral salpingo-oophorectomy
BUN	Blood urea nitrogen

BX	Biopsy	EBV	Epstein-Barr virus
C&S	Culture and sensitivity	ECF	Extended-care facility
CA	Cancer	ECG	Electrocardiogram
CABG	Coronary artery bypass graft	EDC	Expected date of confinement
CABP	Coronary artery bypass	EEG	Electroencephalogram
CAD	Coronary artery disease	EGD	Esophagogastroduodenoscopy
CAPD	Chronic ambulatory peritoneal dialysis	EKG	Electrocardiogram
CBC	Complete blood count	EMG	Electromyogram
CBS	Chronic brain syndrome	ENT	Ear, nose, and throat
CCF	Congestive cardiac failure	EOB	Explanation of benefits
CCPD	Continuous cycling peritoneal dialysis	EOMB	Explanation of Medicare benefits
CCU	Coronary care unit	EPSDT	Early periodic screening, diagnosis, and treatment
CF	Cystic fibrosis		
CHB	Complete heart block	ER	Emergency room
CHD	Coronary heart disease	ESRD	End-stage renal disease
CHF	Congestive heart failure	EST	Electroshock therapy
CL	Chloride	EUA	Examination under anesthesia
CM	Centimeter	EUD	Etiology undetermined
CNS	Central nervous system	F/U	Follow-up
COPD	Chronic obstructive pulmonary disease	FB	Foreign body
CP	Cerebral palsy	FBS	Fasting blood sugar
CPAP	Continuous positive airway pressure	FSH	Follicle-stimulating hormone
CPK	Creatine phosphokinase	FUO	Fever of undetermined origin
CPR	Cardiopulmonary resuscitation	FX	Fracture
CRD	Chronic renal disease	GE	Gastroesophageal
CRF	Chronic renal failure	GI	Gastrointestinal
CRIF	Closed reduction internal fixation	GTT	Glucose tolerance test
CSF	Cerebrospinal fluid	GU	Genitourinary
CT	Computed axial tomography	GYN	Gynecologic
CTS	Carpal tunnel syndrome	H&P	History and physical
CU	Cubic	H/O	History of
CV	Cardiovascular	HBEAB	Hepatitis be antibody
CVA	Cerebrovascular accident	HBEAG	Hepatitis be antigen
CVD	Cardiovascular disease	HBP	High blood pressure
CXR	Chest x-ray	HCT	Hematocrit
D&C	Dilation and curettage	HEENT	Head, eyes, ears, nose, and throat
D&E	Dilation and evacuation	HIV	Human immunodeficiency virus
D/T	Due to	HKAF	Hip, knee, ankle, foot
DHS	Department of Health Services	HKAFO	Hip knee ankle foot orthosis
DJD	Degenerative joint disease	HOSP	Hospital
DM	Diabetes mellitus	HR	Hour
DME	Durable medical equipment	HX	History
DNR	Do not resuscitate	I&D	Incision and drainage
DOA	Dead on arrival	IBS	Irritable bowel syndrome
DOS	Date of service	ICF	Intermediate care facility
DPT	Diphtheria, pertussis, and tetanus	ICP	Intracranial pressure
DT	Delirium tremens	ICU	Intensive care unit
DTT	Diphtheria tetanus toxoid	IDDM	Insulin-dependent diabetes mellitus
DVT	Deep vein thrombosis	IH	Infectious hepatitis
DX	Diagnosis	IHD	Ischemic heart disease
EAC	Estimated acquisition cost	IM	Intramuscular

IP	Inspiratory pressure	NSVD	Normal spontaneous vaginal delivery
IPD	Intermittent peritoneal dialysis	O2	Oxygen
IPPB	Intermittent positive-pressure breathing	OM	Otitis media
IUD	Intrauterine device	OPD	Obstructive pulmonary disease
IUP	Intrauterine pregnancy	OPV	Oral poliovirus
JODM	Juvenile-onset diabetes mellitus	OU	Both eyes
JRA	Juvenile rheumatoid arthritis	OV	Office visit
KAF	Knee, ankle, and foot	OZ	Ounce
KO	Knee orthosis	PAP	Papanicolaou
KUB	Kidney ureter bladder	PC	Professional component
L/S	Lumbosacral	PDR	Physicians' Desk Reference
LAD	Left anterior descending	PERLA	Pupils equal, react to light and accommodation
LB(S)	Pound(s)		
LBBB	Left bundle branch block	PHP	Prepaid health plan
LBP	Low blood pressure	PID	Pelvic inflammatory disease
LCA	Left coronary artery	PIN	Physician Identifier Number
LE	Lower extremity	PKG	Package
LFT	Liver function tests	PO	By mouth
LGI	Lower gastrointestinal	POE	Proof of Eligibility
LLL	Left lower lobe	POS	Place of Service
LLQ	Left lower quadrant	PPN	Peripheral parenteral nutrition
LMP	Last menstrual period	PRN	As occasion requires
LOC	Loss of consciousness	PRO	Professional Review Organization
LP	Lumbar puncture	PROM	Passive range of motion
LSO	Lumbar sacral orthosis	PTT	Partial thromboplastin time
LTC	Long-term care	PUD	Peptic ulcer disease
LUL	Left upper lobe	PVD	Peripheral vascular disease
LUQ	Left upper quadrant	QD	Every day
MEDS	Medications	QID	Four times a day
MG	Milligram	R/O	Rule out
MI	Myocardial infarction	RA	Rheumatoid arthritis
MIN(S)	Minute(s)	RA	Remittance Advice
MM	Millimeter	RBC	Red blood cell
MMIS	Medicaid Management Information System	RDS	Respiratory distress syndrome
		REM	Rapid eye movements
MMR	Measles, mumps, and rubella	RF	Rheumatoid factor
MONO	Mononucleosis	RHD	Rheumatic heart disease
MRI	Magnetic resonance imaging	RLL	Right lower lobe
MS	Multiple sclerosis	RLQ	Right lower quadrant
MVA	Motor vehicle accident	RML	Right middle lobe
MVP	Mitral valve prolapse	RO	Rule out
NA	Sodium	RT	Right
NEC	Not elsewhere classified	RUL	Right upper lobe
NH	Nursing home	RUQ	Right upper quadrant
NKA	No known allergies	RV	Right ventricular
NKDA	No known drug allergies	RVS	Relative value studies
NM	Nuclear medicine	RX	Prescription
NOC	Not otherwise classified	S/P	Status post
NOS	Not otherwise specified	SBO	Small bowel obstruction
NP	Nasopharyngeal	SED	Sedimentation
NSR	Normal sinus rhythm	SEWH	Shoulder, elbow, wrist, and hand

SI	Sacroiliac
SIDS	Sudden infant death syndrome
SLR	Straight leg raising
SMA	Schedule of maximum allowances
SNF	Skilled nursing facility
SOB	Shortness of breath
SOC	Share of cost
SQ	Subcutaneous
SSA	Social Security Administration
SSI/SSP	Supplemental Security Income/State Supplemental Program
SSN	Social Security Number
STD	Sexually Transmitted Disease
T&A	Tonsillectomy and adenoidectomy
TAB	Therapeutic abortion
TAH	Total abdominal hysterectomy
TAR	Treatment Authorization Request
TB	Tuberculosis
TD	Tetanus diphtheria
TMJ	Temporomandibular joint
TOS	Type of service
TPL	Third party liability
TSH	Thyroid-stimulating hormone
TV	Total volume
UA	Urinalysis
UE	Upper extremity
UGI	Upper gastrointestinal
UNI	Unilateral
URI	Upper respiratory infection
UTI	Urinary tract infection
UV	Ultraviolet
VA	Veterans Administration
VC	Vital capacity
VD	Venereal disease
VDRL	Venereal Disease Research Laboratory

Medical Symbols

Y	Urine
u	Urine
/	Defecation
~,%	Male

o,&	Female
8	Goes up (toe signs)
9	Goes down (toe signs)
>	Increased, enlarged, more than
<	Decreased, diminished, smaller than, less than
#	Number or pounds
	Death
*	Birth
c,c	(L. cum) With
$\square$	Without
+	Plus; excess; acid reactions; positive
--	Minus; deficiency; alkaline reaction; negative
$\forall$	Plus or minus; either positive or negative; indefinite
$\square$	Approximately, equals
©	Not less than
Σ	Not greater than
#	Equal to or less than
$\exists$	Equal to or greater than
$\square$	Not equal to
	Degree
%	Percent

Summary

Understanding proper medical and insurance terminology is essential to both the health claims examiner and the medical biller. Without this knowledge, there will be a higher percentage of errors in both the filling out of forms and the payment of benefits.

Assignments

Complete the Questions for Review.
Complete Exercises 14 – 1 through 14 – 4.

Questions for Review

Directions: Answer the following questions without looking back into the material just covered. Write your answers in the space provided.

1. Define adjustment. _____
   _____

2. The amount payable by the plan to a claimant, assignee or beneficiary under each coverage is called a
   _____

3. What does TIN stand for? _____

4. A _____ is licensed to perform any and all medical care or procedures.

5. What does LUQ stand for? _____

If you were unable to answer any of the questions, refer back to that section, and then fill in the answers.

Exercise 14 – 1

Directions: Write the correct title for the following licensing abbreviation in the space provided.

1. DDS _____
2. EMT _____
3. LPN _____
4. MFCC _____
5. OT _____
6. PA _____
7. MD _____
8. DPM _____
9. CA _____
10. DC _____
11. OD _____
12. EdD _____
13. MSW _____
14. MT _____
15. RPT _____

Exercise 14 – 2

Directions: Define the following terms.

1. Eligibility Period _____

_____

2. Family Deductible _____

_____

3. Last Quarter Carry-Over_____

_____

4. Plan Document _____

_____

5. Common Accident Provision _____

_____

6. Exclusions _____

_____

7. Coinsurance _____

_____

8. Assignment of Benefits _____

_____

9. Basic Benefits _____

_____

10. Adjustment _____

_____

11. Beneficiary _____

_____

12. Benefit _____

_____

13. Maximum(s) _____

_____

14. Pre-existing Exclusion _____

_____

15. Subrogation _____

_____

Exercise 14 – 3

Directions: Write the correct definition for the following abbreviations in the space provided.

1. B/P _____

2. CAPD _____

3. DOA _____

4. D&C _____

5. F/U _____

6. ER _____

7. HR _____

8. FB _____

9. LLQ _____

10. LE _____

11. AK _____

12. BK _____

13. RUQ _____

14. OB _____

15. NH _____

16. % _____

17. / _____

18. 9 _____

19. > _____

20. * _____

21. ☐ _____

22. c,c _____

23. o,& _____

24. ∀ _____

25. ☐ _____

26. # _____

27. _____

28. © _____

29. ☐ _____

30. ~,% _____

Exercise 14 – 4

Directions: Match the following abbreviations with their meaning. Indicate your answer in the space at the left of the abbreviation.

_____	1.	ASO	a. The 1984 act which requires that employers with 20 or more employees offer the spouses age 65+, of active employees the same coverage offered to younger spouses.
_____	2.	COBRA	b. A summary of the plan document which is distributed to members of a self-funded plan.
_____	3.	MWH	c. A group of physicians who have negotiated discounted fees, and do utilization review and quality assurance in exchange for a referral of a population of patients or a monthly per capita payment.
_____	4.	EIN	d. The providing of services such as actuarial benefit plan design, claim processing, data recovery and analysis, and other administrative services for a self-funded plan.
_____	5.	HMO	e. The government act which requires employers with 20 or more employees to offer active employees age 65 or over and their spouses of the same age, the same coverage under any group plan that is offered to younger workers.
_____	6.	EOB	f. Testing performed on an outpatient basis prior to admittance to an inpatient facility.
_____	7.	DEFRA	g. The amount determined to be the maximum allowable by the plan, based on the contract provisions, procedure, date of service, and geographical location of the provider.
_____	8.	OOP	h. Doctor's visits to a patient while the patient is hospitalized in a facility.
_____	9.	SPD	i. The government act which governs every aspect of private pension and welfare plans and requires employers who sponsor plans to operate them in compliance with these standards.
_____	10.	ERISA	j. The portion of a health plan that pays benefits at a set percentage, usually subject to a deductible.
_____	11.	TEFRA	k. A statement generated by the claim payer which indicates how the benefits were applied, paid or denied on a particular claim.
_____	12.	PPO	l. An alternative form of health care delivery which refers all patients to a set location and provides a full range of health services.
_____	13.	UCR	m. The government act which provides for continuation of coverage for employees no longer considered eligible for a plan.
_____	14.	MM	n. Applies to expenses such as the deductible and coinsurance which the insured is expected to pay.
_____	15.	PAT	o. A number assigned by the IRS for tax purposes. This number is used by businesses in place of the social security number.

Honors Certification™

The certification challenge for this chapter will be a written test of the information contained in this chapter. Each incorrect answer will result in a deduction of up to 5% from your grade. You must achieve a score of 85% or higher to pass this test. If you fail the test on your first attempt you may retake the test one additional time. The items included in the second test may be different from those in the first test.

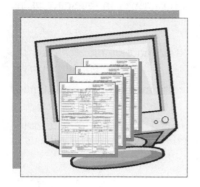

15

Reference Books

After completion of this chapter you will be able to:

- Recognize the *Merck Manual, PDR*, Medical Dictionary, *CPT®* and *ICD-9*, and to explain their use.

Key words and concepts you will learn in this chapter:

Health Care Procedure Coding System (HCPCS) – An index used for billing injections, medication, supplies and durable medical equipment.

International Classification of Diseases--9th Revision Clinical Modification (ICD-9) – An indexing of diseases and conditions.

Medical Dictionary – A book that lists medical terms and their definitions, synonyms, illustrations, and supplemental information.

Physician's Current Procedure Terminology (CPT®) – A systematic listing for coding the procedures or services performed by a physician or provider.

Physicians' Desk Reference (PDR) – A book used to determine whether a pharmaceutical product is a prescription or non-prescription drug.

Reference Book – A source of information to which a reader is referred.

A **reference book** is a source of information to which a reader is referred. In health claims billing, coding, and examining, there are a number of books that are utilized as reference books. These include the *International Classification of Diseases--9th Revision (ICD-9), Physician's Current Procedure Terminology (CPT®), Relative Value Study (RVS), Health Care Procedure Coding System (HCPCS), Physicians' Desk Reference (PDR)*, the medical dictionary, and the Merck Manual. We will discuss each of these books briefly in this chapter. The ICD-9, CPT®, HCPCS, and PDR each have their own chapter to discuss their use in further detail.

ICD-9

The *International Classification of Diseases--9th Revision Clinical Modification* (ICD-9) is an indexing of conditions that serves a dual purpose for health benefits personnel. Mainly, it enables the medical biller and the claims examiner to convert English language descriptions of an illness, injury, or other condition into a numerical code and secondly, it allows for the classification of diseases for statistical purposes. Symptoms, diseases, injuries, and routine services are identified with either a three, four or five digit code, which may be entirely numerical or a combination of alphanumeric.

The ICD-9 consists of three volumes:
- Volume I – A tabular listing of diseases.
- Volume II – An alphabetical listing of diseases by English language description.
- Volume III – A numerical and alphabetical listing of surgical or nonsurgical procedures that may be performed by a physician.

The order of use and the degree of use of these volumes varies.

CPT®/RVS

The *Physician's Current Procedure Terminology (CPT®)* is a systematic listing for coding the procedures or services performed by a physician. Within this text the word "physician" is used generically to apply to any provider of services other than a hospital or other facility. Each procedure is identified with a five-digit numerical code. The purpose of the CPT® is to provide a uniform method of accurately describing medical, surgical, and diagnostic services, which facilitates an effective means of communication among physicians, patients, and claim administrators.

The **Relative Value Study (RVS)** is another reference book used for coding physician services. The RVS preceded the CPT® and was, in fact, the basis on which the CPT® was designed. Consequently, the purpose of the RVS is the same as that of the CPT®. These two manuals are referred to interchangeably even though the rules regarding their usage are somewhat different. Therefore, it is important for the medical biller to know which standard is specified by the plan being processed so that the appropriate rules can be used. The CPT® and RVS each have six major sections:
1. Evaluation and Management – 99201-99499.
2. Medicine – 90001-99199.
3. Surgery – 10000-69999.
4. Anesthesia, CPT® – 0 0100-01999; RVS – 99100-99140 (same as surgery but add anesthesia modifier).
5. Radiology/Nuclear Medicine – 70000-79999.
6. Pathology & Laboratory Tests – 80000-89999.

HCPCS

The *Health Care Procedure Coding System (HCPCS)* was created because of the limitations in the CPT® and RVS for billing injections, medication, supplies and durable medical equipment. These codes are most often used for billing Medicare services, but may also be used for some local carriers. The HCPCS system actually includes three levels of coding:
- Level I – utilizes the current CPT® codes for most procedures.
- Level II – utilizes the HCPCS codes listed in the HCPCS manual.
- Level III – utilizes codes which are specific to the local Medicare carrier.

To properly code using the HCPCS system, you should check Level III codes first. If no code exists for the service or item you are billing, check the Level II codes. Only if there is no Level III or Level II codes should you use the appropriate CPT® code.

Physicians' Desk Reference

The *Physicians' Desk Reference* (PDR) enables a person to determine whether a pharmaceutical product is a prescription or non-prescription drug. This is a very important distinction since most health plans do not cover non-prescription drugs.

The PDR is divided into six sections:
1. Manufacturers' Index.
2. Product Name Index.
3. Product Category Index.
4. Product Identification Section.
5. Product Information Section.
6. Diagnostic Product Information.

The first five sections are used by billing and examining personnel. Each of these sections will be covered in greater detail in the Medications/PDR section of this book.

Medical Dictionary

Medical dictionaries list medical terms and their definitions, synonyms, illustrations, and supplemental information. Numerous medical dictionaries are available. These dictionaries can be very helpful in assisting the biller and examiner to identify diagnoses, their symptoms, prognoses, and common treatment protocols. The use of a dictionary can assist the medical biller in both coding the claim and determining whether or not the diagnosis or service is allowable under a plan.

As a rule, this manual should be used mainly for verifying a diagnosis or affected body area, or checking definitions and the spelling of terms. For greater detail on symptomatology and treatment protocols, the *Merck Manual* is more definitive. As with most dictionaries, entries are arranged alphabetically.

When using the medical dictionary, it is important that you first read through the foreword and any instructions or general guidelines contained in the front of the book. Since each publisher uses different symbols and information, you must read these instructions to understand the symbols and terms and their meanings.

In addition to basic definitions, many medical dictionaries include other information regarding the word or term. These can include the following 14 items:

1. The etymology of the word (i.e., the original language and meaning).
2. The pronunciation of the word.
3. Biographical information on diseases, symptoms, conditions, procedures, or cures that have been given an eponym (named after a person, such as Addison's disease).
4. Synonyms. Often diseases or conditions are known by more than one name. In these instances they are listed as synonyms in the dictionary (i.e., Addison's disease: adrenocortical hypofunction).
5. Abbreviations. If a word or term has a standard abbreviation in the medical community, this abbreviation is often listed in the medical dictionary.
6. Etiology. The causes of the disease.
7. Treatment. Common medical treatments are stated for some diagnoses or conditions. It is understood that this may not be the only effective medical treatment and that specifics of the treatment are not given.
8. Cross-reference. Cross-references for treatments may be included, allowing the user to locate possible drugs or treatments that may prove to be effective.
9. Prognosis. A generalized prognosis for the disease is given. It will sometimes include a prognosis for patients who are not treated and for those that are.
10. Nursing implications. The implications of care of the patient are listed. This may include the need for monitoring of certain conditions or vital signs.
11. Nursing diagnosis cross-reference. Some dictionaries list an appendix of nursing diagnoses and implications. Certain diseases or conditions will be cross-referenced to this section.
12. Subentries. Subentries contain more specific information regarding a term or condition and list some of the different types of conditions that can occur. For example, the subentries under the term "acid" can include acetic a., boric a., citric a., fatty a., and sulfuric a., as well as many others. It is understood that a small letter followed by a period refers to a repetition of the original term or condition. In the example above, the "a." would stand for the word "acid."
13. Illustration cross-reference. An illustration occurs in the dictionary--placed either near the word or under another heading--which illustrates either the term or a portion of the definition. The user is directed to the correct page or term under which the illustration can be found.
14. Cautions or warnings. Certain terms or conditions have a warning placed within the definition. This is most often used with drugs and treatments. This warning can include any side effects or adverse reactions or conditions that can occur from use of the drug or treatment. Often, this caution or warning is in boldface or highlighted within a section to help call attention to it.

When using the medical dictionary it is imperative that the medical biller read through the entire entry. If terms are used in the definition that the medical biller does not understand, the unknown word should also be looked up, either in the medical dictionary (if it is a medical term) or in a standard dictionary (if it is not).

There are numerous diseases, conditions, or terms that are very similar to each other in spelling or pronunciation, but vastly different in meaning. It is important to use the proper term and its proper spelling when billing, and coding a claim.

Merck Manual

Even the most experienced medical biller occasionally has questions regarding the appropriateness of services for a reported diagnosis. The *Merck Manual* is relied on within the medical profession to assist in identifying the symptomatology, prognosis, treatment protocols, etiology, and other miscellaneous information regarding diagnoses.

The *Merck Manual* has two main sections: a listing of diseases and an index. The index is arranged alphabetically by disease. To look something up, simply turn to the index to determine the page the information for a particular disease is located on. The information provided includes the diagnosis, symptoms, prognosis, and treatment.

Summary

The ICD-9, CPT®, RVS, HCPCS, PDR, medical dictionary, and *Merck Manual* are the reference books most commonly used by medical billing and health claims examining personnel.

The ICD-9 is used to code diagnoses and conditions. The CPT® is used to code procedures and services rendered by providers. Use of the PDR assists in determining whether a drug is prescription or non-prescription, and lists some of the properties (i.e., manufacturer, chemical make-up, side effects, appearance) of a specific drug. Medical dictionaries list medical terms and their meanings, and the *Merck Manual* can assist in determining whether a service or procedure is appropriate for a given diagnosis or condition.

Medical billers should familiarize themselves with the use of each of the reference books discussed. Without their proper utilization, delays and denials can result in claims submitted to payors.

Assignments

Complete the Questions for Review.
Complete Exercises 15 – 1 through 15 – 4.

Questions for Review

Directions: Answer the following questions without looking back into the material just covered. Write your answers in the space provided.

1. Which manuals are used for coding diagnoses?_____

   _____

2. Name the two manuals that serve the same purpose and may be referred to interchangeably.

   1. _____

   2. _____

3. The full name of the PDR is _____

4. If you needed to verify a diagnosis, affected body area, or spelling of terms and definitions you would probably refer to the _____

   _____

5. _____ is useful in determining the appropriateness of services for a reported diagnosis.

If you were unable to answer any of the questions, refer back to that section, and then fill in the answers.

Exercise 15 – 1

Directions: Determine the correct reference book needed to answer the following questions then use that reference to find the answer. Do not be concerned if you do not understand all the words in the description or answer.

1. What is the English language description for diagnosis code 460 and 487.1? _____
   _____
   _____

2. Describe diagnosis 1 (code 460) from question 1. _____
   _____
   _____
   _____

3. Define catarrhal._____
   _____
   _____

4. Is fever most commonly a symptom of diagnosis 1 or diagnosis 2? _____
   _____

5. What is a synonym (word with the same meaning) for the common cold? _____
   _____

6. How long is a person contagious with this disease? _____
   _____

7. Name two symptoms or signs of diagnosis 1. _____
   _____
   _____

8. What causes the condition from diagnosis code 1? _____
   _____
   _____

9. What is the incubation period for this disease? _____
   _____

10. What is the procedure code 87060 for and is it appropriate for diagnosis code 460? _____
    _____
    _____

Exercise 15 – 2

Directions: Determine the correct reference book needed to answer the following questions, and then use that reference to find the answer. Do not be concerned if you do not understand all the words in the description or answer.

1. What is the English language description for the procedure code 26535? _____
    _____
    _____

2. What is the English language description for the diagnosis code 345.90? _____
    _____
    _____

3. Is procedure code 26535 a valid treatment for diagnosis code 696.1? _____
    _____

4. Describe the disease from question 2. _____
    _____
    _____
    _____

5. Define paroxysmal disorder. _____
    _____
    _____

6. What is the cause of the disease in question 2? _____
    _____
    _____

7. Name two symptoms or signs of this disease. _____
    _____

8. How effective are anticonvulsant drugs in treating this disease (give percentages of control or reduction of symptoms, if any)? _____
    _____
    _____

9. Can a patient with this disease lead a normal life? _____

10. What book would tell you if a specific drug was considered effective against the given condition? _____
    _____

Exercise 15 – 3

Directions: Determine the correct reference book needed to answer the following questions, and then use that reference to find the answer. Do not be concerned if you do not understand all the words in the description or answer.

1. What do the initials AIDS and HIV stand for? _____

    _____

2. Which of the following is the correct diagnosis code for AIDS? 079.53, V01.7, 042, or 795.71? _____

    _____

3. Describe the disease from question 2. _____

    _____

    _____

4. How is the disease transmitted among adults? _____

    _____

    _____

5. How is the disease transmitted to infants? _____

    _____

6. What is the description of the code 43842 and is it an appropriate treatment for an AIDS patient? _____

    _____

    _____

7. What are the descriptions of the codes 86701, 86702 and 86703, and is any of them an appropriate procedure for a suspected AIDS patient? _____

    _____

    _____

    _____

8. If the patient is a Medicare patient and receives an injection of Interferon, would you use the code J9213 or 90782 and why? _____

    _____

    _____

9. What precautions should medical personnel take when treating someone with AIDS? _____

    _____

    _____

10. What book would tell you if a specific drug was considered effective against the given condition? _____

    _____

    _____

Exercise 15 – 4

Directions: Determine the correct reference book needed to answer the following questions, and then use that reference to find the answer. Do not be concerned if you do not understand all the words in the description or answer.

1. What is the English language description for the diagnosis code 696.1? _____
   _____

2. Describe the disease from question 1. _____
   _____
   _____

3. What are erythematous papules? _____
   _____
   _____

4. What is the cause of the disease in question 1? _____
   _____

5. Name two symptoms or signs of this disease. _____
   _____
   _____

6. Name two possible treatments for this disease. _____
   _____
   _____

7. What is the English language description for the procedure code 97028? _____
   _____
   _____

8. Is procedure code 97028 a valid treatment for diagnosis code 696.1? _____
   _____

9. Should a patient with this disease expose themselves to sunlight? _____
   _____

10. Does smoking affect this condition? If so, in what way? _____
    _____

Honors Certification™

The certification challenge for this chapter will be a written test of the information contained in this chapter. Each incorrect answer will result in a deduction of up to 5% from your grade. You must achieve a score of 85% or higher to pass this test. If you fail the test on your first attempt you may retake the test one additional time. The items included in the second test may be different from those in the first test.

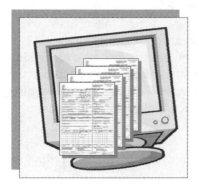

16

ICD-9 Coding

After completion of this chapter you will be able to:

- Discuss the history of the ICD-9 and why it was created.
- Describe the contents of each volume of the ICD-9.
- Describe how each volume of the ICD-9 is arranged.
- State the guidelines concerning ICD-9 coding.
- Describe main terms and how they are used.
- Identify and describe the common signs and symbols used in the ICD-9.
- List the important factors to be aware of when billing using ICD-9 codes.
- Describe how to handle downgrading of codes and concurrent care situations.
- Convert the English-language description of an illness or injury into a numeric ICD-9 code.

Key words and concepts you will learn in this chapter:

ICD-9 – A statistical coding of medical diagnoses and procedures.

Main Term – Identifying names that are the keys by which the ICD-9 is structured. They usually list the type of disease or condition rather than where in the body the disease or condition is located.

Neoplasm – A growth (tumor) that results from abnormal cell activity.

Subclassification – Secondary classifications under a main classification.

ICD-9 refers to the International Classification of Diseases, 9th Revision, Clinical Modification. This is a coding system devised to provide standardization of the coding of diseases, conditions, impairments, and symptoms by the medical and insurance industry.

As our world becomes more and more computerized, new ways have been sought to classify and categorize all types of information. The health care industry is no exception.

History of the ICD-9

The **ICD-9** is a statistical coding of medical diagnoses and procedures that has been around (under different titles) since the early 1900s. It is based on the World Health Organization's (WHO's) International Classification of Diseases (ICD).

The WHO originally created the ICD as a means of compiling data on morbidity and allowing hospitals and clinics to restore and retrieve diagnostic data.

In 1950, The Veterans Administration and the US Public Health Service each began tests on the use of the ICD for hospital indexing. In 1951, New York City's Columbia Presbyterian Medical Center adopted the ICD-6th Revision (with modifications) for use in its medical records department. A few years later the Commission on Professional and Hospital Activities adopted the ICD with similar modifications for the use of hospitals participating in the Professional Activity Study.

Finally, the US National Committee on Vital and Health Statistics (through its subcommittee on hospital statistics) reviewed the ICD and the various modifications and proposed uniform changes.

In 1956, the American Hospital Association and the American Association of Medical Record Librarians (later known as the American Medical Record Association) undertook a study of the efficacies of coding systems for diagnostic indexing. Their study concluded that the ICD provided a good framework for hospital indexing.

In 1977, the National Center for Health Statistics convened a steering committee to provide advice and council on revisions that should be made to the ICD-9. This created the ICD-9CM, which is a clinical modification of the WHO's ICD-9.

Each year the ICD-9 is updated. Upon release of the revised information by the US Department of Health and Human Services, numerous publishing companies print their own version of the information contained in the ICD-9. These versions all contain the same basic information. However, various options are added in an effort to make their book more preferred. These options can include color coding, tabs, numerous symbols, and various instructions and aids.

The decision of which publisher's version of the ICD-9 to use is simply a matter of individual or company choice.

Contents of the ICD-9

The ICD-9CM comprises three volumes:
  Volume I – The tabular or numerical listings, books one and two.
  Volume II – The alphabetic listings, books one and two.
  Volume III – A numeric listing of surgical procedure codes.

Correct ICD-9 coding is important for two reasons:

1. This coding is often used as the statistical basis for clients to review the plan benefits in order to provide the most effective coverage for their members while controlling health care costs.
2. Many computerized claims processing systems use these codes to determine the benefits to pay on a claim. Incorrect coding can lead to incorrect benefit payments.

Volume I

Volume I is structured numerically according to body system. It is used when:
  ▪ An ICD-9 code is provided, but there is no language description of the diagnosis, or
  ▪ A language diagnosis is included, but an ICD-9 code is not indicated and the terms used by the provider cannot be found in Volume II. If you can identify the body system, you may be able to locate an appropriate ICD-9 code.

A number in parenthesis after a code is the page number in Volume II that can be checked to verify the code. Table 16 – 1 shows the organization of Volume I.

Volume II

Volume II is the alphabetical listing of diagnoses. This section is most commonly used first. It is divided into four sections:
1. An alphabetical index of diseases and injuries.
2. A table of drugs and chemicals.
3. An alphabetical index of external causes of injuries and poisonings (accidents) (E codes).
4. A listing of factors affecting the health status of an individual (V codes).

Volume III

Volume III of the ICD-9 is used for coding diagnoses and procedures performed in a hospital. Volume III contains both a tabular listing and index. The tabular listing has procedures arranged according to body sections. The body sections are arranged as follows:
1. Operations on the Nervous System.
2. Operations on the Endocrine System.
3. Operations on the Eye.
4. Operations on the Ear.

5. Operations on the Nose, Mouth and Pharynx.
6. Operations on the Respiratory System.
7. Operations on the Cardiovascular System.
8. Operations on the Hemic and Lymphatic System.
9. Operations on the Digestive System.
10. Operations on the Urinary System.
11. Operations on the Male Genital Organs.
12. Operations on the Female Genital Organs.
13. Obstetrical Procedures.
14. Operations on the Musculoskeletal System.
15. Operations on the Integumentary System.
16. Miscellaneous Diagnostic and Therapeutic Procedures.

The index has procedures listed in alphabetical order. Thus, it is the easiest way to look up a procedure. The medical biller should confirm their choice of code by looking in the tabular listing and checking all referrals, exclusions and notes included.

How to Use the ICD-9

The ICD-9 is structured to move from a general diagnosis to a more specific diagnosis by adding on digits. It uses three, four or five digit codes. Three digit codes are the most general. By adding additional digits, a more precise diagnosis is identified.

The requirements of various processing systems or clients vary. Some may require very precise coding, and the use of five digits would be required. Others may not require such precision, so only three or four digits would be used.

When performing ICD-9 coding, the medical biller should always code to the highest number of digits possible, the highest degree of specificity. This includes four and five digit subclassifications wherever they occur. **Subclassifications** are secondary classifications under a main classification.

General Guidelines

Some basic guidelines should be kept in mind when coding and using the ICD-9. Many of these guidelines were first established by the Health Care Financing Administration (HCFA), which oversees the Medicare Program for the United States. After a recommendation or guideline has been adopted by

Table 16 – 1: Organization of Volume I

Number	Body System/Classification
00 – 13	Infective and Parasitic Diseases
14 – 23	Neoplasms
24 – 27	Endocrine, Nutritional, Metabolic Diseases
28	Diseases of the Blood and Blood-Forming Organs
29 – 31	Mental/Nervous Disorders
32 – 38	Diseases of the Nervous System and Sense Organs
39 – 45	Diseases of the Circulatory System
46 – 51	Diseases of the Respiratory System
52 – 57	Diseases of the Digestive System
58 – 62	Diseases of the Genito-Urinary System
63 – 67	Complications of Pregnancy, Childbirth and the Puerperium
68 – 70	Diseases of the Skin and Subcutaneous Tissue
71 – 73	Diseases of the Musculoskeletal System and Connective Tissue
74 – 75	Congenital Anomalies
76 – 77	Certain Causes of Perinatal Morbidity and Mortality
78 – 79	Symptoms, Signs and Ill-Defined Conditions
80 – 86	Fractures, Dislocations, Sprains and Internal Injuries
87 – 90	Lacerations
91 – 99	Other Accidents, Poisoning and Violence (nature of the injury)
V0 – Y24	Miscellaneous Informative Codings (a particular diagnosis is not indicated)

HCFA or Medicare, private payors and carriers usually adopt the same guidelines shortly thereafter.

Following are general guidelines to keep in mind when trying to locate the proper ICD-9 code:

1. Read through the introduction of the ICD-9 to be sure that you understand any color coding, symbols, abbreviations, and terms that the book uses.
2. Always use both the Index listing (Volume II) and the Numeric Listing (Volume I). Volume II alone will not give you any exclusions, referrals, or instructions for the codes, including the need for four or five digit subclassifications.
3. Always code the principal diagnosis. The principal diagnosis is the condition that is

established as being chiefly responsible for requiring the patient to seek medical care.

    a. Do not code symptoms nor the suspected condition if a final diagnosis is indicated. Symptoms and suspected conditions are usually accompanied by terms such as: "probable," "suspected," "questionable," or "Rule out (R/O)."

    b. It is understood that some conditions will not be fully diagnosed until test results have provided further understanding of the condition; in such cases, code conditions to the highest degree of certainty for the encounter. For example, many codes contain a fourth or fifth digit, which are for "unspecified" conditions or types. Often this will be indicated by the abbreviation NOS for "Not Otherwise Specified." These codes are acceptable if this is the highest level of certainty documented by the physician at this encounter.

    c. The term "Rule-Out" (R/O) is routinely submitted by some providers. This is not a diagnosis and is often not allowable under a plan. Whenever possible, the final diagnosis or the symptoms that prompted the testing should be used for coding.

4. Code only the diagnosis determined by the physician and any complications. Do not list any codes for previous conditions that were previously treated and that no longer exist.

5. Code diagnosis to the highest number of digits possible. For example, do not use only three digits to describe a condition when four and five digit subclassifications exist for that category. Many payors will return such claims requesting additional information.

    Be sure that you follow a category all the way up to the three digit classification. Often, the coding of four and five digits is listed under the main category heading, not under each separate diagnosis or condition.

6. The main diagnosis, condition, or reason for the encounter should be listed first. All other conditions that coexist at the time of treatment and that affect the treatment are to be coded following the main reason. If several conditions equally resulted in the encounter, the doctor or medical biller is free to list whichever they choose first.

7. When a patient is seen for ancillary diagnostic services only, the appropriate V code should be listed first, and the diagnosis or condition that is the underlying reason for the tests should be listed second. If a second code is not listed, delays in claim processing or denial of benefits may result.

    For example, if a chest x-ray is taken (coded V72.5) and no second code is listed, the claim may be denied if there are no benefits for routine chest x-rays. Without the second code the health claims examiner will often assume that the x-ray is for routine screening, not for a specific condition.

8. When a patient is seen for ancillary therapeutic services only, the appropriate V code should be listed first, and the diagnosis or condition that is the underlying reason for the services should be listed second. If a second code is not listed, delays in claim processing or denial of benefits may result.

    For example, if a child receives physical therapy services (code V57.1) due to cerebral palsy (code 343) and no second code is listed, the claim may be denied if there are no benefits for routine physical therapy. Without the second code the health claims examiner will often delay or deny benefits until they receive further information.

9. Diagnosis codes for chronic diseases or conditions may be coded as often as needed when the patient has repeated encounters for the chronic disease or condition.

10. Diagnoses that relate to earlier episodes of care or are chronic and have no bearing on the current treatment are to be excluded.

11. When billing for surgical procedures, use the correct code to indicate the diagnosis or reason for the surgery. If a post-operative diagnosis is different from the pre-operative diagnosis, and the post-operative diagnosis is known at the time the claim is

submitted, you should code the post-operative diagnosis.

12. Adjectives (acute, chronic, and the like) may appear as subterms. For example, the diagnosis of Acute Pelvic Inflammatory Disease may be located in the following manner:

   a. Look up the condition--disease,
   b. Under disease, refer to the subheading (site) of pelvis, pelvic,
   c. Locate the specific condition--inflammatory (female) (PID), and
   d. Finally, locate manifestation, acute--614.3.

13. Cross-reference to synonyms, closely related terms and code categories beginning with "See" and "See also." For example, Pelvic-peritonitis (See also peritonitis, pelvic, female).

14. Carefully read any and all notes under the main term. These can include exclusions, referrals, and examples of diagnoses or conditions.

15. Carefully note any modifiers associated with the main term. Compare these with any qualifying terms used in the diagnosis statement.

16. Watch for subterms listed under a main term. Subterms become more specific the farther down they go.

These guidelines should be memorized and used whenever you are attempting to locate an ICD-9 code. They will ensure a higher degree of accuracy and a higher rate of correct benefit payment on claims.

Main Terms

The Alphabetic Index is arranged by condition, disease, or syndrome. These identifying names are called the Main Terms and are the keys by which this volume is structured. The **Main Terms** usually identify disease conditions rather than locations. The Main Terms may be listed as proper medical terms or as outmoded, ill-defined terms or as eponyms. **Eponyms** are illnesses or conditions named after a person (i.e., Gerhardt's Disease). Certain conditions may be listed under more than one term.

For example, in the following examples, the Main Terms are underlined.

Streptococcal <u>tonsillitis</u>--This can be located in two ways:

- Under tonsillitis (subheading streptococcal)
- Under infection (subheading streptococcal, site--sore throat)

Streptococcal is not a condition; it is the type of organism involved in an infection.

Some other examples include the following:

- <u>Dislocated</u> shoulder,
- Pulmonary <u>edema</u>,
- Pelvic <u>abscess</u>,
- <u>Prolapsed</u> uterus,
- <u>Fractured</u> radius,
- Sick sinus <u>syndrome</u>,
- Chronic <u>hepatitis</u>, and
- External <u>hemorrhoids</u>.

Once you have identified the code in the indexed listing (Volume II), cross-reference your selection with the Tabular listing in Volume 1. This will ensure that you have selected the proper code. It will also allow you to code to the highest degree of specificity.

Be sure to research any exclusions, referrals ("See Also"), and examples to ensure that your code is correct. Also be sure to refer to the three and four digit classification headings. These headings often have further information or list the fourth and fifth digits that apply to all following codes in that classification.

For example, let's use the dislocated shoulder mentioned previously. The index lists the three digit classification for a dislocated shoulder as 831. However, a four digit classification will tell whether the injury is open or closed, and a five digit classification will pinpoint the diagnosis as to the more precise location of the injury. Also, note that a chronic or recurrent shoulder dislocation has an entirely different three digit classification of 718.

Now turn to classification 831 in the tabular listing. You will see that the five digit subclassifications are listed directly below the three digit classification heading. This is followed by the three digit classifications and the four digit classifications.

The reason for this order can be better understood when you look at the codes 800--804. Each of these codes is for a fracture of the skull.

The five digit codes that immediately follow the classification heading can be used with any of the three or four digit classifications that begin with the numbers 800, 801, 803, or 804. The classifications for 804 appear several pages later. This is why it is important to always look back to the four and three digit classification headings when coding.

Exceptions

In some instances, the ICD-9 is organized differently so that the Main Terms do not identify disease conditions. These exceptions include:

1. Obstetric conditions, which are found under "Delivery," "Pregnancy," or "Puerperal." (Puerperal refers to the period immediately following delivery.)
2. Complications of medical and surgical conditions, which are located under "Complications." However, they can also be found under the condition. For example, "evisceration" of an operative wound can be found under evisceration and complication. It is recommended that you look under the condition.
3. Late effects of diseases and injuries, which are under the Main Term "late effects."
4. In some situations, a claim or bill may provide a "diagnosis" that is not a sickness or injury per se. For example, exposure to, history of, problem with, or vaccination are not diagnoses but may be considered appropriate Main Terms.

Appropriate sites and/or modifiers are listed in alphabetical sequence under the Main Terms with further subterm listings as required. For example, the diagnosis of Open Tibia/Fibula Fracture may be located as follows:

See Fracture heading
Locate tibia as a subheading
Site--with fibula
Description--open = 823.92

Neoplasms

A **neoplasm** is a growth (tumor) that results from abnormal cell activity. Selecting an ICD-9 code for a neoplasm involves identifying the following factors:

- The pathologic status of the growth-- benign or malignant,

- The site of the growth--breast, lung, bladder, and
- The cell type (i.e., oat cell).

This information is not always provided on medical reports, claims, or bills. Therefore, as with any other diagnosis, the code selected will be based on the available information. The more information provided, the more specific the code.

For coding growths or tumors, you need to become familiar with the ICD-9 Neoplasm Table (NT) located in Volume II. This table is organized alphabetically by site (location). Since the site is not always known, there is an entry for "unknown site or unspecified."

On the right side of the Neoplasm Table are six columns from which to select an ICD-9 code based on the given diagnosis. The terms used in these columns are defined as follows:

Malignant primary – Primary means that the site of the tumor is the point of origin of the neoplasm. Malignant means that the cancer or growth is growing. Malignant growths will spread throughout the body until they kill the patient.

Malignant secondary – Secondary means that the site of the tumor in question is not where the disease originated. It has spread to this location from the primary site.

Malignant CA in situ – In situ means that the malignant growth is still localized in one area and has not spread.

Benign – Localized growth that does not spread (metastasize) and is not usually terminal.

Uncertain Behavior – Usually a particular type of growth is either always malignant or always benign. There are, however, some growths that may be either. In cases in which the information does not establish which type of manifestation is present and the growth could be either, this coding may be used. As a rule, this column should be used only when the neoplasm's behavior is stated to be uncertain by a pathologist or physician or is listed as such in the Alphabetic Index.

Unspecified – A growth is unspecified when it is not identified as benign or malignant and the type of growth is always one or the other.

The first step in coding growths is to determine whether the growth is benign or malignant. If the status is indicated, go directly to the Table under either the malignant or benign column, according to the site of the growth. Choose the malignant column based on the specifics of the diagnosis---primary, secondary, or in situ.

For example:

DX: Benign Breast Tumor
ACTION: 1. Find "breast" alphabetically.
2. Look at the benign column.
3. The code is 217.

DX: CA in Situ--Uterus
ACTION: 1. Find "uterus" alphabetically.
2. Look under Malignant-CA in situ.
3. The code is 233.2.

DX: Brain Tumor
ACTION: 1. Find "brain" alphabetically.
2. Look under Unspecified.
3. The code is 239.6

If a growth is identified as malignant, but is not further identified as primary, secondary, or CA in situ, assume that it is primary.

The terms CA, cancer, carcinoma, and sarcoma always indicate a malignancy. Other terms, like fibroma and adenoma, require you to check the alphabetical listing (not the Neoplasm Table) of Volume II to determine whether the condition is benign or malignant. Subsequently, the proper column in the Neoplasm Table can be referenced.

For example:

If the diagnosis is:	Look under the Main Term:
Pelvic Fibroma	Fibroma
Adenoma	Adenoma
Adenosarcoma	Adenosarcoma
Papilloma, eyelid	Papilloma
Osteosarcoma	Osteosarcoma

In most cases, looking under the appropriate Main Term will direct you to the correct column in the Neoplasm Table. In some circumstances, however, you will be given a valid ICD-9 code by the provider and you will not need to reference the Neoplasm Table at all.

Sample Exercise I
Locate the appropriate ICD-9 code and write it in the space provided.

Pelvic Fibroma _____

Adenoma _____

Adenosarcoma _____

Papilloma, eyelid _____

Osteosarcoma _____

As you can see, the reference under the Main Term identifies whether the neoplasm is benign or malignant. In the case of adenosarcoma, a valid ICD-9 code (189.0) is given and the Neoplasm Table did not have to be checked.

Remember that M codes are disregarded. Also note that the "See Also" reference, which is usually optional, must be followed in the case of neoplasms.

Over time, you may learn which neoplasms are benign or malignant and may be able to go directly to the Neoplasm Table.

Lesions
Although lesions are similar to neoplasms, they are treated differently by the ICD-9. Lesions should be handled as indicated in the following statements:

If the diagnosis simply states "lesion," look under the Main Term "lesion" alphabetically in Volume II.

If the diagnosis is "benign lesion," look under the Main Term "lesion."

If the diagnosis is "malignant lesion," look under one of the malignant columns in the Neoplasm Table in Volume II.

Sample Exercise II
Locate the appropriate ICD-9 code and write it in the space provided.

Benign Tumor, Foreskin _____

Cancer, Trachea _____

Epithelioma _____

CA in Situ, Uterus _____

Lung Tumor _____

Secondary CA, Pancreas _____

Primary CA, Pylorus _____

Tumor _____

Cancer, Rectum _____

Sarcoma, Skin _____

Fibroadenoma _____

Malignant Tumor Duodenum_____

Sprains/Strains

Sprains and strains are coded according to the site of injury. Strains of the musculoskeletal system are included under the Main Term, Sprain. There is a separate Main Term reference for strains that are not related to the musculoskeletal system (such as eyestrain). If the location of a musculoskeletal strain or sprain is unknown, use code 848.9 (musculoskeletal system). Normally, 848.9 is used as a temporary code while additional information is requested from the provider.

Dislocations

As with strains and sprains, dislocations are coded according to the site of injury. Code 839.8 should be used if the exact injury site is unknown. See previous paragraph.

A closed dislocation includes simple, complete, partial, uncomplicated, and unspecified (type). Open includes infected, compound, and dislocation with a foreign body.

"Chronic," "habitual," "old," or "recurrent" dislocations may be coded as "dislocation, recurrent, and pathologic."

Fractures

As with strains, sprains, and dislocations, fractures are coded according to the site of injury.

Closed fractures include the following descriptions, with or without delayed healing: comminuted, linear, depressed, march, elevated, simple, fissured, slipped epiphysis, greenstick, spiral, impacted, and unspecified.

Open fractures include compound, infected, missile, puncture with or without a foreign body, with or without delayed healing.

Assume that the fracture is closed unless there is wording that indicates otherwise.

When multiple fractures are involved, it is easier to look under the names of the bones involved than to look under "Fracture, multiple."

V Codes

The **V code** listing is a supplementary listing of factors that affect the health status of the patient. Often there are reasons for an encounter that relate to a disease or condition, but do not constitute a diagnosis. There are three main types of occurrences:

1. When a person who is not ill has an encounter with a health care provider for a specific purpose that is not in and of itself a disease or condition. These encounters can include a visit from a person who is getting a vaccination or a check-up, who is acting as an organ or tissue donor to another person, or who wants to discuss a problem that is not considered a disease or condition (i.e., fertility problems, genetic counseling).

2. When a patient with a chronic or recurring condition visits a health care provider for service associated with treatment of that condition. This can include a cast change, dialysis for renal disease, monitoring of pacemaker, and other similar situations.

3. When a situation arises that influences the person's health, but is not a disease or condition. Such situations include exposure to potential health hazards (i.e., tuberculosis, polio), animal bites that require rabies vaccination, and the fact that a person's physiology or family history suggests a factor that should be borne in mind when treatment is received (i.e., carrier of suspected infectious diseases, history of cancer or other diseases, allergies to medicines).

When performing diagnosis coding in circumstances two and three above, the V code should be used as a supplementary code (not the primary diagnosis code). The diagnosis or condition that underlies the reason for the treatment (circumstance two) or that caused the patient to seek medical attention (circumstance three) should be coded as the primary diagnosis. V codes are arranged according to the following headings:

V01 – V09 Persons with potential health hazards related to communicable diseases
V10 – V19 Persons with potential health hazards related to personal and family history
V20 – V29 Persons encountering health services in circumstances related to reproduction and development
V30 – V39 Liveborn infants according to type of birth
V40 – V49 Persons with a condition influencing their health status
V50 – V59 Persons encountering health services for specific procedures and aftercare

V60 – V68 Persons encountering health services in other circumstances

V70 – V82 Persons without reported diagnosis encountered during examination and investigation of individuals and populations

As a medical biller you should examine the V codes and familiarize yourself with the situations they define.

E Codes

The E code listing is a supplementary classification of external causes of injury and poisoning. E codes are used to indicate the cause of the injury, not the injury itself. Therefore, an E code should always be an additional code, not a primary diagnosis code. For example, a patient was a pedestrian struck by a car and suffered a fractured femur. The diagnosis would be fractured femur (code 821.00), and the cause would be pedestrian struck by automobile (E814.7).

To correctly code E codes, consult the index located in section three of Volume II (behind the table of drugs and chemicals). This index is used the same way the index to diseases and conditions is used. First, locate the cause in the index, then turn to the tabular listing to confirm your choice and to ensure correct four and five digit subclassifications.

The beginning of the E code section contains definitions of the terms involved in describing causes. The medical biller should familiarize him or herself with these definitions because they are vital to proper coding. When coding transport accidents, the following headings are used:

- Aircraft and spacecraft (E840 – E845)
- Watercraft (E830 – E838)
- Motor Vehicle (E810 – E825)
- Railway (E800 – E807)
- Other road vehicles (E826 – E829)

If you are coding an accident that involves more than one type of vehicle, the order listed above should be followed. For example, let's code an accident between a car and a streetcar. Since a streetcar is considered a railway vehicle, the car would take precedence. Therefore, you would look under the motor vehicle section to find motor vehicle accident involving collision with train (E810). The four digit subclassification would then

be added to this number to describe the activity of the patient at the time of the accident (see motor vehicle accident section heading).

If you are coding machinery accidents (nontransport vehicles), you should use category E919.x. This allows for a broad description of the type of machinery and activity that made up the cause of the injury. If you wish to provide a more detailed description, the Internal Labor Office has created a Classification of Industrial Accidents According to Agency. However, this classification should be used in addition to the appropriate E code, not in place of it. Some versions of the ICD-9 reproduce this classification listing.

Signs and Symbols Used in the ICD-9

Most coding books have different signs and symbols to alert you to specific situations with codes. However, different versions of the coding books may have different signs and symbols, or none at all.

Listed below are some of the common signs and symbols used in the ICD-9.

- • This code is new to this edition of the ICD-9. It has just been added to the list of ICD-9 codes.
- ▲ This code has been changed from last year's edition of the ICD-9.
- ④ A fourth digit is required to properly use this code.
- ⑤ A fifth digit is required to properly use this code.

Many ICD-9s also have signs or symbols for non-specific codes or unspecified codes. These codes should only be used as a last resort when no other code is appropriate.

Some ICD-9s will also use colors to signify the fourth or fifth digit requirement. For example, a pink box may appear behind the code number.

It is important to understand the meanings of these signs and symbols as they are used in your version of the ICD-9. Without understanding them, your chances of improperly coding a claim can increase greatly.

The details of the signs and symbols used in your version of the ICD-9 should appear in the beginning of the book. You should read this section carefully before beginning coding.

Billing Tips

The medical biller should be aware of a number of factors when entering ICD-9 codes on claims submitted for payment. These factors can cause delays in benefit payments and sometimes even denial of benefits.

However, always remember that to file a false claim is considered fraud, and there are severe penalties for fraud. When taking the following factors into consideration, the medical biller should also remember that the claim should be filled out according to the actual diagnosis or condition that exists and the actual procedure(s) performed. To alter a medical record or a claim just to meet the criteria listed below is to perform a criminal act.

The most important factors to be aware of in billing are:

1. Carefully read through the beginning sections of your ICD-9 book. This will give you a lot of additional information on properly using the book. This is one of your best sources for learning how to use the ICD-9.

2. When coding, the diagnosis coded must support the services rendered. On the CMS-1500, the diagnosis that relates to each procedure performed is placed next to the procedure code. Therefore, each procedure performed should have a diagnosis that substantiates the need for that procedure. If the procedures performed are not supported by the diagnosis (i.e., an x-ray of the foot is taken when the diagnosis is a concussion), benefits for the procedure will be denied. Likewise, claims submitted on a UB-92 may be denied if the diagnosis does not support the need for the goods or services listed in the itemized billing statement.

3. The medical biller is limited to the available number of spaces on the billing form. Only four codes may be entered on the CMS-1500 claim form and ten on the UB-92. If more conditions exist than there are spaces on the form, there are three options:
   a. List only the main conditions up to the number of spaces provided.
   b. On the CMS-1500, if more than six procedures were performed, you may submit on more than one claim form.

   For example, the doctor may treat a patient who was a pedestrian struck by a car. If the patient had multiple injuries, those procedures that were related to the head and upper body injuries could be billed on one claim form and those procedures relating to the lower body injuries could be billed on a second claim form. Both claim forms should contain the correct E code (E814.7), and the date of the accident.
   c. If you strongly believe that additional diagnostic information is needed to process the claim or substantiate the services provided, you may attach a medical report or other supporting documentation to your claim. However, it should be noted that this information may be ignored by the health claims examiner, or it may result in a delay to allow time to review the information.

4. The location of service must be substantiated by the diagnosis and procedures rendered. There are two factors related to this condition:
   a. If the location of service is clearly inappropriate for the services rendered, there will be problems in the payment of the claim. For example, if the diagnosis indicates heart disease and the service provided is a heart transplant, then the location of services cannot be a doctor's office.
   b. Many people will go to a place that is convenient rather than to the place where it is appropriate that they should go. The greatest abuse of this situation is people using the hospital emergency room for situations that are not true emergencies. If the diagnosis listed indicates that the condition was not an emergency, many payors will pay the claim based on the appropriate place of treatment. Since emergency room services cost much more than those same services performed in a doctor's office, this can result in a large discrepancy between the amount billed and the amount received from the payor.

5. The diagnosis must match the level of services provided. When coding procedures, the complexity of the medical condition and the level of service rendered (i.e., minimal, limited, brief, expanded, comprehensive) should be substantiated by the diagnosis listed. If the diagnosis and the complexity of services do not match, often the level of services will be downgraded (see following section on Downgrading of Codes\Benefits) to match the diagnosis.

6. Diagnosis must substantiate service frequency. Often patients need repeated services to alleviate chronic conditions. However, if there is no alleviation of the symptoms or no benefits are received from the continued treatment, payors may deny some or all of the treatments.

Concurrent Care

Often, reimbursement problems arrive when two doctors are seeing a patient at the same time for two unrelated medical conditions. This is known as **concurrent care**. Claims were frequently denied as duplication of services when the patient was seen by two physicians on the same day, when no duplication actually occurred.

Prior to 1992, there was a CPT® modifier (-75) that notated concurrent care. This modifier has since been dropped. Now there are two ways to ensure the greatest possibility of payment from the payor:

1. Submit two separate claim forms, one for each physician, which list two completely separate diagnoses and the related services that were provided.

2. If the separate providers were members of the same medical group and payment is to be made to the medical group, then all services should be submitted on the same claim form. However, two separate diagnoses should be listed, and the procedures performed for each should be substantiated by the referencing of the separate diagnoses next to the procedure.

Downgrading of Codes/Benefits

Diagnoses that do not fit the previously mentioned criteria may cause the health claims examiner to downgrade the codes or the benefits paid. **Downgrading** is a process of reducing a code of a higher value to one of a lower value so that the procedures, locations, and frequency of service are appropriate to the diagnosis given. This can result in the loss of millions of dollars for the health care provider and their patients.

For example, if the diagnosis does not support the level of services provided, a lower level will be assigned. If the diagnosis given does not substantiate the procedures, payment on the procedures will be denied as medically unnecessary. If the location is inappropriate for the service provided, the claim will either be delayed or denied, or the benefits will be paid as if the services were rendered at the appropriate place (as in emergency services being paid at office services rates when no true emergency occurred).

If claims are submitted to Medicare with any of the above-mentioned discrepancies in place, the claim will automatically be returned to the provider without payment of any benefits. The provider must then resubmit a properly completed claim.

If the provider refuses to submit the correct ICD-9 codes, fines may be levied or the provider may be barred from participating in the Medicare program.

ICD-10

Each year the ICD-9 is updated, incorporating new diagnoses and revising or eliminating old ones. However, since these are limited revisions, the book continues to be called the ICD-9. The version is indicated by the year.

Each time there is a major revision of the ICD, it is assigned a new version number. The ICD-9 is for the ninth such revision.

Recently, the American Medical Association developed the ICD-10. This is a major revision of the International Classification of Diseases. Texts have been developed regarding the use of this new coding book; however, the actual book itself is still going through the numerous revision and approval processes necessary before it can be adopted. Since the actual revision itself is not complete, any current manuals give instructions on what they presume the new version will eventually look like. Additionally, while the contents of the ICD-10 will change, the new volume is expected to be used much like the ICD-9. Therefore if you can comfortably use the ICD-9, the transition to the ICD-10 should not prove too difficult.

For these reasons, and since numerous changes are expected prior to the actual introduction of the ICD-10, we have chosen not to include a detailed description of the book here. However, medical billers and health claims examiners should be aware that this text is coming, and, when it is adopted, should be used in place of the current ICD-9.

Summary

The ICD-9 is the primary book used when coding diagnoses on health claims. It is made up of three volumes. Volume I is the tabular listing of diagnoses and conditions. Volume II is the indexed or alphabetic listing of diagnoses and conditions. Volume III is the tabular and alphabetic listing of procedures.

To accurately look up a diagnosis, the medical biller should locate the Main Term for the condition under the indexed listing in Volume II. The numeric code gained should then be checked against the information provided in Volume I, and all referrals, exclusions, and additional digit subclassifications should be consulted to ensure that the right code has been chosen.

The same process is used when coding procedures in Volume III. First, consult the index, then cross-reference the code with the information provided in the tabular listing.

It is vital for the medical biller to understand each of the three volumes of the ICD-9 and how to use them.

It is also important for the medical biller to understand the importance of how diagnosis or ICD-9 codes relate to the other information on a claim form. Diagnoses that do not substantiate services rendered, match the proper location of services, or otherwise conflict with additional information on the claim form will result in delays and denials of benefit payments.

Assignments

Complete the Questions for Review.
Complete Exercises 16 – 1 through 16 – 5.

Correct the exercises upon completion. If you are billing correctly less than 90% of the time, more practice is needed.

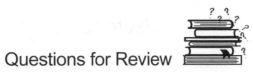

Questions for Review

Directions: Answer the following questions without looking back into the material just covered. Write your answers in the space provided.

1. Volume _____ is the tabular listing of diagnoses.

2. If only a language description of the condition is provided, Volume _____ should be used to locate the numerical listing.

3. Main Terms are used to identify the _____

4. (True or False?) Benign lesions are listed in the Neoplasm Table. _____

5. (True or False?) Always assume fractures are "open," unless otherwise indicated. _____

6. (True or False?) The more digits in the code, the more general the diagnosis. _____

7. (True or False?) Obstetrical related conditions are handled differently than other Main Terms. _____

8. (True or False?) "Rule Out" is a definitive diagnosis. _____

9. Volume II is used in some instances to determine whether a neoplasm is _____

   or _____.

10. One important use of ICD-9 codes by clients is _____

    _____

If you were unable to answer any of the questions, refer back to that section, and then fill in the answers.

Exercise 16 – 1

Directions: Based on the condition, look up the appropriate ICD-9 code and write it in the space provided. Also underline the main term.

Condition	Code
1. Tuberculous Pleurisy	1. _____
2. Nontoxic Nodular Goiter	2. _____
3. Pernicious Anemia	3. _____
4. Bacterial Meningitis	4. _____
5. Tricuspid Valve Disease	5. _____
6. Upper Respiratory Infection (acute)	6. _____
7. Bronchitis	7. _____
8. Acute Bronchitis	8. _____
9. Gangrene Secondary to Diabetes	9. _____
10. Normal Delivery	10. _____
11. Metacarpus Osteoarthrosis	11. _____
12. Apnea	12. _____
13. Exposure to Hepatitis	13. _____
14. Gallbladder Disease	14. _____
15. Acne	15. _____
16. Mexican Typhus	16. _____
17. Endometrium Squamous Metaplasia	17. _____
18. Orbital Melanoma	18. _____
19. Corii Degenerative Melanosis	19. _____
20. Cerebrum Medullomyoblastoma	20. _____
21. Lipoidica Necrobiosis	21. _____
22. Rosacea Acne	22. _____
23. Artificial Insemination	23. _____
24. DTP Inoculation	24. _____
25. Unexplained Night Sweats	25. _____
26. Swimmer's Ear (acute)	26. _____
27. Heart Palpitations	27. _____
28. Paramacular Lesion of the Retina	28. _____
29. Rectal Leukoplakia	29. _____
30. Plasma Cell Leukemia Not in Remission	30. _____

Exercise 16 – 2

Directions: Based on the condition, look up the appropriate ICD-9 code and write it in the space provided. Also underline the main term.

Condition	**Code**
1. Proximal Fibular Open Dislocation	1. _____
2. Gangrene of the Tunica Vaginalis	2. _____
3. Obstructed Gangrenous Hernia	3. _____
4. Hypercholesterolemia	4. _____
5. Dysfunctional Amenorrhea	5. _____
6. SIDS	6. _____
7. Glomerulohyalinosis Diabetic Syndrome	7. _____
8. Gonococcal Salpingo-oophoritis (chronic)	8. _____
9. Bladder Neck Stricture	9. _____
10. Popliteal Thrombophlebitis	10. _____
11. Cooper's Disease	11. _____
12. Superior Mesenteric Artery Syndrome	12. _____
13. Renal Artery Thrombosis	13. _____
14. Recurrent Urethritis	14. _____
15. Enuresis	15. _____
16. Diabetes Mellitus	16. _____
17. Endogenous Obesity	17. _____
18. Essential Hypertension	18. _____
19. Inguinal Hernia	19. _____
20. Tendon Sheath Ganglion	20. _____
21. Borderline Glaucoma	21. _____
22. Glioblastoma of the Forearm	22. _____
23. Ulcerative Gastroenteritis	23. _____
24. Hallux Valgus	24. _____
25. Heart Disease	25. _____
26. Heat Prostration	26. _____
27. Epidural Hematoma of the Brain	27. _____
28. Internal Hemorrhoids	28. _____
29. Familial Hypercholesterolemia	29. _____
30. Endocrine Imbalance	30. _____

Exercise 16 – 3

Directions: Based on the condition, look up the appropriate ICD-9 code and write it in the space provided. Also underline the main term.

Condition	Code
1. Hypothyroidism	1. _____
2. Fetal Alcohol Intoxication	2. _____
3. Diabetic Iritis	3. _____
4. Loss of Appetite	4. _____
5. Embryonal Liposarcoma	5. _____
6. Degenerative Macula	6. _____
7. Necrosis of the Liver	7. _____
8. Ameloblastic Sarcoma	8. _____
9. Septicemic Salmonella	9. _____
10. Squamous Cell Carcinoma of the Skin, In Situ	10. _____
11. Cuboid Infected Fracture	11. _____
12. Recurrent Elbow Dislocation	12. _____
13. Weight Gain Failure	13. _____
14. End Stage Renal Disease	14. _____
15. Thyroid Disease	15. _____
16. Degenerative Nephritis	16. _____
17. Neurofibromatosis	17. _____
18. Cardiovascular Observation	18. _____
19. Tibial Osteosarcoma	19. _____
20. Stirrup Otosclerosis	20. _____
21. Ruptured Spleen	21. _____
22. Skin Sepsis	22. _____
23. Anaphylactic Shock	23. _____
24. Sesamoiditis	24. _____
25. Carotid Artery Stenosis	25. _____
26. Post Status Asthmaticus	26. _____
27. Capsulitis of the Knee	27. _____
28. Glue Ear Syndrome	28. _____
29. Tattoo Removal	29. _____
30. Trichinosis	30. _____

Exercise 16 – 4

Directions: Based on the condition, look up the appropriate ICD-9 code and write it in the space provided. Also underline the main term.

Condition	**Code**
1. Nervous Twitch	1. _____
2. Hurthle Cell Benign	2. _____
3. Pregnant with Twins	3. _____
4. Twisted Umbilical Cord (During Delivery)	4. _____
5. Metastasis to the Pancreas	5. _____
6. Semilunar Cartilage Cyst	6. _____
7. Endometrioid Cystadenocarcinoma of Middle Lobe of Lung	7. _____
8. Premature Heart Contractions	8. _____
9. Severe Sunburn of the Back	9. _____
10. Chemical Burn of Gums	10. _____
11. Struck by a Falling Object	11. _____
12. Deaf Mute	12. _____
13. Cruveilhier's Disease	13. _____
14. Cholecystic Chlamydial Disease	14. _____
15. Alzheimer's Disease	15. _____
16. Fractured Mandible, Open	16. _____
17. Fractured Larynx	17. _____
18. Fractured Femur, Subtrochanteric	18. _____
19. Fractured Tibia and Fibula	19. _____
20. Compound Fx, Trochanter	20. _____
21. Fx Skull with Concussion	21. _____
22. Fx Ribs (Six), Open	22. _____
23. Sprained Ankle	23. _____
24. Strain, Knee	24. _____
25. Sprain, Elbow	25. _____
26. Sprained Foot	26. _____
27. Eye Strain	27. _____
28. Dislocated Joint (Infected)	28. _____
29. Dislocated Jaw, Recurrent	29. _____
30. Dislocated Collar Bone, Open	30. _____

Exercise 16 – 5

Directions: Based on the condition, look up the appropriate ICD-9 code and write it in the space provided. Also underline the main term.

Condition	Code
1. Giant Cell Carcinoma	1. _____
2. Dermatofibroma Protuberans	2. _____
3. Leydig Cell Tumor (male)	3. _____
4. Glomangioma	4. _____
5. Intramuscular Lipoma	5. _____
6. Sebaceous Cyst	6. _____
7. Leukemia	7. _____
8. Oat Cell Lung Carcinoma	8. _____
9. Papillary Hydradenoma	9. _____
10. Mucoid Adenoma of the Auricle	10. _____
11. Juxtaglomerular Tumor	11. _____
12. Malignant Insulinoma	12. _____
13. Basophil Adenoma of the Nose	13. _____
14. Malignant Renal Intraductal Papilloma	14. _____
15. Abdominal Fibromatosis	15. _____
16. Aldosteronoma	16. _____
17. Epithelial Neoblastoma	17. _____
18. Nabothian gland neoplasm (secondary)	18. _____
19. Myxochondrasarcoma	19. _____
20. Plasmacytoma, esophagus	20. _____
21. Bowen's disease	21. _____
22. Papillary intraductal carcinoma, salivary duct	22. _____
23. Carcinomatous cyst of the breast	23. _____
24. Ciliary epithelium diktyoma	24. _____
25. Wrist disgerminoma	25. _____
26. Ependymoblastoma, spinal cord	26. _____
27. Femur Osteofibroma	27. _____
28. Jadassohn's blue nevus	28. _____
29. Hutchinson's melanotic freckle	29. _____
30. Myxofibroma, connective tissue	30. _____

Honors Certification™

The certification challenge for this chapter will be a written test of the information contained in this chapter. Each incorrect answer will result in a deduction of up to 5% from your grade. You must achieve a score of 85% or higher to pass this test. If you fail the test on your first attempt you may retake the test one additional time. The items included in the second test may be different from those in the first test.

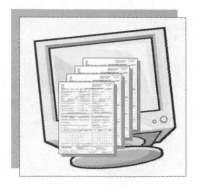

17

CPT® Coding

The **Current Procedural Terminology (CPT®)** is the coding reference manual most commonly used by medical billing personnel. The CPT® provides a listing of descriptive terms and identifying codes for reporting medical services and procedures performed by providers. It uses a five-digit code to identify procedures and services, which not only simplifies reporting but allows for compilation of data by a computer. The purpose of the CPT® is to provide a uniform system that will accurately describe medical, surgical, and diagnostic services.

The CPT® was originally created by the American Medical Association in 1966. Since that time it has undergone extensive revisions. Revisions are made every year with additional updates as needed. Due to the extensive changes that sometimes appear, it is important to use the correct version of the CPT®. Using an outdated CPT® may result in using codes that have been changed or deleted, and may cause a delay or denial of a claim payment.

Inclusion in the CPT® does not constitute endorsement by the American Medical Association or anyone else as to the efficacy of the procedure for a given diagnosis or condition. It also does not imply any insurance coverage or payor provisions of a procedure by its inclusion or exclusion.

The **Relative Value Study (RVS)** is a listing of procedures and their appropriate codes, along with a unit value that has been assigned to the procedure. Often the names CPT® and RVS are used interchangeably. However, the CPT®, not the RVS, should be used when coding procedures. When billing claims, it is important for the biller to understand the difference between the two books and to use the appropriate book when billing claims.

The CPT® and RVS reference books have six major sections:

SECTIONS OF THE CPT® AND RVS

Evaluation and Management		99201--99499
Anesthesia:	CPT®	00100--01999
	RVS	10000 - 69999
		99100--99140
Surgery		10021--69999
Radiology/Nuclear Medicine		70010--79999
Pathology and Laboratory Tests		80048--89356
Medicine		90281—99199
		and 99500—99602

The RVS uses the same codes for anesthesia as for surgery; however, the use of a modifier denotes that services are for anesthesia rather than surgery.

Using the CPT®

To properly code using the CPT®, choose the number code associated with the English-language description of the procedure performed. Sometimes the procedure will be phrased in different terminology (i.e., testectomy is found under orchiectomy even though both are legitimate medical terms). Therefore, it is important to check all related codes and alternate terminology for a procedure. It may also be necessary to consult a medical dictionary for alternate terminology for a specified procedure.

Each section of the CPT® has specific instructions relating to that section prior to the code listing. It is important that you read each of these instructions in order to properly code the procedures contained in that section.

Any qualified provider may bill for any procedure, regardless of the section it is contained in. Therefore, it is important that you become familiar with the entire CPT® book.

Semicolons in the CPT®

Some descriptions in the CPT® are subprocedures of other descriptions. These subheading descriptions will be indented under the main procedure. To properly understand an indented procedure, read the description of the main procedure (the one not indented) up to the semicolon. Next, add the remaining description found in the indented wording.

For example, codes 21208 and 21209 read as follows:

21208   Osteoplasty, facial bones; augmentation
21209   reduction

Therefore, the correct description for 21209 is Osteoplasty, facial bones; reduction. It is important to carefully read the full description of all related procedures before choosing the one which best describes the procedure performed. A slight change in the main description can significantly alter the meaning of the indented procedure.

Signs and Symbols Used in the CPT®

Most coding books have different signs and symbols to alert you to specific situations with codes. However, different versions of the coding books may have different signs and symbols, or none indicated at all.

Listed below are some of the common signs and symbols used in the CPT®.

This code is new to this edition of the CPT®. It has just been added to the list of CPT® codes.

▲ This code has been changed from last year's edition of the CPT®.

( ) This code was deleted. It appears in last year's CPT®, but is not valid for this year. Do not use this code.

+ Add on code. This code must be used with an additional code. This procedure is performed in addition to or in conjunction with another procedure.

⊘ This code is exempt from the use of modifier -51 (modifier -51 indicates multiple surgery).

Many CPT® codes also have signs or symbols for non-specific codes or unspecified codes. These codes should only be used as a last resort when no other code is appropriate.

Some CPT® codes will also use colors to signify the signs and symbols above, or additional code specifications. For example, a pink box may appear behind the code number.

The details of the signs and symbols used in your version of the CPT® should appear in the beginning of the book. You should read this section carefully before beginning coding.

It is important to understand the meanings of these signs and symbols as they are used in your version of the CPT®.

Using the CPT® Index

The CPT® index lists all main procedures, often with a choice of several codes. Again, some procedures are indented, indicating that the unindented procedure listed directly above them is part of the description.

Listings in the CPT® are arranged by the procedure done, then by the site of the procedure. For example, the heading "Amputation" then lists numerous portions of the body which can be amputated, and their related codes. Some portions of the body also have a heading.

Modifiers

Modifiers are two-digit codes that can be added to CPT® codes to denote unusual circumstances. These modifiers more fully describe the procedure that was performed. In addition, modifiers alter the valuation of the procedure by increasing or decreasing the allowed amount.

For example: Modifier -80 denotes the work of an assistant surgeon. Since the assistant surgeon is merely assisting and is not responsible for the primary care of the patient, he is paid substantially less. Most plans allow assistant surgeons at 20% of the UCR value for the surgeon's fee.

Some adjustments to allowed amounts are listed in the CPT® book. However, these adjustments are normally set by the insurance carrier or the plan.

Some commonly used modifiers are as follows:

-22 Unusual procedural services,
-26 Professional component,
-47 Anesthesia by surgeon,
-50 Bilateral procedure,
-51 Multiple procedures,
-52 Reduced services,
-62 Two surgeons,
-80 Assistant surgeon,
-81 Minimal assistant surgeon,
-90 Reference laboratory, and
-99 Multiple modifiers.

Unlisted Codes

Listed at the end of each CPT® section and subsection are **"unlisted codes"** (sometimes called junk codes). These are the codes that end in "99." Procedures that are unusual or new and, therefore, do not have a designated code to describe them are coded by the appropriate unlisted code (based on body section or type of service). These codes are to be used only when no other appropriate code is available.

The following coding sections deal specifically with using the CPT® manual. Only those sections that needed additional explanation are included. Since the CPT® is the main reference manual used by medical billing personnel, it is vitally important that its usage be thoroughly understood. You should also go through the general guidelines listed in the CPT® to assist in coding each section.

Evaluation and Management Codes

Evaluation and management codes designate procedures used to evaluate the patient's condition and to assist the patient in managing that condition.

EVALUATION AND MANAGEMENT CODES	
Office or Other Outpatient Services	99201 – 99215
Hospital Observation Services	99217 - 99220
Hospital Inpatient Services	99221 – 99239
Consultations	99241 – 99275
Emergency Department Services	99281 – 99288
Pediatric Critical Care Patient Transport	99289 – 99290
Critical Care Services	99291 – 99292
Inpatient Neonatal and Pediatric Critical Care Services	99293 – 99296
Intensive (Non-Critical) Low Birth Weight Services	99298 – 99299
Nursing Facility Services	99301 – 99316
Domiciliary, Rest Home, or Custodial Care Services	99321 – 99333
Home Services	99341 – 99350
Prolonged Services	99354 – 99360
Case Management Services	99361 – 99373
Care Plan Oversite Services	99374 – 99380
Preventive Medicine Services	99381 – 99429
Newborn Care Services	99431 – 99440
Special Evaluation and Management Services	99450 – 99456
Other Evaluation and Management Services	99499

The key components in determining the proper code are history, examination, and medical decision making.

Additional components that are considered include counseling, coordination of care, nature of presenting problems, and time.

For further instructions regarding proper coding, see the general guidelines contained in the CPT® book.

The appropriate CPT® section involved is 99201 –99499.

Office or Other Outpatient Services 99201 – 99215

An **office visit** is face-to-face treatment between a physician and a patient in the physician's office, clinic, or outpatient department of a hospital. Any type of licensed professional provider can bill for an office visit. An office visit code does not specify the type of service performed other than that the patient is seen by a physician.

Specialized care such as chiropractic, physical therapy, and psychiatric counseling are located in other coding sections. Specialized care is coded based on the type of treatment provided, not the location of service. The place of the treatment could be anywhere although it is usually in an office.

If care is provided outside of normal office hours, codes 99050 through 99054 are used in addition to the regular office visit code. This allows the provider to obtain extra compensation for the inconvenience of care provided outside the usual business hours.

If the physician does not give a complete language description of the type of visit and does not use a CPT® code, most payors use a designated default code, which is usually either 99211 or 99212. (This is a payor-designated procedure, so it may vary.)

Hospital Inpatient Services 99221 – 99239

Hospital inpatient services is also known as Medical While Hospitalized (MWH). Multiple types of MWH benefits are available. However, regardless of the type of benefit, all are based on the same coding principles.

Coding for these services is based on whether the patient is a new or established patient, the time, and the complexity of the case.

Consultations 99241 – 99275

Usually, a **consultation** is provided by a specialist who has been requested to provide an opinion only. The specialist usually examines the patient at the request of another physician. The specialist may request diagnostic services and may make therapeutic recommendations to the referring physician. However, the specialist does not usually take over the day-to-day treatment or management of the patient. In fact, for the service to qualify as a consultation, the physician cannot be responsible for the regular management of the patient.

If the physician subsequently assumes responsibility for the routine care of the patient, the services should be coded as visits and not consultations. If the consultant is seeing the patient, in addition to the regular attending physician, 99231--99233 should be used.

Second Surgical Opinion Consultations (SSOs) (99271 – 99275) are also a part of this group. A **second opinion** is designed as a benefit to the patient by confirming the need for a surgery.

Many plans provide a special benefit called an SSO benefit, which provides 100% payment for services provided by a second, independent specialist whom the patient consults prior to the scheduling of an elective, non-emergency surgery.

Normally, for an SSO benefit to be payable, the following requirements must be satisfied:

1. The second or third opinion physician must be totally uninvolved with the original recommending physician. Therefore, he cannot be part of the same medical group and will often be picked by the administrator, medical management firm, or payor.
2. The consultation must be completed prior to the scheduling of the surgery.
3. The second-opinion provider cannot perform the recommended surgery.

Depending on the plan, failure to obtain an SSO may result in:

1. Complete denial of all charges for the surgery and related services.
2. Application of a special, reduced coinsurance. For instance, instead of paying 80% of the expenses, 50% would be paid. Noncompliance penalties vary substantially.
3. No change of benefits. In this case, the SSO is considered to be a benefit for the member and is not used to penalize for noncompliance.

Emergency Department Services 99281 – 99288

When a patient goes to the outpatient or emergency department of a hospital, there is usually a physician in attendance who has a contract to provide professional care at the facility. The contracting physician's charges may appear on the hospital bill or may be billed separately.

Many hospitals have two types of outpatient departments: (1) the emergency room (ER); and (2) outpatient medical clinics.

If the patient wants to have his regular physician in attendance and the physician is called in from outside the hospital to provide services, code 99056 should be used.

If the patient visits the outpatient clinic of a facility, regular office visit coding should be used since a clinic is conceptually the same as an office; that is, the same doctors see the same patients, visits are scheduled the same as in an office and the treatment provided is the same as that provided in an office.

Pediatric Critical Care Patient Transport 99289 – 99290

These codes are used to bill for direct face-to-face care by a physician during the transfer of a pediatric patient from one facility to another. The patient must be critically ill or injured and must be 24 months of age or less. These services are coded according to the amount of time spent in transport care, not the specific services required during the time of that care.

Nursing Facility Services 99301 – 99316

A **skilled nursing facility (SNF)** is a specially qualified facility that has the staff and equipment to provide skilled nursing care or rehabilitation services and other related health services.

An individual is often admitted to a Skilled Nursing Facility (commonly referred to as an SNF) from an acute care facility. This may occur because the acuteness of the patient's condition has been stabilized and only time and continued noncritical treatments are required.

Domiciliary, rest Home or Custodial Care Services 99321 – 99333

Custodial care is primarily for the purpose of meeting the personal daily needs of the patient and could be provided by personnel without medical care skills or training. For example, custodial care includes assistance with walking, bathing, dressing, eating, and other activities. Skilled nursing personnel are not required for this nonmedical type of care, which is commonly referred to as "meeting the daily living needs" of the patient. Most plans do not provide coverage for these types of services, and, if they do, payment is limited. If there is a question whether care is custodial or not, copies of the provider's nursing notes or the Admit and/or Discharge Summary reports should be requested.

Home Services 99341 – 99350

As the name implies, **home services** are visits performed by a provider in the patient's home. Today, home visits are extremely rare. The coding of these services is based on the same factors as office visits. In the absence of a proper description, use code 99351.

Preventive Medicine 99381 – 99429

Preventive medicine is, as the name implies, routine, well care provided when there is not an active illness or disease. If there is any credible diagnosis indicated, do not code as preventive. (Some of the services may still be considered preventive and may not be covered, such as immunizations.)

Anesthesia

The CPT® code range for anesthesia is 00100 – 01999. The RVS code range for anesthesia is 10000 – 69999 (same as surgery).

ANESTHESIA CODES

Head	00100 – 00222
Neck	00300 – 00352
Thorax	00400 – 00474
Intrathoracic	00500 – 00580
Spine and Spinal Cord	00600 – 00670
Upper Abdomen	00700 – 00797
Lower Abdomen	00800 – 00882
Perineum	00902 – 00952
Pelvis (Except Hip)	01112 – 01190
Upper Leg (Except Knee)	01200 – 01274
Knee and Popliteal Area	01320 – 01444
Lower Leg	01420 – 01522
Upper Arm and Elbow	01710 – 01782
Forearm, Wrist and Hand	01810 – 01860
Radiological Procedures	01905 – 01933
Burns, Excisions or Debridement	01951 – 01953
Obstetric	01958 - 01969
Other Procedures	01990 – 01999

Anesthesia unit values are listed in the RVS for procedures that require anesthesia administered by an anesthesiologist. Remember that local anesthesia (anesthesia which only numbs a local area) is never allowed separately. Therefore, anesthesia benefits are those that are allowed on procedures that require more than local anesthesia. These units (for all schedules) are used under the following conditions:

- The anesthesia is personally administered by a licensed provider, and
- The provider remains in constant attendance during the procedure for the sole purpose of rendering the anesthesia service.

Anesthesia Base Units

Anesthesia base units are designed to allow for the usual pre- and post-operative care, the administration of the anesthetic, and the administration of fluids and blood incident to the anesthesia or surgery. Remember that the surgical unit values include surgery, local infiltration, digital block, or topical anesthesia.

Anesthesia Time Units

The length of time that a patient is under anesthesia determines the amount of money that will be allowed for the procedure. Anesthesia time begins when the anesthesiologist starts to prepare the patient for the induction of anesthesia in the operating room area (or its equivalent). The time ends when the anesthesiologist is no longer in constant attendance, usually when the patient is ready for post-operative supervision. This time should always be indicated on the claim form when billing for anesthesia services.

Modifiers

All anesthesia services are billed by use of the anesthesia five-digit procedure code plus the addition of a physical status modifier. The use of other optional modifiers may be appropriate.

Physical status modifiers are represented by the initial P followed by a single digit from 1 through 6 as follows:

P1 – A normal healthy patient.
P2 – A patient with mild systemic disease.
P3 – A patient with severe systemic disease.
P4 – A patient with severe systemic disease that is a constant threat to life.

P5 – A moribund patient who is not expected to survive without the operation.

P6 – A declared brain-dead patient whose organs are being removed for donor purposes.

Check the CPT® for optional modifiers which denote special conditions.

Qualifying Circumstances

Many anesthesia services are provided under particularly difficult circumstances because of factors such as extraordinary condition of the patient, notable operative conditions, or unusual risk factors. This section includes a list of important **qualifying circumstances** that significantly impact on the character of the anesthetic service provided. These procedures would not be reported alone, but would be reported as additional procedure numbers qualifying an anesthesia procedure or service. More than one code may be selected.

99100 – Anesthesia for patient of extreme age, under one year or over 70 years.

99116 – Anesthesia complicated by utilization of total body hypothermia.

99135 – Anesthesia complicated by utilization of controlled hypotension.

99140 – Anesthesia complicated by emergency conditions.

Emergency conditions need to be specified. An **emergency** is defined as existing when delay in treatment of the patient would lead to a significant increase in the threat to life or body part.

Surgery

The surgery section of the CPT® book is arranged according to body systems (i.e., integumentary, respiratory). Within each body system, surgeries are arranged according to their anatomic position from the head downward toward the feet.

The RVS lists unit values for surgical procedures, which include the surgery, local anesthesia and the normal, uncomplicated follow-up care associated with the procedure for the time period indicated in the column titled "Follow-up Days."

SURGERY CODES

Integumentary System	10040 – 19499
Musculoskeletal System	20000 – 29999
Respiratory System	30000 – 32999
Cardiovascular System	33010 – 37799
Hemic and Lymphatic System	38100 – 38999
Mediastinum and Diaphragm	39000 – 39599
Digestive System	40490 – 49999
Urinary System	50010 – 53899
Male Genital System	54000 – 55899
Intersex Surgery	55970 – 55980
Female Genital System	56400 – 58999
Maternity Care and Delivery	59000 – 59899
Endocrine System	60000 – 60699
Nervous System	61000 – 64999
Eye and Ocular Adnexa	65091 – 68899
Auditory System	69000 – 69979
Operating Microscope	69990
Cardiac Catheterizations	93501 – 93553

Block Procedures

Block procedures are multiple surgical procedures performed during the same operative session, in the same operative area, usually in the integumentary system. The objective of these codes is to handle multiple repetitions of the same service. A block procedure consists of a primary code and subsequent modifying codes.

For example:
11100 – Biopsy of skin, subcutaneous tissue and/or mucous membrane; single lesion,
11101 – Each separate additional lesion.

11200 – Removal of skin tags, up to 15 lesions
11201 – Each additional 10 lesions

These two are currently the only block procedures listed. These codes are slowly being deleted.

Asterisk Procedures

Asterisk procedures are those surgical procedures denoted by an asterisk (*) to the right of the CPT® code and which require special handling. The asterisk on codes has been eliminated as of the 2004 version of the CPT®. However; they still apply for all procedures performed prior to 1/1/2004. Therefore, we will cover the basics of coding with asterisk procedures here.

If an asterisk follows a CPT® code, the following rules apply:

1. The listed value is for the surgical procedure only.
2. Pre- and post-operative care is to be added on a fee-for-service basis
3. When the (*) procedure is carried out at the time of an initial visit (new patient) and this surgery constitutes the major services for that visit, under CPT® rules, procedure number 99025 is listed in lieu of the usual initial visit as an additional service.
4. When the (*) procedure is carried out at the time of an initial or other visit involving significant identifiable services (i.e., removal of a small skin lesion at the time of a comprehensive history and physical examination), the appropriate visit is coded in addition to the (*) procedure and applicable follow-up care.
5. When the (*) procedure is carried out at the time of a follow-up (established patient) visit and this procedure constitutes the major service at that visit, the service visit is usually not coded separately.
6. When the (*) procedure requires hospitalization, under the CPT®, the appropriate hospital visit is coded in addition to the (*) procedure and its follow-up care.

By Report Procedures

Some procedures are so unusual or variable that it is impossible to determine a standard UCR or unit value allowance. These procedures are called **By Report (BR) procedures**. The RVS may refer to these procedures as Relative Value Not Established (RNE). BR and RNE procedures have to be referred to a professional review unit, a supervisor, or consultant for review to determine the allowance. A copy of the operative report is required for review of these procedures. The anesthesia record may also be needed.

Multiple or Bilateral Procedures

Multiple procedures are more than one surgical procedure performed during the same operative session. **Bilateral procedures** are surgeries that involve a pair of similar body parts (i.e., breasts, eyes). There are two main types of multiple or bilateral procedures:

Same Time, Different Operative Field, Incision, or Orifice

When more than one surgery is performed during the same operative session but through a different orifice (opening) or incision or in a different operative field, 100% of the actual charge or UCR is allowed for the major procedure and 50% of UCR (or actual charge, whichever is less) is usually allowed for each additional procedure.

Bilateral procedures follow the same rules as multiple procedures performed through different incisions.

Same Time, Same Operative Field, Incision or Orifice

Sometimes, when multiple procedures are performed during the same operative session through the same incision, orifice, or operative field, the additional procedures are considered to be incidental.

An incidental procedure is one that does not add significant time or complexity to the operative session. In such a case, the allowable amount would be that of the major procedure only. No additional amount would be allowed for the extra procedures. However, if the additional procedures are not incidental, then the rules for handling multiple procedures explained above would be applied. That is, the major procedure would be considered at 100% of UCR and the lesser at 50%.

For example, let's say that the following bill is received from the provider:

Procedure	Billed Amt	UCR
Tonsillectomy (42821)	$600	$600
Eustachian Tube Inflation (69400)	300	200

Following the rules previously indicated, we would allow 100% of the major procedure plus 50% of the lesser procedure. Therefore, in this example, the allowable amount would be 100% of $600 + 50% of $200 for a Total Allowance of $700.

It is important to understand which procedure is the primary procedure and which is the secondary procedure.

For example, let's look at the same procedures as those just reviewed, billed as follows:

Procedure	Billed Amt	UCR
Tonsillectomy (42821)	$300	$600
Eustachian Tube		
Inflation (69400)	$600	$100
Total	$900	$700

The major procedure is the tonsillectomy, which allows 16.39 units, whereas 69400 is only valued at 1.39 units. Therefore, using the multiple surgery rules but following the doctor's billing the allowed amount would be:

100% of $600 up to the actual charge	$300
50% of $200 or the actual charge, whichever is less	+100
Total Allowance would be	$400

As you can see, incorrect billing would substantially reduce the amount of the claim payment if the insurance company chooses not to use global UCR (comparing the total bill to the total UCR amounts).

Assistant Surgery

As mentioned briefly in the modifiers section, some surgical procedures require an assistant surgeon. When billing for assistant surgeon services, modifier -80 or -81 should be added to the appropriate CPT® code.

Unbundling

Some medical offices practice what is known as "unbundling." The provider is considered to have "unbundled" when he bills separately for procedures that are a part of the primary procedure. For example, a hysterectomy can be performed with or without the removal of the ovaries and/or the fallopian tubes. Therefore, a provider billing for a hysterectomy and removal of the ovaries is unbundling. The maximum allowance is the UCR for the hysterectomy. An extreme example is billing for the removal of a gallbladder and also billing for the repair of the open wound created by the surgery. Of course, the repair is inherently part of the gallbladder surgery.

Follow-Up Days

Follow-up days are days immediately following a surgical procedure for which a provider must monitor a patient's condition in regard to that particular procedure. Surgical procedures include the surgery, local anesthesia, and the normal, uncomplicated follow-up care associated with the procedure for the time period indicated in the RVS.

Complications or other circumstances requiring additional or unusual services concurrent with the procedure or procedures, or during the listed period of normal follow-up care, may warrant additional charges on a fee-for-service basis. However, unless the provider specifically indicates unusual circumstances, it should be assumed that the follow-up care is routine. All visits occurring within the listed follow-up days should be combined with the surgical charge. The following are categories of follow-up care:

Follow-up care for diagnostic procedures (i.e., endoscopy, injection procedures for radiology) includes only care that is related to recovery from the diagnostic procedure itself. Care of the underlying condition for which the diagnostic procedure was performed or other accompanying conditions is not included and may be charged separately in accordance with the services rendered.

Follow-up care for therapeutic procedures generally includes all normal postoperative care. Complications, exacerbations, recurrence, or the presence of other diseases or injuries requiring additional services concurrent with the surgical procedure(s) or during the indicated period of normal follow-up care may warrant additional charges coded and allowable separately.

When additional surgical procedure(s) are carried out within the listed period of follow-up care for a previous surgery, the follow-up periods will run concurrently through their normal termination.

Maternity Expenses

Most plans provide coverage for maternity-related expenses on the same basis as any other illness. Some plans, however, limit or exclude maternity related expenses for either the spouse or the dependent children or occasionally for the subscriber/member. The services normally provided in maternity cases include all routine, antepartum care (prior to delivery), delivery, and all routine, postpartum care (after delivery). The maternity procedure codes are based on this premise unless the specific code indicates otherwise.

Ante-partum care (prenatal) includes:
- Initial and subsequent history,
- Physician's exams, usually one per month for the first eight months, then weekly during the 9th month,
- Weight, blood pressure, urinalysis (monthly or weekly),
- Fetal heart tones, and
- Maternity counseling on food requirements, vitamins and related items.

Delivery includes:
- Vaginal delivery (with or without episiotomy, forceps or breech delivery), and
- Cesarean delivery.

Postpartum care (after delivery) includes:
- Post-delivery hospital visits, and
- Post-delivery office visits (usually one or two routine check-ups) during the first six weeks following delivery.

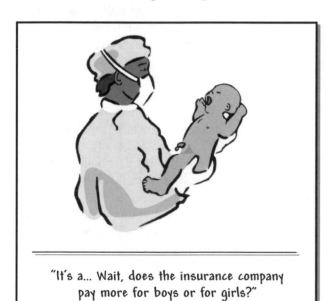

"It's a... Wait, does the insurance company pay more for boys or for girls?"

Other Maternity-Related Procedures

The following are other types of maternity related procedures:

1. **Artificial insemination** is the introduction of semen into the vagina or cervix by artificial means. Some plans consider this a covered expense, and some do not since it is not for the treatment of a disease or injury.

2. **Amniocentesis/chromosomal analysis** are the trans-abdominal perforation of the uterus for the purpose of withdrawing amniotic fluid surrounding the fetus. The chromosomal analysis is the diagnostic study performed on the fluid to study the number and structure of the chromosomes to see whether any abnormalities are present.

An amniocentesis/chromosomal analysis are performed:
- To identify genetic defects of the fetus,
- To determine whether the fetus has attained an adequate state of gestation, and,
- To determine the sex of the fetus.

Charges for amniocentesis and chromosomal analysis are usually covered if the provider can demonstrate the medical necessity of the testing for the patient, such as a family history of specific genetic defects, or maternal age of greater than 35 years. The use of these tests to determine fetal sex alone is not covered by most plans.

In-utero fetal surgery has made it possible to perform surgery on a fetus while it is in the mother's womb; and also to remove the fetus from the womb, perform surgery, and return it back to the womb, with the pregnancy continuing to term. If the surgery is covered, it is often covered as the mother's expense as a complication of pregnancy.

Abortion is a premature expulsion of an embryo or nonviable fetus. There are three different types of abortions:

1. A spontaneous abortion occurring naturally.
2. A therapeutic abortion intentionally induced because the life of the mother would be endangered if the pregnancy were allowed to continue to term.
3. An elective abortion intentionally induced to terminate an unwanted pregnancy.

Coverage for abortions varies greatly from plan to plan. Spontaneous and therapeutic abortions are covered by most plans; however, elective abortions are often excluded. In addition, some plans may pay for certain services for spouses and then exclude these services for dependent children. Therefore, all abortions should be billed to the plan, but the patient should be notified that the insurance carrier may not cover these services.

Cosmetic Surgery

Cosmetic surgery is a surgical procedure performed solely to improve appearance and is usually not covered by benefit plans.

Although some procedures are cosmetic in nature, they may also be performed for functional reasons. For instance, a blepharoplasty is the removal of excessive skin and fat from the eyelids. Certainly, removal of excessive skin and fat improves the person's appearance. However, most plans cover blepharoplasty when the skin overhang is so extensive that it interferes with the patient's peripheral vision. Therefore, the fact that a cosmetic procedure is performed does not necessarily mean that it is considered solely cosmetic.

When the restorative or cosmetic nature of the procedure is not obvious, billers should include documentation to verify the need for services. This documentation often includes:

- Hospital admission history and physical,
- Operative report,
- Pathology report,
- Pre- and post-operative photographs, and
- A narrative report from a referring physician, if available, and
- Pre- and post-operative photographs, if available.

Radiology/X-ray

The radiology section of the CPT® is arranged according to the anatomic position, the body part, starting at the head and moving downward toward the feet. Knowledge of anatomy will make it much easier to locate which area of this section to refer to. This section is divided into four subsections.

RADIOLOGY CODES	
Diagnostic Radiology	70010--76499
Diagnostic Ultrasound	76506--76999
Radiation Oncology	77261--77799
Nuclear Medicine	78000--79999

Diagnostic x-rays are flat or two-dimensional pictures of a particular body part or organ. X-rays are created by sending low-level radiation through the body onto a sheet of film. The image on the exposed piece of film looks like a negative from a roll of camera film. X-rays are most useful for looking at bones and dense tissue since softer tissue is not clearly defined.

Ultrasonography provides a more definitive type of picture than x-rays. Instead of using radiation, sound waves are bounced off the desired structure. The pattern and amount of sound returned constitute what forms a picture of the organ. This type of viewing is less potentially damaging than x-rays. This is why ultrasound scanning can be used during pregnancy, whereas x-rays are not.

Radiation oncology services are the use of radiation to treat a condition. This treatment is used in conjunction with chemotherapy to treat malignant cancers. Normally, radiation therapy is composed of multiple treatments and does not include a "picture" of the body part. It is done for treatment purposes only, not for diagnostic reasons.

Nuclear medicine combines use of radioactive elements and x-rays to image an organ or body part. Certain radioactive elements collect in different organs. Therefore, to see whether an organ is working effectively or to determine whether it is enlarged, a radioactive element is injected into the patient, and pictures are taken of the organ at specified intervals to determine how, where, and how much of the element collects in a specific organ.

CT scans (computed tomography) are 365-degree pictures of specific body areas. This scan provides a three-dimensional picture of the area and is used to help identify tumors and cancers located in an organ. CT scans are much more definitive than x-rays.

Pathology/Laboratory

Laboratory examinations are the analyzing of body substances to determine their chemical or tissue type make-up. Body fluids or tissues are collected and then either run through analyzing machines or viewed under a microscope to identify any abnormal substances or tissues.

PATHOLOGY CODES

Organ or Disease Oriented Panels	80048 – 80076
Drug Testing	80100 – 80103
Therapeutic Drug Assays	80150 – 80299
Evocative/Suppression Testing	80400 – 80440
Consultations (Clinical Pathology)	80500 – 80502
Urinalysis	81000 – 81099
Chemistry	82000 – 84999
Hematology and Coagulation	85002 – 85999
Immunology	86000 – 86849
Transfusion Medicine	86850 – 86999
Microbiology	87001 – 87999
Anatomic Pathology	88000 – 88099
Cytopathology	88104 – 88199
Cytogenic Studies	88230 – 88299
Surgical Pathology	88300 – 88399
Transcutaneous Procedures	88400
Other Procedures	89050 – 89240
Reproductive Medicine Procedures	89250 – 89356

CPT® codes 80048 – 80076 refer to various types of panel tests. Panel tests are composed of multiple tests that are combined and run from one specimen. The number of tests determines which code to use. It is not uncommon today for providers to do what is known as **"unbundling"** when billing. Unbundling occurs when a provider bills separately for each test performed even though all the tests came from the same specimen and were done simultaneously. In this instance, the provider gets significantly more money for doing nothing additional. When a charge slip is received from the provider listing numerous lab tests, the biller should check to ensure that the tests are not all part of a single panel test.

For example, a provider may perform all the following tests during a physical exam:

Bill from MD	CPT® Code	Charge
Calcium	82310	$ 25
Carbon Dioxide	82374	$ 25
Chloride	82435	$ 25
Creatinine	82565	$ 15
Glucose	82947	$ 10
Potassium	84132	$ 15
Sodium	84295	$ 15
BUN	84520	$ 30
Total		$135

In this example, all the billed charges should be combined together and coded under one panel code (80048 – Basic metabolic panel).

Lab Coding Specifics

There are many laboratory tests that are commonly ordered by most providers. The following is a list of some of these services with general coding and billing guidelines.

1. Urinalysis – If unspecified, use code 81000.
2. Glucose – If unspecified, use 82947.
3. Pregnancy testing – Unspecified, use 84702.
4. TB Tine Test (86585) – Often, this test is covered only if the diagnosis is for a respiratory condition (i.e., URI, rhinitis).
5. Lab culture and sensitivity – If billed for a "culture and sensitivity", use codes 87181 – 87190. A lab culture does not usually include a sensitivity study. However, a sensitivity study must include the culture. If the billing is for a culture with no indication of a sensitivity study, use codes 87040 – 87158.
6. Pap smears – Usually, a covered expense if the patient is being treated for a gynecologic condition, i.e., vaginitis, pelvic pain, dysmenorrhea.
7. Handling/collection charges – Normally coded 99000 – 99002. This charge is usually billed when the specimen is obtained in the office but sent to an outside laboratory for analysis.

The remaining subsections of this section are based on the type of analysis being performed. The subsections are as follows:

- Urinalysis 81000 – 81099
- Chemistry and Toxicology 82000 – 84999
- Hematology 85000 – 85999
- Immunology 86000 – 86849
- Transfusion Medicine 86850 – 86999
- Microbiology 87001 – 87999
- Anatomic Pathology 88000 – 88299
- Surgical Pathology 88300 – 88399
- Miscellaneous 89050 – 89399

Component Charges

Whenever a lab or x-ray test is performed, there are two distinct services that are actually completed:

The first service is the taking of the specimen or x-ray. This charge should include the expense for the personnel performing the test and the cost of the necessary equipment. This is called the Technical Component and is denoted by adding modifier -27 to the CPT® code.

The second service is for the interpretation or reading of the results of the test. This is called the Professional Component (PC) and is denoted by adding modifier -26 to the CPT® code.

The plan usually limits payment to 60% of UCR for the technical component and 40% of UCR for the professional component.

Medicine

This area of the CPT® includes non-surgical and medical care services. Nonsurgical services include optometry care, chiropractic care, acupuncture treatment, physical therapy, and hospital care. The CPT® code range for medicine services is as follows:

MEDICINE CODES	
Immune Globulins	90281 – 90399
Immunization Administration for Vaccines/Toxoids	90471 – 90474
Vaccines/Toxoids	90476 – 90749
Therapeutic or Diagnostic Infusions	90780 – 90781
Therapeutic, Prophylactic or Diagnostic Injections	90782 – 90799
Psychiatry	90801 – 90899
Biofeedback	90900 – 90911
Dialysis	90918 – 90999
Gastroenterology	91000 – 91299
Ophthalmology	92002 – 92499
Special Otorhinolaryngologic Services	92502 – 92700
Cardiovascular	92950 – 93799
Non-Invasive Vascular Studies	93875 – 93990
Pulmonary	94010 – 94799
Allergy and Clinical Immunology	95004 – 95199
Endocrinology	95250
Neurology and Neuromuscular Procedures	95805 – 96004
Central Nervous System Assessments/Tests	96100 – 96117
Health and Behavior Assessment /Intervention	96150 – 96155
Chemotherapy Administration	96400 – 96549
Photodynamic Therapy	96567 – 96571
Special Dermatological Procedures	96900 – 96999
Physical Medicine and Rehabilitation	97001 – 97799
Medical Nutrition Therapy	97802 – 97804
Acupuncture	97810 – 97814
Osteopathic Manipulative Treatment	98925 – 98929
Chiropractic Manipulative Treatment	98940 – 98943
Special Services, Procedures and Reports	99000 – 99091

Immunizations 90471 – 90749

Immunizations are considered to be preventive treatment. Therefore, an active illness or disease is usually not present.

Therapeutic Injections 90782 – 90799

These codes are used for **therapeutic injections** which are injections required in the treatment of an illness or disease. They are not routine or preventive injections.

Types of therapeutic injections include:

- Subcutaneous--just below the outermost level of skin,
- Intradermal--just below the second level of skin, the dermis,
- Intramuscular – into a muscle,
- Intra-arterial – into an artery, and
- Intravenous – into a vein.

Allergy injections should be coded 95115 – 95134, unless otherwise directed. Most antibiotics are injected intramuscularly.

Psychiatry 90801 – 90899

Psychiatric services and treatment includes treatment for psychotic and neurotic disorders, organic brain dysfunction, alcoholism, and chemical dependency.

The language description generally indicates psychotherapy, individual therapy or group therapy. The ICD-9 coding is usually in the range of 290.00 to 319.00. The providers of service are usually an M.D. (often a psychiatrist) or a clinical psychologist.

Most benefit plans require a referral by an M.D. if one of the following providers is indicated: MFCC (Marriage, Family, and Child Counselor), LCSW (Licensed Clinical Social Worker), or MSW (Master of Social Work).

These CPT® codes are used only when psychiatric counseling or therapy is provided. If such therapy is not provided, even if the service is performed by one of the above licensed providers, a different code range should be used.

Most plans pay a reduced benefit for this type of treatment. There may be a limit on the number of visits per year or per lifetime, along with a dollar limit per visit or per calendar year. Also, many plans cover only certain provider licensing.

Biofeedback 90901 – 90911

Biofeedback is training a person to consciously control automatic, internal body functions. For instance, through conscious control, some body rhythms that control the constriction of blood vessels and beating of the heart can be increased or decreased. This type of treatment can be used for a variety of illnesses or symptoms. A common use is for the control of intractable pain.

Biofeedback is controversial because its effectiveness is very hard to prove or disprove. In addition, it does not cure anything. Instead, it is used as a tool in dealing with the symptoms of a condition, not in its treatment. Generally, most plans do not cover biofeedback, or if it is covered, it is very limited and only covered for certain diagnoses.

Dialysis 90918 – 90999

Dialysis is a maintenance procedure used for End-Stage Renal Disease when the kidneys cease functioning. Note that this is not really a treatment because it is only handling the functions normally performed by the body. (However, it is still referred to generically as "treatment.") To enable a patient with this disease to survive, the blood-cleansing function must be performed artificially by one of three processes currently available: hemodialysis, CAPD--continuous ambulatory peritoneal dialysis, or transplantation of a new kidney.

Most hemodialysis is performed at private dialysis centers. A small percentage of the patients have a machine in their own home. The fees for dialysis are usually billed on a monthly basis. When coding, the actual dates of service should be indicated, or a monthly from/through date should be used. Normally, the insurance carrier provides coverage only for the first 18 months of treatment. After that time, Medicare becomes the primary payor (refer to the Medicare section for additional information). If the dialysis is performed in an acute facility, the patient may be billed separately for the facility fees and the physician fees. Remember, the CPT® codes are only to be used on physician services.

CAPD is performed by the patient at home. The peritoneum of the stomach is used to cleanse the blood. Surgery is required for the implantation of catheters and the construction of the internal bag (made of the peritoneum) to hold the dialysate fluids.

Transplants are coded in accordance with the surgery section of the CPT®.

Ophthalmology 92002 – 92499

Ophthalmology care is provided by either an optometrist or an ophthalmologist (M.D.). Most health plans do not cover routine vision care services related to the refraction and subsequent prescription of glasses or contact lenses. If they are covered, however, the benefits are usually very limited in both the dollar allowance, and the time restraints and are often provided under a separate vision care plan or benefit. Some vision care is essential for the proper care and treatment of eye diseases.

Orthoptics is a retraining of the muscles that control vision. Some plans allow for this therapy for certain conditions such as strabismus and binocular vision. If the plan does allow the therapy, it is usually very limited and may require a second opinion from an ophthalmologist.

Otorhinolaryngologic Services 92502 – 92700 (Ear, Nose, and Throat)

Otorhinolaryngologic services are for the care and treatment of the nerves of the hearing organs. Some of the services entail regular hearing tests. Other services are very complex diagnostic tests performed when it has been determined that there is a hearing loss but the cause of the loss has not been established. As with vision services, this care is often restricted under many health plans.

Cardiovascular 92950 – 93799

The cardiovascular section is very large, and it is heavily used by the medical biller. Following are some of the more commonly billed services:

- EKG 93000,
- EKG Interpretation and Report Only 93010,
- Cardiovascular Stress Test 93015, and
- 24-Hour EKG Monitoring 93224.

Physical Therapy 97010 – 97799

Physical therapy is the science of physical or corrective rehabilitation or treatment of abnormal conditions of the musculoskeletal system through the use of heat, light, water, electricity, sound, massage, and active, passive or restrictive exercise.

This therapy often follows surgery or an injury to a joint or muscle. When either of these events occurs, the muscles attaching to the affected joint become weak or atrophied. Consequently, to restore full movement, concentrated therapy to the affected area may be required. Physical therapy treatments may include functional activities, mobility training, manipulation, physical modalities, assessment, instruction, and specialized testing or therapeutic exercises.

Although physical therapy is usually performed by a Registered Physical Therapist (RPT), it is not uncommon for chiropractors (DC), podiatrists (DPM) and osteopaths (DO) to also bill for these services.

Occupational therapy is a type of physical therapy. The objective of this treatment is to either restore normal movement, or, in the case of paralysis, to teach the patient alternative ways of dealing with his or her handicap to meet the demands of everyday living. Occupational therapy is normally billed by an Occupational Therapist (OT), a hospital or a rehabilitative facility.

Speech therapy is for the purpose of improving speech and verbal communication skills. It is usually performed by a speech therapist.

Physical Medicine 97010 – 98943

Physical medicine is the manipulation and physical therapy associated with the nonsurgical care and treatment of the patient. The most common form of physical medicine is chiropractic manipulation of the spine. Theoretically, any joint can be involved; the most common is the spinal area.

The chiropractor's scope of practice is limited in most states. For example, in some states chiropractors are not allowed to draw blood or prescribe prescription medicines. The limitations vary by state.

Many chiropractors use an accident diagnosis, 84x.xx series, for billing purposes. If an accident or injury has occurred this should be substantiated with a date, place, and the circumstances of the accident or injury indicated. Otherwise, the coding should be changed to reflect a non-injury skeletal condition, (72x.xx).

Specialist Services

The remaining part of this section of the CPT® is composed of services that are usually billed only by specialists within a given field. It is important to take the time to look through this section and to become aware of what services are listed. A brief

explanation of some of these sections is provided below.

Gastroenterology 91000 – 91299

Gastroenterology procedures are those services related to the digestive system, esophagus, stomach, intestines.

Pulmonary 94010 – 94799

Pulmonary services include treatment and testing of the respiratory system, in relation to lung function.

Allergy and Clinical Immunology 95007 – 95199

This section includes allergy testing and desensitization (allergy shots).

Neurology 95805 – 95999

Neurology includes nerve and muscle testing. These services may be considered lab or medical.

Chemotherapy Administration 96400 – 96549

Chemotherapy includes administration of chemotherapy agents, usually for treatment of cancer. These codes do not include the cost of the chemical.

Special Dermatology Procedures 96900 – 96999

Dermatological Procedures are procedures to treat the skin.

Case Management Services 99361 – 99373

Case management services are services that initiate and coordinate the health care treatment team. These services are only required in very complex cases involving multiple body systems that are covered by several providers.

Special Services, Procedures and Reports 99000 – 99191

This section includes miscellaneous services not covered elsewhere. It also includes critical care services that are usually considered to be hospital or emergency care.

Some sections of the CPT® Medicine section may be considered diagnostic testing (DXL), medical, or surgical (this varies from payor to payor).

Billing Tips

The following are billing tips on using the CPT®.
1. As long as you document the time you spent and the reason why, you can bill for the higher level E&M codes (and receive the higher reimbursement).
2. Make sure the diagnosis code you submit is consistent with the level of the visit you are billing for.
3. Assign a person to re-check all codes, prior to the claims leaving the office.
4. If the code you are submitting is a high-level code or is unusual, include documentation to support the services when the claim is submitted.

Summary

The CPT® is used for coding procedures and services rendered by a provider. It provides a uniform means of reporting and allows for computer compilation of data.

The CPT® reference book has six major sections. The correct code is located according to the section that pertains to the service or procedure performed.

Modifiers are two-digit codes that can be added to CPT® codes to denote unusual circumstances. These modifiers more fully describe the procedure that was carried out.

CPT® coding is one of the most vital functions that a medical biller performs. Without proper CPT® coding, claims may be denied, delayed, or returned for correction.

Assignments

Complete the Questions for Review.
Complete Exercises 17 – 1 through 17 – 10.

If you are getting less than 90% accuracy in your coding, the need for more practice is indicated.

Questions for Review

Directions: Answer the following questions without looking back into the material just covered. Write your answers in the space provided.

1. What are Evaluation and Management codes? _____

2. What is Physical Medicine? _____

3. In what order is the CPT® surgical section arranged? _____

4. When is modifier -80 used? _____

5. (True or False?) Modifier -50 is used when billing for pre-operative care only. _____

If you were unable to answer any of the questions, refer back to that section, and then fill in the answers.

Exercise 17 – 1

Directions: Based on the service description, look up the appropriate CPT® code and write it in the space provided.

Description	Code

1. Office visit, evaluation of established patient medical decision low complexity, expanded problem focused history.

 1. _____

2. Rest home visit, evaluation of new patient, medical decision making moderate complexity, expanded problem focused history and exam.

 2. _____

3. Initial hospital visit, new or established patient, detailed or comprehensive history and exam, straightforward medical decision.

 3. _____

4. Subsequent, hospital care, medical decision of moderate complexity, expanded problem focused history.

 4. _____

5. Admission to SNF, established patient, medical decision of low complexity. Detailed history, comprehensive exam.

 5. _____

6. Limited follow-up care in a convalescent facility, straightforward medical decision, problem focused history and exam.

 6. _____

7. Emergency department care, minimal care, straightforward medical decision, problem focused history and exam.

 7. _____

8. Initial inpatient consultation, new patient, medical decision of moderate complexity, comprehensive history and exam.

 8. _____

9. Complex comprehensive initial consultation, office, medical decision of high complexity.

 9. _____

10. Follow-up minimal consultation, office, straightforward medical decision making, problem focused history and exam.

 10. _____

Exercise 17 – 2

Directions: Based on the service description, look up the appropriate CPT® code and write it in the space provided.

Description	**Code**
1. Diathermy with paraffin bath	1. _____
2. Tar and ultraviolet bath, dermatology	2. _____
3. Manipulation for physical therapy by physician, one area	3. _____
4. Electrocardiogram, complete	4. _____
5. Provocative testing, for allergies	5. _____
6. Heart electroconversion	6. _____
7. Gonioscopy	7. _____
8. Psychoanalysis	8. _____
9. Biofeedback training for high blood pressure	9. _____
10. IV therapy for anaphylactic shock, 1 hour	10. _____
11. Informational book of diabetes care	11. _____
12. Specimen handling fee	12. _____
13. Newborn resuscitation	13. _____
14. Subsequent detailed hospital visit	14. _____
15. Group psychotherapy by a physician	15. _____
16. Emergency department care at hospital, problem focused, tetanus toxoid injection	16. _____
17. Supplies, office	17. _____
18. 25 Minute conference with interdisciplinary health team regarding case management	18. _____
19. Rapid desensitization, 45 min. Allergy immunotherapy	19. _____
20. Cardiopulmonary resuscitation	20. _____
21. F/up consultation for complications of diabetes/inpatient, expanded problem moderate complexity	21. _____
22. Injection of penicillin	22. _____
23. Problem focused initial er exam for severe congestion	23. _____
24. Comprehensive exam for new patient with severe arthritis, office, moderate complexity	24. _____
25. Contact lens prescription	25. _____

Exercise 17 – 3

Directions: Based on the service description, look up the appropriate CPT® code and write it in the space provided.

Description	Code
1. IPPB treatment, initial	1.
2. 45-minute individual psychotherapy	2.
3. Color vision exam	3.
4. Extended f/up visit, critical care, 1 hr.	4.
5. Prosthetic training, 35 minutes	5.
6. Peritoneal dialysis for May, age 35	6.
7. Psychological testing, 5 hours	7.
8. Infusion of calcium, 1.5 Hours	8.
9. SSO, extensive, high complexity	9.
10. Tetanus injection for cut due to rusty can	10.
11. Intermediate ophthalmological exam and evaluation for continued care	11.
12. Pediatric pneumogram	12.
13. Typhoid vaccination	13.
14. Initial comprehensive consultation, office, moderate complexity	14.
15. ER problem focused exam for suture removal	15.
16. Initial hospital visit, normal newborn	16.
17. Allergy injection	17.
18. Allergen serum, 1 vial, single antigen	18.
19. Hearing aid exam	19.
20. Initial problem focused consultation, office	20.
21. Pulmonary stress, testing	21.
22. Emergency department follow-up for suture removal, problem focused	22.
23. Discharge from hospital	23.
24. Detailed office visit; subsequent initial hospital comprehensive Admission and history, low complexity	24.
25. Minimal office visit, established patient	25.

Exercise 17 – 4

Directions: Based on the service description, look up the appropriate CPT® code and write it in the space provided.

Description	**Code**
1. Urinalysis	1. _____
2. Complete chest x-ray	2. _____
3. ECG, complete	3. _____
4. CBC	4. _____
5. MRI of left hip joint	5. _____
6. Lipid panel	6. _____
7. Erythropoietin bioassay	7. _____
8. Cat scan of the abdomen with contrast	8. _____
9. Cardiovascular stress test with exercise, interp. Only	9. _____
10. Cholecystography with contrast	10. _____
11. Streptokinase, antibody	11. _____
12. HIV antigen	12. _____
13. Ultrasound for gestational age, limited	13. _____
14. Doppler EKG, complete	14. _____
15. Facial nerve function study	15. _____
16. Ova and parasites, concentration and identification	16. _____
17. Blood potassium	17. _____
18. Estradiol, ria (placental)	18. _____
19. General toxicology screen	19. _____
20. Cyanocobalamin bioassay (Vitamin B-12)	20. _____
21. Lithium levels, interp. and Report only	21. _____
22. Serum albumin	22. _____
23. Needle biopsy ultrasonic guidance, complete	23. _____
24. Unilateral renal venography, complete	24. _____
25. MRI w/contrast, brain	25. _____

Exercise 17 – 5

Directions: Based on the service description, look up the appropriate CPT® code and write it in the space provided.

Description	Code
1. Wet mount for ova and parasites	1. _____
2. Huhner test and semen analysis	2. _____
3. Platelet survival study	3. _____
4. Intermediate radiology therapeutic treatment planning	4. _____
5. Cat, lumbar spine w/o contrast	5. _____
6. A/p abdominal x-ray, single view	6. _____
7. Intravenous kub, pyelography	7. _____
8. B-scan retroperitoneal echography, limited	8. _____
9. Infusion of radioelement solution	9. _____
10. Salivary gland function study	10. _____
11. Comprehensive metabolic panel	11. _____
12. Serum cholesterol, total	12. _____
13. Blood ethchlorvynol	13. _____
14. X-ray knee, a/p and lateral	14. _____
15. Feces screening for lipids, qualitative	15. _____
16. Ascorbic acid (vitamin C), blood	16. _____
17. Desipramine, assay	17. _____
18. Digoxin, RIA (reduced services)	18. _____
19. Histamine test	19. _____
20. Galactose test (reference laboratory)	20. _____
21. Cephalogram, orthodontic (professional component)	21. _____
22. X-ray hand; minimum of three views	22. _____
23. Duodenography, hypotonic	23. _____
24. Pelvimetry, with or without placental localization	24. _____
25. X-ray forearm, a/p and lateral (professional component)	25. _____

Exercise 17 – 6

Directions: Based on the service description, look up the appropriate CPT® code and write it in the space provided.

Description	**Code**
1. Radiologic exam, hand: two views	1. _____
2. Bone age studies	2. _____
3. Xeroradiography	3. _____
4. Mammography; unilateral	4. _____
5. Echography, spinal canal and contents	5. _____
6. Tuberculosis, intradermal	6. _____
7. Theophylline, assay	7. _____
8. Urinalysis, chemical, qualitative	8. _____
9. Obstetric profile	9. _____
10. Iron binding capacity, serum; chemical	10. _____
11. Radiologic examination, abdomen single view	11. _____
12. Radiologic exam, hip; unilateral	12. _____
13. Glucose tolerance test, 3 specimens	13. _____
14. FSH	14. _____
15. Hepatitis panel	15. _____
16. Entire spine, myelography, super. & inter.	16. _____
17. Cervicocerebral angiography, w/catheter including vessel origin	17. _____
18. Basic dosimetry, radiation therapy	18. _____
19. Laryngography w/contrast super & inter	19. _____
20. Protozoa antibody tube, guide.	20. _____
21. Gases, blood PO_2 by manometry	21. _____
22. Heparin assay	22. _____
23. Hepatitis Be antigen (hbeag)	23. _____
24. Necropsy (autopsy); forensic examination	24. _____
25. Russell viper venom time, diluted	25. _____

Exercise 17 – 7

Directions: Based on the surgery service description, look up the appropriate CPT® code and write it in the space provided.

Description	Code
1. Excision of mediastinal cyst	1. _____
2. Pyelotomy; with exploration	2. _____
3. Repair, laceration of palate; up to 2 cm.	3. _____
4. Resection of external cardiac tumor	4. _____
5. Wedging of clubfoot cast	5. _____
6. Puncture aspiration of cyst of breast	6. _____
7. Removal of foreign body; intraocular, anterior chamber	7. _____
8. Mastoidectomy; complete	8. _____
9. Open treatment of ankle dislocation	9. _____
10. Nipple/areola reconstruction	10. _____
11. Hysterotomy, abdominal	11. _____
12. Cholecystectomy	12. _____
13. Amniocentesis, any method	13. _____
14. Spinal puncture, lumbar, diagnostic	14. _____
15. Acne surgery, removal of comedones	15. _____
16. Routine obstetric care w/antepartum care, vaginal	16. _____
17. Excision of tonsil tags	17. _____
18. Direct repair of aneurysm, carotid--assistant	18. _____
19. Arthroscopy, ankle surgical removal of FB	19. _____
20. Excision of lesion of pancreas - assistant	20. _____
21. Ureterectomy, with bladder cuff (separate procedure)	21. _____
22. Radical abdominal hysterectomy - assistant	22. _____
23. Tenotomy, subcutaneous, toe, single	23. _____
24. Synovectomy, intertarsal	24. _____
25. Pericardiocentesis; initial	25. _____

Exercise 17 – 8

Directions: Based on the service description, look up the appropriate CPT® code and write it in the space provided.

Description	**Code**
1. Excision or curettage of bone cyst or benign tumor, talus or calcaneus	1. _____
2. Removal of permanent pacemaker	2. _____
3. Renal biopsy, percutaneous by trocar	3. _____
4. Partial hymenectomy or revision of hymenal ring	4. _____
5. Myringotomy	5. _____
6. Thoracoplasty	6. _____
7. Repair blood vessel, direct; neck	7. _____
8. Colostomy or skin level cecostomy	8. _____
9. Circumcision, using clamp; newborn	9. _____
10. Salpingo-oophorectomy; complete	10. _____
11. Bronchoplasty, graft repair - assistant	11. _____
12. Tracheoplasty, cervical	12. _____
13. Closed treatment of metacarpal fracture; single w/o manipulation	13. _____
14. Cryotherapy	14. _____
15. Open treatment of distal tibial fracture of fibula only	15. _____
16. Vaginal hysterectomy	16. _____
17. Total ankle replacement	17. _____
18. Tympanotomy	18. _____
19. Angioplasty	19. _____
20. Lithotripsy, extracorporeal shock wave with water bath	20. _____
21. Radial orchiectomy, inguinal	21. _____
22. Repair of cleft plate	22. _____
23. Vulvectomy	23. _____
24. Venous thrombectomy, direct or catheter	24. _____
25. Complete amputation of penis	25. _____

Exercise 17 – 9

Directions: Based on the service description, look up the appropriate **Anesthesia** CPT® code and write it in the space provided.

Anesthesia Description	**Code**
1. Routine obstetric care w/antepartum care, vaginal	1. _____
2. Excision of tonsil tags	2. _____
3. Anoscopy	3. _____
4. Arthroscopy, ankle surgical removal of FB	4. _____
5. Laryngoscopy	5. _____
6. Proctoscopy	6. _____
7. Bronchoscopy	7. _____
8. Ophthalmoscopy	8. _____
9. Femoral artery ligation	9. _____
10. Orchiopexy, unilateral or bilateral	10. _____
11. Biopsy of liver	11. _____
12. Catheterization, urethra; simple	12. _____
13. Treatment of spontaneous abortion	13. _____
14. Adrenalectomy	14. _____
15. Urethroplasty; first stage	15. _____
16. Laminectomy	16. _____
17. Sigmoidoscopy	17. _____
18. Renal biopsy, percutaneous	18. _____
19. Liver transplant (recipient)	19. _____
20. Myringotomy	20. _____
21. Thoracoplasty	21. _____
22. Repair blood vessel, direct; neck	22. _____
23. Pneumocentesis	23. _____
24. Circumcision, using clamp; newborn	24. _____
25. Salpingo-oophorectomy; complete	25. _____
26. Bronchoplasty, graft repair	26. _____
27. Tracheoplasty, cervical	27. _____
28. Treatment of closed metacarpal fracture; single	28. _____
29. Cryotherapy	29. _____
30. Treatment of closed distal tibial fracture	30. _____

Exercise 17 – I0

Directions: Based on the service description, look up the appropriate CPT® and ICD-9 code and write it in the space provided.

Description	ICD-9 code	CPT® code
1. Glaucoma provocative test	1. _____	_____
2. Diabetic minimal check-up, established	2. _____	_____
3. Hearing loss comprehensive testing	3. _____	_____
4. Allergen immunotherapy injection for grass	4. _____	_____
5. Physical therapy for skeletal pain, 45 minutes	5. _____	_____
6. F/up newborn care, in the hospital	6. _____	_____
7. Problem focused f/up visit to shady oaks rest home, advanced senility	7. _____	_____
8. Emergency high complexity admit to Hoag Memorial Hospital, pulmonary edema	8. _____	_____
9. Manipulation with hot packs and traction and ultrasound, physical therapy for low back pain	9. _____	_____
10. Therapeutic phlebotomy for URI	10. _____	_____

Honors Certification™

The certification challenge for this chapter will be a written test of the information contained in this chapter. Each incorrect answer will result in a deduction of up to 5% from your grade. You must achieve a score of 85% or higher to pass this test. If you fail the test on your first attempt you may retake the test one additional time. The items included in the second test may be different from those in the first test.

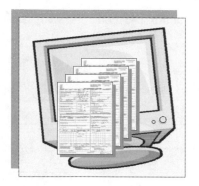

18

HCPCS Coding

After completion of this chapter you will be able to:

- Explain the purpose and use of the Health Care Procedure Coding System (HCPCS).
- Describe the three levels used in HCPCS coding.
- Properly code procedures or items using HCPCS.

Key words and concepts you will learn in this chapter:

Air Ambulance – A helicopter or other flight vehicle used to transport severely injured or ill persons to a hospital.

Base Call Charge – The amount automatically charged for an ambulance to respond to a call even if the patient is not subsequently transported.

Chemotherapy Drugs – Drugs administered to help fight cancer and other serious diseases.

Durable Medical Equipment (DME) – An item that can be used for an extended period of time without significant deterioration (i.e., it can stand repeated use).

Durable Medical Equipment Regional Carriers (DMERCs) – One of four regional Medicare carriers responsible for the processing of Durable Medical Equipment claims.

Emergency Medical Technicians (EMTs) – Emergency medical personnel who render emergency treatment at the scene of the injury or illness and are trained in basic life support.

Enteral Therapy – The administration of nutritional products directly into the small intestines.

Medically Oriented Equipment – Equipment that is primarily and customarily used for medical purposes.

Mobile Intensive Care Unit – A life support vehicle equipped to provide care to critically ill patients who require transportation to a hospital or from one hospital to another.

Orthotics – Devices used to straighten or correct a deformity or disability.

Paramedics – Specially trained emergency medical personnel who render emergency treatment at the scene of the injury or illness and are trained in advanced life support.

Parenteral Therapy – Therapy that involves administering substances to a patient via a tube inserted into a vein. (i.e., medications or nutritional supplements).

Prosthetic Devices – Devices designed to replace a missing body part or to restore some function to a paralyzed body part.

Van Transportation Units – Specially equipped vans that can handle wheelchairs and patients who are unable to get in and out of a regular vehicle.

Procedure coding is a way for providers to report to an insurance carrier the exact service(s) they perform for their patients. The accuracy and precision of a procedure system is a critical element in any claims processing operation because it provides the vehicle to communicate these services and to ensure proper reimbursement of benefits.

While the CPT® covers many of the services provided by providers, it does not cover everything. Medicare carriers consistently needed additional information on certain types of claims. These often included claims for medical equipment and supplies. Additionally, Medicare payors would often request information regarding the drugs being provided to the patient. The CPT® only provides five codes for injectable drugs:

> 90782 – Subcutaneous or intramuscular injection
> 90783 – Intra-arterial injection
> 90784 – Intravenous injection
> 90788 – Intramuscular injection of antibiotic
> 90799 – Unlisted injection

These codes give no indication of the type of drug being injected, or what it is used for (i.e., pain management, alleviation of symptoms, etc.). Medicare needed additional information to process these claims. The Health Care Procedure Coding System (HCPCS) is a listing of codes and descriptive terminology used for reporting the provision of supplies, materials, injections and certain services and procedures to Medicare. With the advent of the HCPCS J codes, the biller can now enter a code to indicate what drug is being given to the patient.

When billing Medicare patients, HCPCS codes should be used. Additionally, many insurance carriers are now insisting on the use of HCPCS codes when no appropriate CPT® code can be given.

General Information

In the early 1980s there were over 120 methods of coding procedures. In an attempt to simplify coding, the Health Care Financing Administration (HCFA) created the Health Care Procedure Coding System (HCPCS).

HCPCS are based on the American Medical Association (AMA) Current Procedure Terminology (CPT®) with additional codes and modifiers developed by HCFA. HCPCS are made up of three coding levels:

1. Level 1: The first level contains only the CPT® codes and modifiers. Maintenance of these codes is the responsibility of the AMA, and updates are done on a yearly basis. There are over 7,000 CPT® codes; however the CPT® is limited in its selections for materials, supplies and injection codes. For example, the code 99070 is used for all supplies.

2. Level 2: The second level includes the HCFA designated codes. These are non-physician services such as Durable Medical Equipment, Prostheses and Orthoses. A few physicians' services that were not found in the CPT® codes were assigned HCFA codes, such as J codes for injections. HCFA codes are alphanumeric beginning with A0000 and continuing through V9999. There are over 2,400 HCPCS codes which are updated yearly.

3. Level 3: This level contain codes local to the individual Medicare carrier and are not found in the first two levels. These codes are also alphanumeric, but are located in the ranges beginning with W, X, Y, and Z. This may include new codes designated by the carrier, or old codes which were deleted from the HCPCS but are still used by the local carrier.

While the acronym HCPCS is technically used to denote all three levels of the coding system, many people commonly use it to denote just the Level 2 and 3 codes which differ from the more commonly used CPT® codes.

Medicare requires the use of HCPCS codes for all services provided to Medicare patients. In some states, HCPCS codes are also required for Medicaid billing. Since there are numerous changes to the CPT® and HCPCS codes every year, it is imperative that the biller use the most current edition of the CPT® and HCPCS manual.

To properly code these claims, remember that Level 3 codes have the highest priority. If no Level 3 code properly describes the procedure performed (or there are no Level 3 codes for your region), then Level 2 codes should be considered. If no Level 3 or Level 2 code is appropriate for the procedure, then the current CPT® code may be used. Using this system, it is not uncommon to find CPT®, Level 2 and Level 3 codes all listed on one claim form.

The HCPCS coding system also includes two digit modifiers at both the local and national level (Level 3 and Level 2). These modifiers may be two letters or a letter followed by a number.

Claims for Medicare patients, if are improperly coded, may be delayed, denied, or payment may be reduced. Continued problems may result in the possibility of receiving audits and fines, or the doctor may be dropped from the Medicare program.

Be sure to check the front of your HCPCS manual for additional information on codes that are not valid for Medicare, services that are not covered by Medicare, and items that have special coverage guidelines. Modifiers are used when billing Medicare; however, not all modifiers are acceptable. The front of your HCPCS book should have guidelines on those modifiers which may be used.

Coding Using the HCPCS Manual

Most versions of the HCPCS manual contain an index in the back. This index lists most of the procedures and/or items that are included in the manual. However, not all items may be included. For example, some HCPCS indexes do not list all the drugs included in the J code section. Since most of these drugs are listed in alphabetical order, it is often not difficult to locate the correct code.

To locate a HCPCS code for an item or service, use the index. The index will provide you with the specific HCPCS code for that item or service. If there is more than one applicable code, the index will list all codes, or may list a range of codes (i.e., L3810 – L3860). However, just looking in the index is not enough. After identifying the code, locate the code in the lettered section and read the information provided. There may be additional information regarding the code, or there may be references to other codes which may be more appropriate.

As with the CPT® and ICD-9, the HCPCS manual uses semicolons. Thus, if a code is indented, the full description of that code includes everything in the unindented code directly above it, up to the semicolon. For example, use your HCPCS manual to locate code L3805. The correct description for this code would be: Wrist-hand-finger-orthoses (WHFO); long opponens, no attachment, custom fabricated.

Sections of the HCPCS Manual

The HCPCS manual is categorized into numerous sections. Each section begins with a letter, and within that section, each code begins with the same letter.

HCPCS codes are categorized into the following sections:

Transportation Services	A000 – A0999
Medical and Surgical Supplies	A4000 – A7509
Miscellaneous and Experimental	A9000 – A9999
Enteral and Parenteral Therapy	B0000 – B9999
Temporary Hospital Outpatient PPS	C0000 – C9999
Dental Procedures	D0000 – D9999
Durable Medical Equipment	E0000 – E9999
Temporary Procedures and Professional Services	G0000 – G9999
Rehabilitative Services	H0000 – H9999
Drugs Administered Other than Oral Method	J0000 – J8999
Chemotherapy Drugs	J9000 – J9999
Temporary Codes for DMERCS	K0000 – K9999
Orthotic Procedures	L0000 – L4999
Prosthetic Procedures	L5000 – L9999
Medical Services	M0000 – M9999
Pathology and Laboratory	P0000 – P9999
Temporary Codes	Q0000 – Q9999
Diagnostic Radiology Services	R0000 – R9999
Private Payer Codes	S0000 – S9999
State Medicaid Agency Codes	T0000 – T9999
Vision Services	V0000 – V2999
Hearing Services	V5000 – V5999

Let's look at each of these sections in more detail.

Transportation Services

These codes are used to report transportation services, including ambulance and air ambulance services. Ambulance expenses are expenses that are incurred to transfer an injured or sick person to a medical facility. These expenses are not considered professional or hospital services.

Benefits are usually payable for transfer to another hospital when medically necessary. For example, if one hospital does not have the facilities to treat the patient's medical condition, the patient may be transferred to the closest hospital with appropriate facilities.

An ambulance expense is covered under the following conditions:

1. The ambulance must be medically necessary and not for the patient's convenience.

2. Transportation is provided by a professional ambulance/paramedic service.
3. Transportation is to the nearest facility capable of treating the patient.
4. Transportation is provided from one facility to another when the necessary treatment cannot be obtained from the first hospital.
5. Transportation to home from a facility is provided if the patient is unable to travel in an upright position. Exceptions such as this vary by plan, so refer to the plan provisions before processing.
6. Charges for ambulance services are covered when either emergency room or inpatient hospital charges are also billed. An exception would be in the case of an insured that is dead on arrival at the hospital.
7. Transportation to a facility if the claimant is dead on arrival, even though no treatment or charges are incurred at the facility.

Many plans designate a maximum allowable amount for each trip based on usual and customary guidelines. Expenses commonly billed by an ambulance service include:

- **Base call charge.** This is the amount automatically charged for the ambulance to respond to a call even if the patient is not subsequently transported,
- **Oxygen** and oxygen supplies,
- **Mileage**,
- **Linens**,
- **Emergency response charge**. This is an extra expense in addition to the base charge, which may be added if the patient's condition is severe enough that resuscitation efforts or other types of stabilization measures are required, and
- **Paramedic response charge**. If paramedics rather than emergency medical technicians (EMTs) are used, an extra expense may be added.

Air Ambulance

An **air ambulance** is a helicopter or other flight vehicle used to transport severely injured or ill person to a hospital. Air medical transport may be covered if:

1. The facility in the area where the patient is injured cannot manage the patient's condition and it is medically necessary to transfer the patient by air to another facility more equipped to treat the patient, or
2. Ground transport time would be prolonged and thus, compromise the patient's medical status.

Coverage is limited to the regular air ambulance charge for transportation to the nearest facility that can handle the case.

Many plans do not cover this service, regardless of the reason required. The cost of air ambulance ranges from a base charge of about $1,200 upward, and is usually based on an hourly rate.

When a person becomes ill while traveling, he or she may want to be transferred to a hospital near home or be treated by a specific specialist in another city, even though the city where he or she is presently located has qualified specialists in the field. In these instances, ambulance expenses are not covered, regardless of whether an air ambulance or a conventional ambulance is used. This is because the transportation is not considered "medically necessary."

Charges for commercial or private airplane transportation, regardless of the reason required, are usually not covered.

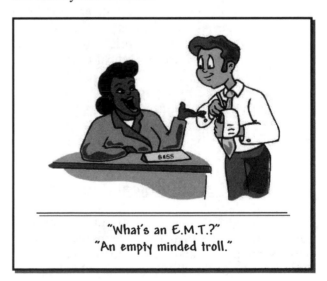

"What's an E.M.T.?"
"An empty minded troll."

Paramedics

Paramedics are specially trained emergency medical personnel who render emergency treatment at the scene of the injury or illness. They are trained in advanced life support, whereas **Emergency Medical Technicians (EMTs)** are trained in basic life support. There are significant differences in educational requirements and certification of a paramedic compared with those of an EMT. Consequently, when a paramedic is required, an additional fee is usually charged.

Paramedic fees may be covered under a Basic ambulance benefit or may be strictly allowable under Major Medical. The plan provisions should stipulate the handling of this expense.

Mobile Intensive Care Unit

A **mobile intensive care unit** is a life support vehicle equipped to provide care to critically ill patients who require transportation to a hospital or from one hospital to another. It is designed to serve as an extension of an intensive care unit at a hospital.

The staffing of this unit usually involves a registered nurse and several other allied health professionals. The fees are in the same range as that for an air ambulance. Such charges may be covered if they are determined to be medically necessary in lieu of regular ambulance services.

Van Transportation Unit

Many companies provide non-emergency transportation of the disabled to doctors' offices or hospital facilities. **Van transportation units** are specially equipped to handle wheelchairs and patients who are unable to get in and out of a regular vehicle. As a rule, it is required that the patient be able to sit in an upright position. The driver may have very basic medical training, such as cardiopulmonary resuscitation (CPR), but is generally not able or equipped to handle acute patients. This type of transportation is not covered by most plans because it is not considered medically necessary.

Medical and Surgical Supplies

Perishable medical and surgical supplies may be covered under the plan if the items can be used only by the patient and are medically necessary in the treatment of the illness or injury. Medical and surgical supplies include:

1. Disposable, nondurable supplies and accessories required to operate medical equipment or prosthetic devices.
2. Necessary drugs and biological items put directly into equipment (such as nonprescription nutrients).

3. Initial and replacement accessories essential for operating medical equipment.
4. Supplies furnished and charged by a hospital, surgical center, or physician as part of active therapy, such as ace bandage, cast, and cervical collar.

Examples of medical supply items include diabetes testing strips, catheters, syringes, ostomy pouch, etc.

Do not include items or supplies that could be used by the patient or a member of the patient's family for purposes other than medical care.

Miscellaneous and Experimental

This section is used to code services which are considered to be experimental or investigational in nature. These services are often not covered by insurance carriers.

Patients who receive these services should be informed ahead of time that the services may not be covered. They can then make an informed decision regarding their care.

If patients are involved in an investigational study (i.e., to study the effectiveness of a drug or procedure), their costs may be covered by the entity that is monitoring the study. In such cases, a separate patient chart should be kept so that the investigational charges are kept separate from other charges.

Enteral and Parenteral Therapy

Enteral therapy involves the administration of nutritional products directly into the intestines. A tube is inserted through the nasal passage into the stomach. This is used for patients who are unable to chew or swallow.

Parenteral therapy involves administering substances to a patient via a tube inserted into a vein. (i.e., medications or nutritional supplements). Nutrition may be given to patients whose digestive system cannot tolerate food.

This section of the HCPCS includes codes for both the equipment used to deliver the therapy, and the nutritional solutions themselves. When coding for these services, be sure to include all codes that apply to the given situation.

Temporary Hospital Outpatient PPS

The codes in this section are used to bill for services that are covered under the **Outpatient Prospective Payment System.** This system uses the **Ambulatory Payment Classifications (APCs)** to bill for outpatient hospital services. This payment classification system will be discussed in detail in the chapter for Hospital Billing.

APCs group several services together under one code. This code is then eligible for a lump sum payment. This payment covers all services provided by an outpatient facility. If the facility is able to treat the patient for less than this amount, they are allowed to keep the full amount. However, if the hospital provides goods and services that amount to more than the APC reimbursement, they must write off any extra amounts.

The codes in this section are temporary. Many of these codes will be added to the official list of APC codes within a year or two. By providing these temporary codes in the HCPCS book, facilities are able to bill for new procedures and services that have not yet been assigned an official APC code. However, it is important to remember that inclusion in the HCPCS manual does not necessarily mean that these services will be covered by Medicare or a private payor.

Dental Procedures

The codes included in this section are comparable with those included in the Current Dental Terminology (CDT) book released by the American Dental Association (ADA).

While most dental procedures are not covered by Medicare, there are times when a procedure may be covered. The reasons include:

- Accident,
- Dental treatment required as a result of a medical procedure, and
- Restorative.

Procedures

Some procedures performed on the mouth or teeth are covered under dental plans, but others may be covered under Major Medical plans. This holds true even though the services were performed by a dentist or an oral surgeon rather than an MD. These can include the following services:

1. Accidental injury to the teeth (see section on dental accidents).
2. Surgery to remove impacted, unerupted, or supernumerary teeth. Major Medical benefits are generally paid in the case of tissue-impacted, partly bone-impacted, or totally bone-impacted teeth.
3. Jawbone surgery.
4. Tumors or cysts within the oral cavity.
5. Nasal, auricular, orbital, or ocular prosthesis.
6. Obturators or repair of the cleft palate.
7. Complex, subperiosteal, or endosseous implants.
8. Lab charges such as urinalysis, hemoglobin, hematocrit, and complete blood count.
9. Repair of fractures of the mandible, maxilla, or facial bones.

If a specific service is covered under the Major Medical portion of the plan, then all related services (such as exams and x-rays) are also covered under the Major Medical plan.

1. **Emergency room benefits**. If emergency services are necessary and a dentist is not available, benefits may be allowable under the medical plan.
2. **Hospital and anesthesia benefits**. If hospital confinement is necessary for dental services, some plans allow Major Medical coverage for the hospital expense. Anesthesia expenses are usually covered for services that require hospitalization. Anesthesia charges are not usually covered for outpatient services. Hospital confinement may be necessary because of the severity of the condition or because of underlying factors. For example, if a patient has a history of hemophilia or unstable diabetes, because of the possible complications arising from the surgery, the hospital benefit is usually paid. When hospital benefits are covered under Major Medical, the physician's or dentist's fees are still covered under the dental plan.
3. **Oral-antral fistulas**. Oral-antral fistulas are unnatural openings between the oral and nasal cavities. If the opening occurs as a result of dental treatment (i.e., tooth

extraction where the root has penetrated the sinuses), then the services would be considered dental. However, if the opening is treated after a 6-week period, it may be considered a medical expense even though the cause was tooth-related. This occurs because the delayed closure is usually the result of disease or infection. If the fistula is not a result of a dental condition, the cause of the fistula should be indicated (i.e., tumor, disease). In such cases, Major Medical benefits usually cover the services.

4. **Gross misalignment of the jaws**. Often, pretreatment study models and an operative report should be requested to assist in the determination of coverage. If the surgery is a covered expense, it is often covered under both medical and dental plans. The claim usually needs to be referred to a supervisor or a medical review committee for determination of coverage.

5. **Other surgical services**. The following surgeries may be covered under dental or medical benefits, depending on the plan: reduction of fractures to the mandible or maxilla, tumors or cysts of the gums or mouth, alveolectomy (due to a non-dental condition), cleft palate or similar medical condition, and non-dental bone surgery.

6. **Cobalt therapy-related services**. Cobalt or x-ray therapy causes damage to the teeth and tissues of the oral cavity. Dental services that are necessary due to cobalt or x-ray therapy are generally covered as medical.

7. **Prescriptions and injections**. Prescriptions and injections that are generally covered for non-dental services are usually also covered when prescribed by a dentist or oral surgeon.

Occasionally, an orthodontic appliance (i.e., banding, braces) is used immediately before or after surgery. This appliance is often used as a splint. In this case, the appliance may be covered as medical. However, care must be taken to ensure that the appliance is being used for splinting purposes and not for orthodontic purposes. Appliances used for orthodontic purposes would not be covered unless specifically indicated by the contract.

If a dental service is covered under Major Medical, some payors convert the ADA codes into the appropriate CPT® or HCPCS codes and then apply the appropriate UCR conversion. The specific company and plan guidelines vary widely regarding Major Medical coverage for dental services and should be consulted prior to claim processing.

Dental Accidents

Many carriers cover accidental injury to permanent natural teeth under medical benefits. For the injury to qualify as an accident, you should be able to place the exact date, time, and place at which the accident occurred. However, damage due to chewing or biting is generally not considered accidental.

Under the provisions of most contracts, the teeth must be permanent natural teeth which were in place prior to the accident. Often dentures, partials, or "non-natural" teeth are excluded. In this case, if there was damage to the pontic and the adjoining abutment teeth, the abutment teeth would be covered but the pontic would not. However, if the teeth were evulsed (knocked out) as the result of an accident, fixed or removable prosthetics may be covered as "required to alleviate the damage." Likewise, deciduous teeth are often not covered since they are not permanent teeth.

Some plans may restrict payment to "sound" natural teeth. The term "sound" natural teeth defines teeth that are in good condition, without substantial restoration, fractures, cracks, extensive decay, or damage due to periodontal disease. The "good condition" clause applies to the crown of the tooth and also to the root structure and the supporting structures of the tooth.

Durable Medical Equipment

Durable medical equipment (DME) is an item that can be used for an extended period of time without significant deterioration (i.e., it can stand repeated use). Therefore, an item that can be rented and returned for re-use would meet the requirement for durability. Medical supplies of a disposable nature, such as incontinent pads and surgical stockings, would not qualify as durable.

Medically oriented equipment is primarily and customarily used for medical purposes (i.e., it is designed to fulfill a medical need). Therefore, it is generally not useful in the absence of an illness or injury. For example, an air conditioner may be used in the case of a heart patient to lower room temperature and reduce fluid loss. However, since the primary and customary use is nonmedical in nature, an air conditioner cannot be considered medical equipment. If the item could be used in a regular manner in the absence of a diagnosis, it is probably non-medical in nature.

DME Billing Procedures

Most plans allow for the purchase or temporary rental of equipment and supplies when prescribed by a physician. However, certain requirements must be satisfied.

Basically, three tests must be applied to items billed as DME in determining whether or not the items may be covered under a plan:

1. Does the item satisfy the definition of DME?
2. Is the item reasonable and necessary for the treatment of an illness or injury or for improvement of the functioning of a malformed body part?
3. Is the item prescribed for use in the patient's home?

Only when all three conditions are met will the item be covered by the plan.

An item may meet the definition of DME and yet not be covered by the plan. Two things to be considered are:

1. **Reasonableness**. This evaluates the soundness and practicality of the DME approach to therapy, including such factors as:
   a. Is the need for the unit based on failures of other less costly approaches?
   b. Have more conservative means been attempted?
   c. What benefits will be derived from the unit?
   d. Do the benefits justify the expense?
2. **Necessity**. Equipment is necessary when it is expected to make a meaningful contribution to the treatment of the patient's illness or injury or to the improvement of the functioning of a malformed body part.

For DME to be purchased or temporarily rented, the equipment must be prescribed for use in the home. Therefore, any facility that meets at least the minimum requirements of the definition of a hospital or skilled nursing facility is usually excluded from consideration.

A patient's home can be considered, but is not limited to:

- His or her own home, apartment, or dwelling,
- A relative's home,
- A home for the elderly, and
- A nursing home.

Oxygen

Many plans cover the use of oxygen under DME benefits. Even though the oxygen itself is not durable, the canister in which the oxygen is contained and transported is durable, and it therefore, falls under the category of DME.

Billing Requirements

All claims for DME should be documented with the following information:

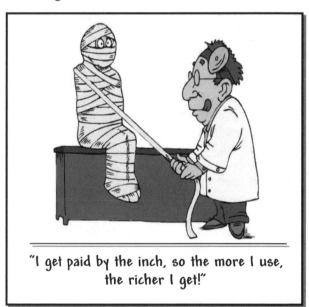

"I get paid by the inch, so the more I use, the richer I get!"

1. A description of the equipment prescribed by the physician. If the item is a commonly used item, a detailed description may not be necessary. However, with new equipment, it is important to try to obtain a marketing or manufacturer's brochure that indicates how the item is constructed and how it functions.
2. A statement of the medical necessity of the equipment. This should be in the form of a prescription showing the imprinted

name, address, and telephone number of the prescribing physician. The related diagnosis should also be indicated.

3. An indication as to whether the item is to be rented or purchased, and the rental or purchase price.

4. The estimated length of time that the equipment will be needed. This information will aid in the analysis of whether a rental or a purchase is more economical.

5. An indication as to where the equipment will be used and for how long.

Rental versus Purchasing Determinations

If the rental fee is greater than the purchase price, rental is allowed up to but not exceeding the purchase price. Purchase of the item is not required. However, the member should be notified that an expense that is higher than the purchase price may not be allowed.

Repairs, Replacement, and Delivery

Repairs are covered when necessary to make the equipment functional. If the expense for repairs exceeds the estimated cost of purchasing or renting new equipment for the remaining period of medical need, payment is limited to the lower amount.

Replacements are usually covered in cases of irreparable damage or wear or when the patient's physical condition has changed. Replacements due to wear or changes in the patient's physical condition must be supported by a current physician's order. Replacements due to loss may or may not be covered, depending on the circumstances. Usually, replacement is not covered when disrepair or loss results from a patient's carelessness.

Charges for delivery of the DME and oxygen are usually covered.

Procedures and Professional Services

The codes listed in this section are often temporary codes set up to identify professional services for which no corresponding CPT® code exists. These are often services which are covered by Medicare, but may or may not be covered by other insurance carriers. For example, flu shots for the elderly or those in need are covered by Medicare. However, most traditional insurance carriers consider these shots to be preventive medicine. If the plan does not

cover preventive medicine, flu shots may not be covered.

Many of these codes are deleted when a corresponding CPT® code is created. Thus, it is important to use the HCPCS book for the current year when coding these services.

Rehabilitative Services

The codes in this section identify rehabilitative services, such as alcohol or drug abuse treatment. These services are often covered under the mental/nervous portion of a health plan.

Many insurance carriers are recognizing the role that drug and alcohol abuse plays in affecting the health of the patient. For that reason, many carriers will reimburse for rehabilitative services. Additionally, many companies will cover the costs for these services if they feel it will help them to retain a good employee.

Many of these codes are specific to a certain type of facility. It is important to determine the type of facility providing the treatment before using the codes in this section.

Drugs Administered Other than Oral Method

This is one of the most frequently used sections when coding for Medicare patients. J codes indicate the type of drug being administered to a patient.

When coding drug usage, it is important to note the dosage amount contained in the code description. This amount is often a standard dosage amount, or portion of a dosage amount. Check the amount, actually administered to the patient. If the amount administered is twice the amount listed in the HCPCS code description, then list the code, but place a "2" in the unit's column to indicate that the dosage was doubled.

It is important to note the method by which the drug was administered. This section of the HCPCS book includes all drugs that are administered other than orally. That can include an injection, inhalation, suppository, insulin pump, etc. Each method of administration can have a different code. In order to properly code, you must take into account the drug used, the amount given, and the administration method.

Some drugs have both a brand name and a generic name. The generic name of the drug is the one listed in the HCPCS book. However, if a common brand name drug is often administered, the HCPCS will list the brand name in brackets [ ] directly behind the generic name of the drug. However, the index in most HCPCS books does not list the brand name of the drug, only the generic name. To locate the generic name for a brand name drug, consult the Physician's Desk Reference (PDR). (For more information on using the PDR, see the Medications and the PDR Chapter.)

While the drugs in this section are somewhat alphabetical, there are many drugs that will appear out of order. They may be in order of their brand name, since that is the name that was first applied to the drug when it first came out (and when the HCPCS code was first assigned). There may also be too many new drugs added to a given section. If no more code numbers are available, a number slightly out of alphabetical order may need to be assigned.

Some drugs also have additional information. These can include items such as the person doing the administration. For example: Code J0270 is for the injection of alprostadil, 1.25 mcg. However there is a note that the code may be used for Medicare when it is administered under the direct supervision of a physician. The code is not to be used for people who are self-administering the drug. For this reason it is important to read the full description included with a code. You should never code from the index alone.

Immunosuppressive Drugs

Immunosuppressive drugs included in this category are for the suppression of the immune system. These drugs may be administered orally.

Patients who have received a transplanted organ need to keep their immune system suppressed or their bodies will reject the new organ. There may also be additional reasons for administering immunosuppressive drugs.

Chemotherapy Drugs

Chemotherapy drugs are those drugs administered to help fight cancer and other serious diseases. These drugs have a toxic effect on the diseased cells (and often on other cells in the body).

The same guidelines regarding checking dosage, brand versus generic names, etc. apply to this section the same as they applied to the section for drugs administered other than orally.

Temporary Codes for DMERCs

This sections contains codes that were temporarily assigned for used by **Durable Medical Equipment Regional Carriers (DMERCs)**.

All Medicare DME claims should be submitted to one of four regional carriers. The proper regional carrier for the claim is dependent upon the residence of the beneficiary, not the point where the DME item was purchased. For a list of the DMERCs and the areas they serve, you can go to the Medicare website at www.medicare.gov. Because DME claims are sent to and processed by different carriers than regular services, it is important not to mix DME and services on the same claim.

These codes will often further define a piece of durable medical equipment that was ordered for a patient. For example, this section will list several additional types of wheelchairs and wheelchair attachments. The codes in this section are often deleted when no longer needed. This can be due to an additional code being created in the regular DME codes (E Codes), or from the equipment no longer being considered valid treatment for a given condition or situation.. These codes should only be used when you are instructed to do so by the DMERC in your area. Otherwise the closest regular DME codes should be used.

Since these codes are temporary, there are numerous changes to this listing every year. For that reason it is important to always use a current HCPCS manual when coding in this section.

Orthotic Procedures

Orthotics is devices used to correct a deformity or disability. They are also used to correct misalignment of the joints, especially the joints used for walking. Orthotics can be as small as a lift placed inside the shoe, or as large as a brace to correct curvature of the spine.

When billing for an orthotic device, you will need to include a copy of the prescription with the complete diagnosis. Some carriers may even require pictures to be taken to document the need for the device. Other carriers may request literature from the manufacturer of the device explaining how the device is used and the benefits to the patient.

Before billing for these items it is best to contact the insurance carrier and ask what their guidelines are. They can inform you of any documentation you will need to submit with the claim. Submitting the documentation at the same time you submit the claim can prevent a delay in processing.

Prosthetic Procedures

Prosthetic devices are designed to replace a missing body part or to restore some function to a paralyzed body part.

Prosthetic devices include the making and application of an artificial part medically necessary to replace a lost or impaired body part or function, such as an artificial arm or leg.

Prosthetics are intended to replace body parts that are permanently damaged. Many carriers will accept the provider's decision that the body part needs to be replaced. If the judgment of the attending physician is that the condition is of long and/or indefinite duration, the test of permanence is met.

Covered expenses associated with prosthetics include:

- Shipping and handling as part of the purchase price,
- Temporary post-operative prostheses, and
- Replacement charges when replacement is due to a change in the patient's physical condition. (Children often need replacement prostheses every 6 to 12 months depending on their growth rate and other factors.) Replacement is not covered for wear and tear.

Medical Services

This section contains very few codes, and most of the included codes are not covered by Medicare or other providers. The reason this section is so small is that most procedures that would be listed here are already listed in the CPT®. Thus, the CPT® would be the main coding manual for these medical services.

Often, the codes that are included in this section are considered new or experimental.

The modifiers included in this section will often designate the type of provider involved. This can include psychologists, clinical social workers, etc.

Pathology/Laboratory

The codes in this section are for pathology and laboratory tests. Many of these codes are not listed in the CPT®.

Some of the codes in this section are for the testing of blood or blood parts (i.e., plasma, platelets), to insure that it is free of disease before being transfused into a patient. There are also codes for the separation of blood into the various specific components that a patient might need.

A few of the tests in this section (i.e., pap smears), can be split into the technical component (the person or facility taking the test or drawing the blood), and the professional component (the person interpreting the test results). If the provider performs the test, but does not interpret the results, it is important to use the modifier –TC.

Temporary Codes

This section is used for creating temporary codes. This list will contain codes that are current, as well as codes that have been superceded by a permanent HCPCS code. Some codes will be superceded by a CPT® code that has been added to the CPT®.

This section includes many different types of procedures and services. Many of these codes pertain to new drugs that have been added to the markct. Thcrc may also bc codes that break an existing code into more specifics (i.e., casting procedures may be broken into the area being cast, the type of cast, and/or the age of the patient involved).

As with the other temporary code sections, the items in this section will be changed frequently, so it is important to use the current HCPCS manual when coding.

Diagnostic Radiology Services

This short section is for recording transportation of x-ray or EKG equipment to a nursing home or other facility. In situations where there is more than one patient to be seen, or where the patient is too fragile to be moved, it is easier to transport the equipment to the patient.

Private Payer Codes

These codes are temporary national codes that have been created by private payors. The codes in this section include drugs, procedures, DME, and numerous other items and services.

There are also numerous codes for indicating services provided in the home. These codes are not valid on most claims, and are not accepted by Medicare. Before using these codes, consult the payor. Many private payors will not accept claims that use these codes.

State Medicaid Agency Codes

The codes in this section were added to the HCPCS book in 2002 to meet the needs of state Medicaid agencies. They often deal with services that are covered by Medicaid, but not by Medicare or many private payors.

The codes included in this section involve services for home care, education, drug or alcohol treatment, or mental/nervous services.

Before using these codes, check with your state Medicaid carrier. Not all states consider these codes to be acceptable for reporting services.

Vision Services

The codes in this section are used to report services performed on or pertaining to the eyes. These can include eyeglasses, contacts, prosthetic eyes, lenses or other items pertaining to the care and use of the eyes or eyeglasses.

The codes in this section can be very specific regarding the type of lenses used in the glasses and other factors. Because of this, special training may be needed to code these services properly.

Any devices ordered in this section must have a prescription written by an authorized provider. A copy of this prescription should be submitted with the claim. Medicare provides coverage for some of these services, though not all.

Hearing Services

The codes in this section are used for reporting services in regards to hearing. This includes hearing testing, as well as devices used to assist those who are hearing impaired (i.e., hearing aids). Other assistive living devices (i.e., telephone amplifier, television caption decoder) are also included in this section. There are also codes for speech-language services such as speech screening.

Any devices ordered in this section must have a prescription written by an authorized provider. A copy of this prescription should be submitted with the claim.

Modifiers

Each section of the HCPCS manual has modifiers that are unique to that section. It is important that medical billers check the modifiers for each section before billing a claim. Without the proper modifiers, claim payment may be delayed or denied. This is especially true in the case of Medicare claims. Not including the appropriate modifier can also cause incorrect reimbursement.

Modifiers in the HCPCS manual are usually two digit letter codes. In some cases, two separate one digit letter codes will be combined to make up a single two digit letter code. For example, in the transportation services section, the first letter indicates where the patient was picked up from and the second letter indicates where the patient was delivered to.

Summary

The HCPCS manual provides additional codes to be used when billing Medicare, or to bill for services or items for which no current CPT® code exists.

The HCPCS includes numerous sections for coding transportation services, dental procedures, vision and hearing services, to name a few.

There are three levels of HCPCS coding
1. Level 1: Contains only the CPT® codes and modifiers.
2. Level 2: Includes the codes found in sections A through V of the HCPCS book.
3. Level 3: Contains codes local to the individual Medicare carrier and are not found in the first two levels. These codes are found in sections W through Z in the HCPCS book.

Assignments

Complete the Questions for Review.
Complete Exercises 18 – 1 through 18 – 2.

Questions for Review

Directions: Answer the following questions without looking back into the material just covered. Write your answers in the space provided.

1. What is the HCPCS book used for? _____

   _____

2. What are the three coding levels of HCPCS?

   1. _____

      _____

   2. _____

      _____

   3. _____

      _____

3. What can happen if you continually use the wrong modifiers when coding Medicare claims?_____

   _____

4. What are the three tests that are applied to DME items to determine if they will be covered under a plan?
   1. _____

      _____

   2. _____

      _____

   3. _____

      _____

5. What is a DMERC? _____

   _____

If you were unable to answer any of the questions, refer back to that section, and then fill in the answers.

Exercise 18 – 1

Directions: Determine the correct HCPCS codes for the following procedures/items.

1. Moisture exchanger, disposable, for use with invasive mechanical ventilation.   1. _____

2. Detailed and extensive oral evaluation - problem focused.   2. _____

3. Application of desensitizing medicaments.   3. _____

4. Injection of calcium gluconate, per 10ml.   4. _____

5. LSO, lumbar flexion (Williams flexion type).   5. _____

6. Cellular therapy.   6. _____

7. Stomach tube-levine type.   7. _____

8. Routine venipuncture for collection of specimen.   8. _____

9. Jaw motion rehabilitation system.   9. _____

10. Dialysis equipment, unspecified.   10. _____

11. Replace quadrilateral socket brim; molded to patient model.   11. _____

12. Cardiokymography.   12. _____

13. Lenticular, nonaspheric, per lens, bifocal.   13. _____

14. Speech screening.   14. _____

15. Platform attachment; forearm crutch.   15. _____

16. Bone replacement graft, first site.   16. _____

17. Collagen skin test kit.   17. _____

18. Injection, tetracycline, 200 mg.   18. _____

19. Ambulatory surgical boot.   19. _____

20. Prosthetic implant.   20. _____

21. Potassium hydroxide (Koh) preparation.   21. _____

22. Transportation of portable EKG to nursing home.   22. _____

23. Infusion of normal saline solution, 250cc.   23. _____

24. Botulinum toxin type A, 2 units.   24. _____

25. Orthodontic treatment (non-contract fee).   25. _____

26. House call.   26. _____

27. Rollabout chair, 6 inch casters.   27. _____

28. Dialysis blood leak detector.   28. _____

29. Imiglucerase injection.   29. _____

30. Mens orthopedic oxford shoes.   30. _____

Exercise 18 – 2

Directions: Determine the correct HCPCS codes for the following procedures/items.

1. Synthetic vascular graft material implant.   1. _____
2. Artificial larynx, BV type.   2. _____
3. Thoracic low profile extension, lateral.   3. _____
4. Azithromycin dihydrate capsules, 1 gm.   4. _____
5. Infusion chemo treatment.   5. _____
6. Triam A injection, 10mg.   6. _____
7. Sterile syringe, 30cc.   7. _____
8. Amalgam, 2 surfaces, primary.   8. _____
9. Tigan Injection, 100 mg.   9. _____
10. UV cabinet, home use.   10. _____
11. Ampicillin sodium injection, 400 mg.   11. _____
12. Dexasone LA injection.   12. _____
13. Assessment for hearing aid.   13. _____
14. Epoetin alpha injection, 1500 units, (non ESRD)   14. _____
15. Low pressure equalization wheelchair pad.   15. _____
16. Cortisone injection, 50 mg.   16. _____
17. Cervical collar molded to patient.   17. _____
18. Celestone soluspan, 3 mg.   18. _____
19. Non-elastic binder for extremity.   19. _____
20. Canal preparation and fitting.   20. _____
21. Pediatric speech aid.   21. _____
22. Fresh, frozen plasma.   22. _____
23. Preparation of vaginal wet mount.   23. _____
24. Gas impermeable contact lens.   24. _____
25. Reverse osmosis water purifyer.   25. _____
26. Reimplantation of tooth.   26. _____
27. Tylenol, non-prescription.   27. _____
28. Duoval PA   28. _____
29. Addition to prosthetic sheath, air seal suction system.   29. _____
30. Insulin injection, 100 units.   30. _____

Honors Certification™

The certification challenge for this chapter will be a written test of the information contained in this chapter. Each incorrect answer will result in a deduction of up to 5% from your grade. You must achieve a score of 85% or higher to pass this test. If you fail the test on your first attempt you may retake the test one additional time. The items included in the second test may be different from those in the first test.

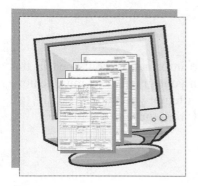

19

Medications and the PDR

After completion of this chapter you will be able to:

- Determine if a pharmaceutical is a prescription or a non prescription drug.
- List the sections of the *Physicians' Desk Reference* and the information each section contains.
- Properly use the *Physicians' Desk Reference*.

Key words and concepts you will learn in this chapter:

Controlled Drugs – Drugs that are more tightly controlled by federal mandates due to their addictive, experimental, toxic, or other highly volatile properties. There are four classifications ranging from the least controlled to the most controlled.

Legend Drug – A drug requiring a prescription. The "legend" always appears on the label.

Medications – Drugs used to treat diseases, symptoms, or discomforts.

Nonlegend Drug – A drug that does not require a prescription.

Over-the-Counter Drug (OTC) – A drug that may be purchased without a prescription. Also known as a nonlegend drug.

Pharmaceuticals – Drugs.

Prescription Legend – A label inscribed as follows: "Caution: Federal (United States) law prohibits dispensing without a prescription."

Proprietary Drug – A drug that is patented or controlled by a manufacturer. The manufacturer copyrights the trade or brand name. This is not the same as the generic name, which identifies the drug's chemical composition.

Medications are drugs (often called **pharmaceuticals**) used to treat diseases, symptoms, or discomforts (i.e., pain medications). Prescription medications are usually covered under benefit plans in one of two ways: (1) under a separate, free-standing plan for outpatient, prescription medicines only, or (2) under Major Medical as any other eligible expense, subject to all applicable deductibles, copayments, limitations, and exclusions.

Generic vs. Brand Name Drugs

When a pharmaceutical company develops a drug, they can file for and may receive patent protection for that particular drug. This allows the pharmaceutical company to exclusively manufacture that drug for a period of time. After that time, any company may manufacture the drug.

A pharmaceutical manufacturer bears the cost of all research, development and testing of a new drug. Therefore, they must recoup the costs of that research and development, as well as, hopefully, make a profit on their work within that time period. Other companies which begin manufacturing the drug after the time period expires do not have the research and development costs associated with the drug. Therefore, they can produce an equivalent drug for a lot less money. These drugs produced by other manufacturers are called **generic drugs**.

When making a generic drug, the manufacturer must provide appropriate safety data to the Food and Drug Administration (FDA). This data includes sufficient proof that the generic product has the identical active ingredient(s) and is as effective as the brand name drug in all aspects. When the generic drug meets these requirements, it is considered "therapeutically equivalent."

Some generic drugs are not the same as their brand name counterparts. They may contain a similar, but different active ingredient, or they may be for a different dosage amount than the brand name drug. In such a case they are not considered to be therapeutically equivalent. For these drugs, an insurance carrier may require the physician to prescribe the generic drug to be covered by a prescription benefit, or they may allow the full benefit for the brand name drug.

Most manufacturers of generic drugs also make brand name drugs. In fact, 70% to 80% of all generic drugs are made by the same manufacturers that make the brand name drugs. The profit made on the generic drugs helps to offset some of the research and development costs of other brand name drugs.

Service Plans

Separate prescription service plans are usually handled by third-party administrative (TPA) organizations, which establish networks of participating pharmacies and then assume responsibility for the claims processing. Such plans usually include some if not all of the following components:

1. The claimant is not required to pay for his or her prescription with a large cash outlay. Instead, a small specified copayment amount, chosen by the group, is paid by the claimant for each prescription (copayments usually range from $2 to $15).
2. The pharmacy accepts an identification card as evidence that payment will be made by the plan; it then bills the plan for the unpaid balance.
3. A claim form is not required from the cardholder. The pharmacy bills the TPA directly.
4. The member is required to go to a participating pharmacy to fill prescriptions. Otherwise, the claimant will be responsible for full payment of the medication, or a reduced percentage may be paid by the TPA. In this case, the claimant would have to submit the prescription to the TPA for payment consideration.
5. Each prescription filled will provide a supply for a specified number of days – usually a 30-day maximum.

Prescription service plans typically exclude the following types of expenses:

1. Devices or medical/surgical supplies of any type such as bandages, gauze, etc.. Hypodermic needles and syringes may be covered for diabetics.
2. Contraceptive drugs, even though the medication may have been prescribed for other than contraceptive purposes.
3. Drugs dispensed while the member is confined in a facility, including those given on the day of discharge.
4. Immunization agents, biological sera, blood, plasma, or other blood agents.
5. Investigational or experimental drugs.
6. Health foods, food supplements, vitamins, and appetite suppressants.

As with most other plan provisions, the covered and excluded charges vary from plan to plan. Therefore, the benefits should be verified.

Physicians' Desk Reference

The **Physicians' Desk Reference (PDR)** is published annually with supplements published as necessary during the year. The manual comprises the following sections:

Manufacturer's Index (white) – arranged alphabetically by manufacturer, then by drug name. The name and address of the manufacturer are included. This section includes prescription and nonprescription drugs.

Product Name Index (pink) – arranged alphabetically by brand name or generic name (if provided). Prescription and nonprescription drugs are included. This section is usually used first to locate the manufacturers name and the page number for further information.

Product Category Index (blue) – arranged alphabetically by drug action category, that is, according to the most common use of the drug. If the drug is an antidepressant, it is listed under the antidepressant category; and if it is an antacid, it is listed under the antacid category.

Product Identification Section (gray) – arranged alphabetically by manufacturer; then by brand name. This section contains the actual size and full-color reproductions. Only the reproductions submitted by the manufacturer are included.

Product Information Section (white) – arranged alphabetically by manufacturer, then by brand name. Most pharmaceuticals are described by indications and usage, dosage, administration, description, clinical pharmacology, supply warnings, contraindications, adverse reactions, overdosage precautions and other miscellaneous information.

Diagnostic Product Information (green) – arranged alphabetically by manufacturer, then by product. This section provides a description of diagnostic products only.

Medical billers use the Product Information Section (white) the most. However, since generic drugs are less expensive than brand name medications, many plans encourage their members to purchase generically and offer increased payment incentives. Therefore, use of the Product Name Index (which includes both brand name and generic names) is increasing. For instance, instead of paying for generic drugs at the plan's regular coinsurance rate of 80%, 100% may be payable. As with all benefits, this varies widely by plan.

Definitions

Controlled Drugs – Drugs that are more tightly controlled by federal mandates due to their addictive, experimental, toxic, or other highly volatile properties. In this group, four classifications range from the least controlled to the most controlled. Even the least controlled of the Controlled Drugs is more highly regulated than regular prescription medications.

Legend Drug – A drug requiring a prescription. The "legend" always appears on the label

Legend, Prescription – The pharmaceutical manufacturer's warning on the label: "Caution: Federal (United States) law prohibits dispensing without a prescription."

Nonlegend Drug – A drug not requiring a prescription.

Over-the-Counter Drug (OTC) – A drug that may be purchased without a prescription. Also known as a nonlegend drug.

Proprietary Drug – A drug that is patented or controlled by a manufacturer. The manufacturer copyrights the trade or brand name. This is not the same as the generic name, which identifies the drug's chemical composition.

Symbols

The following symbols appear in the various sections of the PDR, usually to the right side of the drug name. If nothing appears to the right, the drug is not a legend medication.

OTC – This is an over-the-counter drug. A prescription is not required and it is usually not covered under benefit plans.

Rx – Prescription required for purchase.

CI-CIV – Controlled substance. Prescription always required.

O – Identi-Code symbol. It is a manufacturer's identification code. This symbol does not indicate whether or not a prescription is required. It is placed directly on the medicine (if in pill form).

TM – Registered Trademark.

These symbols should be checked carefully as they can affect the payment of a claim.

Summary

Medications are drugs used to treat diseases, symptoms, or discomforts. The two ways in which coverage is provided for the payment of drugs is under a service plan and under a Major Medical plan. However, drugs that do not require a prescription (over-the-counter drugs) are generally not covered by either plan.

The Physicians' Desk Reference (PDR) can be used to determine whether or not a drug is a prescription drug. In addition, the PDR lists drug manufacturers, product names, product categories, product identification (pictures), specific product information, and diagnostic product information.

Assignments

Complete the Questions for Review.
Complete Exercises 19 – 1 through 19 – 3.

Questions for Review

Directions: Answer the following questions without looking back into the material just covered. Write your answers in the space provided.

1. What are medications? _____

2. Explain what the difference is between a legend and a non-legend drug. _____

   _____

3. Name the six sections of the PDR.

   1._____

   2._____

   3._____

   4._____

   5._____

   6._____

4. (True or False?) Controlled drugs can be purchased over the counter. _____

5. What does Rx stand for? _____

   _____

If you were unable to answer any of the questions, refer back to that section, and then fill in the answers.

Exercise 19 – 1

Directions: Look up the following medications in the PDR. Indicate in the space provided whether or not the drug is prescription by writing in the status symbol. Also, indicate the trade name if the generic name is given; indicate the generic name if the trade name is given. The manufacturer's name is indicated in parenthesis.

	Name	**Symbol**
1. Fluorouracil Cream (Roche)		
2. Proventil (Schering)	NA	
3. Spectazole (Ortho-McNeil)		
4. Fenfluramine Hydrochloride (Robins)		
5. Valium Injectable (Roche)		
6. Klonpin (Roche)		
7. Psyllium Husk Fiber (Proctor & Gamble)		
8. Metaproterenol Sulfate (Boehringer Ingelheim)		
9. Pentazocine Hydrochloride and Acetominophen (Winthrop)		
10. Flonase (Glaxo-Smith-Kline)		
11. Dilantin Injection Parenteral (Parke-Davis)		
12. Sotradecol Injection (Elkins-Sinn)		
13. Aldomet Tablets (Merck)		
14. Mandol (Lilly)		
15. Viagra (Pfizer)		

Exercise 19 – 2

Directions: Write at least one diagnosis that the indicated medication is normally used to treat.

1. Atromid

2. Inderal LA

3. Quibron

4. Ortho-Novum

5. Pro-Banthine Tablets

6. Sus-Phrine Injection

7. Tofranil Tablets

8. Lanoxin Injection

9. Diethylstilbestrol

10. Parafon Forte

Exercise 19 – 3

Directions: List the manufacturer of the following medications as listed in the PDR.

Medication	Manufacturer
1. Xylocaine 2% Jelly	
2. Decadron Tablets	
3. Ganite	
4. Flagyl Capsules	
5. Capoten Tablets	
6. Similac	
7. K-Lor Powder Packets	
8. Bactrim Pediatric Suspension	
9. Wytensin Tablets	
10. Hytrin Capsules	
11. Jevity	
12. Tenex Tablets	
13. Lidocaine 5% Ointment	
14. Sudafed 12 Hour Capsules	
15. Zantac 150 and 300 Tablets	

Honors Certification™

The certification challenge for this chapter will be a written test of the information contained in this chapter. Each incorrect answer will result in a deduction of up to 5% from your grade. You must achieve a score of 85% or higher to pass this test. If you fail the test on your first attempt you may retake the test one additional time. The items included in the second test may be different from those in the first test.

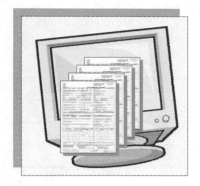

20

CMS - 1500

After completion of this chapter you will be able to:

- Properly complete the CMS-1500 claim form.
- Gain speed and accuracy in completing the CMS -1500 claim.

Key words and concepts you will learn in this chapter:

CMS-1500 Claim Form – A standardized form for use as a "universal" form for billing professional services.

Place of Service Code – A numerical code to indicate the place where the service was rendered.

The CMS-1500 claim form is a standardized form approved by the American Medical Association for use as a "universal" form for billing professional services **(see Figure 20 – 1 and 20 – 2).** This is the only form acceptable for billing Medicare and Medicaid programs for physician's services and/or medical supplies (the UB-92 is allowed for use when billing hospital services).

The following listing will assist in explaining the uses of the various items. It contains the item number along with the name of the item and a brief description of the information needed. The word "same" refers to a description that is the same as the title of the box.

The various sections of the CMS-1500 include information categorized as follows: patient, insured, secondary insurance, third party liability, authorization signature, illness, procedures performed, and provider of services.

Item # and Item Name/Description

Following are the numbers, titles and descriptions of the items found on the CMS-1500.

Information About the Patient
These boxes contain information about the patient.

1 **Medicare, Medicaid, TRICARE (CHAMPUS), CHAMPVA, FECA Black Lung or Other.** Check the box of the organization to which you are submitting this claim for payment if you are submitting the form to one of those organizations listed.
2 **Patient's Name.** Same.
3 **Patient's Birth Date and Sex.** All dates should be recorded as Month/Day/Year. Check the box for the appropriate sex.
5 **Patient's Address and Phone Number.** Same.
6 **Patient's Relationship to Insured.** Same.
8 **Patient's Status.** Check applicable boxes.

PLEASE
DO NOT
STAPLE
IN THIS
AREA

CARRIER

| | PICA | | | HEALTH INSURANCE CLAIM FORM | PICA | | |

1. MEDICARE   MEDICAID   CHAMPUS   CHAMPVA   GROUP HEALTH PLAN   FECA BLK LUNG   OTHER   1a. INSURED'S I.D. NUMBER   (FOR PROGRAM IN ITEM 1)
(Medicare #) (Medicaid #) (Sponsor's SSN) (VA File #) (SSN or ID) (SSN) (ID)

2. PATIENT'S NAME (Last Name, First Name, Middle Initial)

3. PATIENT'S BIRTH DATE   MM | DD | YY   SEX   M   F

4. INSURED'S NAME (Last Name, First Name, Middle Initial)

5. PATIENT'S ADDRESS (No., Street)

6. PATIENT RELATIONSHIP TO INSURED   Self   Spouse   Child   Other

7. INSURED'S ADDRESS (No., Street)

CITY   STATE

8. PATIENT STATUS   Single   Married   Other

CITY   STATE

ZIP CODE   TELEPHONE (Include Area Code)

Employed   Full-Time Student   Part-Time Student

ZIP CODE   TELEPHONE (INCLUDE AREA CODE)

9. OTHER INSURED'S NAME (Last Name, First Name, Middle Initial)

10. IS PATIENT'S CONDITION RELATED TO:

11. INSURED'S POLICY GROUP OR FECA NUMBER

a. OTHER INSURED'S POLICY OR GROUP NUMBER

a. EMPLOYMENT? (CURRENT OR PREVIOUS)   YES   NO

a. INSURED'S DATE OF BIRTH   MM | DD | YY   SEX   M   F

b. OTHER INSURED'S DATE OF BIRTH   MM | DD | YY   SEX   M   F

b. AUTO ACCIDENT?   PLACE (State)   YES   NO

b. EMPLOYER'S NAME OR SCHOOL NAME

c. EMPLOYER'S NAME OR SCHOOL NAME

c. OTHER ACCIDENT?   YES   NO

c. INSURANCE PLAN NAME OR PROGRAM NAME

d. INSURANCE PLAN NAME OR PROGRAM NAME

10d. RESERVED FOR LOCAL USE

d. IS THERE ANOTHER HEALTH BENEFIT PLAN?   YES   NO   If yes, return to and complete item 9 a-d.

READ BACK OF FORM BEFORE COMPLETING & SIGNING THIS FORM.

12. PATIENT'S OR AUTHORIZED PERSON'S SIGNATURE I authorize the release of any medical or other information necessary to process this claim. I also request payment of government benefits either to myself or to the party who accepts assignment below.

SIGNED _____   DATE _____

13. INSURED'S OR AUTHORIZED PERSON'S SIGNATURE I authorize payment of medical benefits to the undersigned physician or supplier for services described below.

SIGNED _____

PATIENT AND INSURED INFORMATION

14. DATE OF CURRENT: MM | DD | YY   ILLNESS (First symptom) OR INJURY (Accident) OR PREGNANCY(LMP)

15. IF PATIENT HAS HAD SAME OR SIMILAR ILLNESS. GIVE FIRST DATE   MM | DD | YY

16. DATES PATIENT UNABLE TO WORK IN CURRENT OCCUPATION   MM | DD | YY FROM   TO   MM | DD | YY

17. NAME OF REFERRING PHYSICIAN OR OTHER SOURCE

17a. I.D. NUMBER OF REFERRING PHYSICIAN

18. HOSPITALIZATION DATES RELATED TO CURRENT SERVICES   MM | DD | YY FROM   TO   MM | DD | YY

19. RESERVED FOR LOCAL USE

20. OUTSIDE LAB?   YES   NO $ CHARGES

21. DIAGNOSIS OR NATURE OF ILLNESS OR INJURY. (RELATE ITEMS 1,2,3 OR 4 TO ITEM 24E BY LINE)

1. ____ . ____   3. ____ . ____

2. ____ . ____   4. ____ . ____

22. MEDICAID RESUBMISSION CODE   ORIGINAL REF. NO.

23. PRIOR AUTHORIZATION NUMBER

24. A DATE(S) OF SERVICE						B Place of Service	C Type of Service	D PROCEDURES, SERVICES, OR SUPPLIES (Explain Unusual Circumstances) CPT/HCPCS MODIFIER	E DIAGNOSIS CODE	F $ CHARGES	G DAYS OR UNITS	H EPSDT Family Plan	I EMG	J COB	K RESERVED FOR LOCAL USE
From MM	DD	YY	To MM	DD	YY											
1															
2															
3															
4															
5															
6															

25. FEDERAL TAX I.D. NUMBER   SSN   EIN

26. PATIENT'S ACCOUNT NO.

27. ACCEPT ASSIGNMENT? (For govt. claims, see back)   YES   NO

28. TOTAL CHARGE $0.00

29. AMOUNT PAID

30. BALANCE DUE $0.00

31. SIGNATURE OF PHYSICIAN OR SUPPLIER INCLUDING DEGREES OR CREDENTIALS (I certify that the statements on the reverse apply to this bill and are made a part thereof.)

32. NAME AND ADDRESS OF FACILITY WHERE SERVICES WERE RENDERED (if other than home or office)

33. PHYSICIAN'S, SUPPLIER'S BILLING NAME, ADDRESS, ZIP CODE & PHONE #

SIGNED _____   DATE _____

PIN#   GRP#

PHYSICIAN OR SUPPLIER INFORMATION

(APPROVED BY AMA COUNCIL ON MEDICAL SERVICE 8/88)   PLEASE PRINT OR TYPE   APPROVED OMB-0938-0008 FORM CMS-1500 (12-90),   FORM RRB-1500, APPROVED OMB-1215-0055 FORM OWCP-1500,   APPROVED OMB-0720-0001 (CHAMPUS)

Figure 20 – 1: Front of the CMS-1500 Claim Form

BECAUSE THIS FORM IS USED BY VARIOUS GOVERNMENT AND PRIVATE HEALTH PROGRAMS, SEE SEPARATE INSTRUCTIONS ISSUED BY APPLICABLE PROGRAMS.

NOTICE: Any person who knowingly files a statement of claim containing any misrepresentation or any false, incomplete or misleading information may be guilty of a criminal act punishable under law and may be subject to civil penalties.

REFERS TO GOVERNMENT PROGRAMS ONLY

MEDICARE AND CHAMPUS PAYMENTS: A patient's signature requests that payment be made and authorizes release of any information necessary to process the claim and certifies that the information provided in Blocks 1 through 12 is true, accurate and complete. In the case of a Medicare claim, the patient's signature authorizes any entity to release to Medicare medical and nonmedical information, including employment status, and whether the person has employer group health insurance, liability, no-fault, worker's compensation or other insurance which is responsible to pay for the services for which the Medicare claim is made. See 42 CFR 411.24(a). If item 9 is completed, the patient's signature authorizes release of the information to the health plan or agency shown. In Medicare assigned or CHAMPUS participation cases, the physician agrees to accept the charge determination of the Medicare carrier or CHAMPUS fiscal intermediary as the full charge, and the patient is responsible only for the deductible, coinsurance and noncovered services. Coinsurance and the deductible are based upon the charge determination of the Medicare carrier or CHAMPUS fiscal intermediary if this is less than the charge submitted. CHAMPUS is not a health insurance program but makes payment for health benefits provided through certain affiliations with the Uniformed Services. Information on the patient's sponsor should be provided in those items captioned in "Insured"; i.e., items 1a, 4, 6, 7, 9, and 11.

BLACK LUNG AND FECA CLAIMS

The provider agrees to accept the amount paid by the Government as payment in full. See Black Lung and FECA instructions regarding required procedure and diagnosis coding systems.

SIGNATURE OF PHYSICIAN OR SUPPLIER (MEDICARE, CHAMPUS, FECA AND BLACK LUNG)

I certify that the services shown on this form were medically indicated and necessary for the health of the patient and were personally furnished by me or were furnished incident to my professional service by my employee under my immediate personal supervision, except as otherwise expressly permitted by Medicare or CHAMPUS regulations.

For services to be considered as "incident" to a physician's professional service, 1) they must be rendered under the physician's immediate personal supervision by his/her employee, 2) they must be an integral, although incidental part of a covered physician's service, 3) they must be of kinds commonly furnished in physician's offices, and 4) the services of nonphysicians must be included on the physician's bills.

For CHAMPUS claims, I further certify that I (or any employee) who rendered services am not an active duty member of the Uniformed Services or a civilian employee of the United States Government or a contract employee of the United States Government, either civilian or military (refer to 5 USC 5536). For Black-Lung claims, I further certify that the services performed were for a Black Lung-related disorder.

No Part B Medicare benefits may be paid unless this form is received as required by existing law and regulations (42 CFR 424.32).

NOTICE: Any one who misrepresents or falsifies essential information to receive payment from Federal funds requested by this form may upon conviction be subject to fine and imprisonment under applicable Federal laws.

NOTICE TO PATIENT ABOUT THE COLLECTION AND USE OF MEDICARE, CHAMPUS, FECA, AND BLACK LUNG INFORMATION
(PRIVACY ACT STATEMENT)

We are authorized by CMS, CHAMPUS and OWCP to ask you for information needed in the administration of the Medicare, CHAMPUS, FECA, and Black Lung programs. Authority to collect information is in section 205(a), 1862, 1872 and 1874 of the Social Security Act as amended, 42 CFR 411.24(a) and 424.5(a) (6), and 44 USC 3101;41 CFR 101 et seq and 10 USC 1079 and 1086; 5 USC 8101 et seq; and 30 USC 901 et seq; 38 USC 613; E.O. 9397.

The information we obtain to complete claims under these programs is used to identify you and to determine your eligibility. It is also used to decide if the services and supplies you received are covered by these programs and to insure that proper payment is made.

The information may also be given to other providers of services, carriers, intermediaries, medical review boards, health plans, and other organizations or Federal agencies, for the effective administration of Federal provisions that require other third parties payers to pay primary to Federal program, and as otherwise necessary to administer these programs. For example, it may be necessary to disclose information about the benefits you have used to a hospital or doctor. Additional disclosures are made through routine uses for information contained in systems of records.

FOR MEDICARE CLAIMS: See the notice modifying system No. 09-70-0501, titled, 'Carrier Medicare Claims Record,' published in the *Federal Register*, Vol. 55 No. 177, page 37549, Wed. Sept. 12, 1990, or as updated and republished.

FOR OWCP CLAIMS: Department of Labor, Privacy Act of 1974, "Republication of Notice of Systems of Records," *Federal Register* Vol. 55 No. 40, Wed Feb. 28, 1990, See ESA-5, ESA-6, ESA-12, ESA-13, ESA-30, or as updated and republished.

FOR CHAMPUS CLAIMS: PRINCIPLE PURPOSE(S): To evaluate eligibility for medical care provided by civilian sources and to issue payment upon establishment of eligibility and determination that the services/supplies received are authorized by law.

ROUTINE USE(S): Information from claims and related documents may be given to the Dept. of Veterans Affairs, the Dept. of Health and Human Services and/or the Dept. of Transportation consistent with their statutory administrative responsibilities under CHAMPUS/CHAMPVA; to the Dept. of Justice for representation of the Secretary of Defense in civil actions; to the Internal Revenue Service, private collection agencies, and consumer reporting agencies in connection with recoupment claims; and to Congressional Offices in response to inquiries made at the request of the person to whom a record pertains. Appropriate disclosures may be made to other federal, state, local, foreign government agencies, private business entities, and individual providers of care, on matters relating to entitlement, claims adjudication, fraud, program abuse, utilization review, quality assurance, peer review, program integrity, third-party liability, coordination of benefits, and civil and criminal litigation related to the operation of CHAMPUS.

DISCLOSURES: Voluntary; however, failure to provide information will result in delay in payment or may result in denial of claim. With the one exception discussed below, there are no penalties under these programs for refusing to supply information. However, failure to furnish information regarding the medical services rendered or the amount charged would prevent payment of claims under these programs. Failure to furnish any other information, such as name or claim number, would delay payment of the claim. Failure to provide medical information under FECA could be deemed an obstruction.

It is mandatory that you tell us if you know that another party is responsible for paying for your treatment. Section 1128B of the Social Security Act and 31 USC 3801-3812 provide penalties for withholding this information.

You should be aware that P.L. 100-503, the "Computer Matching and Privacy Protection Act of 1988", permits the government to verify information by way of computer matches.

MEDICAID PAYMENTS (PROVIDER CERTIFICATION)

I hereby agree to keep such records as are necessary to disclose fully the extent of services provided to individuals under the State's Title XIX plan and to furnish information regarding any payments claimed for providing such services as the State Agency or Dept. of Health and Humans Services may request.

I further agree to accept, as payment in full, the amount paid by the Medicaid program for those claims submitted for payment under that program, with the exception of authorized deductible, coinsurance, co-payment or similar cost-sharing charge.

SIGNATURE OF PHYSICIAN (OR SUPPLIER): I certify that the services listed above were medically indicated and necessary to the health of this patient and were personally furnished by me or my employee under my personal direction.

NOTICE: This is to certify that the foregoing information is true, accurate and complete. I understand that payment and satisfaction of this claim will be from Federal and State funds, and that any false claims, statements, or documents, or concealment of a material fact, may be prosecuted under applicable Federal or State laws.

According to the Paperwork Reduction Act of 1995, no persons are required to respond to a collection of information unless it displays a valid OMB control number. The valid OMB control number for this information collection is 0938-0008. The time required to complete this information collection is estimated to average 10 minutes per response, including the time to review instructions, search existing data resources, gather the data needed, and complete and review the information collection. If you have any comments concerning the accuracy of the time estimate(s) or suggestions for improving this form, please write to: CMS, N2-14-26, 7500 Security Boulevard, Baltimore, Maryland 21244-1850.

Figure 20 – 2: Back of the CMS-1500 Claim Form

Information About the Insured

These boxes contain information on the insured, their insurance and their employment.

1a **Insured's ID Number.** Social Security number, ID number or policy number of insured.

4 **Insured's Name.** Subscriber's Name.

7 **Insured's Address and Phone Number.** Same.

11 **Insured's Policy Group or FECA Number.** Subscriber's Group Number. This number refers to primary insured listed in 1a above.

11a **Insured's Date of Birth.** Same.

11b **Employer's Name or School Name.** Employer or school name of insured party.

11c **Insurance Plan Name or Program Name.** Name of insurance company and/or group plan.

11d **Is There Another Health Benefit Plan?** Check appropriate box. If "YES" is checked, then items 9A-9D must be completed.

Information about the Secondary Insurance

These boxes contain information about a secondary insurance policy (if any), which may provide coverage on this patient.

9 **Other Insured's Name.** Other insured whose coverage may be responsible, in whole or in part, for the payment of this claim.

9a **Other Insured's Policy or Group Number.** Same.

9b **Other Insured's Date of Birth and Sex.** Same.

9c **Employer's Name or School Name.** Employer or School Name of other insured party.

9d **Insurance Plan Name or Program Name.** Name of insurance company and/or group plan for other insured.

Information about Third Party Liability

These boxes contain information on whether a third party may be liable for payment on this claim.

10a **Was Condition Related to: Employment?** If "YES" is marked, then there is Worker's Compensation Insurance involved. If "NO" is marked, then Worker's Compensation is not involved. Circle whether employment is current or previous.

10b **Was Condition Related to: Auto Accident?** If "YES" is marked, then check for an injury date (Item 14) and an injury diagnosis (Item 21). The state the accident occurred in should also be indicated. If "NO" is marked then the claim may not be for an injury.

10c **Was Condition Related to: Other Accident?** If "YES" is marked, then check for an injury date (Item 14) and an injury diagnosis (Item 21). If "NO" is marked then the claim may not be for an injury.

10d **Reserved for Local Use.** Same

Authorization Signatures

These boxes should be signed by the insured, or a permanent release of information and assignment of benefits should be kept on file. If there is a permanent release of information or assignment of benefits on file, the words SIGNATURE ON FILE should be placed in these boxes.

12 **Patient's or Authorized Person's Signature.** Patient's release of medical information.

13 **Assignment of Benefits.** This box should be signed by the patient in order to allow the insurer to pay the physician directly.

Information about the Illness

These boxes contain information about the current illness.

14 **Date of Illness, Injury, Accident or Pregnancy.** All injury claims (i.e., injury diagnosis) must have an injury or accident date. If the patient's condition is a pregnancy, the date of the last menstrual period should be indicated.

15 **If Patient Has Had Same Or Similar Illness, Give First Date.** Same.

16 **Dates Patient Unable To Work in Current Occupation.** Same.

17 **Name Of Referring Physician or Other Source.** If this patient was referred to the current physician by another physician, hospital, or clinic, the referring party should be listed here.

17a **I.D. Number of Referring Physician.** Same

18 **Hospitalization Dates Relating to Current Services.** Same.

19 **Reserved for Local Use.** Leave blank.

20 **Outside Lab.** Was laboratory work performed outside your office? If so, check the yes box and indicate the total of the charges.

21 **Diagnosis or Nature of Illness or Injury.** The diagnosis indicates why the patient visited the provider. Both an ICD-9 code and a description should be indicated.

22 **Medicaid Resubmission Code.** Leave blank.

Information About the Procedures Performed

These boxes contain information about the procedures which were performed.

23 **Prior Authorization Number.** Authorization number for services which were approved prior to being rendered.

24a **Date of Service.** The date service was rendered by the provider. A complete date must be given.

24b **Place of Service.** The location where the services were performed (see following section for further information).

24c **Type of Service.** Leave blank.

24d **Procedures, Services or Supplies.** The 5-digit procedure code as found in the CPT®/RVS and HCPCS manuals. These are codes that have been assigned to each procedure the provider can perform. By selecting the proper code, billers can describe the type of service performed with a few numbers. This eliminates the confusion that used to arise from various abbreviations and descriptions of a procedure. It also allows for easy computer tabulation of the different procedures performed.

24d **Modifier Code.** The two-digit modifier from the CPT®/RVS further describing the procedure code.

24e **Diagnosis Code.** This is used in conjunction with Item 21. The number placed in Item 24E (i.e., 1, 2, 3, 4) refers to diagnosis 1, 2, 3, or 4 in Item 21. In other words, the doctor can perform different services for different illnesses or injuries on different dates and submit them all on one claim form.

24f **Charges.** The charge per line of service.

24g **Days or Units.** The number of times a service was performed

24h **EPSDT Family Plan.** Leave blank.

24i **EMG.** If service was rendered in the hospital emergency room, place a Y in this item. This information should match the service code in Item 24B.

24j **COB.** Are there other insurance policies or plans which may be responsible for payment on this claim? Indicate a Y for yes, an N for no.

24k **Reserved for Local Use.** Leave blank.

28 **Total Charge.** The total charge of the claim.

29 **Amount Paid.** The amount paid by the patient or subscriber.

30 **Balance Due.** The difference between the total charge and the amount paid by the patient or subscriber (if any).

Information about the Provider of Services

These boxes contain information about the provider of services.

25 **Federal Tax I.D. Number.** If the provider of service is a physician or an individual, his/her Social Security or Taxpayer Identification Number should be used. If the provider of service is a facility, an Employer Identification Number should be indicated.

26 **Patient's Account Number.** Same

27 **Accept Assignment for Government Claims.** Refers only to TRICARE or Medicare. Do not use to assign payment on this claim to the provider. Use Item 13 only for your assignment of payment.

31 **Signature of Physician or Supplier of Service Including Degrees or Credentials.** Must be signed by the provider indicating that the said services have indeed been rendered. Degrees or credentials (i.e., M.D., D.O., etc.) should follow the name.

32 **Name and Address of Facility Where Services Were Rendered.** If this information is the same as Item 33, it may be left blank.

33 **Physician's/Supplier's Billing Name, Address, Zip Code And Phone #.** The name, address and phone number of the physician or supplier of service. This is the address that payments will be addressed to if assignment of benefits were made in Item 13.

Item 24B, Place of Service

This is a numerical code to indicate the place where the service was rendered. Place of Service codes are as follows:

00-10 **Unassigned**

11 **Office** (Location other than a hospital, Skilled Nursing Facility (SNF), Military Treatment Facility, Community Health Center, State or Local Public Health Clinic or Intermediate Care Facility (ICF), where the health professional routinely provides health examinations, diagnosis and treatment of illness or injury on an ambulatory basis).

12 **Home** (Location other than a hospital or other facility where the patient receives care in a private residence).

13-20 **Unassigned**

21 **Inpatient hospital** (A facility other than psychiatric, which primarily provides diagnostic, therapeutic (both surgical and nonsurgical) and rehabilitation services by, or under the supervision of, physicians to patient admitted for a variety of medical condition).

22 **Outpatient Hospital** (A portion of a hospital which provides diagnostic, therapeutic (both surgical and non surgical) and rehabilitation services to sick and injured persons who do not require hospitalization or institutionalization.) A patient who is not admitted to a hospital (i.e., one who is under 24-hour supervision) is an outpatient.

23 **Emergency Room -- Hospital** (A portion of a hospital where emergency diagnosis and treatment of illness or injury is provided.) Patients in the emergency room are considered to be facility outpatients. (Remember to also complete box 24I.)

24 **Ambulatory Surgical Center (ASC)** (A freestanding facility other than a physician's office where surgical and diagnostic services are provided on an ambulatory basis.) When this code is used, the facility must be an HCFA-approved ASC.

25 **Birthing Center** (A facility other than a hospital's maternity facilities or a physician's office that provides a setting for labor, delivery and immediate post-partum care as well as immediate care of newborn infants.)

26 **Military Treatment Facility** (MTF) (A medical facility operated by one or more of the Uniformed Services. MTF also refers to certain former U.S. Public Health Service facilities now designated as Uniformed Service Treatment Facilities (USTF).)

27-30 **Unassigned**

31 **Skilled Nursing Facility** (A facility which primarily provides inpatient skilled nursing care and related services to patients who require medical, nursing, or rehabilitative services which does not provide the level of care or treatment available in a hospital.)

32 **Nursing Facility** (A facility which provides skilled nursing care and related services for the rehabilitation of injured, disabled, or sick persons or on a regular basis health-related care services above the level of custodial care to other than mentally retarded individuals.)

33 **Custodial Care Facility** (A facility which provides room, board and personal assistance services, generally on a long-term basis, and which does not include a medical component.)

34 **Hospice** (A facility, other than a patient's home, in which palliative and supportive care for terminally ill patients and their families are provided.)

35-40 **Unassigned**

41 **Ambulance -- Land** (A land vehicle specifically designed, equipped and staffed for lifesaving and transporting the sick or injured.)

42 **Ambulance -- Air or Water** (An air or water vehicle specifically designed, equipped and staffed for lifesaving and transporting the sick or injured.)

43-50 **Unassigned**

51 **Inpatient Psychiatric Facility** (A facility that provides inpatient psychiatric services for the diagnosis and treatment of mental illness on a 24-hour basis, by or under the supervision of a physician.)

52　**Psychiatric Facility Partial Hospitalization** (A facility for the diagnosis and treatment of mental illness that provides a planned therapeutic program for patients who do not need full-time hospitalization, but who need broader programs than are possible from outpatient visits in a hospital-based or hospital-affiliated facility.)

53　**Community Mental Health Center** (A facility that provides comprehensive mental health services on an ambulatory basis, primarily to individuals residing or employed in a defined area. Includes a physician-directed mental health facility.)

54　**Intermediate Care Facility/Mentally Retarded** (A facility which primarily provides health-related care and services above the level of custodial care of mentally retarded individuals but does not provide the level of care or treatment available in a hospital or SNF.)

55　**Residential Substance Abuse Treatment Facility** (A facility which provides treatment for substance (alcohol and drug) abuse to live-in residents who do not require acute medical care. Services include individual and group therapy and counseling, family counseling, laboratory tests, drugs and supplies, psychological testing, and room and board.)

56　**Psychiatric Residential Treatment Center** (A facility or distinct part of a facility for psychiatric care which provides a total 24-hour therapeutically planned and professionally staffed group living and learning environment.)

57-60　**Unassigned**

61　**Comprehensive Inpatient Rehabilitation Facility** (A facility that provides comprehensive rehabilitation services under the supervision of a physician to inpatients with physical disabilities. Services include rehabilitation nursing, physical therapy, occupational therapy, speech pathology, social or psychological services, and orthotics and prosthetics services. There are specific licensing requirements for these facilities.)

62　**Comprehensive Outpatient Rehabilitation Facility** (A facility that provides comprehensive rehabilitation services under the supervision of a physician to inpatients with physical disabilities. Services include physical therapy, occupational therapy, and speech pathology services. There are specific licensing requirements for these facilities.)

63-64　**Unassigned**

65　**End Stage Renal Disease Treatment Facility** (A facility other than a hospital, which provides dialysis treatment, maintenance and/or training to patients or care givers on an ambulatory or home-care basis.)

66-70　**Unassigned**

71　**State or Local Public Health Clinic** (A facility maintained by either State or local health departments that provides ambulatory primary medical care under the general direction of a physician. Such facilities must be physician-directed.)

72　**Rural Health Clinic** (A certified facility which is located in a rural medically underserved area that provides ambulatory primary medical care under the general direction of a physician. Qualified facilities do not bill Part B of Medicare for items or services except for DME and orthotics and prosthetics.)

73-80　**Unassigned**

81　**Independent Laboratory** (A laboratory certified to perform diagnostic and/or clinical tests independent of an institution or a physician's office.)

With the exception of hospital inpatients, the place of service for lab tests will be based on where "drawn" instead of where the test is actually performed. If the physician is billing for a lab service performed in his/her own office, then use the appropriate code for provider's office. If an independent laboratory is billing, show the place where the sample is drawn. An independent laboratory drawing a sample in its laboratory shows the code for independent laboratory as the place of service. If an independent laboratory is billing for a test on a sample drawn on a hospital inpatient, then the appropriate code for hospital inpatient is entered as the place of service. If the independent laboratory is billing for a test on a sample drawn in a physician's office, then the appropriate code is for provider's office.

82-98 **Unassigned**

99 **Other Unlisted Facility** (Other service facilities not identified above.)

Tips on Completing the CMS-1500

Properly completing the CMS-1500 is vital to getting the proper reimbursement for the services that were rendered. The following tips will help to minimize errors and speed processing of a claim.

1. Use all capital letters.
2. Do not go outside the box lines. Many forms are scanned by computer and exceeding the box limits can cause errors.
3. Be sure that all necessary boxes are filled in.
4. Be sure that all diagnoses have related procedures, and all procedures have a related diagnosis.
5. Do not write on the form unless it is for the purpose of signing in box 12, 13 or 31.
6. Do not sign or write in red ink. Many scanners used by insurance carriers are trained to ignore everything in red on the form and just pick up the data. Therefore, anything in red will not be picked up by the scanner.
7. Do not use a highlighter on the form. Some scanners will pick up the highlighter and turn it into a black mark, thus obliterating the information in that item.
8. Handwritten claims should be printed neatly and accurately using black ball point pen.
9. Use only alphabetical letters or numbers. Symbols should not be used (i.e., ", $, #, cc). Omit commas, periods or decimal points.

10. Be sure the printer has sufficient ink to create a strong character.
11. Use only black in Pica, or Ariel 10, 11, or 12 point font, or other font accepted by the insurance carrier.
12. Do not use proportional fonts. The typeface used should have the same width for each character.
13. Use all capital letters.
14. Do not place more than one service or code on each of the service code lines. If more than six procedures were done, use an additional form.
15. Include only CPT and ICD-9 codes. Do not use narrative descriptions of services or diagnoses.
16. Use only letters. Do not use special characters such as periods, parentheses, dollar signs and ditto marks.
17. All items on the form should be typed. Nothing should be hand-written.
18. If it is necessary to add attachments, they should be on paper that is 8.5 by 11 inches. The font should be the same one used to complete the form.

Observing these rules will help ensure that claims are scanned in properly, and decrease the chance of errors and delays.

Summary

The CMS-1500 is the most widely accepted form for billing professional services. It is vital that the correct information be inserted in each item to allow the claim to be processed without delay. While the completion may seem simple, it takes practice to be able to properly fill out the form in the correct manner.

Assignments

Complete the Questions for Review.
Complete Exercise 20 – 1.

Questions for Review

Directions: Answer the following questions without looking back into the material just covered. Write your answers in the space provided.

1. What is the CMS-1500 claim form used for? _____

   _____

2. If the provider of service is an individual, what should be placed in the box entitled Federal Tax ID

   Number? _____

3. Which box denotes that Workers' Compensation is involved in the claim? _____

   _____

4. How would you indicate that the place where services were rendered was an office? _____

   _____

5. What are the boxes at the top of the CMS-1500 form, labeled "Medicare, Medicaid, TRICARE,

   CHAMPVA, Feca Black Lung, and Other" for? _____

   _____

6. What does the term "Assignment of Benefits" mean? _____

   _____

7. On the CMS-1500, what is Item 24I "EMG" for? _____

   _____

8. On the CMS-1500, what does Item 24J "COB" stand for and what does the term mean? _____

   _____

   _____

9. (True or false?) When a physician or provider of service signs a medical billing form, he/she is legally

   stating that the service(s) which they are seeking payment for have actually been performed. _____

10. What is a "Unit of Service"? _____

If you were unable to answer any of the questions, refer back to that section, and then fill in the answers.

Exercise 20 – 1

Directions: Bill the following services on a CMS-1500. In all cases, the provider is Henry Higgins, M.D., 1234 Hyacinth Highway, Dubuque, Iowa 52000. Amounts in parentheses are the amounts the doctor is billing for the procedure. Patient information should be obtained from the patient chart.

1. On 3/4/xx Abby Addison comes in to visit the provider. She has a bad case of the flu and receives a problem-focused office visit ($95), and a therapeutic injection (vitamin B-12) ($30).

2. On 3/3/xx Bobby Bumble visits the provider for treatment of a superficial abscess on his neck. The provider does an incision and drainage of the abscess ($95).

3. On 3/4/xx Cathy Crenshaw visits the provider for treatment of a cut on her arm. The provider performs a moderate complexity office visit with five stitches ($110) and a tetanus injection ($30). On 3/15/xx Cathy comes in to have her stitches removed.

4. On 3/3/xx Daisy Doolittle visits the provider for a refill of her contraceptive prescription. The provider performs a problem focused exam and writes her a new prescription ($95).

5. On 3/3/xx Edward Edmunds visits the provider for pain and swelling in his shoulder. The provider does a moderate complexity office visit ($110) and a urinalysis ($30). The final diagnosis is tendonitis. On 3/10/xx the provider operates to remove the calcium deposits. The operation was done at Commerce Union Medical Center, 1029 Commerce Way, Dubuque, Iowa 52000.

Honors Certification™

The certification challenge for this chapter will be a written test of the information contained in this chapter. Each incorrect answer will result in a deduction of up to 5% from your grade. You must achieve a score of 85% or higher to pass this test. If you fail the test on your first attempt you may retake the test one additional time. The items included in the second test may be different from those in the first test.

21

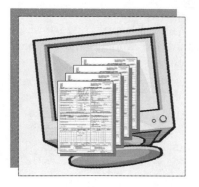

UB-92 Hospital Billing Form

After completion of this chapter you will be able to:

- Describe the purpose of the UB-92.
- Properly code the type of bill.
- Properly identify condition codes, occurrence codes and occurrence span codes.
- Properly complete the UB-92 billing form.
- Identify hospital revenue codes.

Key words and concepts you will learn in this chapter:

Condition Code – A two-digit code used to identify conditions relating to this bill that may affect payor processing.

Occurrence Code – A code and associated date defining a significant event relating to this bill that may affect payor processing.

Occurrence Span Codes – A code and the related dates that identify an event relating to the payment of the claim. These codes identify occurrences that happened over a span of time.

Revenue Codes – A code that identifies a specific accommodation, ancillary service, or billing calculation.

Source of Admission Code – A one-digit code indicating how the patient was referred to the facility.

Type of Admission Code – A two-digit code indicating the priority of the patient when they entered the hospital.

Uniform Bill--1992 (UB-92) – A form used by hospitals or other hospital-type facilities for inpatient and outpatient billing.

Value Code – A code and the related dollar amount that identifies data of a monetary nature that is necessary for processing the claim.

The **Uniform Bill--1992 (UB-92)** is intended to be used by hospitals or other hospital-type facilities for inpatient and outpatient billing **(see Figure 21 – 1 and 21 – 2)**. The data elements and the design of the form were determined by the National Uniform Billing Committee. This form was designed to provide the basic data needed by most payors to adjudicate a large majority of their claims. The objective was to accommodate a wide range of needs while eliminating the need for attachments.

As you use this form, you will become familiar with the various items.

Item # and Item Name/Description

The following list will assist in explaining the uses of the various items. It contains the item number along with the name of the item and a brief description of the information required. The word "same" refers to a description that is the same as the title of the item.

Item #	Item Name/Description

1   **Provider Name, Address, and Telephone Number.** Name, address, and telephone number of hospital or clinic where services were rendered.

2   **Reserved (untitled).** All unlabeled items are reserved for state or national use. Their use may be assigned by either the state or National Uniform Billing Committee.

3   **Patient Control Number.** Patient's account number.

4   **Type of Bill.** Three-digit code providing information regarding what type of bill is being submitted. (See following section for further information.)

5   **Federal Tax Number.** Provider's Identification Number or Social Security Number.

6   **Statement Covers Period.** The dates of service that this billing statement represents. Dates should match those on the itemized billing statement. For services rendered on the same day, both dates should be the same.

7   **Covered Days.** Number of days that services are covered by primary payor.

8   **Noncovered Days (inpatient only).** Number of days services are not covered by primary payor. For Medicare, the reason for non-coverage should be explained by occurrence codes, PSRO items, or in remarks.

9   **Coinsurance Days.** Number of days for which the patient must pay a portion of the costs of services. For Medicare, the inpatient Medicare days occurring after the 60th and before the 91st day in a single spell of illness.

10 **Lifetime Reserve Days.** Under Medicare, each beneficiary has a lifetime reserve of 60 additional days of inpatient hospital services after using 90 days of inpatient hospital services during a spell of illness.

11 **Reserved for State Assignment**

12 **Patient's Name.** Same.

13 **Patient's Address.** Same.

14 **Birth Date.** Patient's date of birth.

15 **Sex.** Patient's sex.

16 **Marital Status.** Patient's marital status (S = Single, M = Married, X = Legally Separated, D = Divorced, W = Widowed, U = Unknown).

17 **Date of Admission.** Date patient was admitted to hospital.

18 **Hour of Admission.** Hour patient admitted to hospital according to a 24-hour clock (i.e., 10:10 p.m. would be written 22:10). 99 = unknown.

19 **Type of Admission.** Numerical code denoting the priority of this admission (see following section for further information).

20 **Source of Admission.** Numerical code denoting the source of this admission (see following section for further information).

21 **Discharge Hour.** Time patient was discharged from inpatient care. Time should be written according to a 24-hour clock. 99 = unknown. This element is not necessary for outpatient care.

22 **Patient Status.** Numerical code denoting the status of the patient as of the statement-through date. This element is necessary only for inpatient care (see following section for further information).

23 **Medical Record Number.** Number assigned by the provider to the medical record.

24–30 **Condition Codes.** Codes used to identify conditions relating to the claim that may affect payor processing (see following section for further information). No specific date is associated with this code.

31 **Reserved for National Assignment.**

32–35 **Occurrence Codes.** The code and associated date defining a significant event relating to this bill that may effect payor processing (see following section for further information).

36 **Occurrence Span.** The code and the related dates that identify an event that relates to the payment of the claim. These codes identify occurrences that happened over a span of time (see following section for further information).

37 **Internal Control Number.** The control number assigned to the original bill by the payor or the payor's intermediary.

38 **Responsible Party Name and Address.** Name and address of person ultimately responsible for insuring payment of the bill. This is usually the patient, or the parent or legal guardian if the patient is a minor.

39–41 **Value Codes and Amounts.** Codes and the related dollar amount that identify data of a monetary nature that is necessary for the processing of this claim (see following section for further information).

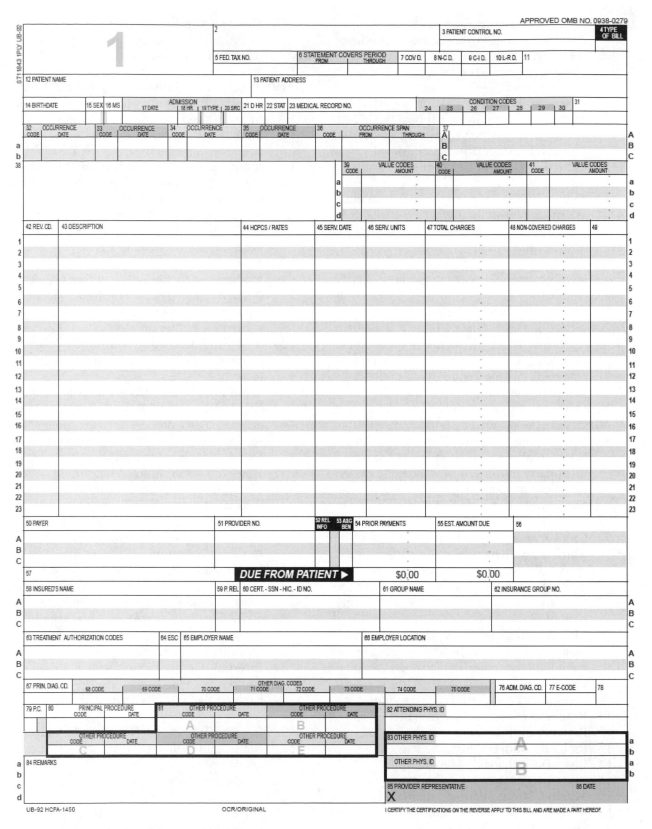

Figure 21 – 1: Front of the UB-92 Billing Form

UNIFORM BILL: **NOTICE: ANYONE WHO MISREPRESENTS OR FALSIFIES ESSENTIAL INFORMATION REQUESTED BY THIS FORM MAY UPON CONVICTION BE SUBJECT TO FINE AND IMPRISONMENT UNDER FEDERAL AND/OR STATE LAW.**

Certifications relevant to the Bill and Information Shown on the Face Hereof: Signatures on the face hereof incorporate the following certifications or verifications where pertinent to this Bill:

1. If third party benefits are indicated as being assigned or in participation status, on the face thereof, appropriate assignments by the insured/ beneficiary and signature of patient or parent or legal guardian covering authorization to release information are on file. Determinations as to the release of medical and financial information should be guided by the particular terms of the release forms that were executed by the patient or the patient's legal representative. The hospital agrees to save harmless, indemnify and defend any insurer who makes payment in reliance upon this certification, from and against any claim to the insurance proceeds when in fact no valid assignment of benefits to the hospital was made.

2. If patient occupied a private room or required private nursing for medical necessity, any required certifications are on file.

3. Physician's certifications and re-certifications, if required by contract or Federal regulations, are on file.

4. For Christian Science Sanitoriums, verifications and if necessary re-verifications of the patient's need for sanitorium services are on file.

5. Signature of patient or his/her representative on certifications, authorization to release information, and payment request, as required be Federal law and regulations (42 USC 1935f, 42 CFR 424.36, 10 USC 1071 thru 1086, 32 CFR 199) and, any other applicable contract regulations, is on file.

6. This claim, to the best of my knowledge, is correct and complete and is in conformance with the Civil Rights Act of 1964 as amended. Records adequately disclosing services will be maintained and necessary information will be furnished to such governmental agencies as required by applicable law.

7. For Medicare purposes:

If the patient has indicated that other health insurance or a state medical assistance agency will pay part of his/her medical expenses and he/she wants information about his/her claim released to them upon their request, necessary authorization is on file. The patient's signature on the provider's request to bill Medicare authorizes any holder of medical and non-medical information, including employment status, and whether the person has employer group health insurance, liability, no-fault, workers' compensation, or other insurance which is responsible to pay for the services for which this Medicare claim is made.

8. For Medicaid purposes:

This is to certify that the foregoing information is true, accurate, and complete.
I understand that payment and satisfaction of this claim will be from Federal and State funds, and that any false claims, statements, or documents, or concealment of a material fact, may be prosecuted under applicable Federal or State Laws.

9. For CHAMPUS purposes:

This is to certify that:

(a) the information submitted as part of this claim is true, accurate and complete, and, the services shown on this form were medically indicated and necessary for the health of the patient;

(b) the patient has represented that by a reported residential address outside a military treatment center catchment area he or she does not live within a catchment area of a U.S. military or U.S. Public Health Service medical facility, or if the patient resides within a catchment area of such a facility, a copy of a Non-Availability Statement (DD Form 1251) is on file, or the physician has certified to a medical emergency in any assistance where a copy of a Non-Availability Statement is not on file;

(c) the patient or the patient's parent or guardian has responded directly to the provider's request to identify all health insurance coverages, and that all such coverages are identified on the face the claim except those that are exclusively supplemental payments to CHAMPUS-determined benefits;

(d) the amount billed to CHAMPUS has been billed after all such coverages have been billed and paid, excluding Medicaid, and the amount billed to CHAMPUS is that remaining claimed against CHAMPUS benefits;

(e) the beneficiary's cost share has not been waived by consent or failure to exercise generally accepted billing and collection efforts; and,

(f) any hospital-based physician under contract, the cost of whose services are allocated in the charges included in this bill, is not an employee or member of the Uniformed Services. For purposes of this certification, an employee of the Uniformed Services is an employee, appointed in civil service (refer to 5 USC 2105), including part-time or intermittent but excluding contract surgeons or other personnel employed by the Uniformed Services through personal service contracts. Similarly, member of the Uniformed Services does not apply to reserve members of the Uniformed Services not on active duty.

(g) based on the Consolidated Omnibus Budget Reconciliation Act of 1986, all providers participating in Medicare must also participate in CHAMPUS for inpatient hospital services provided pursuant to admissions to hospitals occurring on or after January 1, 1987.

(h) if CHAMPUS benefits are to be paid in a participating status, I agree to submit this claim to the appropriate CHAMPUS claims processor as a participating provider. I agree to accept the CHAMPUS-determined reasonable charge as the total charge for the medical services or supplies listed on the claim form. I will accept the CHAMPUS-determined reasonable charge even if it is less than the billed amount, and also agree to accept the amount paid by CHAMPUS, combined with the cost-share amount and deductible amount, if any, paid by or on behalf of the patient as full payment for the listed medical services or supplies. I will make no attempt to collect from the patient (or his or her parent or guardian) amounts over the CHAMPUS-determined reasonable charge. CHAMPUS will make any benefits payable directly to me, if I submit this claim as a participating provider.

ESTIMATED CONTRACT BENEFITS

Figure 21 – 2: Back of the UB-92 Billing Form

42 **Revenue Code.** Revenue code referencing the type of services provided (see following section for further information).

43 **Revenue Description.** A description of the services provided. Abbreviations may be used. Accommodation (room) descriptions must be entered first on the bill and must be in chronologic order of appearance (i.e., 03/01/89 ICU, 03/02/89 semiprivate room).

44 **HCPCS/Rates.** The accommodation rate for inpatient bills, or the CPT® or HCPCS code for ancillary or outpatient services. Outpatient Worker's Compensation and Medicaid require HCPCS coding in this space.

45 **Service Date.** The date the service was provided if this is a series bill where the date of service differs from the from/through date on the bill.

46 **Units of Service.** Quantitative measure of services, days, miles, pints of blood, units, or treatments (i.e., if a patient was hospitalized for three days, a 3 would be placed here).

47 **Total Charges.** Total charges for that line of services.

48 **Noncovered Charges.** The amount per line of service that is not covered by the primary payor.

49 **Reserved for National Assignment.**

50 **Payor Identification.** Name of insurer(s) covered by the patient who may be responsible for payment on this bill. Insurers should be listed in order of Primary Payor, Secondary Payor, and Tertiary Payor(s). If required, numbers identifying each payor organization should be listed.

51 **Provider Number.** The number assigned to the provider by the listed payor.

52 **Release Information.** A Y (yes) or N (no) designation stating whether or not patient's signature is on file authorizing the release of information. An R may also be entered to show that a hospital has restricted authorization to release information. In such a case the authorization should be attached. If no Authorization to Release Information is on file, one must be obtained before sending in the claim.

53 **Assignment of Benefits.** A Y (yes) or N (no) designation stating whether or not patient's signature is on file authorizing the insurer to pay the provider of service directly instead of the patient. If a Y is placed in this item, you must have an assignment of benefits signed by the insured on file in your office. (See following section for further information.)

54 **Prior Payments.** The amount that has been paid toward this bill prior to the current billing date. These can include payments by the patient, other payors, and so on.

55 **Estimated Amount Due.** The amount estimated by the provider to be due from the indicated payor. This is usually the total amount due minus any previous payments.

56 **Reserved for State Assignment.**

57 **Reserved for National Assignment.**

58 **Insured's Name.** Name of the person listed on the insurance forms (subscriber's name). This may be a spouse or parent of the patient.

59 **Patient's Relationship to Insured.** Numerical code designation indicating the relationship between the patient and the insured (see following section for further information).

60 **Subscriber's Certificate Number.** The policy number under which the insured is covered if it is an individual policy. If the insured is covered under a group policy (such as one offered by his/her employer), often the insured's Social Security number is used as the subscriber number.

61 **Insured Group Name.** The name of the group or company that holds the insured's policy. Often this is the employer of the insured. This information is required by Medicare when Medicare is not the primary payor.

62 **Insurance Group Number.** The group number denoting the group policy or plan under which the insured is covered.

63 **Treatment Authorization Code.** A number indicating that the treatment described by this bill has been authorized by the payor.

64 **Employment Status Code.** A code denoting whether or not the employee is currently employed part- or full-time, is retired, or is in active military service (see following section for further information).

65 **Employer Name.** Name of the employer of the insured person.

66 **Employer Location.** Address of the employer of the insured or responsible party.

67 **Principal Diagnosis Code.** ICD-9 code for the diagnosis of the patient's condition. The diagnosis shown should reflect the information contained in the patient's medical record for the dates indicated in Item 6 even if the diagnosis is changed at a later date.

68-75 **Other Diagnosis Codes.** ICD-9, V, and E Codes for any additional diagnosis of the patient's condition.

76 **Admitting Diagnosis.** The ICD-9 code provided at the time of admission.

77 **External Cause of Injury Code (E Code).** The ICD-9 Code for an external cause of injury, poisoning or adverse effect.

78 **Reserved for State Assignment.**

79 **Procedure Coding Method Used.** An indicator code that identifies the coding method used for procedure coding on the claim.
    1-3 Reserved for State Assignment
    4   CPT®-4
    5   HCPCS
    6-8 Reserved for National Assignment
    9   ICD-9CM

80 **Principal Procedure Codes and Date.** CPT® code for principal procedure rendered and the date that procedure was rendered. For Medicare, ICD-9 codes must be entered here and on Item 81.

81 **Other Procedure Codes and Dates.** CPT® code for additional procedures rendered and the dates of those procedures.

82 **Attending Physician ID.** Name and license number of the physician who is primarily responsible for the patient.

83 **Other Physician ID.** Name and license number of secondary physician, assistant surgeon, and so on.

84 **Remarks.** Pertinent data for which there is no other specific place on the form. Often this space is used to record the nature of an accident (i.e., fell and hit head on concrete, 06/09/XX). For Medicaid, required for abortion certification when the attending physician is an employee of the hospital and does not submit a separate bill. Also, multiple visits to the ER on the same day should be recorded.

85 **Provider Representative Signature.** Signature of provider representative. In the case of a hospital billing, it is not necessary for the attending physician to sign, as long as a representative of the hospital signs the form certifying that the information entered is in conformance with the certifications specified on the reverse of the bill. Billers should make sure that the physician's certification is contained in the hospital records.

86 **Date Bill Submitted.** Date the bill was signed and submitted for payment.

The following items needed further description for which space was not available in the above text. Please study the following before completing the billing forms.

Item 4, Type of Bill

The following code structure is to be used to classify the type of bill. Each claim should have a 3-digit code entered in this space that corresponds with the following information.

The following code structure is to be used to classify the type of bill. Each claim should have a 3-digit code entered in the space that corresponds with the following information.

First Digit – Type of Facility
1   **Hospital.**
2   **Skilled Nursing.**
3   **Home Health.**
4   **Christian Science.** Hospital.
5   **Christian Science.** Extended Care.
6   **Intermediate Care.**
7   **Clinic.***
8   **Special Facility.***
9   **Reserved For National Use.**

* If Type of Facility is a Clinic (Code 7), then the Bill Classifications for Clinics Only must be used. If Type of Facility is a Special Facility (Code 8), then the Bill Classifications for Special Facilities Only must be used.

Second Digit – Bill Classification
For All Except Clinics
1   **Inpatient.** Includes Medicare Part A.
2   **Inpatient.** Medicare Part B only.
3   **Outpatient.**

4   **Other.** For hospital referenced diagnostic procedures or home health not under plan of treatment. This is to be further defined at the state level.

5-7   **Reserved For National Use.**

8   **Swing Beds.**

9   Reserved For National Use.

Clinics Only

1   **Rural Health**

2   **Hospital based or Independent Renal Dialysis Center.**

3   **Free Standing**.

4   **Outpatient Rehabilitation Facility (ORF).**

5   **Comprehensive Outpatient Rehabilitation Facility (CORF).**

6-8   **Reserved For National Use.**

9   Other.

Special Facilities Only

1   **Hospice.** Non-hospital-based.

2   **Hospice.** Hospital-based.

3   **Ambulatory Surgery Center.**

4   **Free Standing Birthing Center.**

5-8   **Reserved for National Use.**

9   **Other.**

Third Digit – Frequency of Billing

0   **Nonpayment/Zero Claim.** Claim being submitted for information only. Provider does not anticipate payment on the claim.

1   **Admit through Discharge Claim.** This claim is expected to be the only bill submitted for this course of treatment.

2   **Interim – First Claim.** This is the first claim in a series for the same course of treatment.

3   **Interim – Continuing Claim.** A prior claim has been submitted for this course of treatment or confinement, and a subsequent bill is also expected to be issued.

4   **Interim – Last Claim.** A prior claim has been submitted for this course of treatment or confinement and this is expected to be the last bill issued.

5   **Late Charge(s) Only Claim.** A prior claim or complete set of claims has been submitted to the provider and late charges are being added to the prior billing(s).

6   **Adjustment of Prior Claim.** This claim adjusts a prior claim. Adjustments should be made by altering the prior claim with the addition of an explanation and a credit or additional charge added to the claim.

7   **Replacement of Prior Claim.** This claim replaces a prior claim and that prior claim should be considered null and void.

8   **Void/Cancel Prior Claim.** This bill voids the prior bill that was submitted with the same information. In effect, submitting a bill with this code is the same as submitting a duplicate copy of the claim with the word VOID written across the front. This bill may be followed by a replacement claim.

9   **Reserved for National Assignment.**

For example, claims for the following types of bills would be coded the following way:

Hosp admit through discharge, inpatient	111
Hosp inpatient, replacement of prior claim	117
Hosp ER outpatient claim, only bill	131
Rural Clinic outpatient zero claim	716

Item 19, Type of Admission

This is a one-digit code indicating the priority of this admission according to the following structure:

1   **Emergency.**

2   **Urgent.**

3   **Elective.**

4   **Newborn.** A baby born within the facility.

5-8   **Reserved for National Assignment.**

9   **Information Not Available.**

Item 20, Source of Admission

This is a one-digit code indicating the source of this admission according to the following structure:

Emergency, Elective, or Other Admission Types

1   **Physician Referral.** Patient was admitted or referred by his personal physician. If outpatient, the patient may request services (self-referral).

2   **Clinic Referral.** Patient was admitted or referred by this facility's clinic physician.

3   **HMO Referral.** Patient was admitted or referred by an HMO physician.

4   **Transfer from a Hospital.** Patient was transferred from an acute care facility where he/she was an inpatient.

5 **Transfer from a Skilled Nursing Facility.** Patient was transferred from a Skilled Nursing Facility where he/she was an inpatient.

6 **Transfer from Another Health Care Facility.** Patient was transferred from a health care facility other than an acute care facility or a SNF.

7 **Emergency Room.** Patient was admitted by this facility's ER physician.

8 **Court/Law Enforcement.** Patient was admitted or referred upon the direction of a court, or upon the request of a law enforcement agency.

9 **Information Not Available.** Means of admission or referral not known.

A-Z **Reserved for National Assignment.**

For Newborns

1 Normal Delivery.
2 **Premature Delivery.**
3 **Sick Baby.** A baby delivered with medical complications, other than those relating to premature status.
4 **Extramural Birth.** A newborn baby born in a non-sterile environment.
5-8 **Reserved for National Assignment.**
9 **Information Not Available.**

Item 22, Patient Status

This is a two-digit code indicating the status of the patient at the last date covered by this billing statement.

01 **Discharged to home or self-care.** Routine discharge.

02 **Discharged/transferred to another short-term general hospital (inpatient).**

03 **Discharged/transferred to Skilled Nursing Facility (SNF).**

04 **Discharged/transferred to an Intermediate Care Facility (ICF).**

05 **Discharged/transferred to another type of institution (either inpatient or outpatient).**

06 **Discharged/transferred to home under care of home health service organization.**

07 **Left or discontinued care against medical advice.**

08 **Discharged/transferred to home under care of a Home IV provider.**

09 **Admitted as an inpatient to this hospital.** For use on outpatient Medicare claims.

10-19 **Discharge to be defined at state level, if necessary.**
20 **Expired.**
21-29 **Expired to be defined at state level, if necessary.**
30 **Still a patient or expected to return for outpatient services.**
31-39 **Still a patient. To be defined at state level, if necessary.**
40* **Expired at home.**
41* **Expired in a medical facility, hospital, free-standing clinic, or hospice.**
42* **Expired, place unknown.**
43-99 **Reserved for National Assignment.**

*NOTE: Codes with an asterisk are for use only on Medicare claims for hospice care.

Items 24-30, Condition Codes

This is a two-digit code used to identify conditions relating to this bill that may affect payor processing. There is no specific date associated with this code as there is in Items 32-36. Condition codes should be entered in numeric sequence.

Insurance Codes

01 **Military Service-Related.** Medical condition incurred during military service.

02 **Condition is Employment-Related.** Patient alleges that medical condition is due to environment/events resulting from employment.

03 **Patient Covered By Insurance Not Reflected Here.** Indicates that patient/patient representative has stated that coverage may exist beyond that reflected on this bill.

04 **HMO Enrollee.** Indicates Medicare beneficiary is enrolled in an HMO and provider expects to receive payment from the HMO.

05 **Lien Has Been Filed.** Provider has filed legal claim for recovery of funds potentially due a patient as a result of legal action initiated by or on behalf of the patient.

06 **ESRD Patient in First 18 Months of Entitlement Covered by Employer Group Health Insurance.** Medicare may be a secondary insurer if the patient is also covered by employer group health insurance during the first 18 months of ESRD entitlement.

07 **Treatment of Non-terminal Condition for Hospice Patient.** The patient is a hospice enrollee, but the provider is not treating his/her terminal condition and is requesting regular Medicare reimbursement.

08 **Beneficiary Would Not Provide Information About Other Insurance Coverage.** Same.

09 **Neither Patient Nor Spouse is Employed.** Same.

10 **Patient and/or Spouse is Employed But No Employer Group Health Plan Exists.** Same.

11 **Disabled Beneficiary But No Large Group Health Plan.** Patient is disabled and is not covered by a large group health plan.

12-16 **Payor Codes.** Reserved for payor processing.

Special Conditions

17 **Reserved for National Assignment.**

18 **Maiden Name Retained.** A dependent spouse entitled to a benefit that does not use her husband's last name.

19 **Child Retains Mother's Name.** A child that does not have his or her father's last name.

20 **Beneficiary Requested Billing.** Provider understands services are not covered or excluded, but beneficiary requests determination by payor.

21 **Billing for Denial Notice.** Provider understands services are not covered or excluded, but requests denial notice from payor.

22-25 **Reserved for National Assignment.**

26 **Veterans Affairs (VA) Eligible Patient Chooses to Receive Services in a Medicare Certified Facility.** Patient has chosen a Medicare certified facility rather than a VA certified facility.

27 **Patient Referred to a Sole Community Hospital for a Diagnostic Laboratory Test.** This code is for use by Sole Community hospitals only. It indicates patient was referred for a diagnostic laboratory test. Payment is generally made at 62%. This code should not be used when a specimen only is referred to a hospital.

28 **Patient and/or Spouse's Employee Health Plan is Secondary to Medicare.** Patient has indicated there is employer group coverage through either the patient or the patient's spouse; however, the employer health plan in under a single employer that has fewer than 20 full- and part-time employees or the employer health plan is a multi or multiple employer health plan that has elected to pay secondary to Medicare for employees and their spouses aged 65 or older for those employers who have fewer than 20 employees.

29 **Disabled Beneficiary and/or Family Member's Large Group Health Plan is Secondary to Medicare.** Patient or family members have indicated that one or more is employed and covered by a large group health plan or other employer sponsored health plan, but the large group health plan is a single employer plan and the employer has less than 100 full- and part-time employees or the large group health plan is a multi or multiple employer plan and that all employers participating in the plan have fewer than 100 full- and part-time employees.

30 **Reserved for National Assignment.**

Student Status

This information is required when the patient is a dependent child over age 18. Use only one of the following codes. The one with the lowest numerical value should take precedence.

31 **Patient is Student (full-time--day).** Patient declares that he or she is enrolled as a full time day student.

32 **Patient is Student (cooperative/work study program).** Same.

33 **Patient is Student (full-time--night).** Patient declares that he or she is enrolled as a full-time night student.

34 **Patient is Student (part-time).** Patient declares that he or she is enrolled as a part-time student.

35 **Reserved for National Assignment.**

Accommodations

36 **General Care Patient in a Special Unit.** Patient temporarily placed in special care unit bed because no general care beds available.

37 **Ward Accommodation at Patient Request.** Patient assigned to ward accommodations at patient's request.

38 **Semiprivate Room Not Available.** Indicates that either private or ward

accommodations were assigned because semiprivate accommodations were not available.

39 **Private Room Medically Necessary.** Patient needs a private room for medical reasons.

40 **Same Day Transfer.** Patient transferred to another facility before midnight on the day of admission.

41 **Partial Hospitalization.** Indicates claim is for partial hospitalization services. For outpatient Medicare this may include psychiatric services (i.e., drug and alcohol treatment).

42-45 **Reserved for National Assignment.**

TRICARE/CHAMPUS Information

46 **Non-availability Certificate On File.** Any TRICARE/CHAMPUS beneficiary who lives within forty miles of a military or public health service hospital has provided to the treating facility a certificate of non-availability (DD1251) certifying the fact that medical care was not obtainable from a military or public health hospital.

47 **Reserved for TRICARE/CHAMPUS.**

48 **Psychiatric Residential Treatment Centers for Children and Adolescents.** Indicates the claim is submitted by a TRICARE/CHAMPUS authorized residential psychiatric treatment center for children and adolescents.

49-54 **Reserved for National Assignment.**

SNF Information

55 **SNF Bed not Available.** Patient's SNF admission was delayed more than 30 days after hospital discharge because a SNF bed was not available.

56 **Medical Appropriateness.** Patient's SNF admission was delayed more than 30 days after discharge from a hospital because his/her condition made it inappropriate to begin active care within that period.

57 **SNF Readmission.** Patient was previously receiving Medicare covered SNF care within 30 days of this readmission.

58-59 **Reserved for National Assignment.**

Prospective Payment

60 **Day Outlier.** A hospital being paid under a prospective payment system is reporting this stay as a day outlier. This entry may be made by either the provider or the payor.

61 **Cost Outlier.** A hospital being paid under a prospective payment system is requesting additional payment for this stay as a cost outlier.

62 **Payor Code.** This code indicates the claim was paid under a DRG. This code is for use by payors, not providers.

63-65 **Payor Codes.** These codes are set aside for payor use.

66 **Provider Does Not Wish Cost Outlier Payment.** A hospital being paid under a prospective payment system is not requesting additional payment for this stay as an outlier.

67-69 **Reserved for National Assignment.**

Renal Dialysis Setting

70 **Self-Administered Erythropoietin (EPO).** Home dialysis patient who self-administers EPO.

71 **Full Care in Unit.** Patient who received staff-assisted dialysis services in a hospital or renal dialysis facility.

72 **Self-Care in Unit.** Patient who managed his own dialysis services without staff assistance in a hospital or renal dialysis facility.

73 **Self-Care Training.** For special dialysis services where a patient and his helper (if necessary) were learning to perform dialysis.

74 **Home.** Patient who received dialysis services at home, but where condition code 75 does not apply.

75 **Home 100% Reimbursement.** Patient received dialysis services at home, using a dialysis machine that was purchased by Medicare under the 100% program.

76 **Back-up in Facility Dialysis.** Home dialysis patient who received back-up.

77 **Provider Accepts or is Obligated to Accept Payment by a Primary Payor as Payment in Full.** Provider has accepted or is obligated (by a contractual arrangement or by law) to accept payment as payment in full.

78 **New Coverage not Implemented by HMO.** A newly covered service under Medicare for which the HMO does not pay.

79 **CORF Services Provided Off-Site.** Physical therapy, occupational therapy, or speech pathology services were provided off-site.

80-99 **Reserved for State Assignment.**

Special Program Indicator Codes

This is a code indicating that the services on this claim are related to a special program.

A0 **CHAMPUS External Partnership Program.** Identifies CHAMPUS claims submitted under the External Partnership Program.

A1 **EPSDT-CHAP.** Early and Periodic Screening Diagnosis and Treatment.

A2 **Physically Handicapped Children's Program.** Services provided under this program receive special funding through Title 8 of the Social Security Act or the CHAMPUS Program for the handicapped.

A3 **Special Federal Funding.** This code has been designed for uniform use by state uniform billing committees.

A4 **Family Planning.** This code has been designed for uniform use by state uniform billing committees.

A5 **Disability.** This code has been designed for uniform use by state uniform billing committees.

A6 **PPV/Medicare 100% Payment.** This code identifies that pneumococcal pneumonia vaccine (PPV) services given should be reimbursed under a special Medicare program provision.

A7 **Induced Abortion--Danger to Life.** Abortion was performed to avoid danger to the woman's life.

A8 **Induced Abortion Victim Rape/Incest.** Same.

A9 **Second Opinion--Surgery.** Services requested to support second opinion on surgery. Part B deductible and coinsurance do not apply.

B0-B9 **Reserved for National Assignment.**

PRO Approval Indicator Services

C0 **Reserved for National Assignment.**

C1 **Approved as Billed.** Approved by the PRO/UR as billed (only for cases that have actually been approved).

C2 **Automatic Approval as Billed Based on Focused Review.** Includes categories of cases that the PRO/UR has determined it need not review under a focused review program.

C3 **Partial Approval.** PRO/UR approved of some services but disapproved others.

C4 **Admission/Services Denied.** All services denied by the PRO/UR.

C5 **Postponement Review Applicable.** PRO/UR review will take place after payment.

C6 **Admission Pre-authorization.** The PRO/UR authorized the admission but not the services.

C7 **Extended Authorization.** The PRO/UR has authorized these services for an extended period of time but has not reviewed the services provided.

C8-C9 **Reserved for National Assignment.**

Claim Change Reasons

Enter only one of the following claim change reasons. The codes have been prioritized. Use the first claim change reason that applies.

D0 **Changes to Service Dates.** Same.

D1 **Changes to Charges.** Same.

D2 **Changes in Revenue Codes/HCPCS.** Same.

D3 **Second or Subsequent Interim PPS Bill.** Same.

D4 **Change in GROUPER Input.** Same.

D5 **Cancel to Correct HICN or Provider#.** Same.

D6 **Cancel Only to Repay a Duplicate or OIG Overpayment.** Includes cancellation of an outpatient bill containing services required to be included on the inpatient bill.

D7 **Change to Make Medicare the Secondary Payor.** Same.

D8 **Change to Make Medicare the Primary Payor.** Same.

D9 **Any Other Change.** Same.

E0 **Change in Patient Status.** Same.

E1-W9 **Reserved for National Assignment.**

X1-Z9 **Reserved for State Assignment.**

Items 32-35, Occurrence Codes

The **Occurrence Code** is a code and associated date defining a significant event relating to this bill that may affect payor processing.

Due to the varied nature of occurrence and occurrence span codes, provisions have been made to allow the use of both types of codes within each. The occurrence span code can contain an occurrence code where the "through" date would not contain an entry. This allows as many as ten occurrence codes to be used.

When reporting occurrence span codes, Items 32a through 35a should be used before using Items 32b through 35b. If these spaces have been filled, you may use Items 36a and 36b to report additional occurrence span codes. In such a case, the beginning date is entered and the through date is left off.

Likewise, if there are more than two occurrence codes to report, additional codes may be entered in Items 32a through 36b.

Accident-Related

01 **Auto Accident.** Code indicating the date of an auto accident.

02 **No Fault insurance Involved.** Code indicating the date of an accident (either auto or other) where the state has applicable no fault liability laws (i.e., legal basis for settlement without admission or proof of guilt).

03 **Accident/Tort Liability.** Code indicating the date of an accident resulting from a third party's action that may involve a civil court process in an attempt to require payment by the third party, other than no fault liability.

04 **Accident/Employment-Related.** Code indicating the date of an accident relating to the patient's employment.

05 **Other Accident.** Code indicating the date of an accident not described by the above codes.

06 **Crime Victim.** Code indicating the date on which a medical condition resulted from allegedly criminal action committed by one or more parties.

07-08 **Reserved for National Assignment.**

Medical Condition

09 **Start of Infertility Treatment Cycle.** The date of the start of infertility treatment cycle.

10 **Last Menstrual Period.** Code indicating the date of the last menstrual period; ONLY applies when patient is being treated for a maternity-related condition.

11 **Onset of Symptoms/Illness.** Code indicating the date the patient first became aware of symptoms/illness.

12 **Date of Onset for a Chronically Dependent Individual.** The date the patient/beneficiary became or becomes a Chronically Dependent Individual. This date begins the first month of the three month period prior to eligibility for respite care benefits.

13-16 **Reserved for National Assignment.**

Insurance-Related

17 **Date Outpatient Occupational Therapy Plan Established or Last Reviewed.** Same.

18 **Date or retirement Patient/Beneficiary.** The beneficiary or patient's date of retirement.

19 **Date of Retirement Spouse.** The date of retirement of the spouse of the patient.

20 **Guarantee of Payment Began.** Code indicating the date on which the provider began claiming Medicare payment under the guarantee of payment provision (HIM 10, 402.1, Item 21).

21 **UR Notice Received.** Code indicating the date of receipt by the hospital of the UR Committee's (PSRO or other responsible group's) finding that an admission for further stay was not medically necessary.

22 **Date Active Care Ended.** Code indicating the date on which a covered level of care ended in a general hospital, or date on which active care ended in a psychiatric or tuberculosis hospital. (HIM 10, 402.1, Item 23). Code not required when PSRO/UR approval is completed.

23 **Reserved for National Assignment.**

24 **Date Insurance Denied.** Code indicating the date the denial of coverage was received by the hospital from any insurer.

25 **Date Benefits Terminated By Primary Payor.** Code indicating the date on which coverage (including Worker's Compensation benefits or no-fault coverage) is no longer available to the patient.

26 **Date SNF Bed Available.** Code indicating the date on which a SNF bed became available to hospital inpatient who requires only SNF level care (HIM 10, 405C).

27 **Date Home Health Plan Established or Last Reviewed.** The date a home plan of treatment was established (this code is only to be used by Home Health providers), (HIM 11 402, Item 13).

28 **Date CORF Plan Established or Last Reviewed.** The date a Comprehensive Outpatient Rehabilitation Facility (CORF) plan was established or last reviewed.

NOTE: Codes 27 and 28 should only be used by hospitals with a Home Health (27) or CORF (28) program.

29 **Date outpatient Physical Therapy Plan Established or Last Reviewed.** Same.

30 **Date Outpatient Speech Pathology Plan Established or Last Reviewed.** Same.

31 **Date Beneficiary Notified of Intent to Bill Accommodations.** The date notice was provided to the beneficiary by the hospital to the patient that inpatient care is no longer required. Beyond this date the patient will be billed for accommodations.

32 **Date Beneficiary Notified of Intent to Bill Procedures or Treatments.** The date notice was given to the beneficiary that requested procedures or treatments are not reasonable or necessary under Medicare or CHAMPUS. Beyond this date the patient will be billed for all procedures and services.

33 **First Day of the Medicare Coordination Period for ESRD Beneficiaries Covered by an Employee Group Health Plan.** The first day of the Medicare coordination period during which Medicare or CHAMPUS benefits are secondary to benefits payable under an employee group health plan. This is required only for ESRD patients.

34 **Date of Election of Extended Care Facilities.** The date the patient elected to receive extended care services. This code is used by Christian Science Sanitoria only.

35 **Date Treatment Started for Physical Therapy.** Same.

36 **Date of Inpatient Hospital Discharge for Covered Transplant Patient.** The date of discharge for a hospital stay during which the patient received a covered transplant procedure and the hospital is billing for immunosuppressive drugs. If the patient received both a covered and a noncovered transplant, the covered transplant would take precedence.

37 **Date of Inpatient Hospital Discharge for Noncovered Transplant Patient.** The date of discharge for a hospital stay during which the patient received a noncovered transplant procedure and the hospital is billing for immunosuppressive drugs.

38-39 **Reserved for National Assignment.**

40 **Scheduled Date of Admission.** The date on which a patient will be admitted as an inpatient to the hospital. This code is for use on an outpatient claim.

41 **Date of First Test for Pre-Admission.** The date on which the first outpatient diagnostic test was performed as part of a pre-admission testing program. This code should be used only if a date of admission was scheduled prior to the administration of the test(s).

Service-Related Codes

42 **Date of Discharge.** Only to be used when "through" date in Item 6 is not the actual discharge date and the frequency code in Item 4 is that of a final bill.

43 **Scheduled Date of Canceled Surgery.** The date for which ambulatory surgery was scheduled.

44 **Date Occupational Therapy Treatment Started.** Same.

45 **Date Speech Therapy Treatment Started.** Same.

46 **Date Cardiac Rehabilitative Treatment Started.** Same.

47-49 **Payor Codes.** These codes are reserved for use by the payor.

50-69 **Reserved for State Assignment.**

70-99 **Occurrence Span Codes and Dates.** See following section.

A0 **Reserved for National Assignment.**

A1 **Birth Date--Insured A.** The birth date of the insured individual covered by insurance considered as primary payor.

A2 **Effective Date--Insured A** Policy. The date insurance coverage under the primary payor began.

A3 **Benefits Exhausted--Payor A.** The last date for which benefits are available. No payments will be made after this date by the primary payor. This code is to be used by the payor, not the provider of services.

A4-A9 Reserved for National Assignment.
B0 Reserved for National Assignment.
B1 Birth Date--Insured B. The birth date of the insured individual covered by insurance considered as secondary payor.
B2 Effective Date--Insured B Policy. The date insurance coverage under the secondary payor began.
B3 Benefits Exhausted--Payor B. The last date for which benefits are available. No payments will be made after this date by the secondary payor. This code is to be used by the payor, not the provider of services.
B4-B9 Reserved for National Assignment.
C0 Reserved for National Assignment.
C1 Birth Date--Insured C. The birth date of the insured individual covered by insurance considered as tertiary payor.
C2 Effective Date--Insured C Policy. The date insurance coverage under the tertiary payor began.
C3 Benefits Exhausted--Payor C. The last date for which benefits are available. No payments will be made after this date by the tertiary payor. This code is to be used by the payor, not the provider of services.
C4-I9 Reserved for National Assignment.
J0-L9 Reserved for State Assignment.
M0-Z9 Occurrence Span Codes and Dates. See following section.

Item 33, Occurrence Span Codes and Dates

Occurrence span codes and dates refers to the code and the related dates that identify an event relating to the payment of the claim. These codes identify occurrences that happened over a span of time. Therefore, they have both a beginning and an ending date. See the information contained under the heading for Occurrence Codes for further information.
70 Qualifying Stay Dates. The beginning and ending dates of a hospital stay of at least 3 days that qualifies the patient for Medicare payment of SNF services billed. This code may only be used by skilled nursing facilities.

70 Payor Code--Non-utilization Dates. The beginning and ending dates during a PPS inlier stay for which the beneficiary had exhausted all full and/or coinsurance days, but which is covered on the cost report. This code is for payor use only.
71 Prior Stay Dates. The beginning and ending dates given by the patient of any hospital, SNF, or nursing home stay that ended within 60 days of this hospital or SNF admission (HIM 10, 310.1, Item 12).
72 First/Last Visit. The beginning and ending dates of outpatient services. This code is for use on outpatient bills only where the entire billing period is not represented by the billing statement dates reflected in Item 4.
73 Benefit Eligibility Period (Primary Payor). The inclusive dates during which CHAMPUS medical benefits are available to a sponsor's beneficiary as shown on the beneficiary's ID card.
74 Noncovered Level of Care. The beginning and ending dates of noncovered care in an otherwise covered hospital stay. This should exclude any days reported with the use of occurrence span code 76, 77, or 79.
75 SNF Level of Care. The beginning and ending dates of a hospital stay for which SNF care was provided. This code should be used only when the payor has given approval for the patient to remain in the hospital due to a SNF bed not being available. This code should not be used for swing-bed cases. For hospitals under prospective payment, this code is needed in day outlier cases only.
76 Patient Liability. The beginning and ending dates of a Medicare patient's hospital stay for which the hospital is allowed to charge the Medicare beneficiary. This charge may be used only when prior approval for the stay has been received from the PRO or Medicare intermediary and the patient has been notified in writing at least three days prior to the beginning stay date.
77 Provider Liability Period. The beginning and ending dates of noncovered care for which the provider is liable. Utilization is charged.

78 **SNF Prior Stay Dates.** The beginning and ending dates given by the patient of a SNF or nursing home stay that ended within 60 days of this hospital or SNF admission.

79 **Payor Code.** The code is for payor use only.

80-99 **Reserved for State Assignment.**

M0 **PRO/UR Approved Stay Dates.** The beginning and ending dates of a hospital stay that were approved when the entire stay was not approved. Condition codes 3 should be used in Items 24-30.

M1-W9 **Reserved for National Assignment.**

X0-Z9 **Reserved for State Assignment.**

Items 39 – 41, Value Codes And Amounts

These spaces are for **value codes** and their related dollar amounts that identify data of a monetary nature that is necessary for processing the claim. The value code structure is intended to provide reporting capability for those data elements that are widely used but do not warrant dedicated items. The codes should be written in numerical sequence. Negative numbers are not allowed except in Item 41.

01 **Most Common Semiprivate Rate.** To provide for the recording of the hospital's most common semiprivate rate.

02 **Hospital Has No Semiprivate Rooms.** Entering this code requires entering a 0.00 dollar amount.

03 **Reserved for National Assignment.**

04 **Inpatient Professional Component.** The amount shown is the total inpatient professional component charges combined together. For use on Medicare inpatient bills in which there is no Part A eligibility or Part A benefits have been exhausted. Medicare uses the information for internal processing procedures and also for HCFA notice of utilization, which is sent to the patient to explain the Part B coinsurance portion that applies to the patient.

05 **Outpatient Professional Component Included in Charges and Also Billed Separately to Carrier.** For use on Medicare OP bills and all Medicaid bills if State specifies the need for this information.

06 **Medicare Blood Deductible.** Total cash blood deductible, if appropriate. Enter the Part A blood deductible amount.

07 **Reserved for National Assignment.**

08 **Medicare Life Time Reserve Amount.** Medicare life time reserve charged in the year of admission.

09 **Medicare Coinsurance Amount.** Medicare coinsurance amounts charged in the year of admission. This code is to be used only if 08 is used.

10 **Lifetime Reserve Amount in the Second Calendar Year.** The amount of the Medicare lifetime reserve in the year of discharge. This code is only used when the bill's beginning and ending dates fall into two different years.

11 **Coinsurance Amount in the Second Calendar Year.** The amount of the Medicare coinsurance in the year of discharge. This code is only used when the bill's beginning and ending dates fall into 2 different years.

12 **Working Aged Beneficiary/Spouse with Employer Group Health Plan.** The dollar amount shown is the amount that was paid by an employer group health plan whose payments were primary to Medicare. The provider signifies this amount is being applied toward Medicare covered services on this bill.

13 **ESRD Beneficiary in a Medicare Coordination Period with an Employer Group Health Plan.** The dollar amount shown is the amount that was paid on behalf of an ESRD beneficiary by an employer group health plan whose payments were primary to Medicare. The provider signifies this amount is being applied toward Medicare covered services on this bill.

14 **No Fault Auto/Other.** The dollar amount shown is the amount that was paid by no-fault insurance (including auto and other) whose payments were primary to Medicare. The provider signifies this amount is being applied toward Medicare covered services for a Medicare beneficiary on this bill.

15 **Worker's Compensation.** The dollar amount shown is the amount that was paid

by workers' compensation insurance whose payments were primary to Medicare. The provider signifies this amount is being applied toward Medicare covered services for a Medicare beneficiary on this bill.

NOTE: If benefits were reduced due to the failure to file a proper claim, the provider should indicate the amount for codes 12-15 that would have been paid had the claim been properly completed.

16 **PHS or Other Federal Agency.** The dollar amount shown is the amount that was paid by a Public Health Service or the Federal Agency whose payments were primary to Medicare. The provider signifies this amount is being applied toward Medicare covered services for a Medicare beneficiary on this bill.

NOTE: If the provider is claiming conditional payment from Medicare on codes 12-16, six zeros should be entered in the amount item. Conditional payment signifies that no amount has been collected from the other insurance as yet and the provider will repay to Medicare any amounts that are subsequently paid by the other insurance.

17-20 **Payor Codes.** These codes are for payor use only.

Medicaid Specific Codes

21-24 **Reserved for State Assignment.**

25-29 **Reserved for National Medicaid Assignment.**

Code Structure

30 **Preadmission Testing.** The charge for outpatient preadmission testing. Hospital admission should have been previously scheduled.

31 **Patient Liability Amount.** The amount indicated is approved for the provider to charge the beneficiary for noncovered diagnostic services, accommodations, or procedures.

32-36 **Reserved for National Assignment.**

37 **Pints of Blood Furnished.** Total number of pints of whole blood or units of packed red cells furnished to the patient.

38 **Blood Deductible Pints.** The number of unreplaced blood units furnished for which the patient is responsible.

39 **Pints of Blood Replaced.** The number of blood pints or packed blood cells that have been replaced by and on behalf of the patient.

40 **New Coverage not Implemented by HMO.** This code is used when the bill includes inpatient charges for newly covered services that are not paid by the HMO. Condition codes 4 and 78 should also be reported.

41 **Black Lung.** Amount was paid by a Black Lung payment, which was primary to Medicare.

42 **VA.** Amount paid by a VA payment, which payment was primary to Medicare.

43 **Disabled Beneficiary Under Age 65 with Large Group Health Plan.** Amount shown was paid by a large group health plan whose payments were primary to Medicare.

NOTE: If benefits were reduced due to the failure to file a proper claim, the provider should indicate the amount for codes 41 and 43 that would have been paid had the claim been properly completed.

44 **Amount Provider Agreed to Accept from Primary Payor Which Amount is Less Than Charges but Higher Than Payment Received and a Medicare Secondary Payment is Due.** The amount indicated is the amount the provider was required to accept from a primary payor. When this amount is less than the charges, a Medicare secondary payment is due.

45 **Accident Hour.** Medical treatment is the result of an accident. The time of the accident should be indicated in the amount column. Times should be written according to a 24-hour clock. 99 = unknown.

46 **Number of Grace Days.** The number of days necessary to arrange for post-discharge care for the patient. This number is determined by PRO/UR review.

47 **Any Liability Insurance.** Amount shown is the amount paid by liability insurance whose payments were primary to Medicare. If the provider is claiming conditional payment from Medicare, 6 zeros should be entered in the amount item.

48 **Hemoglobin Reading.** The latest hemoglobin reading taken during this billing cycle.

49   **Hematocrit Reading.** The hematocrit reading prior to the last administration of erythropoietin that was given during this billing cycle.

50   **Physical Therapy Visits.**

51   **Occupational Therapy Visits.**

52   **Speech Therapy Visits.**

53   **Cardiac Rehabilitation Visits.**
NOTE: Whole numbers for items 48-53 should be reported in the dollar portion of the item. Items 50-53 should indicate the number of visits given from the outset of the illness until the last date indicated in the billing period.

54-55   **Reserved for National Assignment.**

56   **Skilled Nurse – Home Visit Hours.**

57   **Home Health Aide – Home Visit Hours.**
NOTE: For 56-57 indicate the number of hours provided during the billing period. Only hours spent in the home are counted (exclude travel time). Round to the nearest whole hour.

58   **Arterial Blood Gas (PO2/PA2).** The arterial blood gas value at the beginning of each reporting period for oxygen therapy.

59   **Oxygen Saturation (O2 SAT/Oximetry).** The oxygen saturation count at the beginning of each reporting period for oxygen therapy.
NOTE: Either code 58 or 59 is required on the initial bill and the fourth month bill for oxygen therapy.

60   **(HHA) Branch (MSA).** Metropolitan Statistical Area in which the Home Health Agency is located. If the branch location is different than the HHA location, report the MSA in which the branch is located.

61-67   **Reserved for National Assignment.**

68   **EPO-Drug.** Number of units of erythropoietin administered during the billing period. Report amount in whole units.

69   **Reserved for National Assignment.**

70-72   **Payor Codes.** Reserved for payor use.

73-74   **Reserved for National Assignment.**

75-79   **Payor Codes.** Reserved for payor use.

80   **Most Common Ward Rate.** The hospital's most common ward rate.

81-99   **Reserved for State Assignment.**

A0   **Reserved for National Assignment.**

A1   **Deductible Payor A.** The indicated amount is assumed by the provider to be applied toward the deductible amount for the indicated payor.

A2   **Coinsurance Payor A.** The indicated amount assumed by the provider to be applied toward the coinsurance amount for the indicated payor.

A3   **Estimated Responsibility Payor A.** The indicated amount is the estimated responsibility for the indicated payor.

A4-A9   **Reserved for National Assignment.**

B0   **Reserved for National Assignment.**

B1   **Deductible Payor B.** (See A1).

B2   **Coinsurance Payor B.** (See A2).

B3   **Estimated Responsibility Payor B.** (See A3).

B4-B9   **Reserved for National Assignment.**

C0   **Reserved for National Assignment.**

C1   **Deductible Payor C.** (See A1).

C2   **Coinsurance Payor C.** (See A2).

C3   **Estimated Responsibility Payor C.** (See A3).

C4-C9   **Reserved for National Assignment.**

D0-D2   **Reserved for National Assignment.**

D3   **Estimated Responsibility Patient.** The indicated amount is assumed by the provider to be the estimated responsibility for the patient.

D4-W9   **Reserved for National Assignment.**

X0-Z9   **Reserved for State Assignment.**

Item 42, Hospital Revenue Codes

Hospital revenue codes identify a specific accommodation, ancillary service, or billing calculation. Subcategory classifications and standard abbreviations are listed below each major category. The correct subcategory classification should be added to the major category number to create a three-digit number. The use of a fourth digit has been approved by the NUBC for possible future needs. These four-digit numbers are thus far unassigned and therefore not in use.

For a list of current hospital Revenue Codes, see Appendix 21 – 1.

Item 53, Assignment of Benefits

This assignment of benefits will not allow you to release information regarding the patient. A written authorization to release information, signed by the patient or patient representative, is needed (see Item 53). Please note the certification procedure on the back of the UB-92 before completing this item.

Although the UB-92 eliminates the need to send an assignment of benefits to accident and health insurers, hospitals may wish to be extremely careful in the way in which they handle claims involving property and casualty insurers. Property and casualty insurers may not be familiar with the UB-92 and may not be aware that the wording on the back of the UB-92 is sufficient notification of assignment of benefits. Hospitals may wish to send a copy of the assignment on auto accident and similar non-health-oriented insurance carrier claims.

Item 59, Relationship

Numerical code indicating that the patient is related to the insured in the following manner:

01   **Insured Party.**
02   **Spouse of Insured.**
03   **Child of Insured.**
04   **Natural Child/Insured does not have financial responsibility for child.**
05   **Stepchild of Insured.**
06   **Foster child of Insured.**
07   **Ward of the Court.** Patient is a ward of the insured as a result of court order.
08   **Employee.** Patient is employed by the insured.
09   **Unknown.** Patient's relationship to the insured is unknown.
10   **Handicapped Dependent.** Handicapped dependent whose coverage extends beyond normal termination age limits.
11   **Organ Donor.** Used in cases where a bill is submitted for care given to organ donor where such care is paid for by the receiving patient's insurance coverage.
12   **Cadaver Donor.** Used in cases where a bill is submitted for procedures performed on a cadaver donor and such procedures are paid for by the receiving patient's insurance coverage.
13   **Grandchild of Insured.**
14   **Niece/Nephew of Insured.**
15   **Injured Plaintiff.** Used when patient claims insurance as a result of injury covered by insured.
16   **Sponsored Dependent.** Individual not normally covered by insurance, but coverage has been specially arranged to include relationships such as grandparent or former spouse that would require further investigation by the payor.
17   **Minor Dependent of a Minor Dependent.** Code used when the patient is a dependent minor of a dependent minor of the insured.
18   **Parent of Insured.**
19   **Grandparent.**
20-99   **Reserved.**

Item 64, Employment Status Code

Employment Status Code is used to define the employment status of the individual in Item 63.

1   **Employed Full-Time**
2   **Employed Part-Time**
3   **Not Employed**
4   **Self-Employed**
5   **Retired**
6   **On Active Military Duty**
7-8   **Reserved for National Assignment**
9   **Employment Status Unknown**

Summary

The UB-92 is the claim form used when billing for hospital services. It was created by the National Uniform Billing Committee to allow for the necessary information to be inserted on a single form, thus eliminating the need for attachments.

You should familiarize yourself with the form and know the necessary information. Completely and accurately filling out the UB-92 will help to ensure proper claim payments without unnecessary delays.

Assignments

Complete the Questions for Review.
Complete Exercise 21 – 1.

Questions for Review

Directions: Answer the following questions without looking back into the material just covered. Write your answers in the space provided.

1. What is the UB-92 billing form used for? _____

_____

2. What does item 17 indicate? _____

_____

3. What are occurrence codes and occurrence span codes and what is the difference between them? _____

_____

_____

_____

4. What would the code 20 indicate in item 21 on the UB-92? _____

_____

5. What would the code 03 indicate in item 72 on the UB-92? _____

_____

6. On the UB-92, what is a "Medicare Provider Number"? _____

_____

7. How would you write the following times on a UB-92?

   1. 9:55 a.m. _____   6. 2:48 p.m. _____

   2. 10:25 p.m. _____   7. 5:56 p.m. _____

   3. 1:18 a.m. _____   8. Noon _____

   4. 8:01 p.m. _____   9. Midnight _____

   5. 12:23 a.m. _____   10. 6:06 p.m. _____

8. What does a "Y" in the "Release Information?" item denote? _____

_____

9. A patient entered the hospital on 12/01/XX with chest pains. He was diagnosed as having a heart attack and admitted. On 12/05/XX the patient developed pneumonia. On 12/10/XX the patient expired due to causes associated with pneumonia. On 12/12/XX you bill the insurance company for services rendered through 12/04/XX. What is the proper diagnosis for the patient? _____

10. Are the source of admission codes the same for a newborn baby as they are for an adult? _____

_____

If you were unable to answer any of the questions, refer back to that section, and then fill in the answers.

Exercise 21 – 1

Directions: Bill the following services on a UB-92. Use the patient data from the patient charts completed in Exercise 5 – 1. In all cases, the hospital is Commerce Union Medical Center, 1029 Commerce Way, Dubuque, Iowa 52000.

1. Abby Addison was brought into the ER of Union Medical Center on 3/7/XX, after losing consciousness at home. Patient states she had seen her provider three days ago and he had instructed her to rest. However she felt she needed to go to work. Her condition has progressed from influenza to pneumonia. Annette Adams was the attending physician. The following hospital charges were incurred by Abby:

Item	# Days or Units	Cost	Total Charge
Room and Board	3	$395.00	$1185.00
Pharmacy	23		845.00
IV Therapy	21		386.15
Med-Surg Supplies	18		224.25
Laboratory	36		727.00
Respiratory Services	3		269.35
EKG/ECG	1		161.53
SUBTOTAL			**$3,798.28**
PAYMENTS/ADJUSTMENTS			**$ 0.00**
BALANCE DUE			**$3,798.28**

2. Bobby Bumble entered the hospital on 3/30/XX with a ruptured appendix. Brett Barron was the attending physician. The following hospital charges were incurred by Bobby:

Item	# Days or Units	Cost	Total Charge
Room and Board	4	$395.00	$1,580.00
Pharmacy	42		1,567.50
Laboratory	23		983.30
IV Therapy	14		561.50
Med-Surg Supplies	39		1,937.25
Pathology Lab	10		110.50
Dx X-Ray	12		898.90
OR Services	8		977.50
Anesthesia	1		882.25
Respiratory Services	2		74.75
Recovery Room	1		241.45
SUBTOTAL			**$9,814.90**
PAYMENTS/ADJUSTMENTS			**$ 500.00**
BALANCE DUE			**$9,314.90**

3. Cathy Crenshaw entered the hospital emergency room on 4/1/XX for treatment of a fractured arm. Carol Carpenter was the attending physician. The following hospital charges were incurred by Cathy:

Item	# Days or Units	Cost	Total Charge
ER	1		$250.00
Pharmacy	2		75.25
X-Ray	4		147.50
SUBTOTAL			**$472.75**
PAYMENTS/ADJUSTMENTS			**$ 0.00**
BALANCE DUE			**$472.75**

4. Daisy Doolittle entered the hospital for treatment of acute pelvic inflammatory disease on 4/1/XX. Deborah Davidson was attending physician. The following hospital charges were incurred by Daisy:

Item	# Days or Units	Cost	Total Charge
Room and Board	3	$395.00	$1,185.00
Pharmacy	31		321.50
Laboratory	9		314.25
Med-Surg Supplies	19		783.15
Path Lab	11		652.70
IV Therapy	4		89.60
Ultrasound	2		685.20
SUBTOTAL			**$4,031.40**
PAYMENTS/ADJUSTMENTS			**$ 0.00**
BALANCE DUE			**$4,031.40**

5. Edward Edmunds entered the hospital for surgery on his shoulder on 3/10/XX. Edward had tendonitis with calcium deposits on his shoulder which restricted movement. The following hospital charges were incurred by Edward:

Item	# Days or Units	Cost	Total Charge
Room and Board	2	$395.00	$790.00
Pharmacy	12		567.50
Laboratory	6		483.30
IV Therapy	3		361.50
Med-Surg Supplies	37		937.25
Pathology Lab	7		95.50
Dx X-Ray	6		298.40
OR Services	1		928.50
Anesthesia	1		875.25
Respiratory Services	4		74.75
Recovery Room	1		236.45
SUBTOTAL			**$5,648.40**
PAYMENTS/ADJUSTMENTS			**$ 0.00**
BALANCE DUE			**$5,648.40**

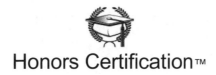

Honors Certification™

The certification challenge for this chapter will be a written test of the information contained in this chapter. Each incorrect answer will result in a deduction of up to 5% from your grade. You must achieve a score of 85% or higher to pass this test. If you fail the test on your first attempt you may retake the test one additional time. The items included in the second test may be different from those in the first test.

Appendix 21 – 1

Hospital Revenue Codes

Major Category Subcategory (Standard Abbreviation)

001 **Total Charges.** To reflect the total of all charges on this bill.

01X **Reserved for internal payor use.**

02X-06X **Reserved for National Assignment.**

07X-09X **Reserved for State Assignment.**

10X **All-Inclusive Rate.** Flat fee charge incurred on either a daily basis or total stay basis for services rendered. Charge may cover room and board plus ancillary services or room and board only.
   0   All-inclusive room and board plus ancillary (ALL-INCL R&B/ANC)
   1   All-inclusive room and board (ALL INCL R&B)

11X **Room and Board--Private (Medical or General).** Routine service charges for single-bed rooms.
   0   General Classification (R&B/PVT)
   1   Medical/Surgical/Gyn (MED-SUR-GYN/PVT)
   2   OB (OB/PVT)
   3   Pediatric (PEDS/PVT)
   4   Psychiatric (PSYCH/PVT)
   5   Hospice (HOSPICE/PVT)
   6   Detoxification (DETOX/PVT)
   7   Oncology (ONCOLOGY/PVT)
   8   Rehabilitation (REHAB/PVT)
   9   Other (OTHER/PVT)

12X **Room and Board--Semiprivate Two-Bed (Medical or General).** Routine service charges incurred for accommodations with two beds.
   0   General Classification (R&B/SEMI)
   1   Medical/Surgical/Gyn (MED-SUR-GYN/2 Bed)
   2   OB (OB/2 Bed)
   3   Pediatric (PEDS/2 Bed)
   4   Psychiatric (PSYCH/2 Bed)
   5   Hospice (HOSPICE/2 Bed)
   6   Detoxification (DETOX/2 Bed)
   7   Oncology (ONCOLOGY/2 Bed)
   8   Rehabilitation (REHAB/2 Bed)
   9   Other (OTHER/2 Bed)

13X **Semiprivate--Three and Four Beds.** Routine service charges incurred for accommodations with three and four beds.
   0   General Classification (R&B/3&4 Bed)
   1   Medical/Surgical/Gyn (MED-SUR-GYN/3&4 Bed)
   2   OB (OB/3&4 Bed)
   3   Pediatric (PEDS/3&4 Bed)
   4   Psychiatric (PSYCH/3&4 Bed)
   5   Hospice (HOSPICE/3&4 Bed)
   6   Detoxification (DETOX/3&4 Bed)
   7   Oncology (ONCOLOGY/3&4 Bed)
   8   Rehabilitation (REHAB/3&4 Bed)
   9   Other (OTHER/3&4 Bed)

14X **Private (Deluxe).** Deluxe rooms are accommodations with amenities substantially in excess of those provided to other patients.
   0   General Classification (R&B/PVT/ DLX)
   1   Medical/Surgical/Gyn (MED-SUR-GYN/DLX)
   2   OB (OB/DLX)
   3   Pediatric (PEDS/DLX)
   4   Psychiatric (PSYCH/DLX)
   5   Hospice (HOSPICE/DLX)
   6   Detoxification (DETOX/DLX)
   7   Oncology (ONCOLOGY/DLX)
   8   Rehabilitation (REHAB/DLX)
   9   Other (OTHER/DLX)

15X **Room and Board--Ward (Medical or General).** Routine service charge for accommodations with five or more beds.
   0   General Classification (R&B/ WARD)
   1   Medical/Surgical/Gyn (MED-SUR-GYN/WARD)
   2   OB (OB/WARD)
   3   Pediatric (PEDS/WARD)
   4   Psychiatric (PSYCH/WARD)
   5   Hospice (HOSPICE/WARD)
   6   Detoxification (DETOX/WARD)
   7   Oncology (ONCOLOGY/WARD)
   8   Rehabilitation (REHAB/WARD)
   9   Other (OTHER/WARD)

16X **Other Room and Board.** Any routine service charges for accommodations that cannot be included in the more specific revenue center codes.
   0   General Classification (R&B)
   4   Sterile Environment (R&B/STRL)
   7   Self-Care (R&B/SELF)
   9   Other (R&B/Other)

17X **Nursery.** Charges for nursing care to newborn and premature infants in nurseries.
   0   General Classification (NURSERY)
   1   Newborn (NURSERY/NEWBORN)
   2   Premature (NURSERY/PREMIE)
   5   Neonatal ICU (NURSERY/ICU)
   9   Other (NURSERY/OTHER)

18X **Leave of Absence.** Charges for holding a room while the patient is temporarily away from the provider.
   0   General Classification (LOA)
   1   Reserved (RESERVED)
   2   Patient Convenience (LOA/PT CONV)
   3   Therapeutic Leave (LOA THER)
   4   ICF/MR--any reason (LOA/ICF/ MR)
   5   Nursing Home (for hospitalization) (LOA/NURS HOME)
   6   Other Leave of Absence (LOA/OTHER)

19X **Not Assigned.**

20X **Intensive Care.** Routine service charge for medical or surgical care provided to patients who require a more intensive level of care than is rendered with the general medical or surgical unit.
   0   General Classification (ICU)

1 Surgical (ICU/SURGICAL)
2 Medical (ICU/MEDICAL)
3 Pediatric (ICU/PEDS)
4 Psychiatric (ICU/PSYCH)
6 Post-ICU (POST ICU)
7 Burn Care (ICU/BURN CARE)
8 Trauma (ICU/TRAUMA)
9 Other Intensive Care (ICU/OTHER)

21X **Coronary Care.** Routine service charge for medical or surgical care provided to patients with coronary illness who require a more intensive level of care than is rendered in the general medical care unit.
0 General Classification (CCU)
1 Myocardial Infarction (CCU/MYO INFARC)
2 Pulmonary Care (CCU/PULMON)
3 Heart Transplant (CCU/TRANS-PLANT)
4 Post-CCU (POST CCU)
9 Other Coronary Care (CCU/OTHR)

22X **Special Charges.** Charges incurred during an inpatient stay or on a daily basis for certain services.
0 General Classification (SPCL CHGS)
1 Admission Charge (ADMIT CHG)
2 Technical Support Charge (TECH SUPPT CHG)
3 UR Service Charge (UR CHG)
4 Late Discharge, Medically Necessary (LATE DISCH/MED NEC)
9 Other Special Charges (OTHER SPEC CHG)

23X **Incremental Nursing Charge Rate.** Charge for nursing service assessed in addition to room and board.
0 General Classification (NURSING INCREM)
1 Nursery (NUR INCR/NURSERY)
2 OB (NUR INCR/OB)
3 ICU (NUR INCR/ICU)
4 CCU (NUR INCR/CCU)
5 Hospice (NUR INCR/HOSPICE)
9 Other (NUR INCR/OTHER)

24X **All-Inclusive Ancillary.** A flat rate incurred on either a daily basis or total stay basis for ancillary services only.
0 General Classification (ALL INCL ANCIL)
9 Other Inclusive Ancillary (ALL INCL ANCIL/OTHER)

25X **Pharmacy.** Charges for medication produced, manufactured, packaged, controlled, assayed, dispensed, and distributed under the direction of licensed pharmacist. This category includes blood plasma, other components of blood, and IV solutions.
0 General Classification (PHAR)
1 Generic Drugs (DRUGS/GENRC)
2 Nongeneric Drugs (DRUGS/ NONGENRC)
3 Take Home Drugs (DRUGS/ TAKEHOME)
4 Drugs Incident to Other Diagnostic Services (DRUGS/INCIDENT OTHER DX)
5 Drugs Incident to Radiology (DRUGS/INCIDENT RAD)
6 Experimental Drugs (DRUGS/ EXPERIMT)
7 Nonprescription (DRUGS/ NONPSCRPT)
8 IV Solutions (IV SOLUTIONS)
9 Other Pharmacy (DRUGS/OTHER)

26X **IV Therapy.** Administration of intravenous solution by specially trained personnel to individuals requiring such treatment.
0 General Classification (IV THER)
2 Infusion Pump (IV THER/INFSN PUMP)

3 IV Therapy--Pharmacy Services (IV THER/PHARM/SVC)
4 IV Therapy/Drug/Supply Delivery (IV THER/DRUG/SUPPLY DELV)
9 Other IV Therapy (IV THERP/ OTHER)
NOTE: Providers billing for home IV therapy should use the HCPCS code that describes the pump in Item 44.

27X **Medical/Surgical Supplies and Devices.** Charges for supply items required for patient care.
0 General Classification (MED-SUR SUPPLIES)
1 Nonsterile Supply (NON-STER SUPPLY)
2 Sterile Supply (STERILE SUPPLY)
3 Take Home Supplies (TAKE HOME SUPPLY)
4 Prosthetic/Orthotic Devices (PROSTH/ORTH DEV)
5 Pacemaker (PACE MAKER)
6 Intraocular Lens (INTRA OC LENS)
7 Oxygen-Take Home (O2/ TAKEHOME)
8 Other Implants (SUPPLY/ IMPLANTS)
9 Other Supplies/Devices (SUPPLY/ OTHER)

28X **Oncology.** Charges for the treatment of tumors and related diseases.
0 General Classification ONCOLOGY
9 Other Oncology (ONCOLOGY/ OTHER)

29X **Durable Medical Equipment (Other Than Renal).** Charge for medical equipment that can withstand repeated use (excluding renal equipment).
0 General Classification (DME)
1 Rental (MED EQUIP/RENT)
2 Purchase of new DME (MED EQUIP/NEW)
3 Purchase of used DME (MED EQUIP/USED)
4 Supplies/Drugs for DME Effectiveness (Home Health Agency Only) (MED EQUIP/SUPPLIES/ DRUGS)
9 Other Equipment (MED EQUIP/ OTHER)

30X **Laboratory.** Charges for the performance of diagnostic and routine clinical laboratory tests.
0 General Classification (LAB)
1 Chemistry (LAB/CHEMISTRY)
2 Immunology (LAB/IMMUNLGY)
3 Renal Patient (Home) (LAB/RENAL HOME)
4 Nonroutine Dialysis (LAB/NR DIALYSIS)
5 Hematology (LAB/HEMAT)
6 Bacteriology & Microbiology (LAB/BACT-MICRO)
7 Urology (LAB/UROLOGY)
9 Other Laboratory (LAB/OTHER)

31X **Laboratory Pathological.** Charges for diagnostic and routine laboratory tests on tissues and culture.
0 General Classification (PATH LAB)
1 Cytology (PATHOL/CYTOLOGY)
2 Histology (PATHOL/HYSTOL)
4 Biopsy (PATHOL/BIOPSY)
9 Other (PATHOL/OTHER)

32X **Radiology--Diagnostic.** Charges for diagnostic radiology services provided for the examination and care of patients. Includes taking, processing, examining, and interpreting radiographs and fluorographs.
0 General Classification (DX X-RAY)
1 Angiocardiography (DX X-RAY/ ANGIO)
2 Arthrography (DX X-RAY/ARTH)
3 Arteriography (DX X-RAY/ ARTER)
4 Chest X-Ray (DX X-RAY/CHEST)
9 Other (DX X-RAY/OTHER)

33X **Radiology--Therapeutic.** Charges for therapeutic radiology services and chemotherapy are required for care and treatment of patients. Included therapy by injection or ingestion of radioactive substances.
- 0   General Classification (RX X-RAY)
- 1   Chemotherapy--Injected (CHEMOTHER/INJ)
- 2   Chemotherapy--Oral (CHEMOTHER/ORAL)
- 3   Radiation Therapy (RADIATION RX)
- 5   Chemotherapy--IV (CHEMOTHERP-IV)
- 9   Other (RX X-RAY/OTHER)

34X **Nuclear Medicine.** Charges for procedures and tests performed by a radioisotope laboratory utilizing radioactive materials as required for diagnosis and treatment of patients.
- 0   General Classification (NUC MED)
- 1   Diagnostic (NUC MED/DX)
- 2   Therapeutic (NUC MED/RX)
- 9   Other (NUC MED/OTHER)

35X **CT Scan.** Charges for computed tomographic scans of the head and other parts of the body.
- 0   General Classification (CT SCAN)
- 1   Head Scan (CT SCAN/HEAD)
- 2   Body Scan (CT SCAN/BODY)
- 9   Other CT Scans (CT SCAN/OTHR)

36X **Operating Room Services.** Charges for services provided to patients in the performance of surgical and related procedures during and immediately following surgery.
- 0   General Classification (OR SERVICES)
- 1   Minor Surgery (OR/MINOR)
- 2   Organ Transplant--Other than kidney (OR/ORGAN TRANS)
- 7   Kidney Transplant (OR/KIDNEY TRANS)
- 9   Other Operating Room Services (OR/OTHER)

37X **Anesthesia.** Charges for anesthesia services in the hospital.
- 0   General Classification (ANESTHE)
- 1   Anesthesia Incident to Radiology (ANESTHE/INCIDENT RAD)
- 2   Anesthesia Incident to Other Diagnostic Services (ANESTHE/ INCDNT OTHER DX)
- 4   Acupuncture (ANESTHE/ ACUPUNC)
- 9   Other Anesthesia (ANESTHE/ OTHER)

38X **Blood.**
- 0   General Classification (BLOOD)
- 1   Packed Red Cells (BLOOD/PKD RED)
- 2   Whole Blood (BLOOD/WHOLE)
- 3   Plasma (BLOOD/PLASMA)
- 4   Platelets (BLOOD PLATELETS)
- 5   Leucocytes (BLOOD/ LEUCOCYTES)
- 6   Other Components (BLOOD/ COMPONENTS)
- 7   Other Derivatives (Cryoprecipitates) (BLOOD/DERIVATIVES)
- 9   Other Blood (BLOOD/OTHER)

39X **Blood Storage and Processing.** Charges for storage and processing of whole blood.
- 0   General Classification (BLOOD/ STOR-PROC)
- 1   Blood Administration (BLOOD/ ADMIN)
- 9   Other Blood Storage and Processing (BLOOD/OTHER STOR)

40X **Other Imaging Services.**
- 0   General Classification (IMAGE SVS)

- 1   Diagnostic Mammography (DIAG MAMMOGRAPHY)
- 2   Ultrasound (ULTRASOUND)
- 3   Screening Mammography (SCRN MAMMOGRAPHY)
- 4   Positron Emission Tomography (PET SCAN)
- 9   Other Imaging Services (OTHER IMAGE SVS)
  NOTE: High-risk beneficiaries should be noted by the inclusion of one of the following ICD-9 diagnosis codes:
- V10.3   Personal History--Malignant neoplasm breast cancer
- V16.3   Family History--Malignant neoplasm breast cancer (mother, sister or daughter with breast cancer)
- V15.89   Other specified personal history representing hazards to health (not given birth prior to 30, a personal history of biopsy proven breast disease). Must be coded to the appropriate 4th or 5th digit.

41X **Respiratory Services.** Charges for administration of oxygen and certain potent drugs through inhalation or positive pressure and other forms of rehabilitative therapy through measurement of inhaled and exhaled gases and analysis of blood and evaluation of the patient's ability to exchange oxygen and other gases.
- 0   General Classification (RESPIR SVC)
- 2   Inhalation Services (INHALATION SVC)
- 3   Hyperbaric Oxygen Therapy (HYPERBARIC O2)
- 9   Other Respiratory Services (OTHER RESPIR SVS)

42X **Physical Therapy.** Charges for therapeutic exercises, massage, and utilization of light, heat, cold, water, electricity, and assistive devices for diagnosis and rehabilitation of patients who have neuromuscular, orthopedic, and other disabilities.
- 0   General Classification (PHYS THERP)
- 1   Visit Charge (PHYS THERP/ VISIT)
- 2   Hourly Charge (PHYS THERP/ HOUR)
- 3   Group Rate (PHYS THERP/ GROUP)
- 4   Evaluation or Reevaluation (PHYS THER/EVAL)
- 9   Other Physical Therapy (OTHER PHYS THERP)

43X **Occupational Therapy.** Charges for teaching manual skills and independent personal care to stimulate mental and emotional activity on the part of patients.
- 0   General Classification (OCCUP THERP)
- 1   Visit Charge (OCCUP THERP/ VISIT)
- 2   Hourly Charge (OCCUP THERP/ HOUR)
- 3   Group Rate (OCCUP THERP/ GROUP)
- 4   Evaluation or Reevaluation (OCCUP THER/EVAL)
- 9   Other Occupational Therapy (OTHER OCCUP THERP)

44X **Speech-Language Pathology.** Charges for services provided to persons with impaired functional communications skills.
- 0   General Classification (SPEECH PATHOL)
- 1   Visit Charge (SPEECH PATH/ VISIT)
- 2   Hourly Charge (SPEECH PATH/ HOUR)
- 3   Group Rate (SPEECH PATH/ GROUP)
- 4   Evaluation or Reevaluation (SPEECH PATH/EVAL)
- 9   Other Speech-Language Pathology (OTHER SPEECH PAT)

45X **Emergency Room.** Charges for emergency treatment to those ill and injured persons who require immediate unscheduled medical or surgical care.
- 0   General Classification (EMERG ROOM)
- 9   Other Emergency Room (OTHER EMER ROOM)

46X **Pulmonary Function.** Charges for tests that measure inhaled and exhaled gases and analysis of blood and for tests that evaluate the patient's ability to exchange oxygen and other gases.
0   General Classification (PULMON FUNC)
9   Other Pulmonary Function (OTHER PULMON FUNC)

47X **Audiology.** Charges for the detection and management of communication handicaps centering in whole or in part on the hearing function.
0   General Classification (AUDIOL)
1   Diagnostic (AUDIOLOGY/DX)
2   Treatment (AUDIOLOGY/RX)
9   Other Audiology (OTHER AUDIOL)

48X **Cardiology.** Charges for cardiac procedures rendered in a separate unit within the hospital. Such procedures include but are not limited to heart catheterization, coronary angiography, Swan-Ganz catheterization, and exercise stress test.
0   General Classification (CARDIOL)
1   Cardiac Cath Lab (CARDIAC CATH LAB)
2   Stress Test (STRESS TEST)
9   Other Cardiology (OTHER CARDIOL)

49X **Ambulatory Surgical Care.**
0   General Classification (AMBUL SURG)
9   Other Ambulatory Surgical Care (OTHER AMBL SURG)

50X **Outpatient Services.** Outpatient charges for services rendered to an outpatient who is admitted as an inpatient before midnight of the day following the date of service. These charges are incorporated on the inpatient bill of Medicare patients.
0   General Classification (OUTPATIENT SVS)
9   Other Outpatient Services (OUTPATIENT/OTHER)

51X **Clinic.** Clinic (nonemergency/scheduled outpatient visit) charges for providing diagnostic, preventive, curative, rehabilitative, and education services on a scheduled basis to ambulatory patients.
0   General Classification (CLINIC)
1   Chronic Pain Center (CHRONIC PAIN CL)
2   Dental Clinic (DENTAL CLINIC)
3   Psychiatric Clinic (PSYCH CLINIC)
4   OB-GYN Clinic (OB-GYN CLINIC)
5   Pediatric Clinic (PEDS CLINIC)
9   Other Clinic (OTHER CLINIC)

52X **Free-Standing Clinic.**
0   General Classification (FR/STD CLINIC)
1   Rural Health--Clinic (RURAL/ CLINIC)
2   Rural Health--Home (RURAL/ HOME)
3   Family Practice (FAMILY PRAC)
9   Other Freestanding Clinic (OTHER FR/STD CLINIC)

53X **Osteopathic Services.** Charges for a structural evaluation of the cranium, entire cervical, dorsal, and lumbar spine by a doctor of osteopathy.
0   General Classification (OSTEOPATH SVS)
1   Osteopathic Therapy (OSTEOPATH RX)
9   Other Osteopathic Services (OTHER OSTEOPATH)

54X **Ambulance.** Charges for ambulance service, usually unscheduled, to the ill/ injured who require immediate medical attention.
0   General Classification (AMBUL)

1   Supplies (AMBUL/SUPPLY)
2   Medical Transport (AMBUL/MED TRANS)
3   Heart Mobile (AMBUL/ HEARTMOBL)
4   Oxygen (AMBUL/OXY)
5   Air Ambulance (AIR AMBUL)
6   Neonatal Ambulance Services (AMBUL/NEONAT)
7   Pharmacy (AMBUL/PHARMACY)
8   Telephone Transmission EKG (AMBUL/TELEPHONIC EKG)
9   Other Ambulance (OTHER AMBULANCE)
NOTE: Units may be either miles or trips.
NOTE: On items 55-58, charges should be reported to the nearest hour.

55X **Skilled Nursing.** Charges for nursing services that must be provided under the direct supervision of a licensed nurse to ensure the safety of the patient and to achieve the medically desired result. This code may be used for nursing home services or a service charge for home health billing.
0   General Classification (SKILLED NURS)
1   Visit Charge (SKILLED NURS/ VISIT)
2   Hourly Charge (SKILLED NURS/ HOUR)
9   Other Skilled Nursing (SKILLED NURS/OTHER)

56X **Medical Social Services.** Charges for services such as counseling patients, interviewing patients, and interpreting problems of social situation rendered to patients on any basis.
0   General Classification (MED SOCIAL SVS)
1   Visit Charge (MED SOC SERVS/ VISIT)
2   Hourly Charge (MED SOC SERVS/HOUR)
9   Other Medical Social Services (MED SOCIAL SERVS/OTHER)

57X **Home Health Aide (Home Health).** Charges made by a home health agency for personnel that are primarily responsible for the personal care of the patient.
0   General Classification (AIDE/ HOME HEALTH)
1   Visit Charge (AIDE/HOME HLTH/ VISIT)
2   Hourly Charge (AIDE/HOME HLTH/HOUR)
9   Other Home Health Aide (AIDE/ HOME HLTH/OTHER)

58X **Other Visits (Home Health).** Charges by a home health agency for visits other than physical therapy, occupational therapy or speech therapy, which must be specifically identified.
0   General Classification (VISIT/ HOME HEALTH)
1   Visit Charge (VISIT/HOME HLTH/ VISIT)
2   Hourly Charge (VISIT/HOME HLTH/HOUR)
9   Other Home Health (VISIT/HOME HLTH/OTHER)

59X **Units of Service (Home Health).** Revenue code used by a home health agency that bills on the basis of units of service.
0   General Classification (UNIT/ HOME HEALTH)
9   Home Health Other Units (UNIT/ HOME HLTH/OTHER)

60X **Oxygen Home Health.** Charges by a home health agency for oxygen equipment, supplies, or contents, excluding purchased items. If a beneficiary has purchased a stationary oxygen system, and oxygen concentrator or portable equipment, revenue codes 292 or 293 apply. DME other than oxygen systems is billed under codes 291, 292, or 293.
0   General Classification (O2/HOME HEALTH)

1   Oxygen--Stationary Equipment, Supplies or Contents (O2/STAT EQUIP/SUPPL/CONT)
2   Oxygen--Stationary Equipment or Supplies Under 1 LPM (O2/STAT EQUIP/UNDER 1 LPM)
3   Oxygen--Stationary Equipment or Supplies Over 4 LPM (O2/STAT EQUIP/OVER 4 LPM)
4   Oxygen--Portable Add-on (O2/ PORTABLE ADD-ON)

61X   **MRI.** Charges for Magnetic Resonance Imaging of the brain and other parts of the body.
0   General Classification (MRI)
1   Brain (including brain stem) (MRI-BRAIN)
2   Spinal Cord (including spine) (MRI-SPINE)
9   Other MRI (MRI-OTHER)

62X   **Medical/Surgical Supplies.** Charges for supplies required for patient care. This code is an extension of code 27X and allows for the reporting of additional breakdown, if needed. Subcategory 1 is for providers who are not able to bill supplies used for radiology procedures under radiology. Subcategory 2 is for providers who are not able to bill supplies used for other diagnostic procedures under diagnostic procedures.
1   Supplies Incident to Radiology (MED-SUR SUPP/INCDNT RAD)
2   Supplies Incident to Other Diagnostic Services (MED-SUR UPP/INCDNT ODX)

63X   **Drugs Requiring Specific identification.** Charges for drugs and biologicals requiring specific identification required by the payor. If you are using HCPCS to identify the drug, the HCPCS code should be entered in Item 44.
0   General Classification (DRUGS)
1   Single Source Drug (DRUG/ SNGLE)
2   Multiple Source Drug (DRUG/ MULT)
3   Restrictive Prescription (DRUG/ RSTR)
4   Erythropoietin (EPO) less than 10,000 units (DRUG/EPO 10,000 Units)
5   Erythropoietin (EPO) more than 10,000 units (DRUG/EPO 10,000 Units)
6   Drugs requiring detailed coding (DRUGS/DETAIL CODE)
NOTE: Revenue Code 636 relates to a HCPCS code. Therefore, the appropriate HCPCS code should be entered in Item 44. The specific units of services to be reported should be in hundreds (100s) rounded to the nearest hundred.

64X   **Home IV Therapy Services.** Charge for IV drug therapy services that are done in the patient's home. For home IV providers, the appropriate HCPCS code must be entered for all equipment and covered therapy.
0   General Classification (IV THER SVC)
1   Nonroutine Nursing, Central Line (NON RT NURSING/CENTRAL)
2   IV Site Care, Central Line, HCPCS related(IV SITE CARE/CENTRAL)
3   IV Start/Change Peripheral Line (IV STRT/CHNG/PERIPHRL)
4   Nonroutine Nursing Peripheral Line (NON RT NURSING/PERIPHRL)
5   Training Patient/Caregiver, Central Line (TRNG PT/CAREGVR/ CENTRAL)
6   Training Disabled Patient, Central Line (TRNG DSBLPT/CENTRAL)

7   Training Patient/Caregiver, Peripheral Line (TRNG PT/ CAREGVR/PERIPHRL)
8   Training Disabled Patient, Peripheral Line (TRNG DSBLPT/ PERIPHRL)
9   Other IV Therapy Services (OTHER IV THERAPY SVC)
NOTE: Units need to be reported in 1-hour increments.

65X   **Hospice Service.** Charges for hospice care services for a terminally ill patient. The patient would need to elect these services in lieu of other services for a terminal condition.
0   General Classification (HOSPICE)
1   Routine Home Care (HOSPICE/RTN HOME)
2   Continuous Home Care (HOSPICE/ CTNS HOME)
3   RESERVED
4   RESERVED
5   Inpatient Respite Care (HOSPICE/ IP RESPITE)
6   General Inpatient Care (Nonrespite) (HOSPICE/IP NONRESPITE)
7   Physician Services (HOSPICE/ PHYSICIAN)
9   Other Hospice (HOSPICE/OTHER)
NOTE: There must be a minimum of 8 hours of care (not necessarily continuous) during a 24-hour period to receive the Continuous Home Care rate from Medicare under code 652. If less than 8 hours of care are provided, code 651 should be used. Any portion of an hour counts as an hour.
    When billing Medicare under code 657, a physician procedure code must be entered in Item 44. Code 657 is used by the hospice to bill for physician's services furnished to hospice patients when the physician is employed by the hospice or receives payment from the hospice for services rendered.

66X   **Respite Care.** Charges for hours of service under the Respite Care Benefit for homemaker or home health aide, personal care services, and nursing care provided by a licensed professional nurse.
0   General Classification (RESPITE CARE)
1   Hourly Charge/Skilled Nursing (RESPITE/SKILLED NURSE)
2   Hourly Charge/Home Health Aide/ Homemaker (RESPITE/HMEAID/ HMEMKR

67X   **Not Assigned.**

68X   **Not Assigned.**

69X   **Not Assigned.**

70X   **Cast Room.** Charges for services related to the application, maintenance, and removal of casts.
0   General Classification (CAST ROOM)
9   Other Cast Room (OTHER CAST ROOM)

71X   **Recovery Room.**
0   General Classification (RECOV RM)
9   Other Recovery Room (OTHER RECOV RM)

72X   **Labor Room/Delivery.** Charges for labor and delivery room services provided by specially trained nursing personnel to patients, including prenatal care during labor, assistance during delivery, postnatal care in the recovery room, and minor gynecological procedures if they are performed in the delivery suite.
0   General Classification (DELIVROOM/LABOR)
1   Labor (LABOR)

2 Delivery (DELIVERY ROOM)
3 Circumcision (CIRCUMCISION)
4 Birthing Center (BIRTHING CENTER)
9 Other Labor Room/Delivery (OTHER/DELIV-LABOR)

73X EKG/ECG (Electrocardiogram). Charges for operation of specialized equipment to record electromotive variations in actions of the heart muscle on an electrocardiograph for diagnosis of heart ailments.
0 General Classification (EKG/ECG)
1 Holter Monitor (HOLTER MON)
2 Telemetry (TELEMETRY)
9 Other EKG/ECG (OTHER EKG/ECG)

74X EEG (Electroencephalogram). Charges for operation of specialized equipment to measure impulse frequencies and differences in electrical potential in various areas of the brain to obtain data for use in diagnosing brain disorders.
0 General Classification (EEG)
9 Other EEG (OTHER EEG)

75X Gastrointestinal Services.
0 General Classification (GASTR-INTS SVS)
9 Other Gastrointestinal (OTHER GASTROINTS)
   NOTE: Use 759 with the procedure code for endoscopic procedure.

76X Treatment/Observation Room. Charges for the use of a treatment room, or observation room charges for outpatient observation services.
0 General Classification (TREATMT/OBSERVATION RM)
1 Treatment Room (TREATMT RM)
2 Observation Room (OBSERV RM)
9 Other Treatment/Observation Room (OTHER TREAT/OBSERV RM)

77X Not Assigned.

78X Not Assigned.

79X Lithotripsy. Charges for using lithotripsy in the treatment of kidney stones.
0 General Classification (LITHOTRIPSY)
9 Other Lithotripsy (LITHOTRIPSY/ OTHER)

80X Inpatient Renal Dialysis. A waste removal process that uses an artificial kidney when the body's own kidneys have failed. The waste may be removed directly from the blood (hemodialysis) or indirectly from the blood by flushing a special solution between the abdominal covering and the tissue (peritoneal dialysis). In-unit lab nonroutine tests are medically necessary tests in addition to or at greater frequency than routine tests that are performed in the dialysis unit.
0 General Classification (RENAL DIALY)
1 Inpatient Hemodialysis (DIALY/ INPT)
2 Inpatient Peritoneal (Non-CAPD) (DIALY/INPT/PER)
3 Inpatient Continuous Ambulatory Peritoneal Dialysis (DIALY/ INPT/CAPD)
4 Inpatient Continuous Cycling Peritoneal Dialysis (DIALY/ INPT/CCPD)
9 Other Inpatient Dialysis (DIALY/ INPT/OTHER)

81X Organ Acquisition. The acquisition of a kidney, liver, or heart for use in transplantation. Organs other than these are included in category 89X. Living donor is a living person from whom kidney is obtained for transplantation.

Cadaver is an individual who has been pronounced dead according to medical and legal criteria from whom organs have been obtained for transplantation.
0 General Classification (ORGAN ACQUISIT)
1 Living Donor--Kidney (KIDNEY/ LIVE)
2 Cadaver Donor--Kidney (KIDNEY/ CADAVER)
3 Unknown Donor--Kidney (KIDNEY/UNKNOWN)
4 Other Kidney Acquisition (KIDNEY/OTHER)
5 Cadaver Donor--Heart (HEART/ CADAVER)
6 Other Heart Acquisition (HEART/ OTHER)
7 Donor--Liver (LIVER ACQUISIT)
9 Other Organ Acquisition (ORGAN/ OTHER)

82X Hemodialysis--Outpatient or Home. A program under which a patient performs hemodialysis away from the facility using his or her own equipment and supplies. Hemodialysis is the removal of waste directly from the blood.
0 General Classification (HEMO/OP OR HOME)
1 Hemodialysis/Composite or Other Rate (HEMO/COMPOSITE)
2 Home Supplies (HEMO/HOME/ SUPPL)
3 Home Equipment (HEMO/HOME/ EQUIP)
4 Maintenance 100% (HEMO/HOME/ 100%)
5 Support Services (HEMO/HOME/ SUPSERV)
9 Other Outpatient Hemodialysis (HEMO/HOME/OTHER)

83X Peritoneal Dialysis--Outpatient or Home. A program under which a patient performs peritoneal dialysis away from the facility using his or her own equipment and supplies. Waste is removed by flushing a special solution between the tissue and the abdominal covering.
0 General Classification (PERTNL/ OP OR HOME)
1 Peritoneal/Composite or Other Rate (PERTNL/COMPOSITE)
2 Home Supplies (PERTNL/HOME/ SUPPL)
3 Home Equipment (PERTNL/ HOME/EQUIP)
4 Maintenance 100% (PERTNL/ HOME/100%)
5 Support Services (PERTNL/HOME/ SUPSERV)
9 Other Outpatient Peritoneal (PERTNL/HOME/OTHER)

84X Continuous Ambulatory Peritoneal Dialysis (CAPD)-- Outpatient or Home. A program under which a patient performs continual dialysis away from the facility using his or her own equipment and supplies. The patient's peritoneal membrane is used as a dialyzer.
0 General Classification (CAPD/OP OR HOME)
1 CAPD/Composite or Other Rate (CAPD/COMPOSITE)
2 Home Supplies (CAPD/HOME/ SUPPL)
3 Home Equipment (CAPD/HOME/ EQUIP)
4 Maintenance 100% (CAPD/HOME/ 100%)
5 Support Services (CAPD/HOME/ SUPSERV)
9 Other Outpatient CAPD (CAPD/ HOME/OTHER)

85X Continuous Cycling Peritoneal Dialysis (CCPD)-- Outpatient or Home. A program under which a patient performs continual dialysis away from the facility using his or her own equipment and supplies. A machine is used to make automatic exchanges at night.
0 General Classification (CCPD/OP OR HOME)
1 CCPD/Composite or Other Rate (CCPD/COMPOSITE)
2 Home Supplies (CCPD/HOME/ SUPPL)

3 Home Equipment (CCPD/HOME/ EQUIP)
4 Maintenance 100% (CCPD/HOME/ 100%)
5 Support Services (CCPD/HOME/ SUPSERV)
9 Other Outpatient CCPD (CCPD/ HOME/OTHER)

86X **Reserved for Dialysis (National Assignment).**

87X **Reserved for Dialysis (National Assignment).**

88X **Miscellaneous Dialysis.** Charges for dialysis services not identified elsewhere. *Rationale*: Ultrafiltration is the process of removing excess fluid from the blood of dialysis patients by using a dialysis machine but without the dialysis solution. The designation is only used when the procedure is not performed as a part of a normal dialysis session.
0 General Classification (DIALY/ MISC)
1 Ultrafiltration (DIALY/ ULTRAFILT)
2 Home Dialysis Aid Visit (HOME DIALY AID VISIT)
9 Miscellaneous Dialysis Other (DIALY/MISC/OTHER)

89X **Other Donor Bank.** Charges for the acquisition, storage, and preservation of all human organs (excluding kidneys).
0 General Classification (DONOR BANK)
1 Bone (DONOR BANK/BONE)
2 Organ (other than Kidney) (DONOR BANK/ORGN)
3 Skin (DONOR BANK/SKIN)
9 Other Donor Bank (OTHER DONOR BANK)

90X **Psychiatric/Psychological Treatments.** Charges for providing treatment for emotionally disturbed patients, including patients admitted for diagnosis and for treatment.
0 General Classification (PSYCH TREATMENT)
1 Electroshock Treatment (ELECTRO SHOCK)
2 Milieu Therapy (MILIEU THER)
3 Play Therapy (PLAY THERAPY)
9 Other (OTHER PSYCH RX)

91X **Psychiatric/Psychological Services.** Charges for providing nursing care and employee, professional services for emotionally disturbed patients, including patients admitted for diagnosis and those admitted for treatment.
0 General Classification (PSYCH SVS)
1 Rehabilitation (PSYCH/REHAB)
2 Day Care (PSYCH/DAYCARE)
3 Night Care (PSYCH/NIGHTCARE)
4 Individual Therapy (PSYCH/INDIV RX)
5 Group Therapy (PSYCH/GROUP RX)
6 Family Therapy (PSYCH/FAMILY RX)
7 Biofeedback (PSYCH/BIOFEED)
8 Testing (PSYCH/TESTING)
9 Other (PSYCH/OTHER)

92X **Other Diagnostic Services.** Charges for other diagnostic services not otherwise categorized.
0 General Classification (OTHER DX SVS)
1 Peripheral Vascular Lab (PERI-VASCUL LAB)
2 Electromyogram (EMG)
3 Pap Smear (PAP SMEAR)
4 Allergy Test (ALLERGY TEST)
5 Pregnancy Test (PREG TEST)
9 Other Diagnostic Service (ADDL DX SVS)

93X **Not Assigned.**

94X **Other Therapeutic Services.** Charges for other therapeutic services not otherwise categorized.
0 General Classification (OTHER RX SVS)

1 Recreational Therapy (RECREA-TION RX)
2 Education/Training (EDUC/TRNG)
3 Cardiac Rehabilitation (CARDIAC REHAB)
4 Drug Rehabilitation (DRUG REHAB)
5 Alcohol Rehabilitation (ALCOHOL REHAB)
6 Complex Medical Equipment--Routine (CMPLX MED EQUIP-ROUT)
7 Complex Medical Equipment--Ancillary (CMPLX MED EQUIP-ANC)
9 Other Therapeutic Services (ADDITIONAL RX SVS)
NOTE: Use 930 with a procedure code for plasmapheresis. Use 932 for dietary therapy and diabetes-related services, education, and training.

95X **Not Assigned.**

96X **Professional Fees.** Charges for medical professionals that the hospitals or third party payors require to be separately identified.
0 General Classification (PRO FEE)
1 Psychiatric (PRO FEE/PSYCH)
2 Ophthalmology (PRO FEE/EYE)
3 Anesthesiologist (MD) (PRO FEE/ ANES MD)
4 Anesthetist (CRNA) (PRO FEE/ ANES CRNA)
9 Other Professional Fees (OTHER PRO FEE)

97X **Professional Fees (continued).**
1 Laboratory (PRO FEE/LAB)
2 Radiology--Diagnostic (PRO FEE/RAD/DX)
3 Radiology--Therapeutic (PRO FEE/RAD/RX)
4 Radiology--Nuclear Medicine (PRO FEE/NUC MED)
5 Operating Room (PRO FEE/OR)
6 Respiratory Therapy (PRO FEE/ RESPIR)
7 Physical Therapy (PRO FEE/ PHYSI)
8 Occupational Therapy (PRO FEE/ OCUPA)
9 Speech Pathology (PRO FEE/ SPEECH)

98X **Professional Fees (continued).**
1 Emergency Room (PRO FEE/ER)
2 Outpatient Services (PRO FEE/ OUTPT)
3 Clinic (PRO FEE/CLINIC)
4 Medical Social Services (PRO FEE/ SOC SVC)
5 EKG (PRO FEE/EKG)
6 EEG (PRO FEE/EEG)
7 Hospital Visit (PRO FEE/HOS VIS)
8 Consultation (PRO FEE/CONSULT)
9 Private Duty Nurse (FEE/PVT NURSE)

99X **Patient Convenience Items.** Charges for items that are generally considered by the third party payors to be strictly convenience items and, as such, are not covered.
0 General Classification (PT CONV)
1 Cafeteria/Guest Tray (CAFETERIA)
2 Private Linen Service (LINEN)
3 Telephone/Telegraph (TELEPHN)
4 TV/Radio (TV/RADIO)
5 Nonpatient Room Rentals (NONPT ROOM RENT)
6 Late Discharge Charge (LATE DISCH)
7 Admission Kits (ADMIT KITS)
8 Beauty Shop/Barber (BARBER/ BEAUTY)
9 Other Patient Convenience Items (PT CONVENCE/OTH)

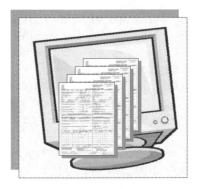

22

Hospital Billing

After completion of this chapter you will be able to:

- Choose the proper form for billing various types of hospital services.
- Describe what personal items are and give examples.
- Describe what APCs are and how they affect payment.
- Explain what DRGs are and how they affect payment on a hospital claim.
- Explain the purpose of a charge description master and the information contained on it.
- Describe the common methods used for entering hospital charges on a patient's bill.
- Discuss how billing can affect other departments in a hospital.
- Discuss the importance of precertification, pre-authorization and utilization review.
- Describe what an ambulatory surgical center does.

Key words and concepts you will learn in this chapter:

Admission Kit – A kit routinely issued to hospital patients that usually includes an emesis basin, carafe, cup, lotion, tissue, and mouthwash.
Ambulatory Patient Classifications (APCs) – Similar to DRGs, but are for patients who are scheduling surgery on an outpatient basis. A single amount is allowed for the procedure, all ancillary services, and any necessary follow-up care.
Ambulatory Surgical Centers (Surgi-centers) – Facilities equipped to allow for the performance of surgery on an outpatient basis.
Bar code – A number that is assigned to a specific item.
Charge Description Master (CDM) – A list of the services and related charges for each procedure provided.
Diagnosis Related Groups (DRGs) – A set amount paid for hospital services based on the type of illness.
Interim Billing – A periodic billing for services prior to the patient being discharged from the hospital.
Itemized Bill – A bill that lists each item, service or supply on an individual line and indicates the cost for that one item.
Personal Items – Those items that are primarily for the comfort of the patient and are not medically necessary.
Prospective Payment System (PPS) – A system set up by Medicare which pays hospitals under APCs rather than on a fee for service basis.
Status Indicators – Indicators that alert the provider to special circumstances that may occur when using certain APCs.

M ost of us have been in a hospital at least once in our lives. At the end of a hospital stay a bill for services usually received.

Hospital billing can be confusing if you do not understand how the process works. However, with basic knowledge and training, competently billing for hospital services should be easily accomplished.

Which Claim Form Is Right?

There are two main forms used for billing insurance carriers; the CMS-1500 and the UB-92. Both claim forms are used in a hospital setting.

CMS-1500 Billing

If you are billing for services provided in a hospital setting by an independent licensed provider other than the hospital, those charges are usually placed on a CMS-1500. These providers may include a surgeon, assistant surgeon, anesthesiologist, radiologist, oncologist, cardiologist, or any number of other professionals.

The one exception to this is charges for nursing staff. The charge for nursing care is included in the overall room and board charges for the hospital.

When billing for provider services, it is important to include the information for the specific provider in box 33 of the CMS-1500. Without this information the insurance carrier will not be able to process the claim. The name and address of the hospital should be provided in item 32.

Some hospitals will have certain providers "on staff." When a provider is on staff it means that he is paid by the hospital for work performed. In this situation the hospital will bill for the provider and the provider's address will be the hospital, or the accounts receivable office of the hospital. The payments made by insurance carriers will be sent directly to the hospital.

If a provider is not on staff, they will usually perform their own billing out of their private office. This office may be their regular practice location, or it may even be their home if they work solely in the hospital setting (i.e., an anesthesiologist).

If the hospital bills for the services, the hospital billing department is responsible for all follow-up on the claim. This includes balance billing the patient, patient accounting, and collections. If the provider does his own billing, the provider or his staff is responsible for all billing issues.

UB-92 Billing

Services rendered by a hospital or hospital employed personnel are billed on the UB-92. This includes all room and board, medications, operating room charges, supplies used by the patient, x-ray fees (for the equipment, supplies and room, though not necessarily for the radiologist, etc.).

Many hospitals use bar coded stickers to assist in billing. A **bar code** is a number that is assigned to a specific item. This number is often represented by a series of thin and fat vertical lines.

In the hospital setting, items will often have a peel-off bar code affixed to them when they are received by the hospital. The bar code is different for each item.

When a patient uses an item, the item is removed from the supply area. The bar code is then peeled off and placed on a special billing page of the patient's chart. This happens for each item the patient uses. Thus, if the patient uses two items, two separate bar codes are peeled off and affixed to the patient chart.

When billing is performed, the item numbers from each bar code are entered into the computer. This is often done using a bar code scanner like the ones seen in many retail and grocery stores. Each number that is entered generates a line item charge on the patient's bill.

Sometimes it can be difficult to determine which charges to put on which form. Some hospitals will even combine the charges and place them on a single form. For example: the hospital may charge one all-inclusive charge for an x-ray. This charge will include not only the equipment, supplies and the room, but also the services of the radiologist.

When bills with all-inclusive charges are submitted to the insurance carrier for payment, the insurance carrier may insist that the charges be itemized according to charges for the facility (equipment, supplies and room) and charges for professional services (the provider).

Itemized Bills

Many hospitals provide their patients with an **itemized bill**. This type of bill lists each item, service or supply on an individual line and shows the cost for that one item. Many patients prefer to receive an itemized bill so that they can understand exactly what they are being billed for. Additionally, facilities in many states are required to provide an itemized bill to any patient that requests one.

Some hospitals will routinely include an itemized bill when billing patients. The markup (the difference between what the hospital pays for an item and what they charge the patient for that same item) can be very high. It is not uncommon for a hospital to charge a patient $10 for a single aspirin.

The increased charge helps to cover the cost of the nurse speaking with the doctor, getting approval for the drug, notating the patient's chart, going to the pharmacy or drug cabinet, placing the required dosage into a paper cup, and then dispensing it to the patient. Additionally, there may be other charges included such as shipping and handling, charges for labeling and inventorying the item, the time it takes for someone to put the information into the computer system, and also the amount of time needed to bill for the item.

Some insurance carriers will also request itemized billings. This allows them to be sure that there are not any non-covered services or items included in the bill. For example, if a patient requests slippers or an extra pillow, these items are not considered medically necessary and are often excluded by the insurance carrier.

Personal Items

Personal items are those items that are primarily for the comfort of the patient and are not medically necessary. The following items are considered to be personal items and are not usually covered by a plan. These charges may need to be coded separately, or they may be combined with other ancillary charges. However, patients should be warned at the time they request such items that they are not usually covered by an insurance carrier.

Personal items can include:
- Barber expenses,
- Personal hygiene kit,
- Videotaping of birth,
- Birth certificate, photos,
- Cot rental,
- Room transfer requested,
- Lotion,
- Television,
- Telephone,
- Toothbrush, toothpaste,
- Guest trays,
- Mouthwash,
- Gift shop expenses , and
- Slippers.

Most hospitals automatically issue an admission kit to incoming patients. An **admission kit** usually includes an emesis basin, carafe, cup, lotion, tissue, and mouthwash. Some plans administratively allow for one kit. Additional kits are usually not covered. This type of kit may also be called a maternity kit, Ob-Gyn kit, hygiene kit, patient comfort kit, and other names.

DRGs

In the early days of health insurance, providers were reimbursed for each procedure they performed. There was no incentive to limit the procedures.

Diagnosis Related Groups (DRGs) were introduced as a means of cost control for insurance carriers (especially Medicare). The idea was to encourage hospitals to help limit some of the costs associated with certain illnesses.

Not all illnesses that a patient receives treatment for are part of a DRG. There is a specific list of DRGs that have been identified by Medicare and also by some other insurance carriers.

When a patient receives treatment for a DRG illness, the billing is handled differently than if the patient is not being treated for a DRG illness. Under a DRG, the insurance carrier (including the Medicare insurance carrier) will pay a set amount for the total care for the treatment. If the hospitals costs are above this amount, they will only receive this set amount. They cannot balance bill the patient for any amount which are not covered by the DRG set amount.

However, if the hospital's charges are less than the set amount, they will still receive the set amount from the carrier. They are allowed to keep the full amount.

It is important for the hospital to note those illnesses which are covered under DRGs. While this notation should not drastically alter patient care, it may remind doctors not to order services or procedures which are questionable.

Ambulatory Patient Classifications

Ambulatory Patient Classifications (APCs) are similar to DRGs, but are for patients who receive services on an outpatient basis. As with DRGs, a set amount is allowed for the procedure, all ancillary services, and any necessary follow-up care.

There are approximately 500 APC codes which cover approximately 5,000 services. However, most providers will only use a few of these APCs on a repeated basis.

APCs are used as part of the Medicare Outpatient **Prospective Payment System (PPS)**. This is a new system set up by Medicare (as of

August 1, 2000) which pays hospitals under APCs rather than on a fee for service basis.

It is important for billers to realize that the services provided by a hospital may cover more than one APC, and multiple APCs may be included on a single claim.

Many of the services covered under Medicare Part B are grouped under APCs. These include radiation therapy, clinic visits, ER visits, diagnostic tests and services, surgical pathology, cancer chemotherapy, etc.

Medicare patients who are covered by Part B but not by Part A may have certain additional services covered under APCs.

When billing using APCs, it is important to remember that the single APC code covers all facility charges and services. However, the professional services of physicians is paid as a separate expense. These providers should continue to bill using a separate CMS-1500 form.

Medicare will often use fiscal intermediaries to group the procedures on a hospital bill into the APC groups. For examples of APC groups, look in the C Codes section of the HCPCS.

Status Indicators

In addition to APCs, the HOPPS system uses **status indicators**. These indicators will alert the provider to special circumstances that may occur when using certain APCs.

The current status indicators include:

S   Significant procedure – The payment for this procedure is not reduced when multiple procedures are performed during the same visit.

T   Significant Procedure, but a reduction applies when this procedure is performed in conjunction with other procedures.

K   Drugs that are eligible for payment separate from the infusion procedure.

X   Ancillary Services.

V   Visit to a clinic or emergency room.

N   Incidental service. This service is incidental and would be packaged with the major procedure. No additional amount would be allowed.

G   Drug/Biological Pass-through.

H   Device Category Pass-through.

Certain services such as diagnostic laboratory services and durable medical equipment are not paid under APC groupings. These items will use the status indicators A, F, P and C.

Excluded Services

Certain services are excluded from APC grouping. These services include ambulance, physical and occupational therapy, speech-language pathology, clinical diagnostic laboratory, durable medical equipment, and non-implantable prosthetic and orthotic devices. These services will be reimbursed at the separate fee-for-service rate.

Additionally, physicians and non-physician practitioners continue to be reimbursed under the fee-for-service basis. Non-physician practitioners include physician's assistants, nurse practitioners, certified nurse midwives and psychologists.

APCs are only for outpatient care. Thus, services that require the patient to be admitted to the hospital are not covered under the PPS system.

Most hospitals are automatically included in the PPS system. This includes rural hospitals with fewer than 100 beds, certain cancer hospitals and children's hospitals. However, these types of hospitals may be exempt from certain reductions in their Medicare payments.

Charge Description Masters

In years past, patients were not expected to understand all the items included on their hospital bill. Many of the items were listed by code number, supply number, or a medical term that was difficult to understand.

Recent legislation has mandated that the information contained on a hospital billing be written in everyday language. This allows the patient to double-check their bill, and to reconcile the statement they receive from the hospital with the explanation of benefits received from the insurance carrier. Thus, hospital billing departments are now required to include descriptions on their line item bills which are written in language that is easily understood.

To comply with this new regulation, each provider is required to have a **Charge Description Master (CDM)**. The CDM is a list of the services and related charges for each procedure provided. A complete service listing includes each of the following components:

Department Name. The name of the department where the charge originated. Each department should have an abbreviated code which designates the department where the code originates from. For example: the Cardiac Intensive Care Unit might be designated CICU.

Department Number. Each department should be assigned their own number. This allows you to quickly verify the department where the charges originated.

Charge Number. Each charge should be given its own individual reference number. This is a unique number assigned by the provider. Charges which originate in a single department often receive similar numbers.

Revenue Code. This is the code which normally appears on the UB-92. (For more information see the UB-92 chapter.)

Description. A description of the charge or service. This description should be specific enough for the patient to understand the service or item they are being charged for.

CPT® Code. If the service has an appropriate CPT® code associated with it, that code should be listed in this field.

HCPCS Code. If the service or item has an appropriate HCPCS code associated with it, that code should be listed in this field.

Charge. The charge for the service. This should be the normal fee which the provider charges for this service.

Descriptions, codes and other parts of the CDM should be checked on a regular basis to insure that they are still accurate and complete. Additionally, the medical biller should become aware of any charges for which the insurance allowed amount is greater than the billed amount. This may indicate a need to increase the amount charged by the provider in order to receive maximum reimbursement from insurance carriers. This information will be included on an Explanation of Benefits (EOB) which is provided by the insurance carrier upon reimbursement of the claim. It is often attached to the check and indicates how the insurance carrier determined the appropriate payment amount.

Providers also need to create an itemized billing form which lists the above items. This will allow the patient to see exactly what they are being charged for and what the cost is.

As a medical biller, you may be responsible for choosing the right charge description for billing the patient, and for creating itemized patient statements for those patients that request them. You may even be responsible for entering new charge descriptions into the master list.

It is important to watch the CDM as you are using it to attempt to spot any errors or items that might seem to be overbilled or underbilled. These errors should be brought to your supervisor's attention immediately.

Entering Charges

There are many people who deal with a patient in a hospital setting. Each of these people may be providing goods or services that need to be billed to the patient. For example, a patient may request pain medication from a nurse. The nurse will contact the doctor with the request. The doctor will prescribe the drugs, and will often be the one to make a note on the patient's chart. The health unit coordinator may be responsible for actually ordering the dosage of medication from the pharmacy. However, a nurse may be responsible for actually handing the drug to the patient.

In such case, there needs to be a specific policy for the recording of information onto the patient chart. If you are responsible for hospital or facility billing, it is important to understand and follow the guidelines for patient billing of the items they receive. Without such a policy there is a chance that many of the drugs or other items dispensed will not be charged to the patient.

There are several common methods for insuring that patients are billed for the services and supplies they use. Some of these methods are as follows:

Bar Coding – Some hospitals place bar codes on every item that they receive into inventory (if the item does not already have a bar code attached). This bar code contains a unique number, and each type of item will receive a different bar code number. A computer billing and inventory system is set up that contains the information to correspond with that bar code number. For example, one number will be used to designate an admit kit and the common charge of $25 for that kit.

When a patient requests or is prescribed an item, the bar code for that item will be scanned into their account. The charge will then appear on their account record in the same way that scanning a bar code rings up your charges in a supermarket.

Some items are too small to receive a bar code (i.e., individual capsules or ills). In such a case the bar code is placed on the outside of the bottle, or on a set of labels nearby. When medicine is dispensed, the appropriate bar code is scanned and the information entered into the patient's account.

Some hospitals choose to use peel off bar codes. When an item is dispensed, the bar code will be peeled off the item and placed on the patient's chart. Then at a later date all the items in the patient chart will be scanned in at the same time. After this is done, the page will be replaced with a new blank page. This prevents scanning an item twice and potentially double billing the patient. In some hospitals the job of scanning items will fall to the health unit coordinator or a nurse. In other hospitals it may be the job of the billing department.

Coding from charts – Some hospitals have billers create claims from the information contained in the patient chart. This information can be in the form of triage reports, operative reports, patient history reports, as well as the day-to-day treatment reports for the patient. It is the responsibility of the hospital biller to obtain the information from the chart regarding the goods and services that were provided.

Combined bar code and chart method – Some hospitals will have some items handled by bar code, and other items will need to be obtained from the patient chart. For example, the goods delivered to the patient may be covered by the bar coding method, but other items such as room and board charges will need to be entered by the biller.

Other methods – While the above situations cover many facilities, other facilities may have their own methods for keeping track of goods and services used by the patient. Therefore, it is important to verify the proper billing procedures with your supervisor before billing hospital claims.

Regardless of the type of billing method used, it is the job of the biller to bill claims in a timely manner. This usually means billing patients as soon as their hospital stay is completed. If a patient is receiving extended care, interim billings may need to be created.

Interim Billings

An **interim billing** is a periodic billing for services prior to the patient being discharged from the hospital.

When creating interim billings it is important to include all charges through a specified date of service on a single claim form. Subsequent claim forms should cover dates after the closing date of the prior interim bill. It is important to include all charges in order to reduce the possibility of confusion for an insurance carrier. If they receive more than one bill with the same date of service, some or all of the charges may be denied as duplicate. For example, if a patient received the same medication at two different times during the day, but each medication is billed on a separate claim, the insurance carrier may determine that the second medication charge is merely a duplicate billing of the first one.

How Billing Affects Other Departments

It is important for billers to realize that the information they enter for patient charges will affect many other hospital departments as well. Each year hospitals will determine their budgets based upon the services and billing of the year before. If billing has been done improperly, a department might have a lower budget than it needs to maintain proficiency.

Additionally, staffing is often allocated based upon the amount of services provided and revenues generated by a specific department. Incorrect billing might cause a specific department to be over or understaffed for the upcoming year.

Supplies are also ordered based upon billing charts. Many computer programs have inventory programs tied to them. These programs will indicate when a certain supply is low and may need to be reordered. If items are billed incorrectly, there is the possibility that the facility may run out of an item needed for patient care. This can lead to extra charges incurred from having to rush order the items, or even lead to a lower level of patient care.

Because of these factors it is vitally important that billers pay close attention to the details of the items being billed. Be sure you are choosing the correct code for the service or item provided.

Pre-authorization, Pre-certifications and Utilization Reviews

One of the most common jobs of the biller is to handle the pre-authorization and pre-certification of services. Many insurance carriers require the hospital to pre-certify services prior to, or within a certain period of receiving the services. Without the proper pre-certification or pre-authorization, the insurance carrier may reduce benefits on a claim, or refuse to pay for the services altogether.

For more information on completing pre-certification and pre-authorization, see the Managed Care chapter. However, you should be aware that managed care insurers are not the only plans that may require pre-authorization, pre-certification or utilization review.

Ambulatory Surgical Centers

Ambulatory surgical centers (surgi-centers) are centers equipped to allow for the performance of surgery on an outpatient basis. These centers may be freestanding or affiliated with a major acute care facility. Surgi-centers provide financial savings by eliminating the need for admission into an inpatient facility. An ambulatory surgical facility is a specialized facility that meets all eight of the professionally recognized standards, indicated below:

1. Provides a setting for outpatient surgeries.
2. Does not provide services or accommodations for overnight stays.
3. Has at least two operating rooms and one recovery room; all the medical equipment needed to support the surgery being performed; x-ray and laboratory diagnostic facilities; and emergency equipment, trays, and supplies for use in life-threatening events.
4. Has a medical staff that is supervised full time by a physician including a registered nurse when patients are in the facility.
5. Maintains a medical record for each patient.
6. Has a written agreement with a local acute care facility for the immediate transfer of patients who require greater care than can be provided on an outpatient basis.
7. Complies with all state and federal licensing and other legal requirements.
8. Is not an office or clinic for any physician.

Usually, plans provide benefits on a global basis, covering the facility room usage charge, supplies (i.e., anesthesia gases, medications, trays) on the same basis as inpatient hospital services.

Summary

Billing in a hospital setting has several differences from billing in a medical office. While medical offices often bill using only a CMS-1500, hospitals may use a CMS-1500 for professional services and a UB-92 for facility charges. Additionally, an itemized bill may be used to provide patients with a list of all goods and services received.

Hospitals will often charge for each individual item received by a patient. Billing is often done using a bar code method, using information from a patient chart, a combination of these two methods, or by some other method. Regardless of the method used, it is important for the biller to ensure that all items used and all services received by the patient are billed for.

In an effort to manage costs, Medicare and other insurance carriers are implementing payment by DRGs and APCs. Payments made under DRG and/or APC provisions reimburse the hospital a set amount for the total cost of treatment for a specified condition, rather than paying for each individual item or service.

Assignments

Complete the Questions for Review.

Questions for Review

Directions: Answer the following questions without looking back into the material just covered. Write your answers in the space provided.

1. What is a PPS? _____

_____

_____

2. What is a DRG and how does it work? _____

_____

_____

3. What are the most common methods used for hospital billing?

_____

_____

_____

4. What is an APC and what type of facility does it apply to? _____

_____

_____

5. How can billing affect other departments in a hospital? _____

_____

_____

_____

If you were unable to answer any of the questions, refer back to that section, and then fill in the answers.

Honors Certification™

The certification challenge for this chapter will be a written test of the information contained in this chapter. Each incorrect answer will result in a deduction of up to 5% from your grade. You must achieve a score of 85% or higher to pass this test. If you fail the test on your first attempt you may retake the test one additional time. The items included in the second test may be different from those in the first test.

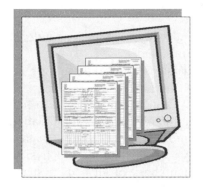

23

Medical Reports

After completion of this chapter you will be able to:

- Explain how medical reports relate to billing forms.
- Recognize a triage report, an operative report, a diagnostic report, and a medical history report and explain their uses.
- Properly create a claim using a medical report.

Key words and concepts you will learn in this chapter:

Diagnostic Testing Report – A transcribed interpretation, "reading", of a laboratory or radiology test.

Operative Report – A transcribed report describing the surgical procedure performed.

Triage – The screening of patients to determine their priority for treatment.

Triage Report – Reports generated at the scene of accidents, in emergency rooms, and in urgent care clinics.

Medical reports are required for virtually every procedure and for all laboratory and radiology examinations. Often medical billers use medical reports to extract the information needed to complete the billing forms. Virtually all information needed on a claim form is included in the medical reports and the patient's medical record.

Of the numerous types of medical reports, the most common that are used by medical billers include triage reports, operative reports, and diagnostic testing reports.

Abstracting From Medical Records

At times the medical biller will be required to create a claim from medical records contained in the patient's chart. The biller will need to abstract the information from medical reports. Triage reports, operative reports and diagnostic tests reports are just a few of the reports that may be included in a patient's chart.

Triage Reports

Triage is the screening of patients to determine their priority for treatment. Often more patients will need treatment than there are medical personnel to care for them. Triage reports are generated to help in allocating treatment resources to patients on the basis of need. It is designed to maximize the number of survivors.

Triage reports are generated at the scene of accidents, in emergency rooms, and in urgent care clinics. For each patient the emergency staff performs a rapid physical assessment, takes vitals signs and a brief patient history. This information is detailed on a triage report, which is used throughout the emergency encounter with the patient. These reports are usually handwritten rather than typed, since often the speed and accuracy of accumulating the information is more important than appearance.

When assessing the need for patient care, first priority is given to establishment of an airway, basic life support measures. Second priority is given to bleeding, neurological trauma and traumatized bones (i.e., fractures, sprains) and tissue (i.e., open wounds, contusions). Patients are reassessed frequently to determine any change of status.

Operative Reports

Operative reports are generated for most surgical procedures performed. The information contained in these reports is often the sole means of information for medical billers. Therefore, it is important that the medical biller understand the basics of an operative report and how to use it to perform medical billing.

Diagnostic Testing Reports

Often, diagnostic testing is performed by an independent laboratory, pathologist, or radiologist. **Diagnostic testing reports** are the "readings" or the interpretation of the tests performed.

Medical billers need to familiarize themselves with the terminology contained within the reports to understand the procedures that were rendered.

Medical History and Physical Examination Reports

Whenever a patient is examined by a physician, a brief history of that exam is kept as part of the patient's permanent file. This history should include the following:

- Date of service,
- Symptoms and complaints,
- Past medical, social and family history,
- Review of systems,
- Current medications,
- Diagnosis,
- Laboratory and x-ray examinations ordered or other referrals, and
- Other miscellaneous medical data.

A complete physical examination is often performed with the initial office visit, the initiation of a major surgical procedure and admission to a health care facility. A complete physical examination a thorough check of all body systems with the results documented in the medical record.

The physician is allowed to bill for the service of compiling a medical history and performing a complete examination on a patient. This code would be considered an E/M (Evaluation and Management) code, since it is not a surgical procedure.

Summary

The four most common medical reports that medical billers use for billing charges are triage reports, operative reports, diagnostic reports, and medical history and physical examination reports.

Medical billers should familiarize themselves with these reports and how the information relates to the standard medical billing forms.

Assignments

Complete the Questions for Review.
Complete Exercises 23 – 1 through 23 – 20.

Each report follows a patient through a single episode of care. Use the information from each of the following reports and the patient charts that were previously completed in Exercise 5 – 1 to complete a claim for each report.

Only after completing the forms should you look at the interpretive information contained in the chapter appendix. Interpretive information is not given for all reports, so that they may be assigned as a class or homework exercise.

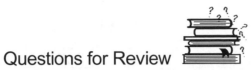

Questions for Review

Directions: Answer the following questions without looking back into the material just covered. Write your answers in the space provided.

1. What are triage reports? _____

   _____

2. What are operative reports? _____

   _____

3. What are diagnostic reports? _____

   _____

4. List six items included on a patient history?

   1. _____

   2. _____

   3. _____

   4. _____

   5. _____

   6. _____

5. In what way does a medical biller use the above reports?_____

   _____

If you were unable to answer any of the questions, refer back to that section, and then fill in the answers.

Exercise 23 – 1

Abby Addison 5678 Any Avenue Alverville, AK 99087	**EMERGENCY SERVICE REPORT**
	ALLERGIES NKA
	CURRENT MEDS: NONE
01/13/xx	**LAST TET. TOX.** **DATE**

ARRIVED VIA: Ambulance ACCOMPANIED BY: Friend	P.M.D. TEL. # NOTIFIED NAME ☐

TRIAGE TIME 14:09 T 98 P 110 R 23 BP 115/82	TIME T P R BP
	SIGN:

DOCTORS ORDERS

TIME	INIT	RESULTS
		RUA:
		CBC: HGB/HCT 10.2/30
		WBC OTHER 14.4
		DIFF: P B M
		E B L
		LYTES:
		Na 140 K 4.5
		CO2 CL
		GLU: 126
		BUN: 23
		CREAT: 0.6
		OTHER LAB
		Beta HCg
		ChL 100
		HCO3 25
		ABG:
		FIO2 BE
		PCO2 PO2
		%SAT pH
		X-RAY: U/S gallbladder and Upper Abd
		EKG:

25 y/o white female with severe abd pain and nausea beginning 1-12-XX. Hematemesis this a.m.
Pt was hospitalized on 1-6-xx with epigastric pain. Pt s/p ERCP on 1-10-xx stone removed. D/C home 1-11-xx.

Pos – dizziness and lightheadedness
Neg – c/p, dyspnea
Neg – dysuria

COMMUNICATION LOG

CONSULT	CALLED	COMMENTS

DISCHARGE IMPRESSION	DR. ORDERS	TIME	SITE	SIGNATURE
	Admit			

| DRAW WOUND IN DIAGRAM
WOUND LENGTH_____
☐ COMPLEX ☐ SIMPLE
☐ PLASTIC DEPTH_____ | INVOLVEMENT
DISTAL ROM
_____OK
DISTAL SENS_____OK
DISTAL CIRG_____OK
TENDONS_____OK | TREATMENT
☐ Y ☐ N BET. PREP
☐ Y ☐ N ANESTH. 1% XYLOC.
DRESSING_____
☐ Y ☐ N SUTURES | TIME OUT:
☐ Y ☐ N IRREG

☐ Y ☐ N SPLINT | ☐ CHARGES
☐ VALUABLES LISTED
☐ NURSES NOTES
☐ AFTER CARE INSTR. GIVEN |

PLAN _ Esophagogastroduodenoscopy

CONDITION: ☐ GOOD **X** FAIR ☐ POOR
DISPOSITION: ☐ HOME ☐ LEFT WITHOUT BEING SEEN **X** ADMIT
☐ LEFT AGAINST MEDICAL ADVICE   ☐ EXPIRED
☐ TRANSFER TO _____   RET TO WORK

Ann Anderson MD _____ M.D. Ann Anderson MD PRINT NAME	_____ M.D. PRINT NAME	*Adrian Adams MD* _____ M.D. Adrian Adams MD PRINT NAME

Exercise 23 – 2

Bobby Bumble 93485 Bumpkiss Court Barkingville, DC 23456 210-938-4756	**EMERGENCY SERVICE REPORT**

ALLERGIES
NKA

CURRENT MEDS:
NONE

06/16/xx

	LAST TET. TOX.	**DATE**

ARRIVED VIA: Ambulance	ACCOMPANIED BY: Friend	P.M.D.	TEL. #

NOTIFIED

NAME ☐

TRIAGE TIME 09:31 T 97.5 P 83 R 23 BP 122/81	TIME T P R BP
	SIGN:

49 y/o male w/injury to Rt wrist. Pt states he was running to catch a bus when his Rt ankle gave way. Pt fell to pavement injuring Rt wrist.

Neg – L.O.C.,
Neg – head trauma
Neg – Dizziness or lightheadedness
Pos – multiple excoriation Rt hand

DOCTORS ORDERS

TIME	INIT	RESULTS
		RUA:
		CBC: HGB/HCT
		WBC OTHER
		DIFF: P B M
		E B L
		LYTES:
		Na K
		CO2 CL
		GLU:
		BUN:
		CREAT:
		OTHER LAB
		ABG:
		FI02 BE
		PCO2 PO2
		%SAT pH
		X-RAY: Rt wrist AP & Lat
		Rt ankle AP & Lat
		EKG:

COMMUNICATION LOG

CONSULT	CALLED	COMMENTS

DISCHARGE IMPRESSION	DR. ORDERS	TIME	SITE	SIGNATURE
Sprain, Rt wrist	F/U with Bill Blake MD re: wrist injury			

DRAW WOUND IN DIAGRAM WOUND LENGTH_____ ☐ COMPLEX ☐ SIMPLE ☐ PLASTIC DEPTH_____	INVOLVEMENT DISTAL ROM _____OK DISTAL SENS_____OK DISTAL CIRG_____OK TENDONS_____OK	TREATMENT TIME OUT:18:01 ☐ Y ☐ N BET. PREP ☐ Y ☐ N IRREG ☐ Y ☐ N ANESTH. 1% XYLOC. DRESSING_____ ☐ Y ☐ N SUTURES ☐ Y ☐ N SPLINT	☐ CHARGES ☐ VALUABLES LISTED ☐ NURSES NOTES ☐ AFTER CARE INSTR. GIVEN

PLAN : Splint Applied
_____

CONDITION: **X** GOOD   ☐ FAIR   ☐ POOR
DISPOSITION: **X** HOME   ☐ LEFT WITHOUT BEING SEEN   ☐ ADMIT
☐ LEFT AGAINST MEDICAL ADVICE   ☐ EXPIRED
☐ TRANSFER TO _____   RET TO WORK

Bruno Ball MD M.D.	M.D.	Benny Barker MD M.D.
Bruno Ball MD PRINT NAME	PRINT NAME	Benny Barker MD PRINT NAME

Exercise 23 – 3

Cathy Crenshaw 9876 Cranbury Lane Crabapple, CT 06192 086-421-3579	**EMERGENCY SERVICE REPORT**

EMERGENCY SERVICE REPORT

ALLERGIES: NKA

CURRENT MEDS:
NPH Insulin, 50U, Glucotrol, Lithium,

11/1/xx	LAST TET. TOX.	DATE

ARRIVED VIA: Car	ACCOMPANIED BY: self	P.M.D.	TEL. #
		NOTIFIED	
		NAME	☐

TRIAGE TIME 07:00 T 98 P 102 R 24 BP 170/90	TIME T P R BP
	SIGN:

DOCTORS ORDERS

TIME	INIT	RESULTS
		RUA:
		CBC: HGB/HCT
		WBC OTHER
		DIFF: P B M
		E B L
		LYTES:
		Na K
		CO2 CL
		GLU:
		BUN:
		CREAT:
		OTHER LAB
		ABG:
		FIO2 BE
		PCO2 PO2
		%SAT pH
		X-RAY:
		U/S Gallbladder/ABD
		EKG:

50 y/o female with c/o N/V x 1.5 wks.

Neg - dizziness
Pos - lightheadedness
Neg - L.O.C.
Pos - icterus

COMMUNICATION LOG

CONSULT	CALLED	COMMENTS

DISCHARGE IMPRESSION	DR. ORDERS	TIME	SITE	SIGNATURE
Jaundice R/O Bile Duct Obstruction	F/u with Dr. Callahan			

DRAW WOUND IN DIAGRAM	INVOLVEMENT	TREATMENT	TIME OUT: 14:22	
WOUND LENGTH_____	DISTAL ROM	☐ Y ☐ N BET. PREP	☐ Y ☐ N IRREG	☐ CHARGES
☐ COMPLEX ☐ SIMPLE	_____OK	☐ Y ☐ N ANESTH. 1% XYLOC.		☐ VALUABLES LISTED
☐ PLASTIC DEPTH _____	DISTAL SENS _____OK	DRESSING_____		☐ NURSES NOTES
	DISTAL CIRG _____OK	☐ Y ☐ N SUTURES	☐ Y ☐ N SPLINT	☐ AFTER CARE INSTR. GIVEN
	TENDONS _____OK			

PLAN _____	CONDITION: ☐ GOOD **X** FAIR ☐ POOR
_____	DISPOSITION: **X** HOME ☐ LEFT WITHOUT BEING SEEN ☐ ADMIT
	☐ LEFT AGAINST MEDICAL ADVICE ☐ EXPIRED
	☐ TRANSFER TO _____ RET TO WORK

Chris Campbell MD		Cindy Carter, MD	
M.D.	M.D.		M.D.
Christopher Campbell MD PRINT NAME	PRINT NAME	Cindy Carter MD PRINT NAME	

Exercise 23 – 4

EMERGENCY SERVICE REPORT

Daisy Doolittle
2345 Daffy Lane
Danbury, DE 19876
098-765-4311

11/26/xx

ALLERGIES	
NKA	
CURRENT MEDS:	
NONE	
LAST TET. TOX.	DATE

ARRIVED VIA: Ambulance	ACCOMPANIED BY: Self
Greenlight Ambulance	

P.M.D.	TEL. #
NOTIFIED	
NAME	☐

TRIAGE	TIME 07:03	T 97	P 92	R 25	BP 125/85

TIME	T	P	R	BP
SIGN:				

34 y/o Hispanic female, LMP 02/20/xx.
c/o Vag discharge with bleeding x 1wk.
Pt feels she is pregnant, but didn't pass tissue.

Neg – dizzy, lightheadedness
Pos – palpable pelvic masses, white vaginal discharge

DOCTORS ORDERS

TIME	INIT	RESULTS
		RUA: 1.008SG
		CBC: HGB/HCT
		WBC OTHER RBC = 1-2
		1-2
		DIFF: P B M
		E B L
		LYTES:
		Na K
		CO2 CL
		GLU:
		BUN:
		CREAT:
		OTHER LAB GC, Wet mount
		Beta HCg
		Gram Stain
		ABG:
		FI02 BE
		PCO2 PO2
		%SAT pH
		X-RAY: Pelvic/low abd
		EKG:

COMMUNICATION LOG

CONSULT	CALLED	COMMENTS

DISCHARGE IMPRESSION	DR. ORDERS	TIME	SITE	SIGNATURE
Dysfunctional uterine bleeding				

DRAW WOUND IN DIAGRAM WOUND LENGTH_____ ☐ COMPLEX ☐ SIMPLE ☐ PLASTIC DEPTH _____	INVOLVEMENT DISTAL ROM _____OK DISTAL SENS _____OK DISTAL CIRG _____OK TENDONS _____OK	TREATMENT ☐ Y ☐ N BET. PREP ☐ Y ☐ N ANESTH. 1% XYLOC. DRESSING_____ ☐ Y ☐ N SUTURES	TIME OUT: ☐ Y ☐ N IRREG ☐ Y ☐ N SPLINT	☐ CHARGES ☐ VALUABLES LISTED ☐ NURSES NOTES ☐ AFTER CARE INSTR. GIVEN

PLAN D/C home. 1.) F/U with Dr. David Day this week.
2.) Use condoms

CONDITION:	X GOOD	☐ FAIR	☐ POOR	
DISPOSITION:	X HOME	☐ LEFT WITHOUT BEING SEEN		☐ ADMIT
	☐ LEFT AGAINST MEDICAL ADVICE			☐ EXPIRED
	☐ TRANSFER TO _____		RET TO WORK	

Doris Dean MD M.D.	M.D.	D.C. Davidson, MD M.D.
Doris Dean MD PRINT NAME	PRINT NAME	D.C. Davidson MD PRINT NAME

Exercise 23 – 5

EMERGENCY SERVICE REPORT

Edward Edmunds
8888 Every Lane
Evanville, CA 90012
123-456-7890

05/09/xx

ALLERGIES
Penicillin
CURRENT MEDS: None
LAST TET. TOX.   **DATE**

ARRIVED VIA: Red Alert Ambulance	ACCOMPANIED BY: Self	P.M.D. TEL. #
		NOTIFIED
		NAME ☐

TRIAGE TIME 06:07	T 97	P 84	R 23	BP 120/80	TIME T P R BP
					SIGN:

66 y/o white male with gunshot wound to both knees.
Pt drove to store. While walking into entrance was struck by bullet which crossed Lt Knee and entered Rt Knee.

Neg – L.O.C.
Minimal pain
Minimal bleeding.

DOCTORS ORDERS

TIME	INIT	RESULTS
		RUA:
		CBC: HGB/HCT
		WBC OTHER
		DIFF: P B M
		E B L
		LYTES:
		Na K
		CO2 CL
		GLU:
		BUN:
		CREAT:
		OTHER LAB
		ABG:
		FI02 BE
		PCO2 PO2
		%SAT pH
		X-RAY L and R Knee:
		EKG:

COMMUNICATION LOG

CONSULT	CALLED	COMMENTS

DISCHARGE IMPRESSION	DR. ORDERS	TIME	SITE	SIGNATURE
Gunshot wound to knee bilaterally	Cirpo 750 Mg	06:30		

DRAW WOUND IN DIAGRAM	INVOLVEMENT	TREATMENT	TIME OUT: 2:58	
WOUND	DISTAL ROM	☐ Y ☐ N BET. PREP	☐ Y ☐ N IRREG	☐ CHARGES
LENGTH ___1"___	_____OK	☐ Y ☐ N ANESTH. 1% XYLOC.		☐ VALUABLES LISTED
☐ COMPLEX X SIMPLE	DISTAL SENS _____ OK	DRESSING_____		☐ NURSES NOTES
☐ PLASTIC DEPTH _____	DISTAL CIRG _____ OK	☐ Y ☐ N SUTURES	☐ Y ☐ N SPLINT	☐ AFTER CARE INSTR. GIVEN
	TENDONS _____ OK			

PLAN D/C to home. Pt to F/U with Dr. Esther Edelman tomorrow	CONDITION: X GOOD ☐ FAIR ☐ POOR
	DISPOSITION: X HOME ☐ LEFT WITHOUT BEING SEEN ☐ ADMIT
	☐ LEFT AGAINST MEDICAL ADVICE ☐ EXPIRED
	☐ TRANSFER TO _____ RET TO WORK

Eric Ericson MD   M.D.   M.D.   Emilio Evans, MD   M.D.

Eric Ericson MD PRINT NAME	PRINT NAME	Emilio Evans MD PRINT NAME

Exercise 23 – 6

Operative Report 1

ARCADIA MEDICAL CENTER
8000 Another Street
Alverville, AK 99188

PATIENT NAME: Abby Addison   PATIENT NUMBER: 33299-08

SURGEON: Albert Adler, MD   PIN: A375201
                  4753 Apple Lane
                  Anderson, AK 99234

DATE OF PROCEDURE: 1-13-xx

PREOPERATIVE DIAGNOSIS: Upper gastrointestinal bleed.

POSTOPERATIVE DIAGNOSIS: Most likely cause of the patient's gastrointestinal bleeding was a Mallory-Weiss tear.

NAME OF PROCEDURE: Upper gastrointestinal endoscopy.

PROCEDURE IN BRIEF: Status post informed consent, the patient was premedicated with Demerol 50 and Versed 2. At this point, an upper GI endoscope was advanced through the esophagus, stomach, and duodenum.

Findings included the following: Normal esophagus, normal stomach, and normal duodenum. There was a slightly raised streak at the GE junction, which was exudative. This was approximately 1 mm x 3 mm. This was consistent with possible Mallory-Weiss tear. No other lesions were appreciated throughout the entire examination. It was also noted that the patient had some mild gastritis consistent with NG tube trauma but no evidence of bleeding.

The overall procedure was tolerated well. The patient was extubated.

          ALBERT ADLER, MD

AA:AA443
d: 1-14-xx
t: 1-14-xx
Document: 448800.aaa

Exercise 23 – 7

Operative Report 2

BRONSON BROTHERS MEDICAL CENTER
9876 Bright Lane
Brighton, DC 23787

DATE:	8/20/xx	PATIENT NUMBER:	9888-0009
PATIENT:	Bobby Bumble	PATIENT DOB:	1/1/44

SURGEON:	Ben Bennett, MD	PIN:	B345678
ADDRESS:	9810 Brock Lane	PHONE:	(000) 123-4567
	Brooklyn, NY 24532	SSN:	005-67-8910

ASSISTANT:	Brian Bradley, MD	PIN:	B189765
	5678 Bastion Way	PHONE:	(000) 789-1234
	Brighton, DC 23789	SSN:	566-12-3456

PRE-OP DX: Chronic Anterior and Lateral Instability of the Right Ankle

POST-OP DX: Same

PROCEDURE: Anterior Lateral Ligamentous Reconstruction of the Right Ankle Using the Peroneus Brevis Tendon

ANESTHESIOLOGIST:	Bertha Blues, MD	PIN:	B316597
	7654 Bluefield Drive	PHONE:	(000) 854-6910
	Brighton, DC 23787	EIN:	58-6143285

ANESTHESIA: Epidural

PROCEDURE: The patient was brought into the room and placed in the sitting position. Dr. Blues did an epidural anesthesia without difficulty. Patient was then placed in the supine position. A lift was placed under the right buttock and a sandbag was placed at the foot area when the knee was bent 90E. The entire right lower extremity was then prepped and draped in the usual fashion. A pneumatic tourniquet was used during the initial stages of the case for 22 minutes. This was during the isolation and dissection of the tissues. A long incision was made over the peroneal tendons halfway up the calf, carried behind the lateral malleolus down to the base of the fifth metatarsal. It was dissected through skin and subcutaneous tissue. The sural nerve was not visualized and was felt to be protected by the posterior skin flap. The sheath of the peroneal tendon was then incised its entire length. The peroneus brevis tendon was isolated from the peroneus longus tendon. The brevis tendon was quite small and therefore decision was made after surgery to use the entire tendon rather than the usual half of the tendon. Muscle tissue was dissected from the tendon at the proper length. After measurement for the eventual coursing of the graft, an incision was made across the tendon. The peroneal brevis tendon was then pulled distally and a Bunnell-type suture was placed into the tendon with a double armed 2-0 Ethibond suture. The needles were then cut and a tag was placed. The dissection of the anterior flap was done so that the anterior talofibular area was dissected free. There was a lot of scarring in this area. Hemostasis was obtained by means of cautery. The tourniquet was deflated at this point.

Further dissection was done into the ankle joint so that it was viewed. It was felt to be fairly normal. A small drill hole was placed on the anterior aspect of the fibula and drilled posteriorly. This was widened with a larger drill. The pin was passed through this tunnel from anterior to posterior and was held quite tightly with the foot in neutral position of dorsiflexion plantar flexion and just slight eversion. It was not maximally everted. Sutures were then placed in the tendon and through the bone with #2 Ethibond.

Once this was secured, sutures were placed into the posterior aspect of the tunnel also with 2-0 Ethibond. The peroneal brevis tendon was then further dissected from its sheath and dislodged from its normal groove and carried anterior so the dissection on the calcaneus could occur. The ridge of the calcaneus was identified, and periosteum was stripped using an elevator. The same drill holes were then made keeping the ridge between the two holes and the distance between the holes was approximately 1   cm. The hole was then widened to the same hole as the fibular hole and the graft was passed from posterior to anterior in the calcaneal tunnel. This was done with the suture ligature passer. This was pulled in quite nicely. There was enough graft to suture the remaining part of the graft back into the position of the anterior talar fibular ligament which was done again with #2 Ethibond.

Once wound was all secured with proper sutures, the drawer sign was negative and patient had slight inversion and could be further everted.

The wound was then irrigated with copious amounts of antibiotic solution. Prior to any drill holes, the superior portion of the wound was closed so that the rest of the tendon that was exposed would not dry out. During the procedure, the tendons were kept constantly moistened with antibiotic irrigation fluid. 2-0 Vicryl was then used for the deep subcutaneous tissue, 3-0 Vicryl for the superficial subcutaneous tissue and staples for the skin. The limb was then dressed sterilely and placed into a Jones compression dressing using cotton and fore and aft plaster splints with bias cut and Ace wrap.

The patient tolerated the procedure from an anesthetic standpoint and was transferred to the RR with stable vital signs under the direction of Dr. Blues. Time under anesthesia: 1 hour, 20 min.

BB: BB77   Dictated and authenticated by: BEN BENNETT, MD
DT: 8-20-xx
T: 8-20-xx
Job#: 8112.B

Exercise 23 – 8

Operative Report 3

CANYON CITY HOSPITAL
4440 CENTER DRIVE
CARSON, CT 06001

PATIENT NAME: Cathy Crenshaw   PATIENT NUMBER: 8779-09

SURGEON: Chung Choi, MD   DATE OF PROCEDURE: 11/12/xx
                  4512 Charley Chan Way   PIN: CC08734
                  Crimson, CT 06010   EIN: 74-5386738
                  (010) 561-4512

PREOPERATIVE DIAGNOSIS: Rule out cause of obstructive jaundice in this patient with a recent cholecystectomy in March 19xx and now with obvious jaundice.

POSTOPERATIVE DIAGNOSIS: No evidence of obvious stones. Stricture at the distal common bile duct, consistent with benign versus malignant disease. Stent placed without difficulty. The patient's pathology report will be reviewed to determine if this is a periampullary carcinoma versus a benign stricture.

NAME OF PROCEDURE:
1. Endoscopic retrograde cholangiopancreatography with biopsy of the ampulla
2. Cytologic specimens from the pancreatic duct
3. Sphincterotomy
4. Placement of an internal stent, common bile duct and the duodenum

PROCEDURE IN BRIEF: Status post informed consent, the patient was premedicated with a total of 150 mg of Demerol, 9 mg of Versed, and 2.5 mg of Glucagon.

At this point, a Pentax upper GI endoscope was advanced through the esophagus into the duodenum and also into the ampulla. The ampulla appeared somewhat erythematous and consistent with the possibility of an infiltrating periampullary carcinoma. A cholangiogram was obtained showing dilatation of the common bile duct with a narrow stricture involving the distal common bile duct. A sphincterotomy was completed at this time and a pancreatogram was also obtained. The pancreatogram appeared normal without any pathology.

A cytologic brush was used to obtain specimens from the pancreatic duct, from the mid body to the ampulla. At this point, with a marked amount of difficulty, the common bile duct was recannulated and a guide wire was advanced into the secondary radicles and a one-step stent was advanced into the common bile duct. This stent was noted to lie between the common hepatic duct and the duodenum with good positioning and good drainage.

The patient also had a biopsy of the ampulla which appeared abnormal, consistent with possible periampullary carcinoma.

CHUNG CHOI, MD

CC:cc33   d: 11-12-xx   t: 11-12-xx   Document: 777.ccc

Exercise 23 – 9

Operative Report 4

DUNCAN DAY HOSPITAL
4499 DOOR WAY
DUNCAN, DE 15678
TIN 38-6915703

Patient:	Doolittle, Daisy	Patient #:	88290499
Date of Surgery:	12/7/xx	DOB:	08/01/59
Surgeon:	Donald Denny, MD*	Assistant:	Diana Dorman, MD*
Anesthesiologist:	Debbie Donovan*	Anesthesia:	General
Pre-operative DX:	Carcinoma of the Cervix	Post-Op DX:	Same

Procedure: Radical Hysterectomy, Partial Vaginectomy, Bilateral Salpingo-oophorectomy, Bilateral Pelvic Lymph Node Dissection, Supra-pubic Cystostomy, Sigmoidoscopy, Cystoscopy

Findings: On examination under anesthesia, the vaginal vault was clear. The cervix showed signs of cancer that was biopsied but it seemed to be confined to the cervix and not into the parametrium. Sigmoidoscopy to 20 cm was clear. The bladder was entirely normal with no evidence of problems. Both urethral orifices were clear. The entire abdominal cavity was explored. Liver and gallbladder were normal. The appendix was absent. There was no evidence of any other diseases within the pelvis. No lymph nodes were palpable in the periaortic common iliac and pelvic lymph nodes. The uterus was anterior freely moveable. Both tubes and ovaries appeared normal. There was a corpus luteum cyst on the left ovary and no evidence of any disease once we opened up the parametrium. Superior vesical space and perirectal spaces were clear.

Procedure: Routine prepping and draping of the perineum, inhalation anesthesia. First, examination was carried out using a disposable sigmoidoscope. We examined the rectum to 20 cm. Finding no disease in that area, the bladder was examined using 30E water cystoscopy unit. Finding no disease in that area, the Foley catheter was placed within the bladder and the abdomen was prepped and draped in the usual manner and opened through a transverse incision through skin and subcutaneous tissue and fascia, muscle and peritoneum. Once the peritoneum was opened, and bleeding was controlled with the Bovie, the above findings were noted.

Some peritoneal washings were obtained. The bowel was packed off by means of laparotomy sponges and Balfour retractor was placed within. The uterus was lifted by Carmalt clamps along the broad ligament. The round ligaments were bilaterally clamped, cut, and ligated with stick ties of 0 Vicryl suture. Retroperitoneal space was then opened exposing the ureter and the external iliac vessels. The ureter was dissected down to the tunnel. The infundibulopelvic ligaments were isolated, doubly ligated and cut. Posterior peritoneum was cut down to the ureter. Bladder flap was developed by sharp dissection to the middle third of the vagina. The tissue off this area was dissected off. Lymph node dissection was carried down to the common iliac, external iliac, obturator fossa and hypogastric vessels bilaterally. Lymph nodes on the right side were suspicious for tumor and so were obtained for frozen section.

The entire area was dissected out and bleeding was contained with the Bovie or with clips. The webb was then taken down by first clamping, cutting, and ligating the uterine vessels and part of the webb was taken down with large Weck clips. Once this was accomplished, our attention was directed to the ureter. The ureter was dissected out of its tunnel, the uterine vessels and parametria being taken over it until we could see the ureter from the pelvic brim down to the bladder. The entire webb was taken down with Bovie or hemoclips. Free ties of 2-0 silk suture.

At this point, the posterior peritoneum was cut. The uterosacral ligaments were taken as far laterally as possible. This was taken down with either large Weck clips or stick ties of 0 Vicryl suture until they were entirely free. The rectum was entirely separated from the vagina. The cardinal and uterosacral ligaments were clamped, cut, and ligated with stick ties of 0 Vicryl suture.

The vaginal vault was then entered and the upper third of the specimen was removed. The vaginal vault was closed with interrupted figure 8 of 0 Vicryl suture. Angles were placed with interrupted 0 Vicryl suture. No bleeding was noted from any of the pedicles. The entire pelvis was irrigated with saline. Retroperitoneal drains were then placed with Jackson-Pratts and these were stitched into the skin with 0 silk suture. Retroperitoneal space was closed with 0 Vicryl suture. Sponge and needle counts were reported as correct. The peritoneum was closed with running 0 Vicryl suture. The fascia was closed with interrupted 0 Vicryl suture. Estimated blood loss was 900 cc.

Total time under anesthesia, 2 hr, 15 min.

DONALD DENNY, MD

DD:DD333
d: 12/7/xx
t: 12/7/xx
Document: 5556.dd

* On staff at Duncan Day Hospital

Exercise 23 – 10

Operative Report 5

EASTWOOD COMMUNITY MEDICAL CLINIC
7854 EAST ROAD, EASTWOOD, CA 98765
(987) 555-6546   TIN: 12-3123152   PIN: E567321

PATIENT NAME:	Edward Edmunds	**PATIENT NUMBER:**	098-000-432EE
PHYSICIAN:	Evelyn Elliot, MD	**ASSISTANT:**	Ernie Escalante
DATE OF OPERATION:	5-10-xx		
PREOPERATIVE DX:	Punctate wounds L knee. FB embedded distal R femur, D/T gunshot wound.		
POSTOPERATIVE DX:	Same		
ANESTHESIA:	General		

OPERATION: Diagnostic and operative arthroscopy, removal of loose and foreign bodies, right knee and partial lateral meniscectomy, right knee.

PROCEDURE: The patient was prepped and draped in the usual aseptic manner under adequate general anesthetic with the patient in the supine position on a flat operating table with a knee post in place. The arthroscope was introduced into the joint through the anteriolateral portal and the arthroscope was passed into the joint and visualization was started in the medial compartment of the joint. The medial meniscus appeared to be intact with ragged frayed edges but none of which appeared to be a significant tear of the meniscus. The intercondylar notch was found to have and intact anterior cruciate ligament. There was an attached loose body in the anterior portion of the intercondylar notch region along the medial eminence at the base of the anterior cruciate ligament. The lateral compartment was then visualized in its entirety and was found to have no loose bodies. The lateral meniscus was found to have a tear at its anterior to middle third junction. With the aid of basket forceps and motorized incisor shaver, this portion of the meniscus was carefully removed, taking care to leave behind a stable rim of meniscus for support of the patient's knee structures. Following this removal, the loose body in the anterior aspect of the knee was carefully removed with the aid of a pituitary rongeur, and a shaver also was used in this region. Visualization was then turned to the posterior compartments of the knee and in the lateroposterior compartment, there was found a penduculated attached loose body in this region, which was carefully removed in a piecemeal fashion with the pituitary rongeur and with a curved motorized suction incisor blade. Following complete removal of this loose body, a small portion was found to have been detached from the main body of this structure and this was carefully removed with the pituitary rongeur. Attention was then turned to the distal right femur. The foreign body was removed with the aid of a pituitary ronguer and a curved motorized suction incisor blade. Following this, all areas were copiously irrigated. Visualization was carried out in the suprapatellar pouch. There was found no loose bodies in this region. The patient's knee was then carefully flushed of all extraneous fragments and debris and then the puncture incisions were closed with 3-0 nylon suture. Following closure of these punctures, three in total, in the anteromedial, anterolateral as well as the suprapatellar area, the joint was then injected with 25 cc of Marcaine with epinephrine for postop analgesia.

Attention was then turned to the left knee. The arthroscope was introduced through the anterolateral portal and passed into the joint and visualization was started in the medial compartment of the joint. The medial meniscus appeared to be intact with no significant damage. All areas were copiously irrigated, followed by closure of the punctate wounds (four). The joint was then injected with 25 cc of Marcaine with epinephrine for postop analgesia. Peripheral pulses were checked prior to removing the patient from the operating room. The pulses were adequate and commensurate with the level they were prior to surgery. The patient tolerated this well and was removed from the operating room in satisfactory condition.

Evelyn Elliot, MD

EE:EE56   D: 5/10/xx T: 5/10/xx DOCUMENT: 77-997.ee

Exercise 23 – 11

Diagnostic Report 1

ARCADIA MEDICAL CENTER
8000 Another Street
Alverville, AK 99188
RADIOLOGY CENTER

Patient: Abby Addison

Patient Number: 33299-08

Referring MD: Ann Anderson, MD

Date: 1-13-xx

Procedure: Ultrasound Upper Abdominal and Gallbladder

Scans of the upper abdomen were performed using 3.5 MHz transducer.

The liver is normal in size, contour, and echogenicity. The pancreatic head appears normal in size and echogenic texture. Both kidneys are normal in size, shape and position with a normal echogenic relationship to the liver. The common bile duct measures 4 mm in size, which is well within normal limits, but is inflamed.

INTERPRETATION: Relatively normal gall bladder and upper abdomen.

Al Alexander, MD
8020 Another Street
Alverville, AK 99188
(000) 555-1111
TIN: 763-76-3763
PIN: A96354

AAA:aa91
d: 1-13-xx
t: 1-14-xx
Document: 77738.aa

Exercise 23 – 12

Diagnostic Report 2

BRONSON BROTHERS MEDICAL CENTER
9876 Bright Lane
Brighton, DC 23787

PATIENT'S NAME
Bobby Bumble

HOSPITAL NUMBER
9888-009

X-RAY NUMBER
80090

ROOM NUMBER
ER

REFERRING PHYSICIAN
Bruno Ball, MD

DATE OF EXAM
6-19-xx

AP & LAT R ANKLE, AP & LAT R WRIST:

INDICATION:
Chronic instability R ankle, injury R wrist,

FINDINGS:
R ankle: There is no evidence of FX or dislocation. There is evidence of tissue swelling.
R wrist: There is no evidence of fx or dislocation. There is evidence of tissue swelling.

INTERPRETATION:
Right ankle: Evidence of tissue swelling. Study limited. Suggest additional studies to correlate physical findings. Suggest MRI to assess tissue damage.
Right wrist: Evidence of tissue swelling.

Beth Brown, MD
Staff x-ray technician

BB:BB95
d: 6-19-xx 1300
t: 6-19-xx 1405
Document: 111122.bbb

Exercise 23 – 13

Diagnostic Report 3

CANYON CITY HOSPITAL
4440 Center Drive
Carson, CT 06001
RADIOLOGY CENTER

Patient: Cathy Crenshaw
Referring MD: Christopher Campbell
Date: 11-1-xx
Procedure: Gallbladder and Upper Abdominal Ultrasound

Scans of the upper abdomen were performed using 3.5 MHz transducer.

The liver is normal in size, contour, and echogenicity. The pancreatic head appears normal in size and echogenic texture. Both kidneys are extremely small consistent with renal failure. There is stricture at the distal common bile duct with some inflammation consistent with benign versus malignant disease

INTERPRETATION: Stricture of the distal common bile duct. Rule out benign verses malignant disease.

.

CHRISTINE CAPLAN, MD
1010 Capital Court, Carson, CT 06010
PHONE: (000) 006-6060
SSN 060-10-0601

CC:CC80   d: 11-1-xx t: 11-1-xx Document: 5566.cc

Exercise 23 – 14

Diagnostic Reports 4

DUNCAN DAY HOSPITAL
4499 DOOR WAY
DUNCAN, DE 15678

PATIENT'S NAME
Daisy Doolittle

HOSPITAL NUMBER
88290499

X-RAY NUMBER
22097222

ROOM NUMBER
ER

REFERRING PHYSICIAN
Doris Dean, MD

DATE OF EXAM
11/26/xx

SITE:
Abdomen

INDICATION:
Dysfunctional uterine bleeding

FINDINGS:
Numerous small masses uterus, cervix & vaginal canal

IMPRESSION:
Carcinoma of the cervix

DAVE DAVIS, MD
Staff x-ray technician
TIN: 31-3253253

DD:DD55
d: 11/26/xx   1130
t: 11/26/xx   1205
Document: 111122.ddd

Exercise 23 – 15

Diagnostic Report 5

EASTWOOD COMMUNITY MEDICAL CENTER
7854 EAST ROAD
EASTWOOD, CA 98765

PATIENT'S NAME
Edward Edmunds

HOSPITAL NUMBER
512555655

X-RAY NUMBER
89898003876

ROOM NUMBER
ER

REFERRING PHYSICIAN
Eric Ericson, MD

DATE OF EXAM
5/9/xx

AP & LAT R & L KNEES:

INDICATION:
Gunshot wound to both knees

FINDINGS:
L knee: No evidence of fracture, dislocation or other significant bone or joint pathology
R knee: FB embedded distal R femur, bone fragments in joint space

IMPRESSION:
Gunshot wound to both knees. Bullet in distal right femur

Eve Ellis, MD
2929 Earle Court
Eastwood, CA 98766
TIN: 865-86-5865
PIN: E764851

EE: EE66
d: 5/9/xx
t: 5/9/xx
Document: 333322.eee

Exercise 23 – 16

Medical History and Physical Examination Report 1

ARCADIA MEDICAL CENTER
8000 Another Street
Alverville, AK 99188

DATE: 1-13-xx
PATIENT NAME: Abby Addison
PATIENT NUMBER: 33299-08
PHYSICIAN: Alfred Ackerman
                   3329 Angels Street
                   Alverville, AK 99230
                   SSN: 332-93-2933
                   PIN: A329083

HISTORY AND PHYSICAL

CHIEF COMPLAINT: Nausea with hematemesis

HISTORY OF PRESENT ILLNESS: This 25-year-old female, who was discharged from Arcadia Medical Center 2 days ago, is readmitted after severe abdominal pain and nausea, followed by hematemesis today. The patient had been hospitalized on 1/6/xx with epigastric pain due to gallbladder disease. There was also evidence for common bile duct obstruction. The patient underwent a laparoscopic cholecystectomy without complications. A gallstone that was blocking the common bile duct could not be retrieved at that time. The patient underwent ERCP on 1-10-xx by Dr. Albert Adler, who successfully removed the obstructing stone. The patient felt relief of abdominal symptoms almost immediately. She was discharged home on 1-11-xx. The next day, the patient began to experience nausea. She had several episodes of vomiting without evidence of hematemesis. However, on 1-13-xx, her abdominal pain worsened and the patient was brought to the hospital by the paramedics. While in transport, the patient vomited bright red blood. She also notes that her stool had been black after hospital discharge. The patient is now admitted and has an NG tube in place.

PAST MEDICAL HISTORY: The patient was hospitalized at Arcadia Medical Center one week ago with gallbladder disease and common bile duct obstruction, as described in the previous section. There is no history of hypertension, diabetes mellitus or heart disease. There are no known allergies.

REVIEW OF SYSTEMS:
Central Nervous System: The patient has felt dizzy during the past 24 hours.
Cardiovascular, Respiratory: There has been no dyspnea or chest pain.
Gastrointestinal: The patient has had severe nausea with vomiting and hematemesis, as described in the history.
Genitourinary: There has been no dysuria.
Musculoskeletal: There have been no joint disturbances.
Vital Signs: Temperature 97.5, pulse 108, respirations 22, and blood pressure 110/80

PHYSICAL EXAMINATION:
General: Well-nourished, well-developed female, alert, somewhat apprehensive. NG tube in place draining coffee-ground material.
HEENT: Pupils are equal, round and reactive to light and accommodation. Extraocular muscles are intact. Fundi are poorly visualized.
Neck: Thyroid not palpable. No jugular venous distention.
Chest: Breath sounds clear to auscultation bilaterally.
Heart: Regular rate and rhythm. No murmurs.
Abdomen: Soft, nontender. Punctate wound, secondary to laparoscopic procedure last week.
Extremities: No pitting edema

LABORATORY RESULTS IN THE EMERGENCY ROOM: WBC 14.4, hemoglobin 10.2, hematocrit 30.1. Sodium 140, potassium 4.5, chloride 100, bicarbonate 25, BUN 23, creatinine 0.6. Random glucose 126.

ASSESSMENT:
1. Upper gastrointestinal bleed; rule out secondary to Mallory-Weiss tear, rule out complications stemming from Problem No. 2.
2. Status post ERCP (endoscopic retrograde cholangiopancreatography) 3 days ago due to Problems 3 and 4.
3. Status post hospitalization last week with gallstones and common bile duct obstruction, secondary to retained stone.
4. Status post laparoscopic cholecystectomy last week, secondary to problem No. 3.

PLAN:
1. Admit.
2. NG tube to low suction.
3. Upper endoscopy by Dr. Albert Adler.
4. Follow-up.

ALFRED ACKERMAN, MD

AA:AA89
D: 1-13-xx
T: 1-14-xx
Document: 5555.aa

Exercise 23 – 17

Medical History and Physical Examination Report 2

BILL BLAKE DOCTORS OFFICE
9000 Broadway Street
Brighton, DC 23787

HISTORY AND PHYSICAL

Patient: Bobby Bumble
          93485 Bumpkiss Court, Barkingville, DC 23456

Date of birth: 01-01-44

Patient #: 44444

Attending: Bill Blake, MD

Date: 08-18-xx

HISTORY OF PRESENT ILLNESS: The patient is a 49-year-old white male with chronic instability of the right ankle. Patient states that 2 months ago he was running to catch a bus and the R ankle collapsed underneath him. He fell to the pavement injuring his R ankle and R wrist. He was transported to Bronson Brothers Medical Center. X-rays showed no evidence of fracture or dislocation to either the ankle or wrist. Patient states that he has had chronic instability of the ankle for "a number of years," possibly relating to a college football injury.

PAST MEDICAL HISTORY: Non contributory

REVIEW OF SYSTEMS:
CARDIO: There has been no history of chest pain, palpitations
PULMONARY: No shortness of breath
MUSCULO: Pain right lower extremity and right hand
CNS: No dizziness, or lightheadedness or paresthesia

PHYSICAL EXAMINATION:
General: Cooperative, pleasant middle aged male who appeared in no acute distress.
HEENT: Mouth---pharynx not injected. Neck---supple without mass or tenderness.
CHEST: Clear with equal breath sounds bilaterally. There was no chest wall discomfort demonstrable on compression.
HEART: Normal S1 and S2 without murmur.
ABDOMEN: benign.
EXTREMITIES: No clubbing, cyanosis. There is non pitting edema to the right ankle Limited range of motion. Pain with flexion. Right lower extremity is positive for drawer test and inversion test.

ASSESSMENT: Chronic instability, right ankle.

PLAN:
1. Admit patient to Bronson Brothers Medical Center
2. Consultation orthopedic specialist; Ben Bennett MD for evaluation and surgical intervention

        Bill Blake, MD
        SSN: 081-89-3081
        PIN: B445544

BB: bbb46
dd: 08-18-xx
dt: 08-18-xx
Document: 77788.bb

Exercise 23 – 18

Medical History and Physical Examination Report 3

CANYON CITY HOSPITAL
4440 Center Drive,
Carson, CT 06001

DATE: 11-6-XX

PATIENT: CATHY CRENSHAW

HISTORY OF PRESENT ILLNESS: Patient is a middle-aged female who presents with jaundice over the past 2 weeks. The patient has had a long history of medical problems, which include: (1) Adult-onset diabetes mellitus, (2) Hypertension, (3) Dialysis, (4) Congestive heart failure and (5) Pneumonia.

The patient's recent medical history started in March, when she presented with gangrene of the left foot. She underwent a left BK amputation, which was eventually converted to a left AK amputation in April. Subsequently, the patient developed cholecystitis in the same hospitalization and underwent a cholecystectomy.

Additional surgical history includes small bowel resection in 2 years ago. Multiple vascular surgeries on the legs, left and right, and she is also status post hysterectomy. Patient discontinued tobacco last year and she has never abused alcohol. Patient was noted to have jaundice in April of this year, but this resolved and she states that she has been tested for Hepatitis B and C at the Dialysis Center and this is now positive.

REVIEW OF SYSTEMS: HEENT: Patient does wear glasses.
CARDIOPULMONARY: Positive for pneumonia, and congestive heart failure related to fluid overload.

SOCIAL HISTORY: History is positive for patient socially being a teacher and she is now retired because of the multiple medical problems. She does occasional part-time work for Creative Creations Corp. making small handicrafts. She has had periodic diarrhea and constipation and also vomiting has started over the past couple of weeks.

PHYSICAL EXAMINATION: Reveals a well-developed, fairly well-nourished female.
PULSE: 88
BLOOD PRESSURE: 150/90
RESPIRATION: 18
WEIGHT: 132 pounds
HEENT: Atraumatic and normocephalic. Obvious scleral icterius is noted.
LUNGS: Clear
CARDIAC: Normal S1 and normal S2
ABDOMEN: Soft, benign, nontender
EXTREMITIES: Without clubbing, cyanosis or edema
NEUROLOGIC: Grossly normal
The patient does not have all of her medications, so we are unable to review all of her medications.

ASSESSMENT: The patient has jaundiced; quite possibly obstructive. Would suggest CBC, PT, PTT, Hepatitis panel to evaluate for the possibility of Hepatitis. Possibility for drug induced vs. viral induced hepatitis. Other considerations include obstructive jaundice, possibly related to common bile duct stone vs. stricture of the common bile duct. Also a possibility that patient may have a neoplasm via periodic jaundice April and now November. Would therefore also suggest ultrasound, endoscopic retrograde cholangiopancreatography.

Impressions:
1. Jaundice; rule out common bile duct obstruction, rule out pancreatic tumor.
2. Leukocytosis; possibly secondary to #1.
3. End-stage chronic renal failure with hemodialysis.
4. Adult-onset diabetes mellitus.
5. Peripheral vascular disease.
6. Left above-knee amputation, 4 months ago secondary to #5.
7. Hypertension.
8. Pregangrenous changes, right foot.
9. Status post aortofemoral bypass graft surgery, 2 years ago.
10. Pulmonary embolism during hospitalization.
11. History of asthma.
12. Surgical correction of small bowel obstruction, 10 years ago.
13. History of polio in childhood with bilateral foot deformities.
14. History of multiple podiatric procedures, secondary to #13.
15. History of recurrent perianal abscesses.
16. History of multiple hospitalizations for psychiatric disorders.

Treatment plan:
1. Surgical evaluation and probable intervention for obstructive jaundice.
2. Laboratory profile.
3. Adjust insulin regimen.
4. Hemodialysis.

CARL CALLAHAN, MD (staff)
CC:CC999 d: 11-6-XX   t: 11-7-XX   Document: 9900099.cc

Exercise 23 – 19

Medical History and Physical Examination Report 4

DAVID DAY M.D.
4508 DOOR WAY
DUNCAN, DE 15678

PATIENT NAME:	DAISY DOOLITTLE	PATIENT NUMBER:	009998
PHYSICIAN:	DAVID DAY, MD	DATE ADMITTED:	11/30/xx

HISTORY AND PHYSICAL

Pt to have surgery at Duncan Day Hospital, 12/7/xx. Procedure to be performed by Donald Denny, MD.

CHIEF COMPLAINT: Dysfunctional uterine bleeding, carcinoma of the cervix.

HISTORY OF PRESENT ILLNESS: Pt went to Duncan Day Hospital on 11/26/xx complaining of abnormal vaginal discharge & bleeding for one week. LMP 02/20/xx.
Abd. x-ray taken. Numerous small masses were found in the uterus, cervix & vaginal canal.

PAST MEDICAL HISTORY: Four NSVD, 2 prior abortions Feb 92, Nov 92. 1 miscarriage requiring extraction, 03/20/xx.

VITAL SIGNS: BP 120/70, Pulse 90, Resp 23, Temp 99.0
PHYSICAL EXAMINATION:
GENERAL: Well-nourished, well-developed 34 y/o H female, cooperative, nervous.
HEENT: Pupils equal, round and reactive to light and accommodation. Extraocular muscles are intact.

NECK: Thyroid not palpable. No jugular venous distention.

CHEST: Breath sounds good to auscultation bilaterally.
HEART: Regular rate and rhythm, no murmurs.
ABDOMEN: Soft, nontender. Positive multiple non-tender palpable masses in RLQ and LLQ.
PELVIC: Vaginal vault clear, cervix showed signs of cancer that was biopsied.
EXTREMITIES: Normal, with good reflexes.

ASSESSMENT: Probable Carcinoma of the cervix

PLAN: Surgical procedure by Dr. Donald Denny
              DAVID DAY MD
              TIN: 11-3093109 PIN: D13093

DD: DD98 D: 11/30/xx   T: 11/30/xx   Document: 999440.ddd

Exercise 23 – 20

Medical History and Physical Examination Report 5

Esther Edelman, MD
5993 Erlich Street
Eastwood, CA 98766

Patient Name: Edward Edmunds   Patient Number: 685947-465   Date: 5-10-xx
The patient is to have surgery on 5/10/xx, to be performed by Dr. Evelyn Elliot, orthopedic surgeon.
CHIEF COMPLAINT: Gunshot wound to both knees

HISTORY OF PRESENT ILLNESS: This 66-year-old male, retired surgeon, suffered a gunshot wound that traversed the left knee and entered the right knee, on the morning of 5/9/xx. There is a bullet lodged in the distal right femur. Apparently wounds to both lt and RT knee were caused by the same projectile. The patient had driven to a store. While walking from his car to the store entrance he was struck by the bullet. The patient saw no one near who appeared to be responsible.

   The patient was seen that day in the Eastwood Community Medical Center ER by Dr. Eric Ericson. An orthopedic surgical consultant, Evelyn Elliot, MD, was called in to discuss possible surgical intervention. Dr. Elliot reviewed the x-ray films taken at Eastwood Community Medical Center. She has recommended surgical intervention to remove the bullet from the distal right femur. Apparently there are bone fragments in the joint space. Since suffering the gunshot wound, the patient has not had severe pain or bleeding. He has been treated with Cipro 750 mg p.o. b.i.d. The patient has not been febrile.

PAST MEDICAL HISTORY: The patient takes no medication on a regular basis. He is not being treated for hypertension, but the patient was given diuretics for about a 2-month period in 19xx. Blood pressure apparently had been elevated at that time. Subsequent measurements of blood pressure have been within normal limits. There is no history of diabetes mellitus. The patient has no frank history of heart disease, but he had an abnormal EKG last year. The record of 03/16/xx, reveals normal sinus rhythm with some nonspecific ST and T wave changes. The patient was seen at that time because of dyspepsia. He has had no chest pain in the past. There has never been dyspnea on exertion, and the patient has not been treated for heart disease. The patient has never previously been hospitalized.

PHYSICAL EXAMINATION:
GENERAL: Well-nourished, older aged male, alert, cooperative.
HEENT: PERRLA. Extraocular muscles intact. Fundi poorly visualized.
NECK: Thyroid not palpable. No jugular venous distention.
CHEST: Breath sounds clear to auscultation bilaterally
HEART: Regular rate and rhythm, no murmurs
ABDOMEN: Soft, nontender
RECTAL: Prostate normal size and symmetrical. Stool brown in color.
EXTREMITIES: Right knee with puncture wound medial aspect; moderate edema. 1+ pitting right lower leg edema. Punctate gunshot wounds on the anterior and medial left patellar area.

ASSESSMENT:

1. Gunshot wound right and left knees with projectile embedded in distal right femur.

2. History of abnormal EKG, nonspecific ST and T wave changes, unchanged since March.

3. History of dyspepsia.

4. Allergy to penicillin.

PLAN:

1. Admit to Eastwood Community Medical Clinic

2. Surgical intervention by orthopedic surgeon, Evelyn Elliot.

ESTHER EDELMAN MD   TIN: 523-52-3523/PIN: E523523
EE:EE77   D: 5/9/xx T: 5/9/xx   Document: 12345678.eee

Appendix 23 – 1

Abstracting from Medical Reports

Triage Report 1

First, transfer the patient identity information from the patient chart and the triage report to the UB-92. This includes name and address information placed in Items 12 and 13.

Next, go through the UB-92 item by item and locate the information that is needed to complete each box.

Item 1 – The name and address of the hospital are not listed. This information would be known by the medical biller, since it would be their place of employment.

Item 4 – The type of bill is 112, since it is for a hospital inpatient, first interim billing. Because additional information is not available, this bill will be for the emergency services only.

Item 5 – The federal tax number is obtained from the provider of service.

Item 6 – Statement period. The patient was admitted to the emergency room on 1/13/xx, and was subsequently admitted to a hospital room. Therefore, the statement ending date should be 1/13/xx.

Items 7 through 10 – Insurance coverage information can found in the patient file which was set up in Exercise 1-1.

Item 14 – The birth date would also be taken from the patient file which was set up in Exercise 1-1.

Item 15 – The patient is female.

Item 16 – The patient's marital status is on the patient information sheet. She is single.

Item 17 – The patient was admitted on 13 Jan xx.

Item 18 – The patient arrived at 14:09.

Item 19 – The patient arrived by ambulance to the ER.

Item 20 – A 1 should be entered here. Seven would not be used for this bill since this bill is for outpatient services only, resulting in a hospital admission. A 7 would be used for the subsequent inpatient bill.

Item 21 – Discharge hour. Since the patient was not actually discharged, this information would be left blank.

Item 22 – Status at time of billing. 09 should be entered in this box because the patient was admitted.

Items 24 through 30 – There are no condition codes related to this billing.

Items 32 through 36 - There are no occurrence codes or occurrence span codes.

Item 38 – According to the patient's chart, the responsible party is the patient. Her name and address should be listed here.

Items 39 through 41 – Should be left blank since there are no specific values listed in the triage report. However, it should be noted that ultrasound scanning of the gallbladder and upper abdomen were taken. Therefore, there would be a professional component involved in reading the ultrasound, so a value would need to be added for patients with Medicare or Medicaid coverage.

Items 42 & 43 – Item 42 should be coded with the appropriate revenue code and 43 with the description. There would generally be a standard charge for the Emergency Room: (450 EMERG ROOM). There should also be codes for medical/surgical supplies used (270 MED-SUR SUPPLIES), for laboratory tests done (300 LABORATORY) and a gallbladder and upper abdominal ultrasound performed utilizing the hospitals ultrasound equipment (402 ULTRASOUND). Enter a total for all charges (001 TOTAL CHARGES). Many hospitals will add a note to the patient and the insurance carrier in this section to indicate these charges are for emergency room and facility charges only. Additional billings may be made for inpatient services or for professional services. Professional services would include not only a physician, but also the x-ray or lab technician, and any other professionals included in the patients care. Such a note helps clarify that additional billings are not a duplicate of this one.

Information given on the triage report would need to be added regarding the standard fees charged by the hospital for triage services to complete the billing form.

Item 50 – The patient chart lists Artin Corporation as the patient's insurance coverage.

Items 52 & 53 – There is no signature on file for release of information or for assignment of benefits. These signatures would need to be obtained prior to filing the claim with the insurance carrier.

Item 54 – If the patient made any payments on the bill, the amount would be entered here. This amount would then be subtracted from the total in 55.

Item 55 – Since it is unknown whether the patient has previously paid her deductible or what amount of coinsurance is due from the patient, it is assumed that the insurance carrier is responsible for the entire amount of the bill.

Items 58 & 59 – The patient is the insured according to the patient chart. Therefore, her name would be entered in Item 58 and the code 01 (self) would be entered in Item 59.

Item 60 – Since no subscriber certificate number has been given, the medical biller should enter the responsible party's Social Security number. This will allow the insurance carrier to verify her policy.

Item 64 – The patient is employed by Artistic Aardvarks. Since there is insurance through her employer, it can be assumed that the patient is working full time. Therefore, her employment status should be listed as 1.

Items 65 & 66 – The patient's employer name, Artistic Aardvarks, and address should be entered here.

Items 67 & 68 – Should contain the diagnosis listed in the Discharge Impression portion of the triage report. However, this patient has been admitted for further study and no diagnosis is given. Therefore, the chief complaint is Hematemesis. This has a diagnosis code of 578.0. The patient also had severe abdominal pain, so code 789.0 would be appropriate for Item 68. The hematemesis code should be listed first as it is an objective diagnosis and the abdominal pain is a subjective diagnosis.

Items 69 through 75 – There were no additional diagnoses associated with the condition

Item 77 – E codes are not needed since this is not an accident and the cause of the hematemesis is unknown.

Items 79 & 80 – An ultrasound of the gallbladder and upper abdominal area were performed. Therefore, 9 should be entered in Item 79, procedure code 88.76 in the first part of Item 80 and the date of 1/13/xx in the second part of Item 80. The information contained in these boxes is used for informational purposes only, not for actual payment. The actual charges for the services would be listed in the itemized billing, which is summarized in Items 42 through 47. For this reason, and because the ICD-9 does not contain codes for lab tests, the individual lab tests performed would not be listed here.

Item 82 – The attending physician information should be taken from the bottom of the triage report. Remember to include any title designations (i.e., MD).

Item 83 – No secondary physician was listed.

Item 84 – It would be appropriate to leave the remarks section blank.

The student should not forget to sign the claim as the hospital representative.

CPT® Codes, descriptions and two-digit numeric modifiers only are copyright 2004 American Medical Association. All rights Reserved.

Triage Report 2

First, transfer the patient identity information from the triage report and the patient chart to the UB-92. This includes name and address information placed in Items 12 and 13, and birth date placed in item 14.

Next, go through the UB-92 item by item and locate the information that is needed to complete each box.

Item 1 – The name and address of the hospital are not listed. This information would be known by the medical biller, since it would be their place of employment.

Item 3 – The patient control number would be the admission number on the triage report and the account number on the patient admitting form. None is listed, so this item can be left blank.

Item 4 – The type of bill is 131 since it is for a hospital outpatient, admit through discharge.

Item 5 – The Federal tax number would be entered here.

Item 6 – Statement period. The patient was admitted on 06/19/xx. Since the discharge time is before midnight, the discharge date would also be 06/19/xx. These same dates would also be the statement period dates.

Item 14 –The patient's birth date is listed on the patient chart.

Item 15 – The patient is male.

Item 16 – The patient chart indicates that the patient is married. Enter an M.

Item 17 – The patient was admitted on 06/19/xx.

Item 18 – The patient arrived at 09:37, so 09 should be entered.

Item 20 – The default code of 1 for "patient self referral" should be used if the referral status is unknown

Item 21 – The discharge hour is 13:01.

Item 22 – Patient's status at time of billing. The patient was sent home, therefore, a 01 should be entered in this box.

Items 32 through 36 – There are no occurrence codes.

Item 38 – According to the admitting form, the responsible party is the patient. His name and address would be entered here.

Item 42 – Should be coded with the appropriate revenue code. There is usually a standard charge for the emergency room and for the wrist and ankle x-rays. The coding would be as follows: 450 Emerg Room, 329 DX XRAY/OTHER. A splint was applied which would create a charge for MED-SUR SUPPLIES (270). TOTAL CHARGES, 001 should be entered at the bottom of the charges.

Information given on the triage report would need to be added regarding the standard fees charged by the hospital for triage services to complete the billing form.

Item 50 – The patient chart lists Bantam Enterprises as his insurance coverage.

Items 52 & 53 – There are no signatures on file for release of information or for assignment of benefits. These signatures would need to be obtained prior to filing the claim with the insurance carrier.

Item 54 – If the patient made any payments on the bill, this amount should be entered here. This amount would then be subtracted from the total in 55.

Items 58 & 59 – The patient is listed as the insured on the patient chart. Therefore, his name should be entered in Item 58 and the code 01 (self) in Item 59.

Item 60 – Since no employee number has been given, the medical biller should place the responsible party's Social Security here. This will allow the insurance carrier to verify his insurance policy.

Item 64 – Since the patient has insurance through his employer, it may be assumed that he is a full time employee. Therefore, a 1 should be entered in Item 64.

Items 65 & 66 – Bobby's employer is listed as Bumbling Bureaucrats. Enter the name and the address.

Item 67 – Should contain the diagnoses listed in the Discharge Impression portion of the triage report: (1) Sprain, R wrist. The diagnosis code is 842.00.

Items 68 through 76 – There are no additional diagnoses associated with the condition.

Item 77 – Since this was an accident, the appropriate E code is E885.

Item 79 – Should indicate a 9 (ICD-9 was used for coding).

Items 80 & 81 – X-rays were taken of the right wrist and right ankle. Enter procedure code 88.23 with the date the x-ray was taken in Item 80 and code 88.28 and the date in Item 81.

Item 82 – The attending physician information can be obtained from the triage report. Remember to include any title designations (i.e., MD).

Item 83 – No secondary physician is listed.

Item 84 – Under remarks, it would be appropriate to write "stumbled while running for bus." to further indicate that injuries were the result of an accident.

Operative Report 1

Step 1
The first step in interpreting and billing the information contained on an operative report is to determine the procedures and services that were utilized.

The operative report is for an operation that utilized hospital operating room and supply services, and the services of a surgeon, an assistant surgeon, and an anesthesiologist.

Since the hospital services and supplies would be contained within a hospital record and would be billed on the UB-92, the medical biller would need the patient's entire file of supplies and services rendered. Since this information is not available from the operative report and patient information sheet (and since the hospital medical billers are

usually separate from those of the surgeon, assistant surgeon, and anesthesiologist), the medical biller would be unable to complete a UB-92 from the information given.

The doctors should bill for their services individually, using a CMS-1500.

Step 2
Transfer the information contained in the header section of the report to the CMS-1500. For example, transfer the information:

DATE:	1-13-xx (to Item 24A)
PATIENT:	Abby Addison (Item 2)
SURGEON:	Albert Adler, MD (Item 33)
POST-OP DX:	Mallory-Weiss tear (Item 21)

Items 1 through 13 – Locate the additional information needed on the patient information sheet (from Exercise 1-1) and transfer it in the same manner. If there is a current valid signature on file for Items 12 and 13, it is appropriate to enter the words "signature on file" on the signature line.

Item 14 – The first date of illness for this episode (1/6/xx) can be obtained from the triage report.

Item 18 – We know that the patient was admitted to the hospital on 01/13/xx, so this date should be placed in the first space in Item 18. Since we don't know when the patient will be discharged, the second space should be left blank.

Step 3
As previously indicated, an operative report is used to determine the procedures actually performed. The next step is to locate the corresponding CPT® code for the procedure performed. The location of the operative area is an Upper gastrointestinal bleed. The procedure is an Upper gastro intestinal endoscopy. As indicated, this procedure involved the upper gastrointestinal tract. Therefore, open the CPT® to the digestive system, gastrointestinal, upper. Code 43235 indicates with or without duodenoscopy.

Item 24E – This procedure is related to diagnosis code 1 (Item 21). Enter a 1.

Item 24G – Charges would need to be obtained from the doctor. Only 1 Upper GI was done. Enter a 1.

Item 24I – Should be N (no) since this procedure was performed after the patient was admitted, not in the emergency room (see triage report).

Item 32 & 33 – The name and address of the hospital would be entered in Item 32 and the name and address of the doctor in Item 33.

Diagnostic Report 1

Step 1
Determine the correct billing form to use. The bill is for provider services. Therefore, the CMS-1500 would be used to bill for diagnostic testing reports.

Step 2
Transfer the information from the diagnostic testing report to the CMS-1500.

Step 3
Transfer the information from the patient information sheet to the CMS-1500.

Step 4
The procedure was a Gallbladder and Upper Abdominal Ultrasound, which has a CPT® code of 76700 (Echography, abdominal, B-scan and/or real

time with image documentation; complete). Be sure to note in **Item 24I** that these services were performed in conjunction with emergency room treatment (see triage report).

Medical History and Physical Examination Report 1

Step 1
Determine the correct billing form to use. The bill is for services rendered by a physician. Therefore, the CMS-1500 would be used to bill for diagnostic testing reports.

Step 2
Transfer the information from the patient history report to the CMS-1500.

Step 3
Transfer the information from the patient information sheet to the CMS-1500.

Step 4
The service provided was an inpatient visit with a history and physical, which has a CPT® code of 99221.

Honors Certification™

The certification challenge for this chapter will be a written test of the information contained in this chapter. Each incorrect answer will result in a deduction of up to 5% from your grade. You must achieve a score of 85% or higher to pass this test. If you fail the test on your first attempt you may retake the test one additional time. The items included in the second test may be different from those in the first test.

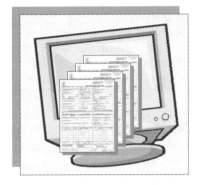

24

Claims Submission Process

After completion of this chapter you will be able to:

- Explain what a clean claim is and why it is important to submit clean claims.
- Explain the reason for the incomplete data master list and the information entered on it.
- Explain what submission time limits are and how they can affect claim payment.
- List the optical scanning guidelines.
- Explain electronic claims submission and its pros and cons.
- List the common billing reports that are used and explain their purpose.
- Explain how to handle denied claims.
- Explain how to handle the resubmission of a claim.
- Explain how to appeal the decision on a claim.
- Explain how to make an adjustment on a claim.
- Discuss the role of the State Insurance Commissioner.

Key words and concepts you will learn in this chapter:

Acknowledgement Report – Reports generated by an insurance carrier indicating claims that were received electronically.

Claim Register – A report that lists for a given time period, all the claims that were printed or submitted by a provider's office to an insurance carrier.

Claim Submission Report – A lists all claims that have been fully completed and are being submitted to the insurance carrier by the provider's office.

Clean Claims – Claims that have all the necessary information to enable them to be processed quickly.

Electronic Claim Submission – Is a process whereby insurance claims are submitted via computerized data (either by data diskette or modem) directly from the provider to the insurance company.

Font – The size of the letters typed on a typewriter or on a computer.

State Insurance Commissioner – This person is responsible for overseeing the insurance companies and their practices within the state.

Type Style – The way the individual characters are formed by a computer or typewriter.

Once the provider has seen the patient and the proper billing forms have been completed, you are ready to submit the claims for payment. There are a number of items which need to be considered before submitting the claims. These include whether or not the claims are considered clean claims, whether the claims are to be submitted on paper or electronically, and whether or not you need to consider any time limits on the claims.

Clean Claims

It is important to be sure that the claims you submit to an insurance carrier are "clean claims." **Clean claims** are claims that have all the necessary information to process them quickly for benefits.

Before submitting a claim for processing, be sure you check it and make sure that all necessary boxes have been filled in. Many times it is assumed that the computer will have filled in all the information. If a field is left blank in the computer, it will probably be left blank on the claim form.

If a claim is submitted for payment with incomplete information many insurance carriers, including Medicare, will often reject it. This can result in numerous claims that are denied, and lots of lost revenues. Additionally, the patient is often requested to make payment for the bill. This can create negative feelings between all parties concerned.

It is important to ensure that all information is complete before creating any claims. Following are several tips that can help you achieve this:

1. Look over the information sheets as soon as they are completed by the patient. If there is information which is incomplete or illegible, ask the patient to clarify the information.
2. When entering data into the computer, note files that contain incomplete data. Often a simple item such as a brightly colored note stuck to the file saying: "Need patient's birthdate" can solve the problem. Be sure to complete the required information before creating any claims.
3. Try to enter patient data while the patient is still at the facility. By doing so you can make a list of any missing information and obtain it before the patient leaves the facility.
4. Use a master list for missing data every time you encounter a file which is incomplete. Check this master list when each patient enters the facility for treatment. If necessary, ask the patient to complete the data at that time.

Incomplete Data Master List

Patient data that is incomplete is a major source of delay in both billing for services, and in payment for those services. Without complete patient data it can be difficult to properly complete a billing form. Additionally, many insurance carriers will refuse to pay a claim that is not completed properly.

Problems of incomplete data often occur because of a discrepancy between the forms the patient completes and the information needed to be input into the computer program.

Having a master list for patients with incomplete data can help an office solve this problem quickly and efficiently.

A sample Incomplete Data Master List is shown in **Figure 24 – 1**. To complete the form, fill in the data in the following fields:

Date: Indicate the date that you first noticed the information was missing.

Patient: Enter the patient's name.

Data Missing: List the data that is missing. Be sure to clearly list all items that are missing. Each piece of missing data should be placed on a separate line.

Why: List the reason why the data is missing. This can alert you to possible problems with your intake forms. For example, if a specific item is consistently overlooked by patients, perhaps it needs to be highlighted.

Disposition: When the information has been obtained, list the date obtained and the means by which the information was obtained.

Comp: Indicate the date the information was added to the computer.

Due to the limited amount of space on the form, standard abbreviations may need to be used. For cxample, the form shown in the example lists several codes. Any standard abbreviations created by the facility should be listed at the bottom of the form. This will eliminate confusion as to the proper abbreviation or its meaning.

Once a month you should send out a letter to all patients included on the incomplete data list. This can be a simple form letter with space at the bottom for them to include the information requested. If a letter is sent, be sure to include a self-addressed, stamped envelope.

Whenever you contact the patient to request the missing information, be sure to indicate that you need it to bill their insurance carrier. When people know that you cannot bill their insurance without it, they are much more likely to take the time to respond to your request.

Having an Incomplete Data Master List can also alert you to information which the computer program needs that is not included on your patient forms. If there are several pieces of data, your facility may want to create an additional form for the patients to complete which requests this information.

Incomplete Data Master List

Indicate below all the patient's whose data is incomplete at the time the patient data is being put in the computer.

Date	Patient/Account	Data Missing	Why	Disposition	Data	Comp
1/1/xx	Kent Wright/12345	Birthdate	IL	PC – 1/10/xx	BD:03/15/63	1/10/xx
		Marital Status	PO	PC – 1/10/xx	Married	1/10/xx

Why Codes:
PO – Omitted or overlooked by patient
IL – Data was completed but is illegible
NI – Not included on forms

Disposition Codes:
PC – Phone Call
LS – Letter Sent
AP – Asked in person while patient was in office.

Figure 24 – 1: Incomplete Data Master List

Submission Time Limits

Many providers require that claims be submitted within a specified period from the date services were rendered. If claims are not submitted within the time limits, payment may be reduced or denied.

Each facility should have a chart indicating the time limits for submission of claims. Additionally, it is best to set a standard of submitting all claims within 10 days of the date services were rendered. Not only does this keep you within the time limits set by most carriers, but it also insures that payment for the services is received as soon as possible.

Optical Scanning Guidelines

Many claims are routinely submitted electronically to insurance carriers. When claims are submitted electronically the claim data is entered directly through the phone lines into the insurance carrier's computer system.

Following are some tips for submitting claims electronically:

1. Be sure you understand the use of capital letters.
2. Be careful about the order of the information on your claims. If the name should be written "last name, comma, space, first name, comma, space, middle initial, period," that is how you need to type the information on the form. If you type the information in the correct order, but omit the comma, the computer program may not be able to distinguish between the first name and the last name. If you type two spaces between the data instead of one, the computer program may consider the space to be the first character of the name. Since data must match exactly with the data in the insurance carrier's computer, mistakes like this can cause a claim to be rejected or denied.
3. Do not type outside the field. Any information that is shown outside the lines of a given field will often not be recognized by the receiving computer. This can cause problems in recognizing the patient information.
4. Use the correct type style. Some computer programs require you to use a specified type

style and/or font. **Type style** is the way the individual characters are formed. **Font** is the size of the letters. If you use an incorrect font the information may be misread by the scanner.

5. If no type style or font is specified, use a common type style such as Times New Roman or Ariel. Be sure to use a large enough font to make the letters clearly distinguishable. This is usually considered to be at least an 11 point font for Times New Roman and a 10 point font for Ariel.
    - This is typed in Times New Roman 11 point.
    - This is typed in Ariel 10 point.
6. Use only black ink for printing or typing. Color inks are often not picked up by the scanner. This is because many scanners have been programmed to ignore everything in red or various shades of red since many forms are printed in red. Since some shades of red can include other colors as well (i.e., yellow or blue depending on the hue), many scanners may also be programmed to ignore these colors.
7. Try to print claims on a black and white printer, not a color one. Many color printers create black by mixing various colors together. What may appear to the human eye as totally black may actually have numerous specks of red and other colors in it. This can create problems for the scanner and cause information to be recorded incorrectly.

If all of the above items are handled properly, there is a much higher chance of creating a claim without problems.

Submitting the Claims

Once you have determined that everything on the claims is correct, you are now ready to submit them for payment.

The first step is to print out the claims that will be submitted on paper. After the claims are printed, check over each one to make sure it fits the definition of a clean claim and that it meets all the requirements for optical character recognition.

Separate the claims by insurance carrier. Some billing programs print the name and address of the insurance carrier on the top of the claims. If your

billing program does not, look at item 11c on the CMS-1500 or item 62 of the UB-92. The information found in this field will usually indicate the name of the insurance plan that covers this patient.

Electronic Claims Submission

Electronic claims submission is a process whereby insurance claims are submitted via computerized data (either by data diskette or modem) directly from the provider to the insurance company. Since some providers (especially hospitals and large medical offices) generate numerous claims per day, this means of submission is much easier than creating numerous pieces of paper, signing, and mailing them.

Claims submitted electronically usually contain fewer errors and since they eliminate the need for data entry personnel to re-enter the information payment is also generated more quickly. In addition, insurance carriers reduce their management and overhead costs by allowing electronic claims submission.

Generally, electronic claims submission is performed on a weekly basis. Once a week the medical biller contacts the insurance carrier using the computer and downloads the information.

If any claims are rejected or if there is a request for further information, the insurance carrier can contact the provider either by telephone, fax, or via computer modem. This allows a medical biller to know immediately if a claim has been rejected or if more information is needed. The claim can then be corrected and resubmitted.

It is important to have the proper equipment and forms before attempting to submit claims electronically. The format of the claim form must be approved by the carrier, and an agreement must also be in place between the provider and the insurance carrier. This agreement contains the basic understanding on the means of submitting data and the correct procedure coding system. Since electronic claims submission does not allow the opportunity for the physician to sign the claims, a physician's signature on the agreement will be accepted in lieu of a signature on the claim form. It is also imperative to have a patient signature on file for Authorization to Release Information and Assignment of Benefits.

Occasionally, some data transmission problems will arise due to systems being incompatible, static or other problems on the telephone lines, or other software or hardware problems. For this reason, always keep a back-up copy of the information transmitted until the claim has been processed. Also, try to submit claims to the insurance carrier early in the morning or late at night. In this way you may miss the peak times, during which your transmission may be interrupted.

If electronic submission is not used, the provider must generate a claim, have it signed, and mail it to the insurance carrier. The insurance carrier must then receive and log the claim, categorize it according to plan and type, screen claims for incomplete information, make a microfilm copy of the claim for future reference, review the claim and make any necessary adjustments, and enter the claim into the computer.

Electronic claim submission not only cuts down on errors, but it dramatically decreases the time needed for payment of the claim and also prevents loss of claims through the mail or other courier service.

Billing Reports

There are a number of reports that can help you manage claims that have been submitted or are in various stages of the process. By generating or running these reports on a daily basis, you can be sure that all services are being billed and all claims are proceeding properly.

The most common of these reports is listed below. Some computer programs have the capacity to generate these reports. If the program does not have a report which specifically covers the information desired, some programs will allow you to create a custom report. If this is not possible, a manual report can always be created.

Following are various reports, information regarding their purpose, and the information generally included in the report.

Transaction Reports

Many medical billing programs allow you to print a report of the claims that were entered or completed on a given day. By printing out this report, you can compare it to the appointment book to insure that all services which were completed during the day have been billed for.

Acknowledgement Reports

Acknowledgement reports are generated by an insurance carrier. They indicate the claims that were received electronically. By comparing this report to the information on your daily journal you can determine if all services that were performed have been billed.

Since claims may be submitted to different insurance carriers, there will be an Acknowledgement Report from each different insurance carrier.

Claims Submission Reports

A **Claims Submission Report** lists all claims that have been fully completed and are being submitted to the insurance carrier by the provider's office. If claims are submitted electronically, this report can be compared to the Acknowledgement Report to insure that all claims were received by the appropriate carriers.

Claims Register

A **Claims Register** is a report that lists for a given time period, all the claims that were printed or submitted by a provider's office to an insurance carrier.

Tracer Claims/Delinquent Claims

If payment is not received within 45 days of billing the insurance carrier, the biller should contact the carrier to determine the reason for the delay. Often the proper forms have not been received. If such is the case, ask which form is missing and who is responsible for sending it.

In many states there is a time limit (often 30 days) in which an insurance carrier must respond to a claim. This response can be payment of the claim, a denial of the claim, or a request for further information.

The insurance carrier may state that they have not received the claim. In such a case, ask if you can fax a copy of the claim to speed up the process. This may be allowed, or some carriers will request that you re-mail the claim. If the claim was sent electronically a copy of your electronic claims submission report or the insurance carrier's acknowledgement report may be helpful in locating the missing claim.

If the carrier is still unable to locate the claim, you can re-submit an electronic claim or re-mail a paper copy.

When speaking with the insurance carrier try to get an idea of when the claim will be paid. Remember that you should attempt to collect payment on services as soon as possible.

Denied Claims

When a claim is denied it is important to determine the reason for the denial. If the claim was denied due to incorrect or incomplete information on the part of the provider's office, re-submit the claim using the procedures in the next section. It is important to correct and re-submit the claim as soon as possible.

If the claim is denied for other reasons, first identify the reason for the problem and then determine the solution needed to fix the problem. If the insurance carrier says the patient is not insured by them, ask what information they used to check for coverage. This is often the name of the insured, their ID number and the policy name or number. If any of these items are different from what is shown in the insurance carrier's records, it can cause the claim to be denied.

Try to determine which piece of information is incorrect. If the information matches what is shown on the forms the patient originally filled out, check the insurance card. You should have made a copy of the insurance card at the time of the patient's first visit. Match the information on the insurance card with what is shown on the claim. If any information is missing or incorrect, correct it in the computer and then re-submit the claim.

If the carrier denies the services as non-covered, request them to identify specifically where in the contract the services are excluded. Be sure to update your files to reflect this information.

Re-submissions

If the claim was denied due to incorrect or incomplete information on the part of the provider's office, it is important to correct the problem and re-submit the claim as soon as possible.

Some insurance carriers require that you get approval to re-submit a claim before doing so. This is because many insurance carriers' claims

processing program is designed to search for duplicate bills. Thus, the program will log the patient information, the date of services, and the services that were rendered. If a claim is sent in with data that matches these items, the computer will automatically flag the claim as a duplicate claim, and the claim may be denied.

To prevent this from happening, be sure to contact the insurance carrier. Make sure that the information that you are correcting on the claim includes the information that caused it to be rejected. There is no reason to re-submit a claim if the required information is not included in the re-submission.

Also, be sure to ask if an approval number needs to be obtained to re-submit the claim. If so, be sure this approval number is included in the appropriate place on the form. This will prompt the computer and/or the claims examiner to know that the claim needs to be reprocessed, not just flagged as duplicate.

Adjusted Claims

At times the insurance carrier will adjust information on your claim. They may bundle together several services, or downcode services they determine were billed inappropriately.

When an adjustment needs to be made to a claim, it is important to perform it as soon as possible.

There are several ways of making adjustments:

Re-create the claim: A new claim can be created which shows only the adjusted information, not the information originally submitted. Because this may cause a discrepancy between what the medical records indicates was done, and what the patient was billed for, the medical record will need to be updated. This can be done by adding in the corrected and/or changed information and indicating that there is an adjustment on the claim. The medical record should indicate exactly what changes were made, and why.

When this type of adjustment is made, you may need to adjust the codes on the original claim, and the amounts for the codes. These types of adjustments may create a need to revise the patient's ledger or statement information, or the medical office's accounting records.

Make an adjustment to the patient account:
The second method is more commonly used. Rather than recreate any documents, an adjustment is simply added to the patient's account. This adjustment should list the items being adjusted, and the reason for the adjustment.

Because this type of adjustment shows up as an adjustment on the medical office's accounting records, there is no need to rerun any accounting reports for previous periods.

Appeals

If you disagree with the denial or adjustment of a claim, you have the right to appeal the decision. Most insurance carriers have a specific process to be used for appeals. This often includes submitting a copy of the claim along with a letter stating the reason you disagree with their decision.

When writing an appeal letter, it is important to be specific regarding why you feel the claim payment, or lack of payment, is incorrect. Simply stating that you do not feel the insurance carrier paid enough on the claim is not enough. You need to state why the payment is incorrect.

If the claim was downcoded to a lower valued procedure, double check your records. If you agree with the downcoding, change it in your records (including the patient's computerized records). If you disagree with the downcoding, submit the claim for appeal. Be sure to attach a copy of the medical records and a letter explaining why the higher code should be allowed.

Balance Billing Patients for Downcoded or Denied Claims

Before balance billing patients on claims that have been denied or downcoded, you need to assess the situation. You may need to adjust the original bill to reflect the downcoded amount. In some cases you may need to remove services from the bill if they have been denied by the insurance carrier. This is especially true in the case of Medicare or Medicaid claims.

If a Medicare or Medicaid claim is denied as not medically necessary, you are not allowed to bill the patient for these services unless the patient was informed prior to services being rendered that

Medicare or Medicaid may not cover the services. If the patient was informed, a Medicare Advance Notice must have been completed prior to the rendering of services. If this notice was not signed before services were rendered, you are not allowed to bill the patient. Any denied services must be written off.

If Medicare has downcoded a claim or service, you must also downcode the claim or service on the bill sent to the patient. For example, if you charged the patient for a high complexity visit and Medicare downcoded the visit to one of moderate complexity, you must downcode the procedure on all billing reports and/or claims. You are only allowed to collect from the patient the amount that would be due from them for the lower coded visit.

State Insurance Commissioner

Each state has a **State Insurance Commissioner**. This person is responsible for overseeing the insurance companies and their practices within the state. If a biller has a repeated problem regarding an insurance carrier not properly paying claims in a timely manner, they can file a report with the State Insurance Commissioner.

The State Insurance Commissioner will assign an investigator to the case if they feel an investigation is warranted. If they find that the insurance carrier is not adhering to state mandates and laws, they can impose sanctions or fines on the insurance carrier.

Because reporting an insurance carrier to the State Insurance Commissioner is a serious situation, you should make all attempts to resolve a situation with the claims examiner or their supervisor first. Then discuss the situation with the provider and allow them to make the determination of whether or not to file a report.

Summary

It is important for the medical biller to properly submit clean claims. This can be done on paper or via electronic (computer) submission.

Regardless of which method you use, it is important to follow the guidelines for that method to insure that the claim can be processed quickly and easily.

If a provider's office has incomplete data on a patient, it is important to obtain that data as quickly as possible. Often, missing or incorrect data can cause delays or denials on claim payment. An incomplete data master list can assist in keeping track of incomplete data if the medical biller is unable to obtain the data immediately.

Many insurance carriers have time limits for submitting claims. Because of this, it is important for the medical biller to submit claims in a timely manner, preferably as soon as services are completed.

If a claim is downcoded or denied, it is important for the medical biller to assess the situation and decide whether they need to accept the decision and create an adjustment, resubmit the claim with additional information, or file an appeal with the insurance carrier.

Assignments

Complete the Questions for Review.

Questions for Review

Directions: Answer the following questions without looking back into the material just covered. Write your answers in the space provided.

1. Describe the purpose of the Incomplete Data Master List. _____

2. What do you do if a claim is downcoded or denied? _____

3. What do you need to file an appeal of a denied or downcoded claim? _____

4. (True or False?) If Medicare has downcoded a claim or service, you must also downcode the claim or service on the bill sent to the patient. _____

5. List and describe the two ways of making an adjustment.

   1. _____

   2. _____

If you were unable to answer any of the questions, refer back to that section, and then fill in the answers.

Honors Certification™

The certification challenge for this chapter will be a written test of the information contained in this chapter. Each incorrect answer will result in a deduction of up to 5% from your grade. You must achieve a score of 85% or higher to pass this test. If you fail the test on your first attempt you may retake the test one additional time. The items included in the second test may be different from those in the first test.

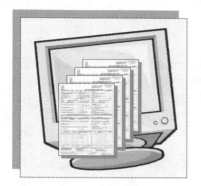

25

Calculator Basics

After completion of this chapter you will be able to:

- Explain the keys and functions of the calculator.
- Properly use the calculator to add, subtract, multiply, and divide numbers.
- Gain speed and accuracy in using the calculator.

Key words and concepts you will learn in this chapter:

Calculator – A machine that computes numbers.

A **calculator** is a machine that computes numbers. It is used to add, subtract, multiply, and divide numbers, as well as compute percentages, square roots, and other mathematical calculations.

Whether you work as a bank teller or an medical biller, you will probably use a calculator every day. Often, there are charges that need to be totaled and amounts that need to be figured. Calculating these sums manually would take many hours. Therefore, it is vital that medical biller master the use of the calculator.

Key Descriptions

Following are the keys most commonly found on a calculator and a description of their functions.

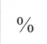 **PAPER ADVANCE KEY** – Advances the paper tape without affecting your calculations.

 CLEAR KEY – Clears the display and the independent add register, pending operations and error/overflow conditions. Reactivates the calculator after an automatic power down.

 PERCENT KEY – Completes multiplication and division operations and shows the result as a decimal.

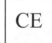 **CLEAR ENTRY KEY** – Clears the last entry only, thus enabling you to enter another number in its place without clearing out all previously entered numbers.

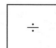 **DIVIDE KEY** – Instructs the calculator to divide the number in the display by the next value entered.

 EQUAL KEY – Completes any pending operation.

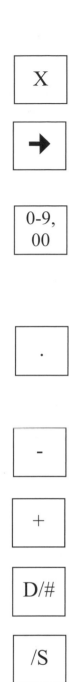

MULTIPLY KEY – Instructs the calculator to multiply the number in the display by the next value entered.

BACKSPACE KEY – Deletes the right-most digit in the display and shifts the remaining digits one place to the right.

NUMBER KEYS – Enter numbers containing up to ten digits. For numbers between one and negative one, a zero automatically precedes the decimal, allowing a maximum of nine digits to the right of the decimal.

DECIMAL POINT KEY – Enters a decimal point. Most calculators have a floating decimal point which allows you to automatically set the decimal point at a given location in the number.

SUBTRACT KEY – Subtracts the number in the display from the independent add register.

ADD KEY – Adds the number in the display to the independent add register.

DATE/NON-ADD KEY – Prints a reference number or date without affecting calculations in progress.

SUBTOTAL KEY – Displays and prints the subtotal in the independent add register. Pressing this key does not affect the contents of the add register.

TOTAL KEY – Displays and prints the total in the independent add register, then clears the register.

MEMORY TOTAL KEY – Displays and prints the value in memory, then clears the memory.

MEMORY SUBTOTAL KEY – **Displays** and prints the value in memory without clearing the memory.

SUBTRACT FROM MEMORY KEY – Prints the number in the display and subtracts it from the value in memory. If a pending multiplication or division operation has been entered, this key completes the operation and subtracts the result from memory.

ADD TO MEMORY KEY – Prints the number in the display and adds it to the value in memory. If a pending multiplication or division operation has been entered, this key completes the operation and then adds the result into memory.

Printer Tape Symbols

Multiple symbols may be printed on printer tapes during calculations. Usually, these symbols will appear to the right of tape entries. Symbols not indicated should be explained in the specific calculator manual.

Symbol	Meaning or Explanation
+	Addition operation
-	Subtraction operation
<>	Subtotal of additions and subtractions
*	Total after "=," "%," or "*/T" is pressed
x	Multiplication operation
÷	Division operation
=	Completion of an operation
%	Percentage
+ *	Percentage add-on
- *	Percentage discount
#	Reference number or date printed in the center of the printer tape
C	Clear key erases all entries

M *	Addition to memory
M-	Subtraction from memory
M <>	Memory subtotal
M *	Memory total
E	Error/overflow condition
IC	**Item Counter Symbol.** When the printer switch is in the IC position, the number of additions to and subtractions from the independent add register is printed above each total or subtotal. The item counter for the independent add register is reset when "*/T" is pressed.

Summary

Proficient use of the calculator is essential for the administrative assistant. Learning the functions of each of the keys and how to use the calculator to achieve the desired results takes practice.

Assignments

Complete the Questions for Review.
Complete Exercises 25 – 1 through 25 – 4.
    Practice gaining speed and accuracy by repeating Exercises 25 – 1 and 25 – 2 until you have mastered the feel of the keys.

Questions for Review

Directions: Answer the following questions without looking back into the material just covered. Write your answers in the space provided.

1. The _____ key completes multiplication and division operations and shows the results as a decimal.

2. What function does the divide key perform? _____

    _____

3. The _____ key completes any pending operations.

4. What is the function of the total key? _____

    _____

5. The memory total key displays and prints the value currently in _____ ,

    then clears the _____ .

If you were unable to answer any of the questions, refer back to that section, and then fill in the answers.

Exercise 25 – 1

Directions: Add each of the following columns of numbers and then subtract the numbers from your total to arrive at zero. Clear the entries from your calculator and subtract the following columns of numbers and total, then add the numbers to your total to arrive at zero. Use the printer tape to check accuracy.

71459	12181	128.49	12.89
28695	57926	321.67	.92
13579	71349	014.89	7.16
58246	02763	906.76	18.21
69021	75396	741.08	267.93
54321	74185	529.63	1234.56
67891	29630	369.25	892.10
83214	36925	801.47	809.13
47986	80147	753.85	693.21
32694	42569	102.36	5679.32
15723	00147	564.12	137.14
38014	73528	321.65	432.78
98752	60413	498.70	6789.50
20361	13311	321.65	1090.17
13979	21769	789.93	578.15
02031	24989	456.89	692.00
11484	67400	999.01	780.29
25763	09121	847.03	566.17

Exercise 25 – 2

Directions: Add each of the following columns of numbers then subtract the numbers from your total to arrive at zero. Clear the entries from your calculator and subtract the following columns of numbers and total, then add the numbers to your total to arrive at zero. Use the printer tape to check accuracy.

54659	46181	645.25	54.65
54165	35164	618.46	.12
41579	87319	614.79	2.76
45126	63453	641.76	78.11
56421	34150	123.08	457.12
20131	78455	469.61	3894.94
78991	23459	849.25	845.79
54164	89925	456.57	209.46
77986	24875	172.85	568.78
12094	23459	501.36	1056.23
12323	57847	841.43	347.51
71014	56748	051.65	351.91
71952	80893	540.71	6519.19
13671	10781	211.65	5056.20
24563	80974	549.93	645.51
63541	43729	635.45	345.48
0.168	89174	333.01	470.00
48567	39874	514.45	456.47

Exercise 25 – 3

Directions: Perform the function indicated for each list of numbers. Try not to watch your hands. Speed is not important at the beginning of performing these exercises. It will come later as you become more familiar with the keys.

1. Add the following numbers.

A.	12	B.	65	C.	44	D.	334
	24		70		69		781
	67		49		26		456
	41		52		73		241
	92		100		84		908
	34		99		35		528
	72		34		21		803

E.	295	F.	4576	G.	54	H.	32.514
	630		8493		835		8.123
	816		90.56		046		61.54
	902		3809		516		123.64
	517		9238		943		543.55
	703		12.98		.0015		999.83
	491		540.5				

2. Enter the first number, then subtract the following numbers.

A.	9999	B.	7654	C.	4329
	45		11		649
	66		92		42
	90		561		631
	1504		341		42
	3535		940		792
	901		52		406

D.	1000.00	E.	564.000	F.	410014
	10.00		.630		.123
	.20		.920		654.456
	341.00		162.000		84.25
	1.78		.789		67.48
	.78		231.000		138.03
	592.00		501.000		486.381

Exercise 25 – 4

Directions: Perform the function indicated for each list of numbers. Try not to watch your hands. Speed is not important at the beginning. It will come later as you become more familiar with the keys.

1. Multiply the following.

A.	231	B.	5482	C.	7602	D.	891
	x 42		x 61		x 201		x 23.61

E.	43.92	F.	24.51	G.	903.45	H.	2503.99
	x.639		x 70%		x 85%		x 90%

I.	492.67	J.	29.16	K.	564465	L.	654.21
	x 75%		x 55%		x 21%		x 75%

2. Divide the first number by the second number in the following equations.

A.	5634	B.	56348	C.	999999	D.	3541
	51		543		.99		66

E.	1000	F.	65430	G.	514623	H.	5100
	.01		125		1523		45

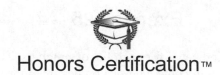

Honors Certification™

The honors certification challenge for this section is a timed test. You will be given several tests with problems similar to those found in Exercises 25 – 1 through 25 – 5 and will be asked to complete the problems and write in your answers. Each incorrect keystroke will result in a 2% deduction from your grade. You must achieve a score of 85% or higher to pass this test. If you fail the test on your first attempt you may take the test one additional time. The items included in the second test may be different from those included in the first test.

There will also be a 5-minute timed test to determine your average keystrokes per minute. You must achieve a speed of 200 keystrokes per minute in order to pass this test. If you fail the test on your first attempt you may take the test one additional time. The items included in the second test may be different from those included in the first test.

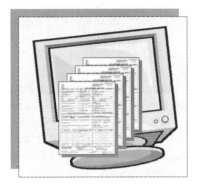

26

General Office Procedures

After completion of this chapter you will be able to:

- Explain how to handle incoming mail.
- Explain how to handle outgoing mail.
- Explain special shipping services that are available.
- Explain the guidelines for ordering office supplies.
- List the main types of office equipment and explain their use.
- Describe a tickler file and explain its use.

Key words and concepts you will learn in this chapter:

Binding Machine – Bind several pages of a document together, often with a strip down the left-hand side of the document.

Certified Mail – Is a package or envelope that must be signed for upon delivery.

Facsimile Machine (more commonly referred to as the fax machine) – Is a machine that transmits pictures over the phone lines by transmitting a series of dot messages.

Multi-line Phones – This means that there is more than one telephone line into the office.

Return Receipt Requested – Upon delivery, a receipt is issued and mailed back to the sender of the package. This allows the sender to have proof of

the delivery and the name of the person who signed for it.

Tickler File – Are often expanding file folders that help you remember items that need to occur on a specific date.

A number of basic procedures need to be followed to help an office run smoothly and to facilitate the organized management of services. Without organization, precious time is lost searching for information or other items. In addition, an unorganized office and unskilled personnel create difficulty and add to the stress level of the patient, since they must wait longer to receive services. The patient may worry that your lack of concern for the office is also reflective of a lack of concern for them.

Mail

Mail can be separated into two types, incoming mail and outgoing mail. Each has its own set of procedures.

Incoming Mail

In any office, it is imperative that the mail be handled properly and routed to the correct person. Generally, one person is designated to handle the incoming mail. Of course every office has its own preferences, so check with your supervisor to see what handling procedures have been established for the company where you are employed. The following are eight general guidelines:

1. Separate mail according to the department or person to whom it is addressed. While separating mail, take note of any mail which was delivered incorrectly to your address. Separating the mail before opening will allow you to return incorrectly delivered mail in the same condition in which it arrived.

2. If mail is to be opened before it is distributed, slit the envelope neatly across the top. Do not tear or destroy the envelope so that any needed information can be preserved. This may include the postmark date, return address, or the city from which the envelope was mailed.

3. Many offices date stamp their mail upon receipt. If this is the case with your company or organization, there are several suggestions which you should follow:

   a. Be sure the date on the stamper is accurate. This may be very important when certain pieces of correspondence need to arrive in a timely manner (i.e., billing department mail when interest or late fees are charged on overdue accounts).

   b. Stamp the date stamper on a piccc of scratch paper to ensure that it has enough ink and that the impression is clear. If the impression is faint, stamp several more times on the ink pad (if it is used) or on a piece of paper (if the stamp is self-inking). This should start the ink flowing again.

   c. When you stamp a piece of correspondence, place the date in an area where it will not cover any writing.

   d. Stamp down once, firmly and securely. Wiggling the stamp back and forth can cause an unclear impression.

   e. Do not stamp checks, business cards, legal documents, or order forms unless your office specifically requests it. Date stamping such items can result in difficultly processing checks, ordering, or complying with legal requirements.

   f. If you have a choice of ink colors, black is best. Other colors are more difficult to photocopy and/or may cause a negative impression. This is especially true of red, since most people associate red ink with a warning.

4. If you receive checks in the mail, be sure they are securely attached to any additional papers (i.e., invoices, statements) which are included. These papers may be the only clue as to which account the check should be credited. Some offices prefer that the account number be immediately written on the check. This insures that the check will be credited to the proper account even if it is separated from its attached documentation.

   If no documentation is attached, check the envelope for additional clues. If the name and address on the check does not match the name and address on the envelope, attach the envelope to the check. This may assist the billing department in locating the correct account.

   Some offices request that the person who opens the checks make an adding machine tape and total the day's receipts. You should always run the tape twice, insuring that the total is the same each time times. Then, take an extra minute to double-check your figures. Often numbers will become transposed, and once a number is in your mind, it is easy for the transposition to occur a second time.

5. When distributing the mail, put urgent looking correspondence on top of the stack. Also be sure to put the mail in a place where the recipient will be sure to see it.

6. If correspondence is received which is marked "Personal and Confidential," leave the envelope sealed and deliver it to the intended recipient unopened.

7. If you receive a document in a "next day" or "urgent" envelope, it should be delivered immediately. This type of document should never sit on your desk for more than five minutes.

Although handling mail may seem like a minor task, it is important to do it properly and efficiently. Mail is the life blood of many offices. Without it, checks and revenues may be lost, patients may not be served, and communication usually breaks down.

Signing for Mail
Some incoming mail requires a signature upon delivery. Before signing, know exactly what you are signing for. Most shipping companies include a notation in fine print stating that your signature is verification that the package was received in good condition and that the contents were not damaged. Also note the number of packages you are signing for. Your signature across four lines of the receipt column is stating that you received four packages. Be sure that the order is complete before signing for it or you or your company may be held liable for any unreceived merchandise or shipments.

It is impossible to tell if the contents are undamaged without opening the box. Take the time to look at the boxes before signing. If the box appears to be damaged, insist on opening it and checking the contents before signing. The delivery person will attempt to have you sign immediately so that he or she can get to the next delivery, but if you do sign, the damaged goods will often not be replaced or paid for by the shipper.

If the contents of the package appear to be damaged, you should note this on the receipt right next to your signature.

Be sure you are authorized to sign for a package. In many offices the authority to sign for packages is limited to a few people, not to any employee in the office.

Returned Mailings
In any company there will be mail which is returned due to improper addressing, lack of postage, or the inability of the postal service to locate the intended recipient.

Mail will usually only be forwarded for one year from the date of the recipient's move. After that time a sticker will be placed on the envelope indicating the new address and the article will be returned to the sender. If a piece of mail is returned because a forwarding address has expired, and the postal service has indicated the new address, the mail should be placed in a new envelope, addressed with the new address and remailed. Be sure to keep the old envelope so that you can update your records.

If a piece of mail is returned with no forwarding address indicated, be sure to delete the name and address from your records. If there is an outstanding balance on an account which has mail returned, be sure the patient's records are also updated. If an outstanding balance or a current patient history does not exist, do not delete the record. Take the time to contact the patient by phone and attempt to locate their new address.

Outgoing Mail

The condition of your outgoing mail is a direct reflection on your office. Therefore, it is imperative that your mail be handled properly. You can imagine the response of a patient who receives a letter bearing bad news which has also been stamped by the postal service "Postage Due."

The first thing is to make sure the mail has been packaged properly. Be sure that the envelope is of adequate size for the material. If there are more than five pages in a document, a #10 (standard sized) envelope should not be used. The thickness of the pages can cause the envelope to become jammed in the postal service's automated equipment. This may result in tearing and loss of the contents. To ensure that envelopes mailed in larger packages arrive in good condition, a thin sheet of cardboard can be placed in the envelope to add resilience.

Before sealing a box, place a letter or other item inside that lists the company's and the recipient's address. This will allow the package to be delivered even if the address shown on the outside is removed or becomes obliterated. Boxes should be sealed with strong packing tape, not string.

All shipping companies, including the postal service, have weight and size limits for the packages they will ship. Most will have a weight limit of 70 pounds per box. The combined length and girth should not exceed 108 inches. To determine the measurement, wrap a tape measure once around the box; then add to the resulting measurement the length of the box. Before shipping, contact the carrier and be sure that you know the exact weight and measurement limits they will allow.

Special Shipping Services

Most companies offer numerous shipping services. These include certification (proof of delivery), return receipt requested, **COD** (cash on delivery), insurance, overnight delivery, and two- or three-day delivery. Additional charges, above and beyond the normal shipping charges, are added for each of these services. Keep any receipts issued to you by the shipper. Without these documents, it is very difficult to trace lost articles or to make a claim for services not delivered.

Certified mail is a package or envelope that must be signed for upon delivery. This provides you with a record of when the item was delivered and the name of the person who signed for it. To send an envelope by certified mail, fill out the certified mail slip provided by the shipping company. The basic information requested is the name and address of the recipient. This tag is attached to the envelope or package to the right of the return address. The tag has a tracking number printed on it. The top portion of the tag is torn off at the perforation and kept as a receipt. If the envelope or package does not arrive, a tracer can be put on it by using the tracking number.

With **return receipt requested**, upon delivery, a receipt is issued and mailed back to the sender of the package. This allows the sender to have proof of the delivery and the name of the person who signed for it. This procedure is usually used with certified mail. The recipient's name and address are placed on one side of the card. The sender's name and address are placed on the reverse of the card. The card is then attached to the envelope or package on the front, or, if there is not sufficient room, on the back. When the article is delivered, the recipient signs the card and the date of delivery is listed. If requested (and an additional fee is paid), the recipient's address will be provided. The sender may also choose to restrict delivery only to the person or persons to whom the article is addressed.

When mailing a shipment of merchandise that the recipient must pay for, COD is often requested. This means that the shipper will collect payment for the item at the time of delivery. When shipping COD, you must specify whether cash, check or cither is acceptable and the amount to be collected. Add any shipping charges to the amount if the recipient is to pay for shipping.

You may wish to purchase insurance for items being shipped. This insurance will pay for lost or damaged items. With many shippers, the first $100 of insurance is included in the cost of shipping a package. Any amount over this must be requested and paid for prior to shipping. The fee is usually nominal, between $.50 and $.75 for every $100 of insurance.

If you need an envelope or package to arrive overnight, it is possible to request this service. Articles can be scheduled for either an afternoon delivery or, for an additional charge, a morning delivery. The delivery area is limited, usually to within the continental United States. In addition, articles must be picked up or delivered to the shipper prior to a specified time to qualify for next-day delivery. This time varies according to your location and the shipper. You must also complete special address labels that request the sender's and receiver's name, address, and phone number, as well as the specific services requested. Many carriers require you to use special packaging and may provide this packaging free of charge upon request.

There is also a special charge for two- or three- day delivery, and delivery is usually limited to the continental United States. There are also similar labels and packaging requirements. Check with your shipper for specific details.

In large cities, it is possible to have a package delivered by courier or messenger. The courier comes to your office, picks up the article, and hand delivers it to the recipient. These services are expensive and are used only for important documents.

Ordering Supplies

Every office needs a certain amount of supplies to run efficiently and smoothly. These supplies may include minor purchases like paper and pens, or major purchases such as office equipment and machinery.

Often the medical biller is required to order supplies, if not for the company, then at least for his or her own use. Therefore, it is important to know basic ordering guidelines. Although many offices have their own procedures, the following are 11 general guidelines to follow:

1. Know what you need before you need it. It does not help to order supplies two days after you have already run out of things. This means going through your desk and any supply cupboards and looking to see what is needed. If you are running low on something, put it on the order list. It is far

better to have a little extra than to run completely out of something. However, do not order more than you can use in three or four months. Having money tied up in supplies decreases the amount available to the company for other operating costs or emergencies.

2. Order everything at once. Numerous small orders are much more difficult to handle and keep track of than one large order. Also, many supply companies offer volume discounts or free delivery or gifts if your order exceeds a certain amount. Be aware of what these levels are. For example, you could save your company money if you were to order $5 more in supplies rather than pay a $10 shipping charge.

3. Know the company from which you are ordering office supplies. Many companies have dealt exclusively with one office supplier for years. The company has established a rapport with the supplier and will purchase only that supplier's products, regardless of whether another supplier offers the same supplies at a lower rate. At times an alternative relationship is set up where you support the supplier's business and they support yours. At other times it is merely a matter of personal loyalty to a company that has treated your company well in the past. Regardless of the reason, it is best to purchase all supplies from the supplier your company has chosen.

4. Be sure you know the payment procedures before ordering. Some companies bill you and allow payment within 30 days. Others demand payment upon receipt. If the supplies are shipped COD, you do not want to have to unexpectedly come up with a check when no one is around to sign it.

5. Fill out the order form completely and accurately. Print or type the information requested, using black ink. Double-check all figures and all order numbers. Proofread the form before sending it out. You do not want to end up with 200 of the wrong item and go through the hassle of sending it back and trying to get the right item.

6. Before sending in an order, make a copy of it for your records. This allows you to check your order against the items you receive when the order arrives.

7. If you are ordering by phone, write out the order before you place the call. This helps keep everything accurate and helps the ordering process run smoothly. It also gives you a permanent record of what you ordered so that you can compare it to the packing slip and the invoice when they arrive.

8. Check the shipment and the packing slip as soon as an order comes in. Make sure that everything is either in the box or is listed on the packing slip as a back-ordered item. If an error occurs in the shipment, first double check your order form. Was the mistake your fault or the supplier's? Then, call the office supplier immediately. If the error was your fault, admit it and resolve the problem. Most suppliers have no problem with exchanging an item. If the fault was theirs, be understanding. Mistakes occur and no one is perfect. If you receive supplies that you did not order, do not open them. Once an item has been opened, many suppliers will not accept a return on it.

9. If the entire shipment is received correctly, make a brief note to that effect on the packing slip and initial it. Then, put the supplies in their appropriate place.

10. Often the invoice will arrive at a later date. When the invoice arrives, check it against the packing slip and the original order. If there are any discrepancies, contact the supplier immediately. If not, turn it over to the person who pays the bills.

11. Finally, if you are aware that finances are a consideration for your company and that a different company offers supplies of the same quality at a lower price, do your homework first. Order catalogs from both companies and compare the costs on the items that you purchase the most. Read the fine print and compare items of the same quality. Also, consider payment options and credit interest rates. If the savings is substantial enough that your company might change, talk to a supervisor and show him or her the differences. It is your supervisor's job to approach the company leaders with a possible change.

Office Machines

In every office, you will use a number of machines nearly every day. These include the telephone, fax machine, and copy machine.

The Telephone

Virtually every company in existence has a telephone and uses it extensively during the working day. The telephone is often more important than the mail in communicating with customers and helping with the running of the office. Therefore, it is important that you understand how to properly use the telephone.

Most companies have **multi-line phones**. This means that there is more than one telephone line into the office. However, the number of these phone lines is limited. If all of the lines are being used, the customer or caller will hear a busy signal and their call will not be connected. For this reason you should keep your call as brief as possible.

Multi-line phones often work similar to single-line phones, with a few exceptions. Most multi-line phones have a single number (i.e., 555-1234) with each additional line numerically increased by one (i.e., line two is 555-1235; line three is 555-1236). The caller needs only to dial the original number (555-1234) and, if that line is busy, the call will automatically roll over to the first available line.

When placing an outgoing call on a multi-line phone, many times you will need to choose a line by pushing a button. Prior to picking up a line, make sure that it is available. Usually, a small lighted button indicates whether the line is currently in use.

Multi-line phones often give you the option of placing callers on hold by depressing a hold button. When transferring a call, speaking with a co-worker or interrupting a conversation for any reason, it is best to put the caller on hold rather than to hold your hand over the mouthpiece or set the phone down.

Different types of phones and phone systems have different ways of transferring calls and returning to a held call. These procedures will need to be described to you by someone who is familiar with the phone or system. It is important to know these procedures prior to needing them so that you do not delay or disconnect a caller.

The Facsimile Machine

The **facsimile machine** (more commonly referred to as the fax machine) is a machine that transmits pictures over the phone lines by transmitting a series of dot messages. This allows for nearly instantaneous transmission of a letter, picture, or other document from one place to another.

The invention of the fax machine has made life easier in offices and has taken some of the stress out of having to mail documents early so that they can be received on time. Although the fax machine is a wonderful invention, it is not perfect. Documents can be lost in transmission and they are generally not as clear as printed material. The special paper used in many fax machines is thinner than normal paper and also bruises or leaves an imprint if it is pressed on. For these reasons, it is important that you always follow up a faxed copy with a hard copy of the document sent through the mail.

The ease of transmitting using the fax machine has often led to using it for nonessential situations. Always remember that a fax transmission is not as clear, and therefore, not as professional looking as something that is directly from a typewriter or printer. Also, remember that when transmitting long distances, you are using a phone line. Therefore, a charge will appear on the telephone bill the same as if you had spoken over the phone.

If the company you are faxing to has several different departments, there may be several fax machines. A fax cover sheet should always be included with the fax. A cover sheet should include the following information:

- The date and time the fax is being sent,
- The name and telephone number of the person sending the fax,
- The name of the person to whom the fax is directed and his/her department or company,
- The number of pages being sent, and
- Sufficient space for messages to be conveyed to the receiver.

The Copy Machine

The copy machine is possibly one of the most widely used office machines. There are always numerous reasons for needing a second copy of a document.

Copy machines can be one of the easiest machines to operate if you understand the basic principles. The first item of importance is the placement of the original. The original should be placed face down on the glass. The exact placement is usually indicated by markings running along the left-hand side of the glass or the bottom. The cover should be closed before making a copy.

To begin the copy process, push the button marked start. Do not lift the cover or remove the original until the copying is complete. To do so will cause a blurred or darkened image on the copy.

Many copiers have special features, such as reduction or enlargement of the original, special paper sizes or types, and collation of the copies. To **collate** copies means to place them in order. For example, if you are making two copies of a document that is three pages long, the machine will turn the pages out in the order of 1, 2, 3, 1, 2, 3. In documents that are not collated the pages would be done in order of 1, 1, 2, 2, 3, 3.

These special features are usually selected by the push of a button.

Since copiers vary according to style and brand name, it is important that you be shown the exact features and the correct operating procedures for the copier that your company uses.

Other Office Machines

A number of other machines may be used in a medical office setting. These can include the postage meter, postage scale, binding machines, folding machines, coffee makers, and vending machines.

Binding machines bind several pages of a document together, often with a strip down the left-hand side of the document. There are numerous types of binding machines, and numerous brands for each type. Generally, the bindings fall into one of three categories: comb binders (have a plastic strip with projecting teeth), spiral binders (have a curved plastic strip with rounded teeth forming an enclosed circle), and spiral wire binders (have a single continuous piece of wire wound through successive holes from top to bottom of the document).

Folding machines are used to fold numerous pieces of paper. The folding guides can be adjusted to various lengths to handle different sizes of paper and different folds. Due to the strength and speed of most folding machines, care should be taken that jewelry, loose clothing, and long hair are not allowed to enter the machine.

Many offices provide free or low-cost cups of coffee to their employees. However, the responsibility often falls to one or more of the employees to keep the pots filled. All coffee machines require the addition of fresh coffee grounds, and some require the addition of water. Care should be taken to keep the pots cleaned on a regular basis. Also, never set an empty or near-empty glass pot on a heated burner. The glass will shatter when it reaches a certain temperature.

Vending machines are available in many offices. Most are stocked and serviced by outside vending companies that are also in charge of handling the monies received. Many vending companies return a portion of the proceeds to the company that has allowed space for the machine, and the vending company should be called if the machine has run out of items or if service is needed.

Tickler Files

The tickler file system is used by a number of people in numerous office settings. **Tickler files** are often expanding file folders that help you remember items that need to occur on a specific date. Basically a tickler file helps tickle your memory.

A tickler file usually consists of the following folders:

- 12 folders labeled with each month of the year.
- 31 folders labeled with the numbers 1 through 31.

To use a tickler file, place the folders numbered 1 through 31 into the folder for the current month (i.e., if today's date is May 5th, place all the numbered folders inside the May folder). Place all folders in front of the current month (i.e., January through April) behind the December folder at the back of the group. Then place all numbered folders for the days prior to the current one into the folder following the current month (i.e., if the date is May 5th, the numbered files for days 5 – 31 would be in the May folder and the folders for days 1 – 4 would be in the June folder). Now your tickler file is ready to use.

To use your tickler file, simply file each item into the folder for the day it needs to occur on. For example, if you need to sign up the provider for a conference by June 1, then place the information on the conference in the folder numbered 1, which should be in the June folder.

On each day, simply look in the folder for that day. Those are the items that you need to accomplish before the day is out.

If you have items that require your attention several months in the future, simply place them in the folder for that month. At the beginning of each month, take the items in that month's folder and insert them into the proper folder for the day of the month they need to be taken care of.

As each day passes, place the folder for that day into the folder for the next month.

By using a tickler file, you can always remember to accomplish the things that require your attention in the future. You will always be reminded of that call you were supposed to return when someone returned from vacation or that conference to sign up for, etc.

Tickler files can be especially important in a medical office if you are requesting information or items from outside vendors or providers. For example, if the provider needs to have lab results returned to the office before the patient's next scheduled visit, place a note in the correct folder several days before the appointment. If the lab results have not been received at that time, contact the lab and ask them to forward the results to you. Be sure to place the reminder to contact the lab in the folder for several days ahead of the appointment. That will provide sufficient time for the lab to finish running the results in case they have not done so yet.

Summary

Although each office has its own procedures to follow, it is important to understand the basic procedures that govern incoming mail, outgoing mail, special shipping services, ordering supplies, and dealing with office machines.

Without basic knowledge of the equipment and how to use it, it is impossible for the medical biller to do their job properly.

Assignments

Complete the Questions for Review.

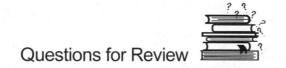

Questions for Review

Directions: Answer the following questions without looking back into the material just covered. Write your answers in the space provided.

1. What is the best ink color to use when date stamping incoming mail?_____

   _____

2. (True or False?) When signing for receipt of a package, your signature certifies that the contents were received undamaged and in good condition._____

   _____

3. Name five special shipping services that you can purchase.

   1. _____

   2. _____

   3. _____

   4. _____

   5. _____

4. When dialing out on a multi-line phone, what is the first thing you should check before picking up the phone? _____

_____

5. What are six guidelines of time management?

    1. _____

    2. _____

    3. _____

    4. _____

    5. _____

    6. _____

If you were unable to answer any of the questions, refer back to that section, and then fill in the answers.

Honors Certification™

The certification challenge for this chapter will be a written test of the information contained in this chapter. Each incorrect answer will result in a deduction of up to 5% from your grade. You must achieve a score of 85% or higher to pass this test. If you fail the test on your first attempt you may retake the test one additional time. The items included in the second test may be different from those in the first test.

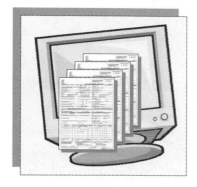

27

Customer Service/ Patient Relations

After completion of this chapter you will be able to:

- Explain positive and negative recognition and give examples of each.
- Discuss the importance of a first impression.
- List the primary customer service and patient relations functions in the medical billing arena.
- List ten items that are important to the art of listening.
- List and describe the steps necessary for problem resolution.
- List and explain the guidelines for dealing with angry or irate customers/patients.
- Discuss the guidelines or items that convey professionalism when dealing with a customer/patient.
- List and explain proper telephone techniques.
- Describe items important to proper telephone etiquette.

Key words and concepts you will learn in this chapter:

Closed-ended Question – A question that limits or restricts a response, usually to a yes or no answer or other brief response.

Customer Service – To service the customer or patient.

Empathy – Being able to participate in another person's feelings or perceptions.

Etiquette – The practices and forms prescribed by convention or by authority. In essence, etiquette is manners.

Open-ended Question – A question that cannot be answered with a "yes," "no," or other brief response.

Standing Appointment – Is any appointment, which happens on a regular basis.

Summary – A brief statement of information covered.

Verification – Repeating information and asking if you have understood it correctly.

Customer service and patient relations are some of the most vital functions your office will provide. Without it, the facility may lose customers and patients. Without customers or patients, the facility may cease to exist.

Whenever you speak with a customer or patient, either on the phone or in person, or write to them, you are performing a customer service function. Many times the medical biller is the only contact that the person will have with the facility. Therefore, to that person you are the company. The image you convey will be what the person believes is the facility's attitude toward him. Accounts have been won and lost based solely on a customer/patient's experience with customer service personnel. Even a single encounter can be enough to win or lose a customer/patient. This chapter is designed to help the medical biller in developing a more professional and positive approach to customer/patient relationships.

Understanding Needs

To respond appropriately to the needs of your customers/patients, you must be able to look beneath the surface or the behavior they exhibit to examine the factors that motivate their actions.

An individual's ability to tolerate problems, disappointments, or frustrations is influenced by the many needs he experiences. Those needs include such things as sleep, food, comfort, love, self-esteem, and achievement. All behavior grows out of need and is directed toward meeting those needs. Needs that have not been met can alter normal behavior.

When experiencing negative emotions such as pain, anxiety, frustration, discomfort, fear, guilt, concern, or worry, the customer/patient's behavior can be difficult to deal with. What would usually be perceived as an insignificant or minor problem can become an important issue to a person whose needs have not been met.

When dealing with customers/patients, bear in mind that their primary concern is that their needs are met. If you assist them in meeting their needs in a pleasant and friendly way, their opinion of you, and thus, the company, will be greatly enhanced. Likewise, if you allow their reaction to a situation to influence you in a negative manner, their opinion of the facility will be a negative one.

Attitudes and Feelings

Attitude is defined as "the manner of acting, feeling or thinking that shows one's disposition or opinion." Therefore, an attitude is the way you think and your view of the world. You may not always be able to choose your situation, but you can always choose your attitude about the situation. The way you think shapes what you become and how your environment is formed. Complete **Exercises 27 – 1** and **27 – 2** to assist you in understanding your current attitude. After completion of the exercises, compare your answers with the answers given by the three people in the second exercise and complete the questions in **Exercise 27 – 3**.

Feelings come into play whenever people interact. Like our attitudes, our feelings strongly influence our actions if we let them. However, in customer service the only acceptable attitude is a positive one. Therefore, it is important to make sure that only positive feelings and attitudes influence your actions.

Every time you have contact with someone you are, in effect, recognizing this person. This recognition can be verbal or nonverbal (such as nodding or smiling at someone).

Recognition can be either negative or positive. When someone compliments you on the way you did something, this is **positive recognition**. When someone says your idea is stupid, this is **negative recognition**. If you imply, through your tone of voice, that your customer's/patient's question is stupid, this is negative recognition. If you provide the information in a cheerful way, this is positive recognition.

In other words, negative recognition makes us feel bad and positive recognition makes us feel good. Both kinds of recognition influence whether or not we do things again, as well as the attitude we adopt toward that act. Consequently, if the amount of positive recognition is increased and the amount of negative recognition is decreased, future behavior is influenced positively.

Following are some examples of positive and negative recognition. Which have you used recently?

Examples of Positive Recognition
- A smile.
- Returning calls as promised.
- Direct eye contact with a person.
- Greeting those you work with daily.
- Speaking in a pleasant tone of voice.
- "Good afternoon, Mrs. Smith."
- "May I place you on hold while I check that for you?"
- "You're well organized."
- "Thank you!" (with a smile).
- "How do you feel about it?"
- "That was very thoughtful of you."
- "You're always so reliable."

Examples of Negative Recognition
- Not greeting someone you know.
- Ignoring a customer/patient or co-workers.
- Grumbling and complaining.
- Looking grouchy.
- Sounding bored.
- Refusing to hurry.
- Not speaking to someone.
- "Stupid. Don't you ever listen?"
- "That idea is ridiculous."
- "Another area handles that type of problem."
- "Don't complain to me."
- "That's not my job."

The way someone receives recognition from others can be positive and negative, too! We are all familiar with the person who has a difficult time accepting a compliment. Instead of saying, "thank you," they respond by belittling or contradicting the compliment. This is negative recognition. How do you respond when someone gives you recognition?

First Impressions and Image

First impressions are a vital part of creating how a customer/patient feels about a person, company, or facility. This impression is usually formed within four minutes of the first meeting. Four minutes is not a long time, but it is long enough for someone to form an impression that may remain with him throughout the life of the relationship.

The kind of first impression a person makes on another person is often made without anyone recognizing it. Everything communicates something. For example, the first thing people use to form an impression about you is your appearance. This consists not only of your clothing and general appearance, but also of your posture, gestures, facial expressions, and the way you move.

The next largest impact is made by your vocal communication. This includes your tone of voice, the volume and pitch, and the speed at which you speak.

Last is your verbal communication. This includes not only the words you speak, but also the terminology you use and the way you speak. Because of this it is important to use terminology that will be understood by the person to whom you are speaking and to speak distinctly and clearly.

Ways to Make a Good First Impression

If your experiences are typical you will meet approximately 10,000 people in your lifetime. This is a lot of chances to make a terrific first impression. Next time you meet someone new use some of the following gestures:

- Extend your hand and give a firm handshake.
- Smile and make eye contact.
- Learn and use the other person's name.
- Be a good listener.

Another point to remember is that when meeting new people in a busy situation (like at a restaurant networking function), avoid letting your gaze wander around the room while others speak.

Focus your attention on the individual, and listen for details that you can use to promote conversation.

Characteristics of Client Relations

It is vital to keep customer service and patient relations a high priority. The personnel who deal with customers and patients must possess highly disciplined personality characteristics. The following characteristics should be demonstrated in each and every client interaction in order to be good at customer service and patient relations:

- Thorough job knowledge.
- Good telephone techniques.
- Knowledge of privacy guidelines and their importance.
- A positive attitude.
- The ability to listen well.
- Knowledge of the business and its practices.

Customer Service Job Functions

As a medical biller your primary customer service and patient relations functions include, but may not be limited to the following:

1. Using computerized or manual files to answer inquiries from customers and patients or potential ones. These inquiries may include numerous topics, such as the dispensation of an order, contractual interpretations, or general questions regarding the facility.
2. Promoting positive customer and patient relationships through positive interaction.
3. Handling written correspondence. Strong letter-writing skills are required to articulate the facility's position.
4. Meeting with walk-in customers and patients and handling their questions concerning services and costs.
5. Detecting and handling the initial investigation of potentially fraudulent activities.
6. Advising supervisors of adverse trends or issues noted through contact with customers and patients, client representatives, and others, and maintain an accurate activity log that documents these trends or issues.
7. Recording comments and reactions (both positive and negative) of customers and patients regarding the services provided.

The Art of Listening

Listening is one of the most important skills a person can learn, especially in the area of customer service. **Listening** is defined as making an effort to hear. Without effort, true listening does not occur. This means that your entire focus should be on what the person is saying, not on any errands you may have to run, other items you may have to get done, or people you would rather be with. The following ten ideas should be learned and practiced:

Limit your own talking. It is almost impossible to talk and listen at the same time.

Try to put yourself in the customer's/ patient's place. Their problems and needs are important to them and should, therefore, be important to you. You can understand and retain their concerns better if you listen to their point of view.

Ask questions. If you do not understand something or if you need clarification, there is nothing wrong with asking questions. In fact, asking relevant questions helps the customer/patient to feel you are listening closely.

Do not interrupt. A pause does not always mean the person has finished speaking. Very often people pause when they are trying to formulate a sentence in their mind. Do not rush them. If you allow a pause of at least five seconds between sentences, it will give the person time to add any other points they wish to make.

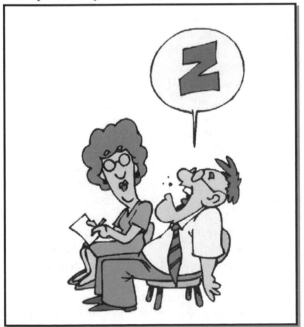

Concentrate. Focus your mind on the conversation, shutting out all outside distractions. If you find your mind wandering, get it back on track.

Take notes. This will help you remember important points in the conversation. However, do not try to write down every word. Note only key words that are relevant to the problem and which will help you to remember the issues at a later time.

Interjections. An occasional, "Yes," "I see," or "I understand," shows the person that you are still tuning in to their words. Just be careful not to overdo it. Too many interjections will make the person feel you are constantly interrupting.

Keep your words and thoughts concise. Personal concerns and stories of what happened to you or someone else waste time and may confuse the person. In addition, it does not help to move the conversation toward resolution of the person's problem.

React to the problem or concern, not to the person. Do not allow yourself to become irritated at things the person says or the way in which he says them.

Do not jump to conclusions. Do not assume you know what the person is about to say. Also, do not finish their sentences, either mentally or verbally. Let the person finish completely before you offer a solution or suggestion.

Listening With Empathy

Empathy means being able to participate in another person's feelings or perceptions, and to try to sense and understand how another person is feeling and what he is experiencing. In customer service and patient relations, this is a critical part of the listening process.

Empathetic listening, on its own, may resolve your customer's or patient's problem. Often giving people a chance to verbally express their problem may clarify their understanding of the situation. It also often provides emotional release and allows them to gain a more logical point of view. Since it gives people a chance to voice their opinions, it can reduce tension and hostility. When people feel you are truly interested in them as well as their problems, thoughts, and opinions, they respect you and are more willing to cooperate with you toward a resolution of problems. Thus, empathetic listening promotes communication, which is essential in the business world. Often communication breaks down because neither party is willing to listen.

Problem Resolution

Listening skills are used throughout the entire problem resolution process. However, there are also specific steps that will bring you and the customer/patient to the resolution of a problem or concern. Following are the six basic steps necessary for a resolution:

- Greet the person.
- Acknowledge the problem.
- Question the person to determine the best way to proceed toward a resolution of the problem.
- Verify the information received from the person and any further actions agreed-upon.
- Counsel the person regarding the steps he or she will need to take toward a resolution of the problem.
- Close the conversation.

Greet the Customer/Patient

The way you greet a person and begin a conversation sets the tone for the entire encounter. This depends not so much on the words you say, but on the tone of your voice and the way you say the words. A pleasant greeting can defuse an angry customer/patient and improve the outlook of their concern. Your voice should communicate pleasantness, caring, and concern from the first word.

To better prepare yourself for customer and/or patient calls, practice greeting them in a pleasant, happy voice. Before you answer the phone or turn toward a customer/patient, take a moment for a quick breath and a smile. Focus your attention on them, not on the task in front of you or any other thoughts. If your mind is not focused, the person will hear your distraction in the tone of your voice.

When a customer or patient enters the office, it is important to greet them as soon as you see them. If you are on the phone or are unable to give your full attention, smile and say, "I'll be with you in just a moment." Then get to them as quickly as you can.

Acknowledge the Problem

Acknowledging your customer's or patient's concern or problem opens the line of communication and lets them know that you are interested in helping to find a solution. It also lets them know that they are important. They will recognize that you empathize with their concern, and that you want to resolve the problem or prevent it from occurring again.

Example:

Medical Biller: "This is John Doe. How may I help you?"

Customer/Patient: "I just got a notice from your office saying that I haven't paid my bill and it is 90 days past due. I paid this bill three months ago."

Medical Biller: "I can understand why you might be upset, sir. If I can ask you a few questions, we can resolve this quickly."

Notice that the response should not be an apology or an admission of error. It also should not accuse or place the blame on the customer/patient. Your primary goal is to acknowledge that a problem or situation exists and that you are willing to work with the person to find a solution. Your voice should remain soft and slow, not allowing the person's anger to seep into your own voice.

In the following exercise, choose the statement that best reflects complete acknowledgment:

1. _____It's no problem to issue you another statement. Let me get your full name and address so I can send it right out.
2. _____Well, you can't pay your bill if you don't know how much it is, can you?
3. _____We'll have to give you a new statement. Hopefully you won't lose this one as well.

Question the Customer/Patient

Questioning is a learned skill. It is used to clarify the reason for an inquiry and to gain information needed to work toward a resolution of the person's concern. There are two kinds of questions: open-ended and closed-ended.

Open-ended questions are those that cannot be answered with a "yes," "no," or other brief response. These questions encourage people to respond freely. They usually begin with words such as "tell me," "why," or "what." Examples of open-ended questions include:

- "Why were you sent here?"
- "What kind of problem do you have?"
- "What happened that you feel that way?"

Closed-ended questions limit or restrict the client's response, usually to a yes or no answer or other brief response. These types of questions usually begin with words like "who," "are," "did," "what," and "which." Therefore, a closed-ended question brings about a specific, narrow response.

Closed-ended questions should be used when you need specific information, need to take more control of the conversation, or need to confirm or verify your understanding of the situation. Examples of closed-ended questions include:

- "What is your account number?"
- "When did you come in for treatment?"
- "Was the item a purchased at a pharmacy?"

Both types of questions are usually necessary in a conversation. They will allow you to resolve the problem quickly while retaining the best possible interrelationship. Too many closed-ended questions may make the person feel as if he is being interrogated. Too many open-ended questions may allow the conversation to wander. Regardless of the type of questions used, listen carefully for the answer in order to resolve the situation. Think through the meaning of the answer before you consider what your next step or your next question should be.

Verify the Information

Verification means repeating the information and asking if you have understood it correctly. It is important to make sure that you have understood the person's concerns and the answers to your questions, especially when you are speaking to someone with an accent. Minor mispronunciations in language can lead to big misunderstandings. For example, consider the ramifications of misunderstanding the following two sentences: "Call me tonight", and "Kill me tonight." As you can see, a mispronounced vowel can change the meaning of a statement.

By using verification, you can make sure that you and the person are saying the same thing and have the same understanding of the situation. Verification also builds a stronger rapport with the person, since the person will realize that you are trying to understand and are truly listening to what she is saying. Verification sentences often begin with phrases such as:

- "If I understand you correctly ..."
- "May I repeat this back to you to make sure I understand?"
- "So you mean ..."
- "Then you want us to ..."

If you believe the person does not understand, question him or her to find out what is unclear. For example:

- "You seem unsure, Mr. Brown; what concerns you?"
- "Specifically, what part is unclear to you, Mrs. Hall?"
- "Is there anything that you would like explained again, sir?"

When repeating information for a second time, it is often better to rephrase it than to repeat it word for word. If there still seems to be a problem, try using examples.

It might also be helpful to offer any resource material that is available. This may include pamphlets, copies of documents, or other material.

Counsel the Customer/Patient

Now you are ready to move on to the counseling step. Counseling may not be necessary in all encounters. When a short or simple answer is required, simply answer the question and conclude the conversation. For example:

- "Yes, Mrs. Minor, we have your appointment listed at 2 o'clock on Tuesday."
- "Yes, Mr. Sampson, the check for that account was received Monday."

However, counseling can be invaluable when the response is lengthy or complex. For example:

- "According to our records we never received payment for Dr. Jordan's claim. May I suggest you talk with the insurance carrier and find out when the claim was paid? If it has been longer than two weeks, ask them if they would like us to resubmit the claim."

Counseling is also helpful when the response requires that you take further action. For example:

- "I need to check our records to see if your account has been paid. Are you able to hold a moment while I pull up the file?"

Finally, counseling assists when the response requires a delay before the problem can be resolved.

- "I need to contact the corporate office for a copy of the records. It will probably take a few days. When I receive it, I'll call you back. You should hear from us by Monday, Mr. Smith."

Counseling entails explaining the situation and then explaining both what the person should do next and what you will do next. In the previous examples the following occurred:

- The patient was expected to contact the insurance carrier's office and you would wait for their response.
- You would check the records and the client would hold.
- You would contact the corporate office and the customer would expect your call by Monday.

Counseling allows a clear picture of the situation and the actions to be taken. In this way each person is clear about what the next step should be in helping to bring the situation to a successful resolution.

Close the Conversation
Once a plan of action has been agreed upon or the person's questions have been answered, it is time to close the call. The important thing to bear in mind is that the encounter should not be considered finished until the person is as satisfied as possible.

When you feel the person is satisfied, use the following steps to close the call:

1. **Summarize the outcomes.** A **summary** is a brief statement reminding the person of what you have agreed to and how it will help or solve his concern. It needs to be clear and concise, and stated in a positive way. For example:
   - "Good, then I'll send that report out right away, Mrs. Phillips, and if you have any questions about it, just give me a call."
   - "So, you'll call the corporate office at the toll-free number I just gave you and find out why they've rejected your application. You'll also ask them what they need to review in your application. If you still have a concern after you've talked to them, just give us a call. Thank you for calling. Goodbye, Mrs. Smith."

2. **Thanking the customer/patient.** Do not forget to thank the customer/patient. If people feel unappreciated they may take their business elsewhere. The two words "thank you" may be the easiest and one of the most important ways to keep your customers and patients and your job.

Occasionally, a customer or patient may want to continue to chat after a resolution has been

reached. In such a case, summarizing the agreed-upon actions in a succinct way will send the message that the conversation is concluding. With determined persons, it may be necessary to firmly but kindly let them know that you have other matters that need your attention. You can explain that while you would love to chat, you need to get back to work.

The use of these basic steps in problem resolution will bring positive results and will help your customer/patients to feel important and appreciated. This is what customer service and patient relations is all about.

To help assess your strengths and weaknesses in the areas just discussed, complete **Exercise 27 – 4** at the end of this chapter.

Handling Difficult Clients

Occasionally, you will receive a call from or be forced to meet with a customer/patient who is irate, tearful, unprepared, or who cannot seem to figure out what to say. The following information will help you to handle people who generally pose the greatest problem for customer service personnel.

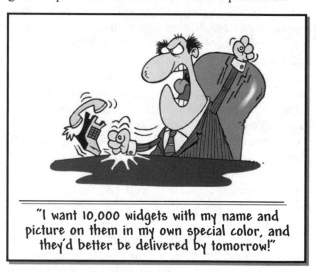

"I want 10,000 widgets with my name and picture on them in my own special color, and they'd better be delivered by tomorrow!"

Irate Customer/Patients
Most people you deal with will be polite, kind, and courteous. Occasionally, however, you will have to deal with a customer/patient who is irate and has no qualms about taking out his anger on you. Remember that your behavior influences the behavior of others. Instead of becoming irate yourself, consider this type of person a challenge. See how long it takes you to get the person calmed down and the problem resolved.

Most irate people perceive themselves as victims who have been wronged by someone. By providing a listening, sympathetic ear, you can let them know that they are important to your business and that their concerns do matter to you. Remember that the person may have a legitimate complaint that needs to be resolved, even if it was not your fault.

Start by listening to what they have to say. Let them vent their anger for a bit and finish what they have to say without being interrupted. Try to understand their point of view.

If they use offensive or abusive language, ignore it. Always try to remember that they are angry with the company and the circumstances, not with you. Ignore the hurt the words cause. If you cannot do this, you have lost control of the situation. If it happens often, you may lose your job.

If they continue with abusive language, try asking if you have done something to personally offend her. This often helps to calm the person and begin moving the situation toward a resolution.

If you are dealing with an abusive caller and this approach does not work, (and if your employer allows you the option of terminating such calls) interrupt the caller and firmly but politely say, "Excuse me, but I prefer not to hear such language. If you do not stop, I am going to have to end this conversation." Say this two times, the second time a little more forcefully than the first. If the language or abuse continues, say, "I am sorry but I need to terminate this call. Please call back when we can discuss this problem in a calm manner." Then hang up immediately. On terminating such a call, inform your supervisor immediately. This type of caller nearly always calls back. Most of the time the caller is apologetic and you can work toward resolving the problem. If the caller is still irate and abusive, the call should be transferred to your supervisor.

If a phone caller is a screamer, let him vent to allow the release of pent-up emotions that you do not want to have to deal with later. However, if the person is facing you in person, especially if other people are around, you need to try to calm the person down as soon as possible.

With either type of people (on the phone or in person), try not to interrupt. This will usually make them angrier. Your voice and actions should show that you understand and accept their feelings, regardless of whether or not you agree with them. Use statements such as "I can see why you are upset." or "I understand that you are angry. Let's see what we can do to resolve the problem." Usually, letting them know you understand and care and are offering to work with him to resolve the problem will defuse the anger. Then try to resolve any problems without transferring them or referring them to another person. If you cannot help them and you need to transfer or refer them, be sure to explain why and give all the information that they need to contact the person to whom you are referring them.

Do not make excuses. It does not help to resolve the situation or help them feel better. If errors have been made, apologize for them without placing blame. Promise to do what you can to resolve the situation, and then do it.

If the caller insists on speaking with your supervisor, put him on hold and briefly explain the situation so that the caller will not need to repeat everything a second time. Before transferring the call, inform the caller of your supervisor's name and that you have briefed him on the situation.

If your supervisor is unavailable, inform the caller of this, and attempt to handle the problem. If you cannot handle the problem, take down the caller's name and telephone number and let her know that you will have the supervisor return the call as soon as possible. This delay often allows the caller to "cool down" and to be able to discuss the situation more calmly when the supervisor returns the call.

Remember the following 11 guidelines in dealing with irate or angry customers/patients:

Remain calm. Remember that the customer/patient is angry at the situation, not you. If you become upset, the discussion will become an argument.

Ask questions. Direct, open-ended questions help to define the problem. However, questions that begin with "Why" are best avoided since they can sometimes be construed as threatening.

Listen carefully to what the person is saying. Do not try to match wits with the person. Allow the person time to vent his feelings. Even angry people will give you valuable information by what they say and how they say it. Let the person know you are listening and are interested by saying "I see" or "Yes, sir." If you are speaking with the person face to face, maintain good eye contact, nod, and keep an attentive facial expression and an open body position.

Be prepared. Be well informed regarding your company and your department. If a person is upset about a policy that cannot be changed, explain how the policy was designed to protect them, you, or the company.

Avoid giving customers/patients the run-around. Try to avoid transferring them to someone else. If at all possible, resolve the problem yourself.

Accept criticism without becoming angry. People who are angry are often looking for a fight to justify their anger. Your pleasant demeanor can be disarming to an angry person.

Agree with the person. Find something in the person's remarks with which you can agree. This will help them to feel you are an ally rather than an enemy. However, never agree to anything that can be misconstrued as a promise of what you or the company will do. Do not place blame. You do not want them to like you and dislike the company.

Avoid defensive behavior. Do not make excuses such as "We are short-staffed," "I am new here," or "It is not my job."

Offer choices. Whenever possible, allow them to choose a plan of action by offering several options. Or ask them how he or she would like you to resolve the problem. This way, they will feel in control of the situation and will take responsibility for the outcome.

Be personal. Introduce yourself and learn the person's name. Say the name as often as it is appropriate during the conversation.

Remember that the more friendly, pleasant, and helpful you are, the more helpful, responsive, and satisfied your customers/patients will be.

Unprepared Customers/Patients

An unprepared customer/patient may not have sufficient information for you to answer questions. Sometimes the person has not taken the time to formulate thoughts, and it may be difficult to determine exactly what the question is. Be patient. Explain what information you need and why you need it. Assure them that you will be happy to be of assistance when the information is provided.

Customer service means serving the customer/patient. However, do not allow yourself to be taken advantage of or talked into performing functions that are not the responsibility of you or your company. Once a person begins taking advantage of you it usually continues, leaving you little time to accomplish your assigned tasks.

Long-winded or Tearful Customers/Patients

Long-winded or tearful customers/patients try to make you feel sorry for them in an attempt to get their way. Sometimes they call or come in simply because they are lonely and want someone to talk to or because they need reassurance. Both types of people have a tendency to try to continue the conversation after their questions have been answered.

It is important with these types of people to maintain a professional attitude. Show your concern, but do not allow yourself to become overly sympathetic.

Question the person to be sure that she is satisfied with your answers. Verify that there are no further questions, and then try to terminate the conversation by politely but firmly explaining that there are other matters that require your attention.

Handling Unwanted Callers

At some point in your career you will probably be asked to screen calls for your supervisor. There will always be people who are put through immediately, and those that your supervisor does not want to speak with. Handling calls under these situations can be very stressful.

As a general rule, no one likes to be rude. However, if all calls are put through, your boss may not have time to complete that important project sitting on his desk.

The best method is to ask your boss what calls should be put through. Find out which people he does not want to speak with, and what to do with people who are not listed in these groups.

If your supervisor is screening a large number of calls, use a simple phrase such as, "Let me see if he's available. May I tell him who is calling?" If he chooses not to accept the call, say to the caller, "He is not available at the moment, may I take a message for him (or may I send you to his voice mail?)?" This way the caller at least feels that he can let the boss know that he called and that he is not being completely ignored.

If the call is from someone you have never heard of, and the boss has asked you to screen out sales calls, ask, "May I tell him who is calling and what this is regarding?" This will usually give you (or your boss) enough of a response to determine if the caller is a sales person or a long lost client.

If there is a caller the boss refuses to speak with, the following tactics often work the best:

1. Do not beat make up excuses. Politely tell the caller that the boss prefers not to accept his call.
2. If you know your boss is under a deadline, try to help the caller yourself, or transfer him to someone else who can help him. This not only makes the person feel important, but it prevents them from calling back at a later date.

Dealing With Sales People

Sales people can be among the most persistent callers to a company. Often they are offering products or services for which you do not have a need. In such cases, the following suggestions can help to eliminate such calls.

If it is a sales person and he requests to send information on his products or services, first determine whether or not you or the company would be likely to use this person's services in the future. If the answer is no, tell the salesperson that you do not think your company would have a need for their products or services, but thank the caller for considering your company. If they persist, decline to give out your address. If they continue to persist, have them send the information to you, then simply drop it in the wastebasket.

If a sales person requests to call back and it is a product or service that your company may have a need for, tell the sales person that your company does not accept unsolicited calls and suggest instead that they send you some literature. Have it addressed to you so that you can evaluate it before passing it on to the appropriate person.

Ask the sales person to remove your company from their calling and/or mailing list. In most states this requires the sales person to remove you or to add you to a "Do Not Contact" list.

If you seem to be getting a lot of calls, ask the sales person where they got your company's information. Many company's names will suddenly end up on a list that is sold to advertisers. If you can find out where the company got your name, you can contact the company selling your information and insist on being removed from their list.

Do not be afraid. Sales people often have forceful personalities. They will try their utmost to get to the person who can immediately say "yes" to a purchase of their products. By telling them that you screen all products or insisting that they send in material, you are thwarting their process. Sales people are not clients, and they have their own interests in mind, not yours. Do not be afraid to be forceful; however, you should not be rude.

Professionalism

In customer service and patient relations, it is very important to use language that conveys a professional attitude. Slang, rudeness, and other discourteous ways of speaking should not be allowed to creep into your vocabulary. Following are 11 comparisons between professional and unprofessional language:

Use courtesy rather than rudeness or sarcasm: "Do you have/need a copy of your contract to refer to?" rather than "Haven't you read your contract?"

Use patience rather than rushing the person: "I can explain that for you," rather than "Will you let me answer your question?"

Use a calm and composed voice rather than reacting personally: "Yes, an error was made," rather than "Don't take it out on me. I didn't do it."

Sound concerned rather than bored or bothered: "How can I be of help?" rather than "What do you want me to do about it?"

Be reassuring rather than uncaring: "That's okay. In your situation it doesn't matter," rather than "I don't care about that."

Use acceptance rather than implying blame:
- (Internally) "It was billed incorrectly," rather than "The biller did it wrong."
- (Externally) "Our record shows no payment date, but I can check," rather than "Your insurance carrier didn't pay it."

Suggest rather than demand: "You might want to ...," rather than "You have to ..." or "We need from you ...," rather than "You have to send ..." or "May I suggest ..." rather than "You must ...."

Restrict your conversation to business rather than discussing personal experiences or opinions: "I can understand this must be an inconvenience for you," rather than "I know someone with that problem who saw a lawyer ...."

Use business-like language rather than slang or nicknames: "Ma'am/sir" rather than "Honey/Dear/Sweetie" or "That is correct," rather than

"You got it." "Your file is complicated," rather than "Your file is screwed up." "I'm doing my best," rather than "Get off my case." "It might not be best," rather than "You're getting ripped off." "Request prompt attention," rather than "Get them on the stick."

Try to sound knowledgeable and logical rather than confused or uninformed: "I don't have an immediate answer to your question but let me find out for you," rather than "I have no idea."

Respect the client rather than imply that you have superior knowledge. "The figure on your form, located in the fourth column, indicates the amount," rather than "I don't see why you don't understand—it's right there on your statement."

To practice, complete **Exercise 27 – 5** at the end of this chapter.

Telephone Techniques

Medical billers conduct a large percentage of their business over the telephone. Therefore, proper telephone etiquette is very important.

Answer Promptly
When your telephone rings, make a point of answering it before the third ring, whenever possible. Prompt answering helps avoid irritation and builds a reputation for efficiency.

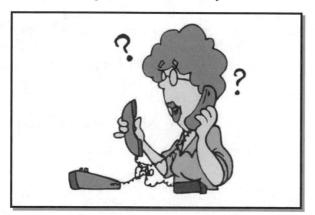

Identify Yourself
Let the caller know whom he is speaking with. It establishes a rapport and lets the caller know that you are a person, as opposed to a computer, and are willing to work to resolve the problem or concern.

Be Friendly
Your tone of voice conveys your willingness to help and makes the customer/patient feel that the

problem is important to you. Make your voice pleasant and control the speed at which you speak. Make the client feel that you are eager to be of assistance. To accomplish this:

1. Be a good listener so that the caller will not have to repeat things.
2. Indicate that you are interested. Use the caller's name whenever possible (but use the last name, not the first name).
3. Be sincere and genuine, and let this come through in your voice.
4. Give your full attention to the caller. A discussion with others while a caller is waiting on the line is inconsiderate and irritating.
5. Avoid interrupting the caller.

Returning to the Line
When you must leave the line to get information, be courteous. Ask if the caller is able to hold or if it would be more convenient for you to call back. Do not automatically assume that the caller has the time or inclination to wait on the line. Here are some suggestions:

1. If the caller agrees to hold, use the hold button. If this is unavailable on your phone, set the phone down gently. Bear in mind that the customer/patient can overhear conversation when the phone is not placed on hold. Be careful not to say anything that might be overheard or misunderstood.
2. If it takes longer than anticipated to obtain the information, update the caller on your progress. If it is going to be more than a couple of minutes, tell the caller that you will contact him as soon as you can get the information. Give the caller an estimate of how long it will take, and keep your promise to call back.
3. When you return to the line let the caller know you have returned. For example, say, "Thank you for waiting."

Transferring Calls
Try to take care of the caller's concern yourself. It is irritating for the caller to be transferred from one person to another. If the caller has a simple problem that is not your responsibility (i.e., change of address, request for an application or material), write the information and give it to the person who is responsible for that function. When it is necessary to transfer a call, take the following four steps:

1. Explain why you need to transfer the call ("I'm unable to assist you with that. However, Mr. Gonzales can help you. May I transfer you?").

2. Wait for the caller's response. If the person does not wish to be transferred, write down her name and phone number and tell the caller that someone will call her back ("I'll have Ms. Smith call you back with the information.").

3. If the caller agrees to be transferred, be careful not to disconnect the call. To be safe, always give the caller the name of the person you are transferring them to and their extension or phone number. Then if the caller is accidentally disconnected, he can call that person directly.

4. Finally, briefly explain the situation or problem to the person to whom you are transferring the call, along with the caller's name. Be concise, but convey enough information that the caller will not need to repeat everything a second time.

Closing the Call

Summarize the conversation to be sure it is closed and to note any follow-up action required of either party. Try your best to say good-bye in a way that will leave the caller feeling satisfied that her problem will be handled correctly. Let the calling party hang up first.

Telephone Tips

In addition to the previous points, here are 14 more suggestions that may be helpful:

1. If your call is going to be lengthy, make an appointment with the client for a date and time for the extended call. In this way, your call will have a better chance of being answered, and your customer/patient will have a better chance of having the time needed to resolve the situation.

2. Outline the topics you need to discuss before placing the call; then stick to the list of topics.

3. Before placing the call try to picture the other person in your mind, and smile at that person. This will put you in a friendly frame of mind.

4. Be kind to whoever answers the phone, even if it is not the person with whom you wish to speak. This person may be your only link to the person you want.

5. If you are unable to reach the person you need, leave a message and make sure the messenger also takes down your phone number. This increases the chances for your call to be returned.

6. Make sure the person has a few minutes to speak to you. A simple, "Do you have a moment to speak with me?" can help a lot. If the answer is "no," ask when the best time would be for you to call back.

7. Most callers find it unnerving to be asked what their call is about. If you are unable to answer your own phone, instruct those who answer for you not to ask this question.

8. Avoid doing other things (i.e., writing or typing) while you are on the phone.

9. Complex information is best handled in person or in writing, especially if it contains critical information or details.

10. Make sure that your caller is satisfied and fully understands before closing a conversation. You cannot see a confused expression over the phone, so listen for it in the caller's voice.

11. If you are taking a message for someone else, do not tell the caller when this person will call back. If the caller is unable to reach the person at that time, he may become upset.

12. Never slam down the receiver, no matter how upset you may be with the caller.

13. Do not eat, drink, chew, or smoke while on the phone. The telephone receiver can magnify these sounds, and they can be very annoying to the caller.

14. Always terminate a call pleasantly and politely.

Phone Calls

The following are general guidelines regarding phone usage. Since these guidelines may vary from company to company or even between departments in a company, be sure you understand your company's policies.

1. **Collect call policy**: Some companies accept collect calls from customers/patients; however, others do not. If you are going to be handling inquiry calls, it is important that you know your company's policy prior to accepting collect calls, not after.

2. **Long distance**: Long distance calls to customers/patients are usually permitted if the information requested in the call is necessary for business purposes. You should organize your thoughts and write down your questions prior to making the call so that you spend as little time on the call as possible. This will drastically reduce the overhead costs of the company.

3. **Telephone system**: Telephone systems can vary greatly from one company to another. Be sure you know how to properly answer a call, transfer a call, and place a caller on hold. Nothing is more irritating to a caller than to be disconnected after being on hold for a long period of time.

Telephone Etiquette

It is important to use proper etiquette on the phone. The word **etiquette** is defined as the practices and forms prescribed by convention or by authority. In essence, etiquette is manners.

While using the telephone, etiquette includes your tone of voice, some basic telephone manners, speaking on the level of the caller, controlling the conversation, and making the appropriate verbal responses.

Tone of Voice
Your tone of voice is the single most important factor in conveying your willingness to help a client. Be pleasant and professional. Pay attention to the other person and respond to her questions in a sincere manner. If you smile while on the phone, this smile will usually come across in your voice.

Working in a customer service area can be demanding, frustrating work. Many callers are angry, irritated, or tired. But the difference between a good customer service person and a poor one is that a good customer service person is always pleasant and kind to each customer, no matter how the person comes across. You cannot allow the person's feelings to influence your own.

Be natural and use simple straightforward language. Use a normal volume that can be heard easily, but is not too loud. Talk at a moderate rate, neither too fast nor too slow.

In many geographic areas there are high concentrations of non-English-speaking or English-as-a-second-language speaking persons. If you do not speak the caller's language and they do not speak English well, it is important to speak slowly and to pronounce words correctly. Do not yell. These callers are not deaf; they just have difficulty with the language. If possible, find someone in your office who speaks the caller's language. If that is not possible, take the time to work with the caller. If necessary, spell out words. Many people have a higher understanding of written language than of spoken language. Above all else, be patient and do not try to rush the situation.

Telephone Manners
Every call is important to the caller and should be treated as such. When the caller feels that you are giving individual attention to the call, rather than routine consideration, he or she will have more confidence in you and the company.

Be tactful. When you must refuse a request because of company policy, give a full and sympathetic explanation. A comment such as "If you will submit your request in writing, we will be glad to give it consideration" sounds more tactful than, "You have to send it to us in writing to get an answer."

Apologize for errors or delays, even if they are not your fault. Things may not always go right, but a little courtesy can help defuse anger. However, be sure your apologies are genuine; otherwise they will sound insincere.

Take time to be helpful. It only takes a little more effort to make your phone contacts pleasant, and it can brighten your day as well as the caller's. Remember that it is better to spend a few minutes trying to keep a client happy than months trying to regain her business.

If you are having a bad day and all your clients seem to be angry or defensive, consider that the problem might be you. People respond to what they think they hear in your voice. If there is irritation, it may make them irritated and can begin a downward spiral. Turn things around by changing the way you are talking or your tone of voice. This simple change may turn your day around.

Speak at the Callers Level
As a customer service representative, you will receive calls from people with varying degrees of education and knowledge. Listen to the way the caller pronounces words and the type of words they use. Then use words on a similar level that the caller can understand. Regardless of the level of the caller, you should avoid the use of technical words that the caller may not understand.

Controlling the Conversation
Your primary goal should be to give the client complete satisfaction in the least amount of time. The following six suggestions can help you accomplish this:

1. Find out as soon as possible what the question or problem is. Have the caller tell you exactly what he wants to know. Do not try to guess. You may guess wrong and provide unwanted or incorrect information or you could bring up questions the caller may not have thought of.
2. Obtain specific information immediately. This may include information such as:
   - What is the account number?
   - What is the client's name?
   - What was the date of the purchase?
   - What was the purchase amount?

3. Answer all questions and make sure the caller understands the issues. Before closing the call, ask whether there are other questions.
4. Do not bring up issues or claims unrelated to the caller's questions.
5. Do not chitchat with the caller. Be polite, but keep the conversation centered on the business at hand.
6. Choose your words and tone of voice carefully. If the caller becomes angry or irritated, the call will take longer.

After the caller's questions have been answered or the requested information has been given, politely close the conversation.

Appropriate Verbal Responses

If a question requires a simple yes or no, it is appropriate to answer as such. However, be aware of questions with which disclaimers should be used. These can involve questions such as, "Does the doctor perform this type of surgery?" or "Does my insurance provide surgical coverage?" Answers to these questions should include disclaimers such as, "Yes, for most patients who are not at high risk" or "Yes, with certain restrictions. Cosmetic surgery is not covered, or a second opinion may be needed to verify the need for some surgeries." Explain that without proper information from the doctor or medical documentation, you cannot tell the caller whether his or her particular procedure will be performed or covered and whether other conditions might need to be taken into consideration.

Many insurance companies have a pre-authorization process, which allows the provider of service to submit documentation regarding the case and suggested procedures prior to the performance of these procedures. This information is reviewed and a qualified approval may be given. This is similar to obtaining an estimate before car repair work is done, but here the estimate covers not how much it will cost, but how much the insurance carrier will cover. If the procedure falls into a gray area, the medical biller should suggest that a pre-authorization review be performed prior to the services being rendered.

If the caller is presenting a hypothetical question, the variables may range too widely to give an answer. Without documented facts it is difficult to make a decision regarding any situation. If the caller insists that you give an answer, explain that your reply is based on the information given and that the answer could vary greatly when the written documentation is received.

If you are unsure about the answer to a question, do not guess. Inform the caller that you are not sure but that you will find out the answer and call him or her back.

When verifying benefits, all facts of coverage should be checked. This includes the diagnosis, the eligibility status, current coverage, dependent eligibility, age limits, and others.

Most calls can be handled using your knowledge, common sense, and patience. Remember never make any promises you can not guarantee. Actually, the only promise you should ever make is to follow through in handling the situation.

Maintaining an Appointment Calendar

A well maintained appointment calendar can make the difference between having a chaotic or calm day. By simply looking at your calendar at the beginning and end of each day, you will know where your free time slots are. If you practice the habit of keeping an orderly calendar, you can decide when the best time would be to do your various tasks. Following are a few tips on how to maintain a calendar:

Put the day and date on the calendar. Make sure the day and date are prominently displayed at the top of each page. With most appointment calendars this information is preprinted. However, if you are using a weekly or monthly planner, the day and date may be displayed anywhere on the page.

A person's name should be on the calendar. If you have calendars for more than one person, put the name of the person the calendar applies to prominently on the top of the calendar. This will help prevent you from writing an appointment on the wrong calendar.

Give your boss a copy of the calendar. If you keep a calendar for your boss, on a periodic basis put a copy of their calendar for the upcoming day or week on their desk. This allows them to know when they need to arrive in the morning, and to plan out their day.

Keep your old calendars. Invariably there will come a time when you are filling out your expense report or other documentation and someone asks "What date were you in Dallas?", or "When did you meet with so-and-so?" By keeping the old appointment calendars you can find this information quickly and easily. The rule of thumb is to keep old calendars for at least 18 months. This allows the information to be available for preparing tax returns or for other purposes. However, if the calendar is the only source for obtaining or verifying information that was used for a tax return, the calendar should be kept for at least four years.

Appointment Setting

Administrative assistants are often asked to set appointments for their supervisors. They are sometimes handed an appointment calendar, and the request is made, without the assistant having any idea of how to go about the task.

Appointment setting is easy if you follow a few basic rules; however, not following these rules can cause a lot of trouble. Following are some of the main appointment setting rules to keep in mind:

Insert standing appointments. Start by putting in any standing appointments. **Standing appointments** are any appointments which happen on a regular basis (i.e., board meeting every second Tuesday at 8 a.m.). Block out the hours you (or the person the calendar pertains to) are usually not in the office, and also any regularly scheduled lunch hours. Many appointment calendars have extended hours, indicating the way work is often done. They may start with space for 6 a.m. or 7 a.m. appointments. If the person you are setting an appointment for usually reaches the office at 9 a.m., shade out the hours before 9 a.m.

A gray or dull colored highlighter often works well for this. So if you need to schedule appointments for these times you can write over the highlighter and still see the information.

Set appointments during a time that is beneficial to your schedule. Unless you want to start meeting people from the first moment you walk in the door, try not to schedule anything for the first half hour after you arrive. This will allow you to make or return phone calls, get a cup of coffee, take off your jacket, etc. It also allows time for you to look over those things that may have been placed on your desk after you left the previous day, and allows you a buffer in case you come in later than expected.

Additionally, a half hour of down time immediately after lunch for your boss can solve a multitude of problems and can also help you catch up if you are running late.

Most people like to organize everything and clean off their desk before leaving for the night. If possible, block out a half hour at the end of the day for this.

By not making appointments at these times, you can relieve some of the stress on yourself.

Write appointments down. Write an appointment in the calendar as soon as you receive it. Do not put it off to do later, regardless of how busy you are. Appointment information is often written on small pieces of paper that are easily lost. Be sure to include the name of the appointment, the location, and the phone number of the person whom the appointment is with. Then shade out or draw a vertical line through any remaining lines corresponding to the time of the appointment. For example, if your calendar has a line for each quarter hour, and Mrs. Smith wants a meeting for two hours, write her name, phone number and the location of the appointment on the first three lines, and then draw a vertical line through the remaining five lines to indicate that the appointment will continue through that time.

Differing appointment times on the calendar. If appointment times differ from the preprinted lines on the calendar, indicate the time of the appointment in parentheses (i.e., if the appointment calendar has a line for every 15 minutes and someone wants a 20 minute appointment). This can prevent you from overlapping the appointments and causing you to fall behind.

List phone numbers with appointments. Put any phone numbers with the appointments. Then if you need to cancel an appointment or reschedule, you do not have to go hunting all over to try and find a phone number. This can be very important if you suddenly have an emergency and you ask someone else to cancel all your appointments. This would not be the time to stop and locate the phone numbers for all of your afternoon appointments.

Do not schedule appointments without the calendar. Do not schedule an appointment if you are not able to verify that the time requested is available. You may think you know what times are open, but without the calendar in front of you, you may not be aware of changes that have been made.

Do not schedule appointments that have not been approved. Do not schedule any appointments if you are not told to do so. This is especially important if you are scheduling appointments for a boss. You do not want to find that someone else has a second calendar or even worse, that you have scheduled an appointment for someone the boss refuses to see.

Be on time. Be on time for all of your appointments. If you schedule a meeting, set a time to visit with a client, or tell a friend you will meet them for a working breakfast, you must be there at the time you set or you may lose their respect. Being on time is just a common courtesy, and it will really help you or your employer to maintain a professional relationship.

By following these simple rules, appointment setting can be accomplished easily and with a minimum of hassle. However, not following the rules can lead to stressful problematic situations.

Summary

Customer service and patient relations are some of the most vital functions that medical billers perform. Without good service customers and patients may go elsewhere. Although it takes hard work, patience, and a good disposition to perform good customer service functions, it is well worth the time and effort.

Following are the most important topics discussed in this chapter, and they should always be kept in mind when dealing with your clients:

- Greet the customer/client promptly.
- Identify yourself by giving your name and title.
- Write down the customer/patient's name and account number as soon as identification is provided.
- Be professional in voice and choice of words.
- Listen to what the person has to say. If the person is angry, let her get the anger out.
- Do not react to a person's hostility with hostility of your own.
- Give out accurate information. If you do not know the answer to a question, take the caller's name and phone number and tell them that you will investigate the matter and will call them back.
- Stay informed concerning all policies and procedures and know the procedures of the company you work for.
- Be patient with the customer/patient. She might not be familiar with your procedures.
- Always be supportive of your peers and your company. Acknowledge when a mistake has been made but do not make derogatory remarks about other personnel or company policies or procedures,
- Be empathetic.
- When necessary, use appropriate disclaimers.

By following the simple rules given, appointment setting can be accomplished easily and with a minimum of hassle. However, not following the rules can lead to stressful problematic situations.

Assignments

Complete the Questions for Review.
Complete Exercises 27 – 1 through 27 – 7.

Questions for Review

Directions: Answer the following questions without looking back into the material just covered. Write your answers in the space provided.

1. What is an attitude? _____

   _____

2. What is positive recognition? _____

   _____

3. (True or False?) A person's positive or negative impressions about another person or an organization are formed within two minutes. _____

4. Define empathy. _____

   _____

5. What are the basic steps that will bring you and the client to the resolution of a problem or concern?

   1. _____

   2. _____

   3. _____

   4. _____

   5. _____

   6. _____

If you were unable to answer any of the questions, refer back to that section, and then fill in the answers.

Exercise 27 – 1

Directions: Rate the following statements as to how often you say or feel that way. 1 = Never, 2 = Seldom, 3 = Sometimes, 4 = Often, 5 = Always.

1. _____   I can't remember people's names.

2. _____   I'm not good on the telephone.

3. _____   I have very little control over my moods.

4. _____   I often think of my job as a chore.

5. _____   What's the use? Nobody cares!

6. _____   I don't seem to have much patience.

7. _____   These clients drive me nuts!

8. _____   If my boss were more understanding, I wouldn't be so upset all the time.

9. _____   I just can't seem to get going in the morning.

10. _____   I don't have as much energy as I used to.

What other statements do you often make or think about yourself? _____

_____

_____

_____

_____

Exercise 27 – 2

Directions: Ask three people who know you well or who are around you often to rate you on the following statements. 1 = Never, 2 = Seldom, 3 = Sometimes, 4 = Often, 5 = Always.

1. _____   He/she can't remember people's names.
2. _____   He/she isn't good on the telephone.
3. _____   He/she has very little control over his/her moods.
4. _____   He/she often thinks of his/her job as a chore.
5. _____   He/she often says or gives the impression that he/she feels "What's the use? Nobody cares!"
6. _____   He/she doesn't seem to have much patience.
7. _____   Clients drive him/her nuts!
8. _____   If his/her boss were more understanding, he/she wouldn't be so upset all the time.
9. _____   He/she just can't seem to get going in the morning.
10. _____   He/she doesn't have much energy.

What other statements does this person often make or seem to think about him/herself?

_____

_____

_____

_____

_____

_____

_____

_____

_____

_____

Exercise 27 – 3

Directions: Refer to the previous two exercises and answer the following questions.

1. In what ways are the answers the same? _____
   _____
   _____

2. In what ways do they differ? _____
   _____
   _____

3. Is this the attitude you wish to have and/or to project to people? Why or why not? _____
   _____
   _____

4. What can you do to change your attitude? _____
   _____

Exercise 27 – 4

Directions: Answer the following questions and write your answers in the space provided.

1. Of the ten steps covered in "The Art of Listening," which is your strongest? _____
   _____

2. Which of these steps do you need to pay more attention to? List all that apply. _____
   _____
   _____

3. Specifically, list three actions that you can take to improve your techniques listed in the previous
   question. _____
   _____

Exercise 27 – 5

Directions: Review the following statements and write an improvement in the space provided.

1. "He's on break." _____
   _____

2. "She's busy. Call back." _____
   _____

3. "Sorry. We're getting ready to close." _____
   _____

4. "I don't know where your file is."_____
   _____

5. "I can't do that for you now. Come back later." _____
   _____

Exercise 27 – 6

Directions: Successful people know their strengths as well as the areas that need improvement. Complete the following questions.

1. Identify three strengths you currently possess which contribute to positive customer service/patient relations.

   1. _____
   2. _____
   3. _____

2. Identify three areas that you would like to grow in to be more effective in customer service/patient relations.

   1. _____
   2. _____
   3. _____

3. Specifically, what actions or steps can you take to improve in the previous three areas?

   1. _____
   2. _____
   3. _____

Exercise 27 – 7

Directions: Read the following statements and rate yourself on how you feel you handle customers. Be honest. This is the only way you can recognize your strengths and weaknesses and work toward improving your weaknesses. Use the following numbers to answer the questions: 1 = Never, 2 = Seldom, 3 = Sometimes, 4 = Often, 5 = Always.

Scoring: Add the total for each question and then compute your score. The following scale gives an analysis of your client service quotient.

68 - 75	Excellent! Your behavior and attitudes set examples for others to follow.
59 - 67	Good. You have a high awareness of how important your role is in customer service.
50 - 58	Moderate. You may be allowing your own biases and feelings to affect your customer service.
41 - 49	Needs definite improvement. Time to get in touch with the obstacles between you and the quality service you should be providing.
Below 40	Poor. You need to make a concentrated effort to turn your attitudes and values around. Change may be slow.

1. _____   I want the service I provide to leave an excellent impression, so I constantly look for ways to improve it.

2. _____   I put the customer's needs first since (s)he is my ultimate boss.

3. _____   I accept people without judging them.

4. _____   I am aware that my attitudes and moods affect the way I respond to customers.

5. _____   I show patience and courtesy regardless of the customer's behavior.

6. _____   I do not allow myself to become irritated or lose my composure when dealing with angry customers.

7. _____   I have developed the habit of following up on all complaints that are brought to my attention.

8. _____   I understand the customer and see his/her problem as most important, and I do all I can to resolve it.

9. _____   I treat all customers equally, regardless of their position, rank, color, clothes, accent or other distinguishing features.

10. _____   I recognize it is perceptions that count when dealing with customers, so I do not allow my frustrations or irritations to show.

11. _____   If something the customer says offends me, I focus on what the client is feeling, not on getting even.

12. _____   I use professional language in my dealings with customers.

13. _____   I use proper telephone techniques and always identify myself to the caller.

14. _____   I make sure the customer is satisfied before terminating the conversation.

15. _____   I do not transfer a call unless it is absolutely necessary to resolve the customer's problem.

_____   Total

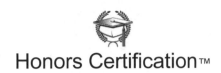

Honors Certification™

Person to Person Customer Service and Patient Relations

The certification challenge for this section consists of a role play situation. You will be asked to role play a situation, providing good service to a customer who may not always be friendly or polite. The number of times you raise your voice, say something inappropriate or react in a negative manner will be recorded. You must have less than three inappropriate responses to the customer's behavior.

If you fail the test on your first attempt you may retake the test one additional time. The items included in the second test may be different from those in the first test.

Telephone Etiquette

The certification challenge for this section consists of a role play situation. You will be asked to role play a telephone conversation, providing good service to a customer who may not always be friendly or polite. The number of times you use incorrect grammar, raise your voice, say something inappropriate or react in a negative manner will be recorded. You must have less than five inappropriate responses to the customer's behavior.

If you fail the test on your first attempt you may retake the test one additional time. The items included in the second test may be different from those in the first test.

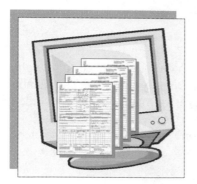

28

Computer Basics

After completion of this chapter you will be able to:

- List and describe the items that will help to make you faster and more accurate when using the computer.
- Describe the three different machines that make up a computer.
- Describe the keyboard and its five components: Typewriter Keys, Numeric Keys, Editing and Cursor Control Keys, Function Keys, and Status Lights.
- List and describe the eight techniques that can help you achieve frustration free computing.
- Recognize and define computer terms.
- List the tips for properly maintaining your computer files.

Key words and concepts you will learn in this chapter:

Brightness Control – A knob which changes the brightness of the image on the screen.

Central Processing Unit (CPU) – The rectangular box that houses the memory and functional components of the computer.

Computer Disk Drive – A place for the storage of information.

Contrast Control – A knob which turns the contrast up and down between varying fields.

Cursor – The small-lighted symbol on the monitor screen that indicates where you are in the program or document.

Hard Drive – Provides space (memory) for information to be stored within the computer itself.

Keyboard – The primary means of communicating with your computer.

Power switch – A control which turns the computer or the monitor on or off.

As with most other industries, the majority of businesses are automated. The computer has, therefore, become an indispensable tool.

Only time and usage will make the medical biller accurate and fast on the computer. However, the following information may assist you when entering data:

Familiarity. Become familiar with the processing program you are using. If you know the fields (spots where specific information is entered), input rates will significantly increase since less verification and decision-making will be required.

Visual Coordination. When learning to use the computer, watch either the video screen or the document you are inputting. Every effort should be made not to watch your fingers, since it is a difficult habit to break.

Preparation. Prepare your documents so that less shuffling of papers is required (i.e., unstaple, arrange by date).

Comfort. A comfortable chair that is adjusted to the correct height decreases fatigue.

Hands Free of Objects. Both hands should be free for typing in data. Pens, pencils, and other tools should not be held while entering data.

The computer is actually a combination of three different machines, the central processing unit (CPU), the monitor, and the keyboard.

The Computer

The **central processing unit (CPU)** is the rectangular box that houses the memory and functional components of the computer. A tremendous amount of studying is required to understand all the inner workings of the computer. However, you should become familiar with a few components, such as the power switch, the reset button, and the disk drives.

The power switch is the on/off switch for the computer. It can be located anywhere on the computer, but is often found toward the back.

The reset button is often found on the front of the computer. Pressing this button clears the screen and "reboots" or restarts the system. In other words, it achieves the same function as turning the computer off and then on again. Use caution with this button. If you do not save your data prior to pressing this button, it may be lost.

A **computer disk drive** is simply a place for the storage of information. Usually, a computer contains a "hard drive" within it. The **hard drive** provides space (memory) for information to be stored within the computer itself.

If there is insufficient memory in the hard drive or if there is a need to make data transportable to another computer or to make a copy of the data, you may record the information on disks.

In the front of most computers is a slot (or several slots). These are alternate floppy disk drives. If the data you are using is stored on a disk, slide the disk into the slot to retrieve it.

At no time should a medical biller be required to repair the computer (unless this is their job). If something is wrong with the equipment, a computer repair technician should be called for on-site repair or the computer should be returned or taken to a computer service center. However, first make sure that all connections are in place at the back of the unit. This is similar to making sure that a television set is plugged in before calling a repairman.

There are a number of connections between the computer and its various components, the power source, and peripheral units (i.e., modems, fax machines). To ensure that all connections are in place, turn off the computer, and simply look at the back of the computer. If any cords or cables are disconnected, they may be the source of the problem. However, be sure that you know where to plug in the cable before attempting to slide it into any of the slots. Plugging in a cord or cable incorrectly can destroy your machine, your programs, or the machines and programs of others whose computers are attached to yours.

The Monitor

The **computer monitor** is the screen that is connected to the computer. It is this screen that allows you to see the programs and the data you are working with. There are four items you should be familiar with on the computer monitor: the power switch, the contrast control, the brightness control, and the cursor.

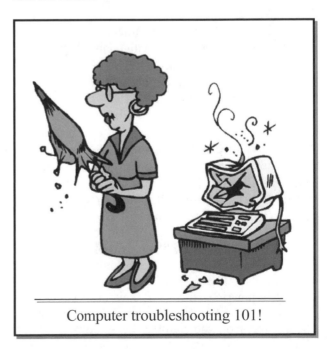

Computer troubleshooting 101!

There is a **power switch** on the monitor like the one on the computer, which turns the monitor on and off. When the monitor is not in use for an extended period of time, the power switch should be turned off to prevent the image from burning into the screen. Be aware that turning off the monitor does not turn off the computer. Therefore, the data and information you were working on are still there. You simply cannot see it.

The **contrast control** turns the contrast up and down between varying fields. This control is usually used to provide more or less contrast between those sections in a document that have been bolded or highlighted and those that have not.

The **brightness control** changes the brightness of the image on the screen. Adjust this knob so that you can read the screen without difficulty or glare.

The **cursor** is the small-lighted symbol on the monitor screen that indicates where you are in the program or document. Depending on the system, this symbol may look like a bright straight line, a bright blinking line, or a blinking or solid box.

The Keyboard

The **keyboard** is your primary means of communicating with your computer. The input commands and data are typed in through the keyboard. Its layout roughly resembles that of an ordinary typewriter. To describe the keyboard more clearly, we will divide it into six parts, each with its own function:

- Keyboard angle adjustment,
- Typewriter keypad with control keys,
- Numeric keypad,
- Editing and cursor control keys,
- Function keys, and
- Three-status lights.

Keyboard Angle Adjustment
You can adjust your keyboard to two different positions for your typing comfort. To adjust, push on the adjustable leg handles on both sides and turn them to the desired position.

Typewriter Keypad With Control Keys
The typewriter area of the keyboard looks and behaves a lot like a standard typewriter keyboard. Like a typewriter, the Shift key produces capital letters. To type the special characters shown above the numbers on the number keys, hold down the Shift key and press the appropriate key. For example, the Shift key with the number 1 produces an exclamation mark (!).

The computer keyboard also includes several special control keys specifically associated with computer operations, including Esc, Ctrl, Alt, and Enter. Here is a brief explanation of some important keyboard and control key functions:

CAPS LOCK – With this key you can type uppercase letters without holding down the Shift key. When Caps Lock is engaged, the indicator light in the upper-right-hand corner of the keyboard lights up. The Caps Lock key only affects the 26 letters of the alphabet. To type special symbols, you still need to press the Shift key.

ENTER – these key acts as both the Return key and the Enter key. As a Return key it ends the line being typed and advances the cursor to the next line. As the Enter key, it is used to execute commands you have typed.

SHIFT – For uppercase letters, punctuation, or symbols, either one of the two Shift keys can be pressed. When the Caps Lock key is engaged, the Shift key acts as an "Un-Shift" key, allowing you to type lowercase letters.

SPACE BAR – Moves the cursor one position to the right. It will also erase characters to the right replacing them with blanks if the computer is in the type over instead of insert mode.

BACKSPACE – This key erases one character to the left of the cursor.

TAB – Moves the cursor to the next tab stop. In some programs the Tab key will act as a margin release to the left if the Shift key is depressed, or will move the cursor one tab spot to the left.

ESC – The Escape key has different functions depending on the program.

ALT – Like the Shift key, Alt performs no function on its own. It is used in combination with other keys. The function of Alt varies, depending on the application being used.

CTRL – This key performs no function on its own. Like the Shift and Alt keys, the control key (Ctrl) is used only in combination with other keys. Ctrl performs many different functions depending on the application being used.

Pressing two or three keys simultaneously can be used to perform a series of unique program control and screen control functions as shown in the following:

KEYS	FUNCTION DESCRIPTION
Ctrl/Break	Terminates the execution of a program and identifies the line where it stops.
Ctrl/Alt/Del	This function resets the computer.
Shift/Print	Causes all data on the screen only to be printed.

To produce the function indicated, press and hold down the first (and second if it is a series of three) key(s) and press the last key. This is by no means a comprehensive list of the functions available.

Numeric Keypad

The numeric keypad is located separately from the alphabetic keys. It is usually on the right-hand-side of a computer keyboard. The keypad performs a dual function.

With the Num Lock key engaged (indicated by the status light in the upper-right-hand corner of some keyboards), the keypad can be used for the rapid data entry of numbers. With Num Lock disengaged, the keypad can be used to move the cursor or to perform special editing features.

A 101 key enhanced keyboard provides a separate keypad for cursor control and editing (located immediately to the left of the numeric keypad). For this reason, most users will find it convenient to leave the Num Lock key on, thus allowing for the rapid entry of numbers. If your keyboard is not a 101 enhanced keyboard, you will probably not want to leave the Num Lock key on.

The following keys operate the same regardless of whether or not the Num Lock key is on or off:

ENTER	Works the same as the Enter key on the typewriter keypad.
+	Displays the Plus symbol.
-	Displays the Minus symbol.
*	Displays the Asterisk, used for multiplication.
/	Displays the Slash, used for division.

The following keys perform differently depending on whether the Num Lock key is turned on or off.

KEY	NUM LOCK ON	NUM LOCK OFF
1 End	1	END – Moves the cursor to the end of the line.
2 ↓	2	↓ – Moves the cursor down.
3 Pg Dn	3	Pg Dn – Moves the cursor down one page, or 25 lines.
4 ←	4	← – Moves the cursor to the left.
5	5	No function.
6 →	6	→ – Moves the cursor to the right.
7 Home	7	HOME – Moves the cursor to the beginning of the line.
8 ↑	8	↑ – Moves the cursor up.
9 Pg Up	9	Pg Up – Moves the cursor up one page, or 25 lines.
0 Ins	0	INS – This key toggles (turns on and off) between Insert and Type over Mode.
. Del	Decimal	DEL – (Delete) Erases one character at the position of the cursor.

Editing and Cursor Control Keys

The 101 key enhanced keyboard contains a separate set of editing keys usually located between the Typewriter and Numeric keypads.

HOME – Moves the cursor to the first character of the line.

CURSOR UP – Moves the cursor up one line for each keystroke.

CURSOR DOWN – Moves the cursor down one line for each keystroke.

CURSOR RIGHT – Moves the cursor to the right one character position for each keystroke.

CURSOR LEFT – Moves the cursor to the left one character position for each keystroke.

END – Moves the cursor to the right of the last character on the current line.

DELETE – Deletes characters at the cursor. All characters to the right will be moved left. If this key is held down it will erase each character as it reaches the cursor.

INSERT/TYPEOVER – On "Insert", characters typed will be inserted before previously typed text, pushing the existing text to the right. On "Type over", existing characters will be typed over.

PAGE UP – Moves the cursor up one page, or 25 lines.

PAGE DN – Moves the cursor down one page, or 25 lines.

SCROLL LOCK – When the Scroll Lock key is pressed, the Scroll Lock light will be illuminated on the keyboard. Once the Scroll Lock light is on, it can be turned off by pressing the Scroll Lock key again, which will also turn off the Scroll Lock mode of operation. Refer to the computer application program manual for more details on this key.

PRINT SCREEN – When the Print Screen key is pressed; the data displayed on the screen will be printed (if the computer is connected to a printer). If the Ctrl key is pressed and held while this key is pressed, the printer function will be disabled or enabled.

PAUSE BREAK – This key suspends the program execution until another key is pressed. When used with the Ctrl key, the program being run will be terminated.

Function Keys
Along the top half of the keyboard or on the left side of some keyboards are 12 function keys that allow complex program commands to be performed with a single keystroke.

Different software programs use function keys for different purposes. Therefore, to properly use these keys, the program-specific user's guide must be referred to. It is highly advisable not to use the function keys without referring to the program instructions, since they may delete data or cancel parts of a program.

Three Status Lights
The three status lights are usually located in the upper-right corner of the keyboard. They are labeled NUM LOCK, CAPS LOCK and SCROLL LOCK. The **Num Lock** light, when lit, signifies the Num Lock function is engaged, thus causing the keys on the numeric keypad to act as numbers rather than cursor movement keys.

When the **Cap Lock** light is on, it signifies that all letters typed on the keyboard will appear as capital letters.

Scroll Lock is a feature that only works with some computer programs. When the **Scroll Lock** is used in these applications, the cursor is locked onto whatever line it is on when the Scroll Lock button is pushed, and the entire page will move around it. For example, if your curser is halfway down the page when you hit the Scroll Lock button, your cursor will remain halfway down the page. When you hit the arrow down key, the entire document will move up one line, but the cursor will remain in the center of the screen.

Frustration Free Computing

According to Murphy's Law, anything that can go wrong will go wrong. However, a number of techniques will help to eliminate the frustration of losing computer-stored information. The following eight techniques should be learned and should become a daily part of your computer life:
1. Save your data often and make back up copies while working on it. A second copy of the data should be saved to a second file when you are finished. A power surge or brief break in the power supply can erase your entries in less than one second.
2. Keep a back up copy in a different location. A second copy of important data should be stored in a different room or, if possible, a different building. This preserves the data in case of fire, destruction of the building, or water damage.
3. Always date the copies of your files so that you can retrieve the latest disk easily.

4. Use permanent disks or tapes to store copies of financial and confidential records and keep them in a secure, fireproof location.

5. Maintain a notebook or log which shows what you have stored in the computer and the file name it is located under.

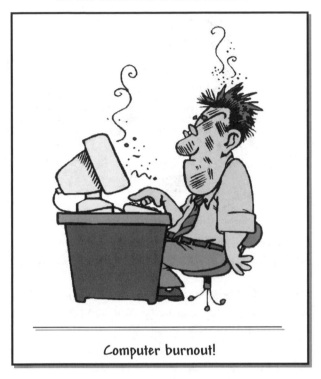

Computer burnout!

6. Set up a system for naming documents so that they will be easily accessible even if you do not have the log.

7. Handle data diskettes properly. This includes the following:

   a. Never touch the magnetic media housed inside the plastic cover. There is a hole in the plastic through which the computer reads the information. On the 3.5-inch disk, this hole is covered by a piece of sliding metal.

   b. Store all disks inside plastic or paper covers to protect them from damage. Insert and remove the disk carefully from the cover to prevent scratching the magnetic media.

   c. Never fold, spindle, or mutilate your disk.

   d. Keep diskettes stored at temperatures between 50 and 125 degrees F. Never leave a data disk exposed to sunlight.

   e. Keep all magnets away from your data disks. Information stored on a magnetic medium can be erased when it comes in contact with a magnet. This includes the magnet contained in office supplies such as paper clip holders.

   f. Before touching a data disk, discharge any static electricity you may have picked up by touching a piece of metal or an antistatic mat. Static electricity also demagnetizes and can erase the data contained on a disk.

   g. When carrying disks across a carpeted area, place the disk inside its protective sleeve and inside another object such as a disk storage box or between the pages of a book. This will prevent erasure by any static electricity that you may pick up by walking across the carpet.

   h. To prevent any changes to information stored on a data disk, slide the button on the disk designed for this purpose. To change the data at a later date simply slide the button back to the original position.

   i. Do not write on a disk label with a ballpoint pen or pencil; use a felt-tip marker. The pressure applied when writing with a pen or pencil may cause indentations on the magnetic media, which may damage the diskette.

8. If you accidentally delete or are unable to retrieve information, immediately remove the disk from the computer. Do not save anything on the disk. Many computer files can be reconstructed with the proper programs, but only if the information has not been written over.

Remember that it is far easier to retrieve data that has been stored properly than to recreate it. Taking proper care of your data will ensure that it will be retrievable when you need it.

Computer Terms

There are a number of terms used in the computer industry that can be confusing to those who have never dealt with computers. The following terms are those most commonly used by medical billers and other computer users.

Bit – (Contraction for binary digit) a single binary digit, either 0 or 1. A bit is the smallest unit of data stored in a computer; all other data must be coded into a pattern of individual bits.

Boot (or bootstrap) – the process of starting up a computer.

CD-ROM – a compact disc format used to hold text, graphics and hi-fi stereo. Basically, it is like an audio CD, but it uses a different format for data. You will need a CD-ROM drive for most new software, since it is a lot easier and quicker for developers to distribute and for you to install software in this format.

Chip or **Silicon Chip** – another name for an integrated circuit, a complete electronic circuit on a slice of silicon crystal only a few millimeters square.

Computer Graphics – use of computers to display and manipulate information in pictorial form.

Central Processing Unit (CPU) – the CPU or processor is considered the brain of the computer. The CPU makes everything else perform, and it is one of the major factors that determine the computer's overall speed. The faster the CPU, the faster the computer can execute your instructions.

Data – facts, figures, and symbols, especially as stored in computers. The term is often used to mean raw, unprocessed facts, as distinct from information, to which a meaning or interpretation has been applied.

Database – a structured collection of data, which may be manipulated to select and sort desired items of information.

Desktop Publishing – use of microcomputers for small-scale typesetting and page makeup.

Disk – a common medium for storing large volumes of data. A magnetic disk is rotated at high speed in a disk-drive unit as a read-write (playback or record) head passes over its surfaces to record or read magnetic variations that encode the data.

Download – to load a file from the Internet or another source onto your computer.

DOS – acronym for disk operating system, a computer operating system specifically designed for use with disk storage; also used as an alternate name for a particular system, MS-DOS.

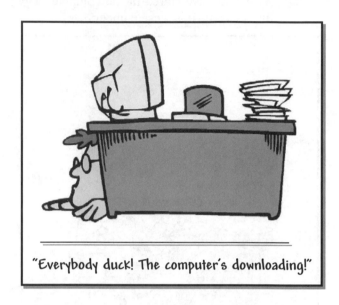

"Everybody duck! The computer's downloading!"

Electronic Mail – or email, is a system that enables the users of a computer network to send messages to other users.

Gigabyte – a measure of memory capacity, equal to one billion bytes. It is also used, less precisely, to mean 1,000 megabytes.

Hacking – unauthorized access to a computer, either for fun or for malicious or fraudulent purposes.

Hard Drive – is the storage place on a computer. It stores information in your computer. You will need a lot of hard drive space to hold all the information you want on your computer.

Hardware – the mechanical, electrical and electronic components of a computer system, as opposed to the various programs which constitute software.

Interface – the point of contact between two programs or pieces of equipment.

Joystick – an input device that signals to a computer the direction and extent of displacement of a hand-held lever.

Keyboard – an input device resembling a typewriter keyboard, used to enter instructions and data.

Laptop Computer – a portable microcomputer, small enough to be used on the operator's lap.

Light Pen – a device resembling an ordinary pen, used to indicate locations on a computer screen.

Megabyte – a unit of memory equal to 1,024 kilobytes. It is sometimes used, less precisely, to mean 1 million bytes.

Memory – the part of a system used to store data and programs either permanently or temporarily. There are two main types: immediate access memory and backing storage. Random Access Memory (RAM) is what your computer and operating system uses to perform functions. RAM is considered a temporary storage area for particular pieces of information required by the computer at any given moment. The more RAM you have, the faster your computer will perform.

Microprocessor – complete computer central processing unit contained on a single integrated circuit, or chip.

Modem – (acronym for modulator/demodulator) device for transmitting computer data over telephone lines.

Mouse – an input device used to control a pointer on a computer screen.

Operating System – a program that controls the basic operation of a computer.

Printer – an output device for producing printed copies of text or graphics.

Procedure – a small part of a computer program that performs a specific task, such as clearing the screen or sorting a file.

Screen or Monitor – an output device on which the computer displays information for the benefit of the operator.

Software – a collection of programs and procedures for making a computer perform a specific task, as opposed to hardware, the physical components of a computer system.

Speech Recognition – or voice input, any technique by which a computer can understand ordinary speech.

Spreadsheet – a program that mimics a sheet of ruled paper, divided into columns and rows.

Touch Screen – an input device allowing the user to communicate with the computer by touching a display screen.

Virtual Memory – a technique whereby a portion of the computer-backing storage memory is used as an extension of its immediate-access memory.

Virtual Reality – advanced form of computer simulation, in which a participant has the illusion of being part of an artificial environment.

Virus – a piece of software that can replicate itself and transfer itself from one computer to another without the user being aware of it. Some viruses are relatively harmless, but others can damage or destroy data.

Word – a group of bits that a computer's central processing unit treats as a single working unit.

Word Processing – storage and retrieval of written text by computer. Word-processing software packages enable the writer to key in text and amend it in a number of ways.

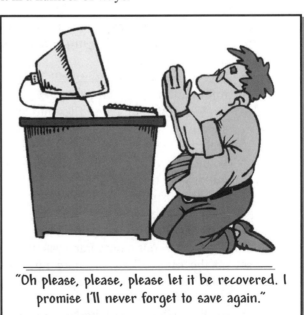

"Oh please, please, please let it be recovered. I promise I'll never forget to save again."

Workstation – high-performance desktop computer with strong graphics capabilities, traditionally used for engineering, scientific research, and desktop publishing.

Zip Drives – are like floppy disk drives, except they hold the equivalent of about 80 floppy disks. You could also use a zip drive for backup purposes.

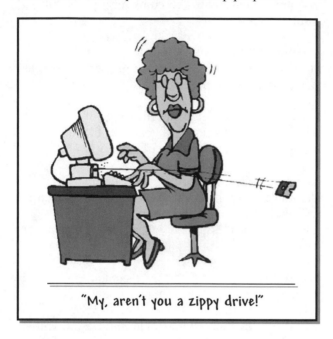

"My, aren't you a zippy drive!"

Maintaining Your Computer Files

Following are several tips for maintaining your computer files:

1. Make sure your paper systems are uncluttered and well structured by adhering to the following:

   a. Throw out old or marginally useful information.

   b. Divide remaining paper files into three classes: working, reference, and archives. Arrange the working files to be nearest you, and the archives to be out of your office.

   c. Create a subject filing structure for each of these classes of paper by mapping out your key functions.

2. Now go into your computer system and set up the same filing structure for your electronic documents. The closer your paper and electronic systems parallel each other, the easier it will be to remember where to file things and where to search for them.

3. If you use email, especially in a corporate environment, you may have hundreds, or in extreme cases, even thousands of messages in your Inbox. Begin deleting them, starting with the oldest.

4. Messages you want to save should be put into the electronic folders or directories you set up in step two.

5. Now do the same with word processing or spreadsheet files.

6. If you need to recapture space on your hard drive, organize your electronic archive system with the same categories you established in step one and transfer your files from your hard drive to floppies or another storage medium.

7. Go through your hard drive and determine if there are any programs you are not using. If so, delete or transfer these to another storage medium.

8. If you are in a corporate environment, or on the Internet and are being swamped with messages, remove yourself from these distribution lists.

9. Go through your documentation and clear out manuals for programs you are no longer using.

10. In the future, establish a certain time each day to process both your paper and email. Do it daily so your files do not build up in your system.

Summary

Computers have infiltrated all aspects of business life. Using the computer saves time and produces neater and cleaner reports, reduces errors and allows for the electronic submission of data.

Learning to use a computer program quickly and accurately and learning the proper means of storing information will provide the medical biller with a valuable skill.

Assignments

Complete the Questions for Review.

Questions for Review

Directions: Answer the following questions without looking back into the material just covered. Write your answers in the space provided.

1. The numeric keypad is used for the _____ _____ when the Num Lock is on.

2. The space bar performs two functions. What are they?

   1. _____

   2. _____

3. What two functions does the Enter key perform?

   1. _____

   2. _____

4. Function keys perform what function? _____ _____

5. The cursor is _____ _____

If you were unable to answer any of the questions, refer back to that section, and then fill in the answers.

Honors Certification™

The certification challenge for this chapter will be a written test of the information contained in this chapter. Each incorrect answer will result in a deduction of up to 5% from your grade. You must achieve a score of 85% or higher to pass this test. If you fail the test on your first attempt you may retake the test one additional time. The items included in the second test may be different from those in the first test.

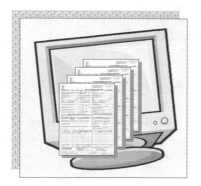

29

Correspondence for the Medical Office

After completion of this chapter you will be able to:

- List the three basic components of effective written communications.
- Write an effective letter and memo.
- Discuss how to properly handle correspondence containing negative content.

Key words and concepts you will learn in this chapter:

Body – The place in a correspondence where you present the purpose of the communication.

Clarity in Writing – Exactness of language.

Coherence in Writing – Information that flows logically from one idea to the next.

Correspondence – Written communication between two people.

Effectiveness in Writing – Being able to evoke the type of response you want your reader to have, whether you want the reader to subscribe to a magazine or to purchase a product or service.

Memo – Short for memorandum, it is a letter intended for distribution within a company.

Correspondence is written communication between two people and it has become an integral part of the business world. Without effective written communications it is almost impossible for a company to succeed. Written communications have permeated every aspect of the business world, from interoffice memos, to correspondence with clients, and from filed reports, to email messages.

Therefore, one of the most important skills that a medical biller can have is the ability to write clearly and effectively. No one wants to read a dull, boring letter, no matter how short. The dullest subject can be made inviting and exciting with effective writing techniques. Remember that the reader will judge you and your company by the type of correspondence received. Learn to use effective language which is clear, concise, and interesting. Your correspondence should also be grammatically correct and properly punctuated.

Before you begin writing think of who your audience is going to be. Are you writing a personal letter to a single person or a newsletter that will be distributed to many people? It will be easier to tailor your writing when you have a clear picture of the reader.

Effectiveness in writing means being able to evoke the type of response you want your reader to have, whether you want the reader to call to schedule an appointment, or pay a bill. Before beginning to compose a letter, ask yourself the following questions:

1. Is this correspondence really necessary? If the answer is no, eliminate it.
2. Could this information be easily expressed over the phone? Would it save time? If the answer is yes, pick up the phone and call.
3. Has this information been expressed in previous correspondence? If so, perhaps a copy of the previous material or a short note referencing it will suffice.
4. Is it vital that the information be written "for the record?" If so, it must be written.

No one wants to waste time reading through information that is not necessary or that has already been covered. Too many communications of this sort may cause your reader to pay less attention when an important piece of correspondence arrives. If the information must be written, follow these points:

1. Determine what you want to say before you begin to write.
2. Determine what action or response you are seeking from the reader.
3. After the correspondence has been written, proofread it carefully for clarity, proper spelling, and proper grammar.
4. Finally, make sure that the correspondence conveys the message you intended.

One trick is to read the correspondence aloud. This often illustrates punctuation and grammar errors that might not have otherwise been caught. You are accustomed to speaking, and passages that are awkward to say aloud usually signal that something is wrong with the way it is written.

There is no prescribed length for a letter. It should be long enough to say what you need in clear concise language and short enough that your reader does not get lost among the words. When you have completed your idea and made it clear to the reader, your correspondence is complete. Do not delete information just because you want to keep the correspondence brief. If the subject matter is pertinent and has been presented in an interesting manner, it will be read regardless of the length.

Let your writing reflect your personality. The most effective way to write correspondence is to write the way you speak. It provides a human link between the writer and the reader. Be concise, simple, direct and professional, but be yourself.

Most correspondence is composed of three parts: the opening, the body, and the closing.

The Opening

The first paragraph and the first sentence of your correspondence are critical. You must gain your reader's attention, interest him in reading further, and make the reader receptive to your ideas. Without the reader's attention you cannot hope to gain the response you are seeking.

Remember that your reader's first interest is usually herself. The reader automatically defines the correspondence according to the personal benefits it will bring. Therefore, you must involve the reader or you run the risk of losing him.

The two principal purposes of the **opening** are to attract attention and to develop interest. Therefore, do not try to say too much in the opening. To be successful, the opening must invite sufficient interest to draw the reader into the body of the correspondence.

The Body

The **body** of the correspondence is where you present the purpose of the communication. Here, you let the reader know what you wish to obtain, if anything. If it is succinct enough any additional information that is needed to verify the request or purpose should also be included here. If it is not, a copy of the information should be attached and a reference should be included in the body of the letter (i.e., see accompanying account statement).

Be sure to provide enough information for the reader to understand your purpose, but not so much that it is overwhelming. Keep the information concise and move the correspondence forward.

Clarity and Coherence

Clarity in writing means exactness of language. It results in the reader understanding what you intended to say. If the meaning is not clear the entire message has failed, no matter how eloquently it was stated. Remember that your reader cannot respond appropriately if he cannot figure out what you want.

After writing a piece of correspondence, take a moment to put yourself in the reader's place and read the letter as if you were seeing it for the first time. Ask yourself, "Does this say what I intended it to say?" If not, it needs to be rewritten.

Coherence means "sticking together." **Coherence in writing** means that the letter or information flows logically from one idea to the next. Being coherent requires that you do not cram too many ideas into a single piece of correspondence. Eliminate any ideas that are not necessary.

If all the information is necessary and the correspondence is still lengthy, consider inserting headings to help the reader determine when you are moving from one thought to another. If your document is not clear and coherent, you will have failed in your attempt to get a message across to your reader and it is not worth sending.

Grammar, Sentence Structure, and Paragraphs

Make sure your grammar and sentence structure is accurate. The impression your letter creates will be a reflection of you and the provider you work for. The last thing you want is your patients thinking they are patronizing an unprofessional facility.

Paragraphs should be kept short and to the point. A paragraph should end when a thought is complete. The only exception is when you add a transitional thought to the end of the final sentence. A **transitional thought** segues into the topic of the next paragraph.

The Closing

The **closing** is the final chance to make your point. It should be a brief summary of the major points contained in the body of the correspondence. Also include a congratulatory or consolatory note if the body of the letter contains good or bad news. Your closing should be fresh, and state in a new and interesting way what the recipient should do, thus enticing him to carry out your wishes.

Correspondence Containing Negative Content

When writing letters that contain negative content (i.e., letters of denial), say "no" as graciously as possible. Your success in keeping this person as a client depends on your saying "no" nicely. Use positive words and phrases to develop a positive feeling within your reader.

Never give bad news in the first paragraph. The reader may stop reading without understanding the reasoning behind the decision. You will have lost the reader without getting the reasons and rationale across in a manner that creates mutual understanding.

Clearly state the reasons for the decision and, if possible, refer the reader to any applicable information to support the provider's decision (i.e., a copy of the contract provisions, a statement of her account). If appeals procedures are applicable, include all the necessary information regarding appeals in your correspondence. This will eliminate unnecessary phone calls at a later date.

Due to time constraints and financial considerations, it may be necessary to respond to your client with a form letter. If the form letter is written in a pleasing tone and uses specific references, you reduce the chances that your reader will think of it as just another form letter. If the letter has been photocopied and is obviously a form letter, consider adding a personal note to the margin that will soften the message.

Format of the Letter

For correspondence to be taken seriously it is important for it to look professional. There are numerous books available that show various styles and formats for letters. Each company has a preferred style, and this style should be used for all correspondence.

Listed below are the three main styles of letters: block style, modified block style and semi-block style. Each of these styles has specific rules regarding formatting of the letter. It is not considered acceptable to mix two or more styles in a single letter or communication.

Legend for **Figure 29 – 1:**
1. **Return Address:** If your stationery has a letterhead, skip this. Otherwise, type your name, address, and (optionally) phone number. These days, it is common to also include an email address.
2. **Date:** Type the date of your letter two to six lines below the letterhead. Three lines are standard. If there is no letterhead, type it where shown.

Figure 29 – 1: Block Style Letter

[Your Name]
[Address]
[City, State, Zip]
[Phone]
[Date Today]
[Re: To What This Letter Refers]

[CERTIFIED MAIL]
[PERSONAL]

[Recipient's Name]
[Company Name]
[Address]
[City, State, Zip]

Dear [Recipient's Name]

[Subject]

The main characteristic of a full block letter is that all typed information is flush with the left-hand margin. The margins are 1.5 inches on the left and the right. The letter is centered up and down, with at least a 1.5 inch margin. There is a double space between paragraphs.

If there is more than one page, the complimentary closing, typist's initials, enclosures, and cc's are placed only on the last page.

Full block is considered to be the most formal style of letters.

Sincerely,

[Signature]

[Your Name]
[Title]

[Typist Initials]
Enclosures: [#]

Cc: [Name of Copy Recipient]
[Name of Copy Recipient]

3. **Reference Line:** If the recipient specifically requests information, such as a job reference or invoice number, type it on one or two lines, immediately below the **Date (2)**. If you are replying to a letter, refer to it here. For example:
   - Re: Job # 625-01
   - Re: Your letter dated 1/1/2005

4. **Special Mailing Notations:** Type in all uppercase characters, if appropriate. Examples include:
   - SPECIAL DELIVERY
   - CERTIFIED MAIL
   - AIRMAIL

5. **On-Arrival Notations:** Type in all uppercase characters, if appropriate. You might want to include a notation on private correspondence, such as a resignation letter. Include the same on the envelope. Examples are:
   - PERSONAL
   - CONFIDENTIAL

6. **Recipient's Address:** Type the name and address of the person and/or company to whom you are sending the letter, three to eight lines below the last component you typed. Four lines are standard.

7. **Salutation:** Type the recipient's name here. Type Mr. or Ms. [Last Name] to show respect, but do not guess spelling or gender. Some common salutations are:
   - Ladies:
   - Gentlemen:
   - Dear Sir:
   - Dear Sir or Madam:
   - Dear [Full Name]:
   - To Whom it May Concern:

8. **Subject Line:** Type the gist of your letter in all uppercase characters, either flush left or centered. Be concise and only use one line. If you type a **Reference Line (3)**, consider if you really need this line. While it is not really necessary for most employment-related letters, examples are below.

- SUBJECT: RESIGNATION
- LETTER OF REFERENCE
- JOB INQUIRY

9. **Body:** Type two spaces between sentences. Keep it brief and to the point.

10. **Complimentary Close:** What you type here depends on the tone and degree of formality. For example:
   - Respectfully yours (very formal)
   - Sincerely (typical, less formal)
   - Very truly yours (polite, neutral)
   - Cordially yours (friendly, informal)

11. **Signature Block:** Leave four blank lines after the **Complimentary Close (10)** to sign your name. Sign your name exactly as you type it below your signature. Title is optional depending on relevancy and degree of formality. Examples are:
   - John Doe, Manager
   - S. Smith
   - Director, Technical Support
   - J. J. Jones - Sr. Field Engineer

12. **Identification Initials:** If someone typed the letter for you, he would typically include three of your initials in all uppercase characters, then two of hers in all lowercase characters. If you typed your own letter, just skip it since your name is already in the **Signature Block (11)**. Common styles are below.
   - AAA/dd
   - AAA:dd
   - Ddd

13. **Enclosure Notation:** This line tells the reader to look in the envelope for more items. Type the singular for only one enclosure, plural for more. If you do not enclose anything, skip it. Common styles are below.
   - Enclosure
   - Enclosures: 3
   - Enclosures (3)

14. **cc:** Stands for **courtesy copies** (formerly **carbon copies**). List the names of people here to who you distribute copies, in alphabetical order. If addresses would be useful to the recipient of the letter, include them. If you do not copy your letter to anyone, skip it.

Figure 29 – 2: Modified Block Style Letter

[CERTIFIED MAIL]
[PERSONAL]

[Your Name]
[Address]
[City, State, Zip]
[Phone]
[Date Today]
[Re: To What This Letter Refers]

[Recipient's Name]
[Company Name]
[Address]
[City, State, Zip]

Attention [Recipient's Name]

Dear [Recipient' Name]

[Subject]

The main characteristic of a modified block letter is that all typed information is flush with the left-hand margin. The margins are 1.5 inches on the left and the right. The letter is centered up and down, with at least a 1.5 inch margin. There is a double space between paragraphs.

If there is more than one page, the complimentary closing, typist's initials, enclosures, and cc's are placed only on the last page.

Modified block letter is not as formal as full block letter.

Sincerely,

[Signature]

[Your Name, Title]

[Typist Initials]
Enclosures: [#]

Cc: [Name of Copy Recipient]

Legend for **Figure 29 – 2:**

1. **Return Address:** If your stationery has a letterhead, skip this. Otherwise, type your name, address, and (optionally) phone number, five spaces to the right of center or flush with the right margin. Five spaces to the right of center is common. These days, it is also common to include an email address.

2. **Date:** Type the date five spaces to the right of the center or flush with the right margin, two to six lines below the letterhead. Five spaces to the right of the center and three lines below the letterhead are common. If there is no letterhead, type it where shown.

3. **Reference Line:** Same as Block Style

4. **Special Mailing Notations:** Same as Block Style

5. **On-Arrival Notations:** Same as Block Style

6. **Inside Address:** Same as Block Style

7. **Attention Line:** Same as Block Style

8. **Salutation:** Same as Block Style

9. **Subject Line:** Same as Block Style

10. **Body:** Same as Block Style

11. **Complimentary Close:** Type this aligned with the Date (2) Same as Block Style

12. **Signature Block:** Align this with the **Complimentary Close (11).** Same as Block Style

13. **Identification Initials:** Same as Block Style

14. **Enclosure Notation:** Same as Block Style

15. **cc:** Same as Block Style

Figure 29 – 3: Semi-Block Style Letter

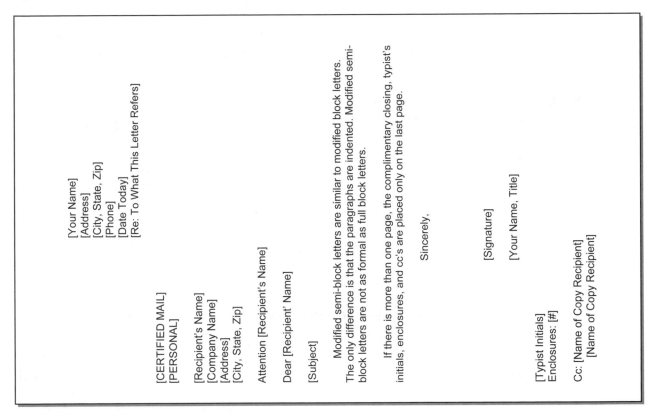

Legend for **Figure 29 – 3:**

1. **Return Address:** If your stationery has a letterhead, skip this. Otherwise, type your name, address and (optionally) phone number, five spaces to the right of center or flush with the right margin. Five spaces to the right of center is common. These days, it is also common to include an email address.

2. **Date:** Type the date five spaces to the right of the center or flush with the right margin, two to six lines below the letterhead. Five spaces to the right of the center and three lines below the letterhead are common. If there is no letterhead, type it where shown.

3. **Reference Line:** Same as Block Style

4. **Special Mailing Notations:** Same as Block Style

5. **On-Arrival Notations:** Same as Block Style

6. **Inside Address:** Same as Block Style

7. **Attention Line:** Same as Block Style

8. **Salutation**: Same as Block Style
9. **Subject Line:** Same as Block Style
10. **Body:** Same as Block Style
11. **Complimentary Close:** Type this aligned with the **Date (2)**. Same as Block Style
12. **Signature Block:** Align this block with the **Complimentary Close (11)**. Same as Block Style
13. **Identification Initials**: Same as Block Style
14. **Enclosure Notation:** Same as Block Style
15. **cc:** Same as Block Style

Tips

Use the following tips when writing letters:

1. Replace the text in brackets [ ] with the component indicated. Do not type the brackets.
2. Try to keep your letters to one page.
3. How many blank lines you add between lines that require more than one, depends on how much space is available on the page.

4. The same applies for margins. The standard for margins is one and one-half inch (108 points) for short letters and one inch (72 points) for longer letters. If there is a letterhead, its position determines the top margin.
5. If you do not type one of the more formal components, do not leave space for them. For example, if you do not type the **Reference Line (3)**, **Special Mailing Notations (4)** and **On-Arrival Notations (5)**, type the **Inside Address (6)** four lines below the **Date (2)**

Business Letter Envelope Components

This sample business letter envelope **(see Figure 29 – 4),** includes formal components, some of which are optional for typical, employment-related business letters.

The graphic below represents the United States Postal Service automation guidelines for a standard business envelope that is 4-1/8 x 9-1/2 inches.

Figure 29 – 4: Sample Business Letter Envelope

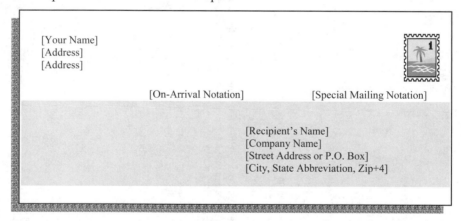

Tips

Use the following tips when creating envelopes:

1. Replace the text in brackets [ ] with the component indicated. Do not type the brackets.
2. If your envelope does not have a preprinted return address, type it in the upper-left corner, in an area not to exceed 50% of the length and 33% of the height of the envelope. Leave a little space between your return address and the top and left edges. How much space will depend on the margin limitations of your printer or typewriter. For example, laser printers typically require margins of at least 1/8 inch (9 points). However, 1/4 inch (18 points) to 1/2 inch (36 points) looks good.

3. Type the **Special Mailing Notation** under the postage area. It does not have to line up perfectly with the stamp as shown, but it looks professional. Type the notation in all uppercase characters, if appropriate. Examples include:
   - SPECIAL DELIVERY
   - CERTIFIED MAIL
   - AIRMAIL

4. Type the **On-Arrival Notation** so that its right edge lines up with the left edge of the recipient's address. This is not a post office requirement, but rather standard formatting. Type the notation in all uppercase characters, if appropriate. You might want to include a

notation on private correspondence, such as when mailing a resignation letter. Examples are:

- PERSONAL
- CONFIDENTIAL

5. The gray shaded area is where the OCR (optical character reader) at the post office scans for the recipient's address. Type the recipient's address within the shaded area, below other information. Do not type anything to the left, right or below the recipient's address. It is a good idea to include a line or two of space below non-address information (such as the notations shown), before typing the recipient's address. This makes it easier for the OCR to distinguish the address.

6. You need special software to print a barcode. It is not required for typical, employment-related letters, but if you want to get fancy, and have a later version of Microsoft Word® or WordPerfect®, they will print barcodes.

Memos

If a message needs to be communicated to a number of people within a company a memo is often written. A **memo** (short for memorandum) is a letter intended for distribution within a company **(see Figure 29 – 5).**

Companies often write memos to share information internally, such as a change of policy or a new method of performing a task. However, memos can be written about any subject.

There are usually three main reasons for disseminating a memo:

1. It is easier to reach a large number of people with a memo, especially if some of them are out of the office. A memo can be left on a desk, ensuring that more people will see it, rather than rely on word of mouth.

2. The memo contains information that a number of recipients need to read (such as a policy change), or information they may need to refer back to at a later time.

3. A memo provides a tangible medium of communication in a documented form.

While typing a memo may seem like a minor part of an administrative assistant's day, memos can be an important part of keeping a company running smoothly.

Many companies will set or change company policies, then notify the personnel by creating a memo and circulating it among the office employees. Employees are then expected to read it and follow the new guidelines. If necessary, the memo should be filed with other important papers so the employee may refer to it at a later date.

For these reasons it is important that memos be written in a clear and easy to understand manner. Be careful of the tone you use when writing a memo, as memos often become a permanent part of a company's or an individual's record.

Additionally, morale can be boosted by a well-written, positive memo, or significantly lowered by a negative one. In fact, a memo praising a certain group of employees and sent to all other employees in the company is one of the easiest and least expensive ways to make people feel important.

Writing a memo of praise lets people know you appreciate their work. It can also motivate others to become involved in future projects.

Memo Format

Most companies have a specific format for their memos. This usually consists of printing them on company letterhead, beginning with a header, then the body of the memo.

The Header

The header usually consists of four items: TO:, FROM:, SUBJECT: and DATE:.

TO: The TO: header is usually typed in capital letters. The name of the recipients may also be in capital letters, or may be in upper and lower case, depending on the policy of the company. Often company memos are addressed to groups of people rather than to individuals. For example, a memo may be designated "TO: All Managers." When a memo is for several people who are not of a designated group (i.e., all managers), the names of the recipients are typed one after another with a comma and space separating the names. Often these people are listed in order of rank (i.e., partners, managers, general staff), or in alphabetical order.

FROM: The FROM: header is also typed in capital letters, with the name of the person creating the memo in either all uppercase or uppercase and lowercase letters, depending on company policy. Usually if one item (i.e., TO: FROM: or SUBJECT:) is in all uppercase, then all items will be in all uppercase. As with the TO: field, this field may also be from a single person or from a group of people (i.e., The Partners).

SUBJECT: The SUBJECT: header is typed in all capital letters (also written as RE:, short for regarding) and is a one line sentence or topic for the memo. Since memos are often filed among other company papers, two or more subjects of importance are not often covered in the same memo. Instead two (or more) separate memos are issued. This allows people to file the memo according to the subject matter, which then makes it much easier to locate and retrieve when necessary.

DATE: The DATE: header is also typed in all capital letters. The date should be given as the date the memo will be distributed. This allows people to track the memos and determine which is the most recent. This can be especially important with memos that alter a company policy or institute a new company policy.

The Body

On most memos, a line or a row of asterisks follows the header information. This separates the header from the body of the memo.

The body of the memo is then typed without a salutation (i.e., Dear Managers), or closing (i.e., Sincerely, The Partners).

Be sure to write clearly and concisely, including all pertinent information. However, extraneous information, which is often included in a formal letter, is not included (i.e., How are you?). Memos usually state the important facts in as few lines as possible. It is very rare for a memo to be longer than one page unless it covers a major policy change.

Once the memo has been typed the person who initiated the memo should approve it. Their approval is usually given by having them initial the original next to their name in the header section. This initialed original is then photocopied and copies are given to each person to whom the memo is addressed. If you issue two or more conflicting memos regarding the same subject on a single day, the subject line should include information that this memo changes or alters the previous memo issued.

Figure 29 – 5: Sample Memo

COMPANY LETTERHEAD

TO: ALL EMPLOYEES

FROM: ANNA ABLEBODY

RE: COMPANY DINNER

DATE: JANUARY 2, 2005

****

I would like to take this opportunity to express my appreciation to all those who helped put together a wonderful New Year's Eve party for the company.

I'm sure you all agree that the Food Committee, consisting of Ginny Gourmet and Terri Tidbit did an excellent job of finding a superb caterer and choosing a wonderful menu.

The decorations created by Winnie Wallpaper, Daniel Décor and Orville Ornaments made the lunchroom an enticing place to be and created a festive atmosphere that set the tone for a wonderful party.

The exciting program, which I'm sure we all enjoyed, was prepared and performed by Rita Recital, Patty Presentation, Peter Performance, Annie Appearance and Sally Staging.

And of course we can't forget the much-appreciated efforts of the cleanup crew: Wally Wiper, Betty Broom and Tracy Trash.

Without the efforts of each and every one of these people we would not have enjoyed such a wonderful party. Please take a moment to thank each of these people personally.

In addition, if more than two memos are issued in a single day with conflicting instructions or changes, the time of the second memo should be placed next to the date. For example, if you issue a memo, then realize you forgot the word "not" in the sentence "On Thursday you should park in the parking garage." The second memo should include the time next to the date. Additionally, the subject line should read something like "Correction of memo re: Parking" to indicate that something on the original memo has been changed.

Postal Abbreviations

There are a number of official abbreviations which the United States Postal Service uses. Following are abbreviations for the most common states and territories:

AL   Alabama
AK   Alaska
AS   American Samoa
AZ   Arizona
AR   Arkansas
CA   California
CO   Colorado
CT   Connecticut
DE   Delaware
DC   District of Columbia
FL   Florida
GA   Georgia
GU   Guam
HI   Hawaii
ID   Idaho
IL   Illinois
IN   Indiana
IA   Iowa
KS   Kansas
KY   Kentucky
LA   Louisiana
ME   Maine
MD   Maryland
MA   Massachusetts
MI   Michigan
MN   Minnesota
MS   Mississippi
MO   Missouri
MT   Montana
NE   Nebraska
NV   Nevada

NH   New Hampshire
NJ   New Jersey
NM   New Mexico
NY   New York
NC   North Carolina
ND   North Dakota
OH   Ohio
OK   Oklahoma
OR   Oregon
PA   Pennsylvania
PR   Puerto Rico
RI   Rhode Island
SC   South Carolina
SD   South Dakota
TN   Tennessee
TX   Texas
UT   Utah
VT   Vermont
VA   Virginia
VI   Virgin Islands
WA   Washington
WV   West Virginia
WI   Wisconsin
WY   Wyoming

Other abbreviations:
Aly   Alley
Ave   Avenue
Blvd   Boulevard
Br   Branch
Byp   Bypass
Cswy   Causeway
Ctr   Center
Cir   Circle
Ct   Court
Cts   Courts
Cres   Crescent
Dr   Drive
Expy   Expressway
Ext   Extension
Fwy   Freeway
Gdns   Gardens
Grv   Grove
Hts   Heights
Hwy   Highway
Ln   Lane
Mnr   Manor
Pl   Place
Plz   Plaza
Pt   Point
PO   Post Office
Rd   Road
R   Rural
RR   Rural Route

Sq	Square
St	Street
Ter	Terrace
Trl	Trail
Tpke	Turnpike
Via	Viaduct
Vis	Vista

Summary

Correspondence is written communication between two people. Regardless of the content of the letter or the response you wish to evoke, the main purpose of correspondence is to communicate your thoughts, ideas, and desires to another person. To achieve this, be sure that the correspondence is necessary, formulate your ideas before beginning to write, and determine the action you wish the recipient to take.

Written correspondence should always contain an opening, a body, and a closing. It should also be clear, concise, coherent, and grammatically correct. Combining all these elements will help to achieve effective written communications

A **memo** is a way of communicating important information within a company as quickly and easily as possible. Memos usually follow a specified format, with a header including TO:, FROM:, SUBJECT:, and DATE: headings.

Assignments

Complete the Questions for Review.
Complete Exercises 29 – 1 through 29 – 2.

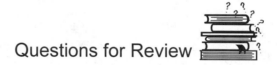

Questions for Review

Directions: Answer the following questions without looking back into the material just covered. Write your answers in the space provided.

1. Before you begin writing a piece of correspondence you should _____
   _____

2. What is the purpose of the opening in a letter? _____
   _____

3. The body of the letter explains the _____

4. If information must be written in the form of a letter, what four points should be followed?
   1. _____
   2. _____
   3. _____
   4. _____

5. If you are writing a letter of denial, should you give the bad news in the first paragraph? _____

6. What are the three main reasons for disseminating a memo? _____
   _____
   _____
   _____

7. What is the usual format for a memo? _____
   _____

8. What four items does the header section usually consist of? _____
   _____

9. (True or False?) Headers are usually typed in lowercase letters. _____

10. (True or False?) Approval of a memo is given by signing one's name at the bottom of the memo.
    _____

If you were unable to answer any of the questions, refer back to that section, and then fill in the answers.

Exercise 29 – 1

Directions: Write a letter for each of the following items. Be sure to use appropriate style, structure and grammar.

1. Write a block style letter to your instructor commending them on their excellent teaching skills.
2. Write a semi-block style letter for your boss, Mr. Harry Hamlet, 555 Hughes Hwy, Hanger, HI 05052, to Medical Billing Supply Warehouse, 2323 Kenneth Road, Kriers, KY 54541. The letter should ask whether the store carries patient billing forms, and if so the cost. Specifically, inquire as to whether they carry the CMS-1500 and UB-92.
3. Prepare envelopes for the above two letters.

Exercise 29 – 2

Directions: Write a letter for each of the following scenarios. Addresses and personal information are contained in the patient files that were set up in Exercise 5-1.

1. Write to Abby Addison's insurance company and request her individual deductible amount and coinsurance limit.

2. Write a letter to Bobby Bumble's insurance carrier to inquire as to whether biofeedback is covered under his plan.

3. You have not received payment from Cathy Crenshaw for services on 11-6-xx for a history and physical. The charge for the service is $125. Write a letter to Cathy to request payment.

4. Daisy Doolittle did not bring in verification of her Medicaid eligibility. She had surgery on 12-7-xx. You need her to bring in or mail a copy of her Medicaid card for December. Let her know that if she does not provide the requested information she will have to personally pay for the services.

5. Edward Edmunds has asked you to write Medicare to find out if removal of a birthmark is a covered service.

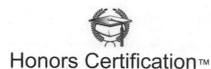

Honors Certification™

Letters

The certification challenge for this section consists of a written test. The instructor will give you a topic along with sender and receiver addresses and ask you to compose a letter in block, modified block, or semi-block style. You must create and print out a letter in the correct style, as well as create an envelope. Spelling, grammar and punctuation count, as well as correct style. The letter should have no errors in it. Each error will result in a deduction of up to 5% from your grade, depending on the type of error. You must receive a score of 85% or higher to pass this test. You are not allowed to use any reference materials when taking the test.

If you fail the test on your first attempt you may retake the test one additional time. The addresses, subject matter, and style may be changed for the second test.

Memos

The certification challenge for this section consists of a written test. You will be required to create a memo in the correct format using the header information and topic supplied to you by your instructor. Spelling, grammar and punctuation count, as well as correct style. The memo should have no errors in it. Each error will result in a deduction of up to 5% from your grade, depending on the type of error. You must receive a score of 85% or higher to pass this test. You are not allowed to use any reference materials when taking the test.

If you fail the test on your first attempt you may retake the test one additional time. The items included in the second test may be different from those in the first test.

Address Abbreviations

You will be given a list of states or other address indicators. You must provide the correct abbreviation for each item. You must score 85% or higher to pass this test.

If you fail the test on your first attempt you may retake the test one additional time. The items included in the second test may be different from those in the first test.

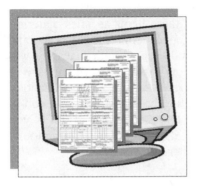

30

Job Search Preparation

After completion of this chapter you will be able to:

- Determine your marketing objectives.
- List and discuss the five items that should be included on a resume.
- Prepare a top-notch resume.
- List and describe the five things to avoid when preparing a resume.
- Exhibit proper interviewing techniques and appropriate mannerisms and dress.
- Write an effective cover letter requesting a job.
- List and describe the four basic components to the interview process.
- Describe the most common misconceptions regarding how a salary should be determined.

Key words and concepts you will learn in this chapter:

Cover Letter – Is an introductory letter to your resume.
Resume – A summary of employment experience and qualifications.

Regardless of the career path you have chosen, all the education in the world is worthless if you do not have good job-hunting skills. Without them, you may never gain employment.

Gaining successful employment requires you to look for a job, and also to market yourself. This works for direct mail advertising companies around the world, and it can work for you too. It is important to start with a set of written objectives, know what separates you from the competition, and familiarize yourself with your target audience.

Job Search Objectives

First, determine your job search objectives. What responsibilities do you want in the position you are looking for? Is there a specific title for such responsibilities? What type of work environment do you desire (i.e., office, hospital, restaurant, outdoor work)? What can you reasonably expect, both in the way of title and salary? Writing down your objectives can help solidify them in your mind and help you formulate a plan of action.

Uniqueness

Most available job openings have numerous people applying for the position. You need to emphasize your uniqueness and the talents that you can bring to the job. What sets you apart from your competitors? Do you have a special talent or area of expertise? Call attention to it. What about a skill you can share with other employees? Highlight it. Let prospective employers know how you can help to train co-workers, saving the company time and money while helping the operation run smoothly.

Do you have contacts in a particular industry that might allow your employer to expand? Tell prospective employers these details to set you apart from the competition.

Target Audience

Success at finding the right job depends not only on the previous two areas discussed, but also on looking in the right place. You would not go to a restaurant to find a job as a typist. Likewise, you would not go to a typing pool to find a job as a waiter. Much depends on where you look for a job.

After deciding on the particular organizations offering the best opportunities, find out who the decision makers are. Who would be the best person for you to contact regarding employment? Get the person's title and name. Find out as much as you can about the person who makes the decisions at the companies you are targeting. What are their professional affiliations (i.e., AFL-CIO, AMA)? What is their career background? What are their job-related concerns and corporate responsibilities? The answers to these questions will help you establish rapport with the person and help you bring out your commonalities.

Build Your Database

Once you have established your target audience, make an organized collection of information about the companies and possible job prospects. Your collection needs to keep track of potential employers, professional contacts, and resources.

Keep detailed and well-organized notes on everyone you speak with that can help you reach your objectives. Always write down the person's name, title, the company or organization name, address, phone and fax numbers, any professional affiliations, the date you spoke or met, how you reached them, what follow-up you should make, and any other relevant information.

Build a file on each company from all the resources available to you. This can include job banks, trade publications, executive search firms, civic groups, alumni associations, social networks, colleagues or co-workers, former employers, and anyone else who can help you. You will be surprised at how many people you know when you start to write them down.

The Resume

Now you are ready to develop your resume and cover letter. Think of these items as sales materials for your career. The cover letter should invite and interest your target audience enough that they will read your resume. Your **resume** is a summary of employment experience and qualifications, essentially the marketing brochure that gets you in the door. Both need to proclaim the benefits you offer to an employer. Sample resumes can be found at the end of this chapter.

A First-Class Resume

A resume can be your best friend or your worst enemy. A first-class resume is one of the most important items you can have in your job search and can open doors for you. A bad resume will slam them shut. In essence, a resume is your personal representative. It tells the company not only who you are, but the type of person you are. No one would welcome an employee who is sloppy and disorganized. Likewise, your resume should not be full of errors or difficult to read. Your resume is a direct reflection of you. Its goal is to get you an interview and help you to land that great job.

The initial screening of a resume occurs very quickly; sometimes it is merely scanned for a few seconds. Your format should keep this in mind. The purpose of this quick scan is to weed out the resumes that have obvious typographic errors, are poorly organized, or are substandard in reproduction. If the author of a resume was not careful enough to proofread and correct his own resume, why should an employer think the person would be any more conscientious at work? If your resume is hard to read or difficult to file (because of odd-shaped paper), it will undoubtedly end up in file 13, also known as the trash can.

Before you write your resume, do a little research. Find a current book on resume writing. This type of book will give you a wealth of information and good resume samples.

The Basics

Your resume should typically be no longer than one page. It should be printed on white or off-white 8.5 x 11 inch paper. Do not use bright or fancy colors. Professionals in the Human Resources area prefer one-page resumes. One-page resumes are easier to read and yet provide enough information to introduce you and your experience. Do not jeopardize your job opportunities by being long-winded or by listing every minute detail about your professional history.

Always be concise and do not abbreviate any words. The chance of being misunderstood is not worth saving the space.

The following five items should be included on your resume:

1. **Name, address, and telephone number:** you would be surprised at how many people leave off one or more pieces of this vital information. Make sure that all the information is correct. Do not cut corners. Your address should include an apartment number and the zip code, and your phone number should include the area code. The easier it is for an employer to contact you, the better.

2. **Objective statement:** some employers and resume writers consider an objective statement to be optional. However, if you have a specific direction, include it. It lets the prospective employer know what your goals are. If you are interested in several different jobs, you might want to replace the objective statement with a qualifying statement. In this way, you will not have to prepare separate objective statements (and resumes) for each job title. Make sure that your resume shows that you have some direction. Your cover letter should also reinforce this.

3. **Qualifying statement:** a qualifying statement is a way to toot your own horn. It sells you as a potential employee and lists your abilities and experiences. You can get ideas for your qualifying statement in the want ads. See what skills and characteristics are desired (i.e., excellent written and verbal communication skills, ability to handle a variety of tasks, and excellent organizational ability). These are exactly the types of statements that should go into your qualifying statement.

4. **Work experience:** there are a variety of ways to state your experience. The most common approach is to list your employment history in reverse chronological order, putting your most recent job first. However, if you have had numerous job changes or a gap in employment, you do not necessarily want to emphasize this. Therefore, you might consider using the functional format resume. This lists together all related experiences rather than listing according to date.

5. **Education:** if you have education or training beyond the high school level you will want this

fact to stand out. Find a way to highlight this so that even when your resume is scanned quickly, additional education can be noticed. The simplest format is to list the degree or certificate, followed by your major or course of study. Follow this with the name and location of the school and year in which you graduated (i.e., Certificate of Completion, Administrative Assisting, Los Angeles College, Los Angeles, CA, 2001). Education and training should be listed in reverse chronological order. See sample resumes at the end of this chapter.

Optional information, if you have room at the bottom, should include special skills, personal notes, hobbies, and references.

Professional Services

If you need additional help, a number of professional resume services are available. It is essential that your resume look professional. This includes the use of a word processor and a letter quality printer. If you do not have access to this type of equipment, it may be a good investment to hire someone to type and print it for you.

Edit and Proofread

You must edit and proofread your resume very carefully. Remember that this single sheet of paper can either help or hurt you in getting a job. It is a direct reflection of you. Before you send it to a potential employer, get a friend to check it for errors and content. Another person often spots things that you have missed.

What to Avoid

Some of these items may seem obvious, but a surprising number of people make these errors on their resumes. The following seven items are things to avoid when you are composing your resume:

1. Never send a carbon copy or an inferior quality copy of your resume to a prospective employer.

2. Never use abbreviations; this includes the term "etc." Anything important enough to be stated should be written out. Write it out or leave it out.

3. Do not waste time and space detailing mundane, entry-level jobs that have no bearing on your present job search.

4. Do not list a desired salary. Discussions of this sort should be saved for the interview. If you ask for too high of a salary, you may not be granted an interview. If you ask for too little, a

prospective employer may wonder what you are worth.

5. Consider the importance of salary, job location, and position desired before you limit yourself. Ask yourself if any of these are more important than a chance for advancement.

6. Do not include information on your age, marital status, religion or race.

7. Do not put "References available on request" because this just annoys prospective employers.

Words to Use in Your Resume

Use an active voice in your resume. Action verbs and specific nouns are best when describing your job duties and accomplishments. Following are words to use in your resume:

Accomplish	Achieve	Act
Adapt	Administer	Advertise
Advise	Aid	Analyze
Apply	Approach	Approve
Arrange	Assemble	Assess
Assign	Assist	Attain
Budget	Build	Calculate
Catalog	Chair	Clarify
Collaborate	Communicate	Compare
Compile	Complete	Conceive
Conciliate	Conduct	Consult
Contract	Control	Cooperate
Coordinate	Correct	Counsel
Create	Decide	Define
Delegate	Demonstrate	Design
Detail	Determine	Develop
Devise	Direct	Distribute
Draft	Edit	Employ
Encourage	Enlarge	Enlist
Establish	Estimate	Evaluate
Examine	Exchange	Execute
Exhibit	Expand	Expedite
Facilitate	Familiarize	Forecast
Formulate	Generate	Govern
Guide	Handle	Head
Hire	Identify	Implement
Improve	Increase	Index
Influence	Inform	Initiate
Innovate	Inspect	Install
Institute	Instruct	Integrate
Interpret	Interview	Introduce
Invent	Investigate	Lead
Maintain	Manage	Manipulate
Market	Mediate	Moderate
Modify	Monitor	Motivate
Negotiate	Obtain	Operate

Order	Organize	Originate
Oversee	Perceive	Perform
Persuade	Plan	Prepare
Present	Preside	Process
Produce	Program	Promote
Propose	Provide	Publicize
Publish	Qualify	Raise
Recommend	Reconcile	Record
Recruit	Rectify	Redesign
Reduce	Regulate	Relate
Renew	Report	Represent
Reorganize	Research	Resolve
Review	Revise	Scan
Schedule	Screen	Select
Sell	Serve	Settle
Solve	Speak	Staff
Standardize	Stimulate	Summarize
Supervise	Support	Survey
Synthesize	Systematize	Teach
Train	Transmit	Update
Write		

Resume Tips

The following tips will help you to create a top-notch resume:

Put a brief description of yourself at the top that highlights your strengths. For example, "A seasoned veteran that is responsible for overseeing three branch offices in three states." Most employers spend only a few seconds on each resume, so get your selling points up front.

Try several different formats. Do not limit yourself to a standard chronological format. Experiment with a functional format, grouping your past activities under headings such as "Team Coordination" or "Supervisory Activities" with applicable experience listed under each. If you have a strong specialty that a prospective employer may need, this format may highlight that trait more effectively than a list of jobs held.

Stick to one or two fonts. Do not try to show off your computer skills by including a multitude of fonts in your resume. This often ends up looking messy and disjointed.

The Cover Letter

Your resume provides a potential employer with your qualifications. The **cover letter** is an introduction to your resume. It invites the potential employer to read further. Your cover letter should be concise and to the point. What you are really trying to say with the cover letter is that you are enclosing your resume and are available for an interview at the prospective employer's convenience. The cover letter should be neatly typed on white or off-white 8.5 x 11 inch paper. See a sample cover letter at the end of this chapter.

Letter Writing Do Nots
The following are items you should avoid when writing your cover letter:

1. Do not include anything in your letter that cannot be substantiated in your interview.
2. Do not try to force an interview by using sympathy or any sense of urgency.
3. Do not load your cover letter with unnecessary information; just present the important facts. The cover letter should be an addendum to your resume.
4. Do not address your letter to a company or a title. Find out the name of the person who holds that title and address it to that person. If you cannot, address it to the department or division that will supervise your work.
5. Do not mail a resume without a cover letter.
6. Do not forget to request an interview in your cover letter.
7. Do not forget to proofread your cover letter, checking for appearance, grammar, and spelling errors.

Marketing Yourself

When marketing your skills, keep in mind the following things:

- segment your audience
- prepare your portfolio
- professionally market yourself

Let's discuss each item individually.

People respond to various things differently. Salespeople know this and segment their audience accordingly. You also need to segment your audience to be sure you are presenting the right benefit (talent) to the right market in the right tone. This often means you have to write several different resumes and cover letters. It is worth it if you want to get the right job. Just be sure your objectives, experience, and message are appropriate to the segment you are trying to sell.

You might also consider creating a portfolio on yourself. This portfolio could include your resume, letters of reference, graphs or charts supporting your accomplishments, samples of previous work, and other informational material. Present the information neatly. A handsome presentation folder conveys a stronger impact than a cover letter and resume alone. Its very size commands more attention. Just do not overload it with too much extraneous information. Present only the best of what you have to offer.

Depending on the situation, it can often be best to present your portfolio during the interview rather than including it with your resume.

Searching for a job is not enough. Instead, you must professionally market yourself. Take charge of the situation and of your career. Job hunters take what comes along; marketing yourself means more. It means going out and searching for the job you want, then selling yourself until you get it.

Develop a plan that will make things happen. Assemble your resources. Present yourself with purpose, professionalism, and positive energy. Not only is this more effective, but it is better for your morale than just starting another dreaded job search!

The Job Interview

The job interview can be one of the most frightening experiences a potential employee faces. Add to this the knowledge that most working adults make an average of ten career changes in their lifetime, each requiring a number of job interviews. That is a lot of stress to go through, but with knowledge can come the power to take control of the interview and turn fear into success.

Part of being prepared for an interview is having your directions, questions, interview agenda, and information about the company prior to the interview, so do your homework! If prepared properly you (the applicant) will know exactly where you stand and how you did by the end of the interview.

Keep in mind that the key to getting hired is chemistry. If someone likes you, they will go out of their way to make you fit.

Your goal should be to get a job offer or at the very least get to the next step, which is another interview. Remember you can turn any offer down but not if you do not have it!

Dress

How you dress and present yourself is also very important. Men should wear a gray or dark blue suit, a white shirt with contrast tie, and polished black shoes. Women should wear a conservative suit with a plain blouse that has a conservative neckline, and low-heeled shoes. Both men and women should make sure their hair is neat and trimmed, and that their hands and nails are clean. Wear little or no jewelry, and no perfume or cologne; you never know what the interviewer might be sensitive to. Give a firm handshake, smile, and make eye contact. Display interest, energy and confidence.

The Application

When you arrive you will frequently be given an application to fill out. This application is very important because whatever information you put on it is what the employer will be verifying (i.e., salary, reasons for leaving, education). Remember, keep it simple. Take a black pen to fill out your application. This color of ink photocopies well.

In the section for "Salary Desired" write the word "open" or "negotiable." NEVER write a dollar amount!

Remember when filling out the area "Reasons for Leaving" that once you put this information on an application it becomes a permanent record. You have signed to have this information verified by the potential employer. Companies do not typically give information beyond salary, start and end dates, and voluntary or involuntary termination (involuntary could be layoff or fired). Whatever you write should be as positive as possible. Employers look for patterns (i.e., job changes due to disagreement with boss, laid off more than once, conflict with other employees, disagreements with management decisions, etc.). When found, good or bad, they feel they get the picture of the applicant. While you want to be honest you also want to keep these reasons neutral if possible.

Be accurate with your education. State the correct degree you earned and the year you received it. This is the easiest information on your application to verify.

Interviewing

Interviewing research indicates that there are four basic components to the interview process:
- The first four seconds.
- The next five minutes.
- The main portion.
- The end or closing.

It is important to fully understand each of these components so that you can control them and reap the best rewards from the interview process.

The First Four Seconds

First impressions are very important. They can put you off to a good start, or they can strike a mark against you that will be hard to erase if an interviewer forms a negative impression.

Eighty percent of a first impression is based on your appearance. For that reason, it is suggested that you dress more formally than you might dress on the job. Keep your appearance conservative; flashy styles can be risky.

The handshake is a symbolic gesture of trust. A firm, brief handshake and direct eye contact indicate self-confidence and trustworthiness.

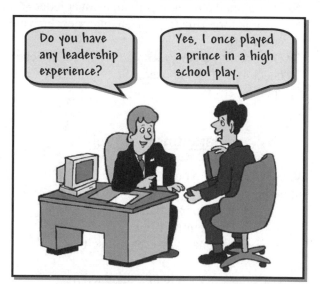

The Next Five Minutes

The next five minutes of an interview can often determine whether you get a job offer or not. Studies reveal that interviewers often form an opinion within this five-minute period. They then seek information that will validate this initial impression. Thus, their opinion influences their decision to either hire or reject the candidate. If the impression was negative, one study reveals, 90% of the time the applicant was not hired. If the opinion was positive, the candidate received a job offer 75% of the time.

Therefore, your primary goal during this time should be to make sure the initial impression is positive. The following suggestions have been found to be the most important:

1. Keep the tone of your voice calm but interested. You should be careful to speak clearly in a voice that is loud enough to be heard, but not so loud that it is annoying.
2. Make direct eye contact with the interviewer. It gives the impression that you are open and honest and have nothing to hide. Eye contact can actually be equal in power to the sound and tone of the voice.
3. Your posture conveys a large message while you are sitting as well as standing. Remaining straight and tall with shoulders back will convey confidence. Leaning forward slightly in your chair will convey interest.
4. Never underestimate the power of a smile for opening the lines of communication.

The Main Portion

After the important amenities have been taken care of, the general questioning will begin. Listen carefully to the questions and focus your answers on the job requirements and on highlighting your strengths. Look for any specific problems that the organization may have. Highlight your skills and work history as they relate to the employer's needs. Remember that if they did not have a need, they would not be interviewing you. Make them believe they need you.

Try to find out as much as possible about the company, the job, and the people. A good interview is a two-way, give-and-take situation. Interviewers expect you to ask questions. Therefore, strong well-directed questions help to create a positive impression. Be sure to listen carefully to the response, and use the information to strengthen your position.

The personality trait that attracts an interviewer the most is enthusiasm. If you like what you have heard about this company, or what you are hearing in the interview, do not be afraid to let the interviewer know. Be comfortable about revealing your personality and the kind of person you are, but do it with interest, awareness, and energy. Many studies have indicated that individuals are often hired based more on their personality than on their skills.

The middle portion of the interview can present some of your greatest difficulty. Be aware of the hidden agenda behind each question. Is the interviewer trying to find out about your skills, your education, or your background?

If an interviewer continually returns to a specific topic, especially in your past, they are unconsciously telling you that they are questioning the response or that they discern a weakness. Remember to control your responses. Frame your experiences in a positive light and focus on the positive aspects that will most benefit the company.

There is probably at least one situation in your history which you would rather not have come out in the open. This may be a termination, a misdemeanor or felony conviction, or a similar problem.

First, determine whether the information will come up during the normal course of the interview, or during the background check. Most companies run a preliminary check on their prospective employees. This may include a brief phone call to previous employers and a check of police records.

Research has shown that negative aspects are seen much more negatively when they are revealed bit by bit. The impression is that you may have other things wrong if they ask the right questions to bring them out.

Take control of this situation by disclosing any negative information briefly and forthrightly before you are asked. In this way you can place the best possible light on the situation. Even a termination can be turned from a negative into a positive by sincerely and honestly discussing what you have learned from the experience and what you will do differently, if you are given the opportunity.

The Closing

Finally, you have reached the closing moments of the interview. Many people begin to lose concentration and relax at this point. Do not! Keep yourself focused. A strong finish may be the difference between you and someone else in a tight race. Show the interviewer you are still excited about the job, especially now that you know more about it and the company.

Make a strong final note by succinctly summarizing your positive points as they relate to the job. There is nothing wrong with asking when a decision on the candidates will be made. When you have the answer, show your enthusiasm by letting the interviewer know that you will call back the afternoon of the decision.

Interviewing is much like a game. If you make all the right moves, you will win the job. If you make errors, you will not. In the end, it is all up to you and the way you play.

Getting Paid What You Are Worth

The issue of salary will undoubtedly come up, either during the interview or before. Salary is probably the most important issue among workers today. Nevertheless, the way in which salary is determined is often one of the least understood aspects when it comes to evaluating your worth. Far too many people see their salary as an extension of themselves and how much they are worth. Often, their point of view is totally unrealistic according to the marketplace.

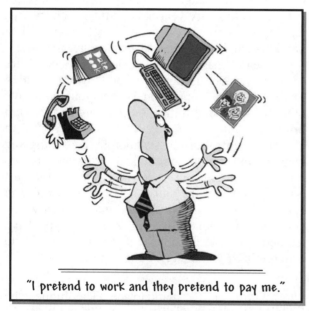

"I pretend to work and they pretend to pay me."

Let's review four of the most common misconceptions regarding how a salary should be determined:

1. **Seeing your monetary compensation as a reflection of your worth as a person.** It is not. Your salary is based on your objective value in the marketplace. If your skills are in high demand you will be paid more than if they are not. This is perhaps the single most common mistake employees make. Their pride tells them that they are too good of a person to work for such meager pay. If you are one of these people you need to face the fact that the laws of supply and demand determine your market worth, not

you. If everyone were able to set their own salary at what they felt they were worth, inflation would increase drastically. You would be making $450 per hour, but a loaf of bread would cost $50.

Bear in mind that when supply and demand chooses a market value for your work, at least it is an objective value, not a subjective one determined by others. So do not take it personally.

2. **Expecting your pay to be determined by your needs.** This is the second most common complaint, and we have all heard it. Employees making comments like: "My partner is out of work, and we cannot pay our bills on my salary alone." "I'm a single parent with children to feed." "I have to put my children in private school." "This salary barely covers the cost of rent and bills every month. What am I supposed to eat on?"

The fact is that no employer can afford to pay an employee based on their needs. People are funny characters. When they have money, they tend to spend it. In the end, you will probably always need more money than you are presently making. Keep your professional dignity by never basing a request for a raise on these types of appeals.

3. **Expecting the length of your employment to determine your market value.** No matter how long you have worked at a particular position, if you can offer nothing more than the person who has worked at the job for a year, then both of you will be paid at approximately the same level. Many employees expect automatic annual raises. This works fine until a company decides that it is less expensive to terminate the older employee and hire a new one at a lower salary. Then the policy does not sound so good anymore.

Recognize that your pay reflects the value of the work you do. Granted, more experience usually leads to a higher quality of employee, and often the pay reflects this. However, the lowly box boy in the supermarket, no matter how great a box boy he is, will never earn as much as the supervisor of a department.

4. **Expecting your pay to go up as the company's profits go up.** This concept ignores a fundamental concept: Employees are not shareholders. They are not taking risks with

their money. Those who expect their pay to increase when the company's profits increase almost never suggest that they should take a pay cut when the company has a bad year. Yet one is exactly the same as the other. If an employee wishes to share in a company's profits and if the company is publicly held, the employee should purchase company stock. However, these employees, like the current shareholders, will then run the risk of losing their money if profits fall.

If you, as an employee, recognize these misconceptions about salary, you are less likely to base your request for a raise on unsound reasons. Next, take into consideration what would be a valid reason for requesting a raise.

First and fundamentally, you need to make some personal decisions. Ask yourself: "Am I in the right job?", "Do I enjoy what I am doing?" Regardless of your answer, the next question should be, "Is it more important for me to have money or to be happy?" The truth is that it takes a lot of money to compensate someone for being miserable. And if you are miserable in your job, you are probably not putting forth your best effort. Lack of effort is definitely not going to get you the raises you would like. So what do you do? First, find the right job for you.

The next important principle is that the laws of supply and demand will prevail. If you want to increase your market value, you must increase your worth to the company, usually by increasing your skills and abilities.

The following suggestions can help you increase your value to the company:

1. Adopt an active mentality, not a passive one. No one is going to increase your skills and abilities for you; you have to do it yourself and it takes work.
2. Never stop learning. Do not be satisfied with knowing your job inside and out. After you have mastered that, begin learning the other jobs in the company, preferably those of the next step up the ladder. Ask questions, read books, or take classes. Make sure that you become a valuable asset to the company and that you are ready for advancement and promotion when the opportunity arises.

3. Make long-range plans rather than waiting for life to just happen to you. Those who sit around rarely go anywhere.
4. Finally, realize that very often a significant change in salary comes from changing jobs, either within your present company or by moving to a different employer. We have all heard comments like "If I were working at the company down the street, I could make more than this!" The obvious response is, "If that is true, then why don't you work at that company?" If the bosses hear you make such a comment, they may assist your transfer to the company down the street by firing you.

Many employees cannot accept the fact that it is either true that their current pay is below market, or it is not. If it is true, why not move on? If it is not, change your market value.

Summary

To find the right job takes more than just a passive look at the classified ads. You must first determine your objectives, your uniqueness, and your target audience. With these topics firmly in mind, write an effective resume and cover letter that will introduce you to a prospective employer.

When you have been granted an interview, keep in mind that the first four seconds are the most critical, followed by the next five minutes.

However, the body of the interview and the closing are also important in determining whether you get a second interview and/or a job offer.

When it comes to salary, your pay is based on your worth to the marketplace. The higher the demand for your skills, the more value will be placed on them and the higher salary you will be paid. Salary is not determined by your worth as a person, your needs, your length of employment, or the company's profits.

Assignments

Complete the Questions for Review.
Complete Exercise 30 – 1. The more prepared you are, the better your job interview will be.

Questions for Review

Directions: Answer the following questions without looking back into the material just covered. Write your answers in the space provided.

1. What three points should your written marketing plan cover?

   1. _____

   2. _____

   3. _____

2. To determine your _____, consider the responsibilities you want on your next job, the industry in which you want to work, and what you can reasonably expect in the way of title and salary.

3. Your _____ should show your target audience that you are worthy of their _____.

4. What is your resume? _____

5. (True or False?) Never use an active voice or concise phrasing in your resume. _____

6. A _____ is a way to toot your own horn.

7. (True or False?) Do not put anything in your cover letter that you cannot substantiate in an interview. _____

8. You should not job-hunt but instead _____ yourself.

9. Working adults normally make how many career changes in a lifetime? _____

10. (True or False?) The only way to achieve a significant increase in pay is to change jobs. _____

If you were unable to answer any of the questions, refer back to that section, and then fill in the answers.

Exercise 30 – 1

Directions: Complete the following items.

1. Fill out the Resume Questionnaire on the following pages.
2. Using the resumes on the following pages as examples, create your own resume.
3. Using the following cover letter as an example, create your own cover letter.

Resume Questionnaire

First Name _____ M.I. _____ Last Name _____

Street _____

City _____ State _____ Zip _____

Day Phone _____ Eve. Phone _____ Soc. Sec. # _____

Position Objective: In the spaces below, enter the Occupational Titles of those positions which you feel you would be best qualified to fill. Opposite each position, enter the total years experience you have. Then indicate your minimum acceptable annual salary. "OPEN" is unacceptable. (Salary information is for your use and should not be included on an application.)

	Years Experience	Desired Annual Salary
Occupational or Professional Title(s)		
_____	_____	$_____
_____	_____	$_____
_____	_____	$_____
_____	_____	$_____

Experience Summary: Please summarize briefly your overall experience and accomplishments.

_____
_____
_____

Education: Type of Degree, Diploma, Certificate, or Years completed: (i.e., HS Diploma, # year(s) College, AA/BA) Highest Level: Type: _____ Major _____

Name of School, College or University _____

Additional Courses/Seminars Taken, and/or Awards: _____

_____
_____

U.S. Citizenship: Yes ____ No ____

Type of Employment: ____ Full Time ____ Part Time ____ Temp ____ Contract _____

Geographic Area: ____ Open to Any Area   Area Desired _____

Skills/Abilities: Include any skills and abilities that may be of benefit to an employer. _____

_____
_____
_____
_____
_____

Work History: Under each position title, describe your duties, responsibilities, and accomplishments. Be sure to list your present or last employer first.

From/To (Mo/Yr) _____ Company Name _____

Location (City & State) _____

Position Title _____ Salary $ _____

Type of Firm or Industry _____

Responsibilities/Accomplishments: _____

_____

From/To (Mo/Yr) _____ Company Name _____

Location (City & State) _____

Position Title _____ Salary $ _____

Type of Firm or Industry _____

Responsibilities/Accomplishments: _____

_____

From/To (Mo/Yr) _____ Company Name _____

Location (City & State) _____

Position Title _____ Salary $ _____

Type of Firm or Industry _____

Responsibilities/Accomplishments: _____

_____

Other Experience/Accomplishments: List briefly any additional experience or accomplishments that you would consider significant. _____

_____

_____

Industry Experience: Please indicate the industries in which you have experience and specify type(s) (i.e., agriculture, construction). _____

_____

_____

_____

Foreign Language(s): _____

I hereby certify that all of the information contained herein is complete and accurate and I agree to report any changes promptly.

Signature: _____ Date: _____

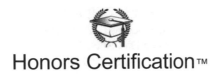

Honors Certification™

Resume and Cover Letter

Create a perfect resume and cover letter. This is a pass/fail item. You must be sure that there are no errors in either the cover letter or the resume. If any errors are found you must correct them before this item will be considered complete. When finished, your resume and cover letter should be printed on nice paper. You may take as long as necessary to complete this challenge.

Interview

You will be interviewed by your teacher or one of your classmates. The interview will take place in front of your class. You must dress appropriately for the interview and conduct yourself as you would in a real interview situation. This is a pass/fail situation. Whether you pass or fail will be determined by whether a majority of your classmates would give you a job based on your interview. If 85% of the class would hire you, you pass.

If you fail the test on your first attempt you may retake the test one additional time. However, 90% of the students must give you a passing score on the second interview.

SALLY STUDENT
12345 SUMMER STREET
SANDY, SC 20000
(803) 555-1234

OBJECTIVE:
To obtain a position in the medical industry which will enable me to use my billing and communications background, supervisory experience, administrative skills, and creative talents.

QUALIFYING STATEMENT:
I am hard working and have excellent verbal and communication skills in both English and Spanish. I also have the ability to handle a variety of tasks and have good organizational skills.

EXPERIENCE:
Medical Biller/Receptionist -- Spring Street Medical Offices, 1234 Spring Street, Sandy, SC, 20001. Duties included: Billing for services using HCFA-1500 and UB-92 billing forms, billing Medicare and Medicaid patients, maintaining medical records, setting appointments, answering phones, typing correspondence, greeting clients, ordering supplies. Job was an internship for completion of requirements for Medical Billing Certificate from The Suburban School. 2/02 - present

Waitress -- The Scrumptious Supper, 4567 Sister Street, Sandy, SC 20030. Duties included: Taking orders, serving customers, cashiering, assisting with making of desserts and other items, bussing tables, acting as hostess. 9/00 - 2/02

Cook/Server -- McStephens Fast Hamburgers, 98765 Stale Street, Sandy, SC 20002. Duties included: Taking orders, serving customers, receiving moneys, keeping an accurate cash drawer, cooking foods (including hamburgers and fries), preparing and maintaining salad bar and condiments bar. 4/98 - 9/00

EDUCATION:
Medical Billing Certificate, The Suburban School, 8765 Sullen Street, Sandy, SC 20022. Maintained a 3.95 GPA and graduated among the top in the class.

Sandy Adult Community School, 84756 Seashore Street, Sandy, SC 20007. Took classes and seminars in Computer Basics, Creative Writing, Working with DOS, Windows, and Word.

Diploma. Sandy High School, 3456 Sunset Street, Sandy, SC 20012. GPA 3.75 Perfect attendance certificate, 1995, 1994. Also took two business courses.

SKILLS:
Computer literate in PowerPoint, Word, Quicken, type (50 wpm), 10 key (6,000 kph), understand medical terminology, knowledgeable in proper business correspondence. Speak and write in both English and Spanish. Hobbies include writing and learning computer programs.

Holly Hopeful
4536 Hammer Way
Hollywood, CA 90611
(818) 555-1772

Sample Cover Letter #1

January 2, 2005

Steve Springer
Personnel Supervisor
Stupendous Supports
102938 Sports Street
Sandy, SC 20020

Dear Mr. Springer:

Please consider me for an administrative assistant position with your firm.

I recently completed my education at The Suburban School, where I received a certificate in administrative assisting. I completed the course with a 3.95 grade point average and was among the top students in my class. The course covered everything an administrative assistant should know, including using reference books, time management skills, legal issues, general office procedures, computer basics, calculator basics, typing, speedwriting, proofreading, correspondence writing, Word, PowerPoint, basic office accounting, customer service, event planning and travel arrangements. I am familiar with the use of Quicken Accounting and Billing, type 50 words per minute and can enter 6,000 keystrokes per hour on the ten key.

I also completed a three-month internship at Spring Street Offices in conjunction with this course, which utilized the knowledge that I had learned. During this internship I completed administrative assistant, billing and receptionist duties for an office that staffed eight professionals and had over 7,500 customers.

I am a conscientious, enterprising person who works very hard to turn in a good performance. I enjoy being creative and industrious. I learn quickly and am more than willing to take on the challenge of learning new things. I am dependable and loyal, and have had perfect attendance at my jobs for the past three years. I also get along well with co-workers and supervisors.

Thank you for taking the time to consider my resume. I would be happy to interview with you at your convenience.

Sincerely,

Holly Hopeful
Holly Hopeful

RESUME

NAME: Holly Hopeful

ADDRESS: 4536 Hammer Way
                   Hollywood, CA 90611

PHONE: (818) 555-1772

EDUCATION: Certificate – Administrative Assisting - 2004, Success School

EXPERIENCE: 2003 - present – Program Assistant. In charge of data entry, answering telephones, typing, and creating files, flyers and circulars. I also took care of sign-in logs and scheduling appointments.

2002 - 2003 -- Office Manager for Sam's Shoe Store. Assisted with running the office, hiring and firing duties and maintained and ordered the stock/inventory. I also scheduled employees and handled financial records.

2001 - 2002 -- Sales Clerk for Sarah's Sweet Shoppe. I assisted customers, maintained the cash drawer, and maintained and ordered stock. I also handled customer service and dealt with returns and dissatisfied customers.

Ivana Job
4646 Jessup Court
Jacobs, IL 60911
(815) 555-0101

Sample Resume #3

OBJECTIVE: A challenging position utilizing my administrative assisting skills and experience.

QUALITIES: Excellent organizational and problem solving abilities. Effectively handle multiple priorities and working under pressure. Skilled with people. Computer literate. Intelligent, accurate, goal-oriented and self-motivated. Superior work ethics.

SUMMARY OF EXPERIENCE: Over 15 years experience in accounting and office work with an emphasis in managing personnel for a large drug store and pharmacy.

WORK HISTORY:
2003 - Present   STORE MANAGER: Responsible to CEO for overall operation of drug store. Administered all human resource functions including hiring, employee relations, payroll and work scheduling. Supervised and set operating procedures for numerous departments. Assisted accounting department with accounts payable, accounts receivable, general ledger and collections. Responsible for multi-account bank reconciliations, tax returns and monthly financial statements. Wrote employee policy and training manual.

2002 - 2003   BUYER: Extensive purchasing and merchandising responsibilities including vendor negotiations, inventory controls and setting displays. Handled advertising, sales and promotions. Improved level of customer service.

1998 - 2002   PHARMACY TECHNICIAN: Assisted pharmacists in fulfilling prescriptions. Coordinated activities of pharmacy personnel. Obtained broad technical knowledge of drugs and medical terminology. Voted employee of the month three times.

EDUCATION, LICENSES: Certificate, Administrative Assisting.
Savemore School, Sandy, SC
State of SC Pharmacy Technician License #TCH 000000

EXERCISES IN MEDICAL BILLING

Exercises in Medical Billing, one of our most popular texts, can be used as a workbook to the <u>Guide to Medical Billing</u>. The first of our Real Life™ series, this text contains an innovative simulated work program which allows students to "work" for the billing department of a large health conglomerate, billing claims and handling numerous real life situations. Medisoft training is also provided.

Using this text, students will gain practical experience with the coding and billing of numerous different types of claims.

Table of Contents:
Understanding the Medical Office and Computer
Computers – A Quick Review
Understanding the Computer Program
Using Medisoft
Simulated Work Program
Documents
Petty Cash and Window Payments
Patient File Forms

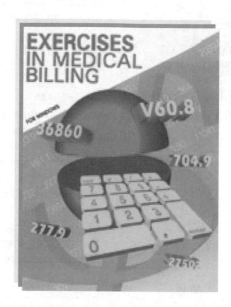

Exercises in
Medical Billing
ISBN: 1-88159-11-6

ICDC Publishing specializes in textbooks and workbooks with a difference!

To **order** this book, or for a list of all our titles, and to see complete **Tables of Contents** and **Sample Chapters**, visit our website at:

www.icdcpublishing.com